AF781796

Diseases of Feedlot Cattle

Diseases of Feedlot Cattle

Rue Jensen, D.V.M., Ph.D., V.Sc.D.

Vice President for Research
Colorado State University
Fort Collins, Colorado

Donald R. Mackey, D.V.M.

Practitioner
Greeley, Colorado

SECOND EDITION

191 Illustrations

LEA & FEBIGER · 1971 · PHILADELPHIA

ISBN 0-8121-0361-0
Copyright © 1971 by Lea & Febiger. Copyright under the International Copyright Union. All rights reserved. This book is protected by copyright. *No part of it may be reproduced in any manner or by any means, without written permission from the publisher.*

Library of Congress Catalog Card Number 74-157468

Printed in the United States of America

PREFACE

From 1961 through 1970 some major trends for the cattle feeding industry developed. In the United States the average annual consumption of beef per person changed from 85 pounds in 1960 to 114 pounds in 1970, an increase of 34%. Furthermore, the estimate for 1980 is approximately 125 pounds annually per person. To meet the demand for quality beef the number of marketed fed cattle doubled, and the proportion of cattle fed to total cattle marketed increased from 52% in 1960 to 73% in 1970. In addition to higher demand for beef, the nature of the cattle feeding enterprise changed. From 1962 through 1968, the number of cattle fattened in feedlots having a capacity of less than 1,000 animals increased 22%, while the number of cattle fattened in feedlots having a capacity of more than 1,000 animals increased 211%. These changes suggest that during the 1970's the number of beef cattle will increase and that most of the slaughtered animals will have been fattened in feedlots where vast numbers of cattle are assembled in crowded conditions.

Under these circumstances, the prevalence of disease may increase and augment the need for disease prevention and treatment programs. Some vaccines will need improvement, and the use of effective immunizing products will need more general acceptance and application. Infectious diseases of the respiratory and digestive systems, while prevalent, should diminish because of preventive measures, but metabolic disorders, such as acute indigestion, may increase in incidence because of the economic need to fatten cattle as rapidly as possible by changing the diet during a short period from roughage to concentrate.

The assemblage of large numbers of cattle for fattening results in the accumulation of tremendous quantities of animal wastes which may pollute water, soil, and air, and contribute to public health hazards and to human discomforts in urban and suburban areas. Although the public demands an adequate supply of beef, it also requires protection of natural resources against pollution.

This book describes some of the health and management problems of the feedlot industry. The volume may help practicing veterinarians in preventing, diagnosing, and treating diseases; feedlot operators in understanding, accepting and planning health programs; and students in perceiving the problems and solutions to problems that may confront them in the veterinary specialty of cattle feedlot practice.

We wish to acknowledge the generous assistance from many colleagues in assembling information and to express sincere gratitude to Millie D. Jensen for manuscript reading and to LaVerne M. Carpenter for the typing.

Fort Collins, Colorado Rue Jensen
Greeley, Colorado Donald R. Mackey

CONTENTS

1

Preconditioning cattle for the feedlot

The production of quality beef involves two kinds of enterprise: the breeding herd and the feedlot. The breeding herds annually produce and sell a crop of calves, and the feedlots purchase, fatten and resell the animals for slaughter. The total process of production from birth of cattle to slaughter requires 1 to 2 years. In the United States approximately 35 million cattle are annually produced and slaughtered for human food; of these animals about 26 million are fed cattle.

Usually the two types of enterprise are geographically separated. Breeding herds are located on pasture and range land, but the feedlots tend to develop near communities, often cities, near large sources of feed concentrates. The separating distance requires transportation of cattle by rail or truck from the location of the breeding herds to the location of the feedlots. Frequently the movement is interstate and may be hundreds of miles in distance. For example, cattle may be produced in Idaho or Wyoming and fattened in Illinois or Iowa.

The breeding herd, consisting of cows and bulls and usually numbering 500 or more per enterprise, uses large areas of pasture land and/or range land for cattle grazing. Depending on the availability and use of the land, the annual crop of calves is sold to feedlots at different ages and sizes. Some operations use all land for maintaining the breeding animals and, consequently, sell the calves at weaning age when most individual animals weigh less than 550 pounds. Other ranches may use part of the land for grazing and maintaining the calves for a year beyond weaning when individual animals weigh more than 550 pounds. At the time of sale and shipment the 6-month-old cattle weighing less than 550 pounds are more susceptible to respiratory, and possibly other, diseases than are the 18-month-old animals weighing more than 550 pounds. Both size categories of cattle, however, require preparation for successful transporting and fattening. At the time of sale, the obviously sick and unthrifty animals are usually excluded. Sales may be through private negotiations with feedlot owners or by auction at large public stockyards with one or more intermediary dealers acting between producer and feedlot operator.

The physical facilities of a feedlot enterprise consist of pens, alleyways, concentrate and roughage feeds, equipment for storing, compounding and distributing feed to the pens, loading and unloading facilities and cattle capable of efficient fattening. Cattle are crowded into pens with an average of 400 square feet per animal. Opportunities for exercise are minimal. Within a pen all cattle use common feeding and drinking facilities. These circumstances facilitate the transfer of contagious diseases among cattle of a pen. Fattening must be accomplished in as little time as possible. Cattle having beginning weights less than 550 pounds usually complete fattening in 300 to 330 days, while animals having entering weights greater than 550 pounds fatten in 90 to 160 days.

For efficient and profitable fattening, cattle must be healthy and fully adjusted to feedlot conditions. The animals must be weaned, castrated, dehorned and accustomed to eating from a bunk and drinking from tanks or other containers; in addition, they must be immunized against certain prevalent feedlot diseases, and freed from excessive external and internal parasites. The application of these preparatory processes at the location of the breeding herd is referred to as "preconditioning" and their application at the feedlot is known as "arrival conditioning."

Review of Literature. The hazards of bovine respiratory diseases associated with transporting cattle from the breeding herd locations to the feedlots have been generally recognized by the cattle industry and veterinary medical profession. The average economic loss associated with shipping have been estimated at $10 to $20 per animal transported (Herrick, 1967). In an effort to obtain information about the management of calves during transit from the breeding herd to feedlot, records of ownership and movement were examined. Of 10,832 calves in one study 8,882 were sold at public auction, and of these, only 8% were traceable through all movements to the feedlot. Of the remaining, 1,950 animals sold at private sale, 38% were traceable to destination. Of 231 calves that developed respiratory disease, only 12 (0.5%) had been weaned at least 30 days before shipment, while 219 (99.5%) had been weaned less than 30 days when shipment occurred (Bristol, 1966). With this kind of information, incomplete as it was, a procedure for preconditioning animals was perceived for abating losses and advocated for general practice. The program applied primarily to cattle weighing less than 550 pounds and consisted of weaning, castrating, dehorning, administering appropriate vaccines and treating for external and internal parasites, at the breeding herd location not fewer than 30 days before shipment. In addition, the program recommended that each animal be identified by an appropriate ear tag and accompanied to destination by a record of all treatments and movements (Herrick, 1967). Later an attempt was made to measure the cost of preconditioning and to determine efficacy of the program. One-hundred-sixteen cattle were included in the study. Some of the animals were preconditioned at the breeding herd location. The cost of preconditioning in labor, vaccines, and veterinarians' time, varied from $1.31 to $3.08 per animal. Feedlot performance of the preconditioned cattle evinced no measurable advantage over control cattle (Meyer, Judy and Armstrong, 1970).

Preconditioning. Preconditioning, the preparation of young cattle for the feedlot before shipment from the breeding herd location, applies to animals weighing less than 550 pounds. The program is flexible to meet varying practices of management. In general, all temporarily stressing procedures of the program are performed approximately 2 to 4 weeks before shipment. Surgical operations, such as castration and dehorning, are performed sufficiently in advance for healing to occur. Weaning allows animals to adjust to eating solid feed from a bunk and to drinking water from a tank. Essential immunizations are for viral bovine rhinotracheitis, parainfluenza-3, and leptospirosis. Less essential and optional immunizations are against bacterial diseases, such as clostridial infections, pasteurellosis, and salmonellosis. Vaccination against viral bovine diarrhea should be postponed until need is clearly established. All animals should be treated for external parasites and grubs by dipping or spraying and for internal parasites, if necessary by medication. Each preconditioned animal is identified by an ear tag number, and a record of all treatments and movements accompanies the animal to destination.

On arrival at the feedlot, preconditioned cattle can move rapidly into the fattening process. During the first 14 to 21 days the animals rest and recuperate from the fatigue of travel and are given palatable grass hay or alfalfa, grain to the extent of 0.5% of body weight and fresh water. Beginning about the fifteenth to twenty-second day the diet consists of roughage in the form of equal parts of hay and corn silage to the extent of 2.5% of body weight and of corn or other grain in the amount of 1% of body weight. The roughage is gradually decreased and the concentrate gradually increased until the average daily consumption of grain is approximately 2% or more of the body weight. Thereafter, as the animals grow in size, the grain is increased to a maximum of 20 to 25 pounds of daily concentrate.

The validity of preconditioning is supported by logic. During transit the stressed animals are commonly exposed to numerous pathogens, especially those causing respiratory diseases. The need for protective immunization may be greater during shipment than during any other time. The cost of labor and materials for administering procedures of preconditioning is the same whether performed at the breeding herd location or at the feedlot. Whichever enterprise performs the service bears the cost. Establishing preconditioning as a widely accepted practice requires a scientific demonstration that a measurable benefit accrues to both the breeding herd producer and the feedlot operator.

Arrival Conditioning. Regardless of advocation and acceptance of preconditioning, some young cattle weighing less than 550 pounds will escape the practice and arrive at the feedlot unprepared for fattening. In addition, older animals weighing more than 550 pounds will not have received special processing.

On arrival at the feedlot, the young cattle should be carefully examined. All sick individuals should be isolated and properly treated. The balance of the herd should rest for 2 days with free access to grass or alfalfa hay and fresh water. Within 36 to 48 hours, the animals should be vaccinated against viral bovine rhinotracheitis, parainfluenza-3, and leptospirosis. If nutritional deficiences are evident, they should also receive injectable forms of vitamins A, D and E. The administration of antibiotics or sulfonamides in feed should be deferred for a week and then used if necessary. Within 7 to 10 days the animals should be treated for external parasites and grubs by spraying or dipping and for internal parasites by administering the anthelmintic mixed in the diet as a single feeding or by individual medication. After 3 to 4 weeks any other needed vaccines, such as clostridial bacterins and bovine viral diarrhea vaccine, may be applied. All vaccines should be applied as recommended by the manufacturer. Gradual adaptation to a full diet of concentrate should be performed as recommended for preconditioned calves.

As they arrive at the feedlot, older cattle, weighing more than 550 pounds, should also be examined for special needs. All sick animals should be isolated and appropriately treated. During the first 2 days of rest and adjustment, the animals should be given access to palatable grass or alfalfa hay and fresh water. After 36 to 48 hours the entire herd should be vaccinated against viral bovine rhinotracheitis, leptospirosis, parainfluenza-3 and bacterial diseases such as clostridial infections. In some areas bacterins against salmonellosis and bacillary hemoglobinuria may be needed. After 7 to 10 days the animals should be treated for external parasites and grubs by spraying or dipping and for internal parasites, if needed, by administering the anthelmintic mixed in the diet as a single feeding or by individual medication. Vaccination against bovine viral diarrhea should

TABLE 1 *Summary of diet schedule in feedlots*

Cattle Weights	*Days in Feedlot*	*Diet*
Less than 550 lbs.	1–21	Grass or alfalfa hay. After second day grain to extent of 0.5% of body wt.
	22–	Roughage consisting of equal parts of hay and corn silage in amount of 2.5% of body wt. Corn or other grain in amount of 1% body wt. Gradually decrease roughage and increase concentrate until daily consumption of grain is 2% or more of body wt.
More than 550 lbs.	1–2	Grass or alfalfa hay.
	3–14	Roughage consisting of equal parts of hay and corn silage in amount of 2.5% of body wt. Corn or other grain in amount of 1% of body wt. At 2–3 day intervals decrease roughage and increase concentrate until daily consumption of grain is 2% or more of body wt.

TABLE 2 *Summary of health treatments in feedlots*

Cattle Weights	*Days in Feedlot*	*Vaccinations or other treatments*
Preconditioned; less than 550 lbs.	1	Remove and treat sick animals.
		Administer any necessary but omitted treatments as below.
Arrival conditioned; less than 550 lbs.	1	Remove and treat sick cattle.
	1–2	Vaccinations: viral bovine rhinotracheitis, parainfluenza-3, leptospirosis. Bovine viral diarrhea, if on arrival some animals show clinical signs of the disease. Injectable vitamins, if needed, A, D, E.
	7–10	Antibiotics and/or sulfonamides, if needed, in feed. Dip or spray for external parasites and grubs. If needed, treat for internal parasites with anthelmintic in single feed or by individual medication.
	21–28	If needed, vaccinate for clostridial diseases and bovine viral diarrhea.
Arrival conditioned; more than 550 lbs.	1	Remove and treat all sick cattle.
	1–2	Vaccinations: viral bovine rhinotracheitis, parainfluenza-3, leptospirosis, and if necessary, for clostridial diseases and salmonellosis.
	7–10	Dip or spray for external parasites and grubs. If needed, treat for internal parasites with anthelmintic in single feed or by individual medication.
	14–21	If necessary, vaccinate for bovine viral diarrhea.
	100–150	Revaccinate for viral bovine rhinotracheitis animals to be in feedlot for 300 or more days.

be avoided unless attack by the disease is anticipated because of disease prevalence in the area. In the latter case, vaccination may be performed 2 to 3 weeks after arrival or earlier if necessary.

Adaptation of the older cattle to a diet of concentrate is gradual over 2 to 4 weeks. On the third day, the daily ration is changed to roughage consisting of equal parts of hay and corn silage in the amount of 2.5% of body weight and corn or other grain in the amount of 1% of body weight. At 2- to 3-day intervals the roughage is decreased, and the grain is increased until the daily concentrate consumed is 2% of body weight. A common feedlot practice is to let animals reach a full diet of concentrates in 2 weeks, but equally good performance with fewer cases of digestive illness, such as rumenitis, founder and acidosis, is achieved by letting animals use 4 weeks to convert the diet to a full feed of concentrate.

References

Bristol, R. F.: Preconditioning of Feeder Cattle Prior to Interstate Shipment. Proc. U.S.L.S.A., (1966): 166–172.

Herrick, J. B.: Report of the Committee on Infectious Diseases of Cattle. Proc. U.S.L.S.A., (1967): 133–135.

Meyer, K. B., Judy, J. W. and Armstrong, J. H.: Economic Analysis of a Feeder Cattle Preconditioning Program. JAVMA, *157* (1970): 1560–1563.

2

Diseases caused by viruses

Viral Bovine Rhinotracheitis

(INFECTIOUS BOVINE RHINOTRACHEITIS; RED NOSE; NECROTIC RHINITIS)

Viral bovine rhinotracheitis, an acute and contagious upper respiratory disease, is clinically characterized by fever and dyspnea and pathologically by rhinitis, sinusitis, laryngitis, and tracheitis. Even though primarily a respiratory disease, less serious infections in feedlot cattle of the genitalia, fetus, conjunctiva, and brain are significant complications that add to economic importance of the disease. Losses result from reduction of live weight, prolonged fattening period, expensive treatment, preventive programs, and mortality. Respiratory diseases are the most important single group of feedlot maladies, and viral bovine rhinotracheitis along with shipping fever and calf diphtheria form the big triumvirate of respiratory infections.

Review of Literature. Since 1950 viral bovine rhinotracheitis has been recognized as a clinical entity. The first published account, reporting observations of the disease in dairy cattle of California, mentioned economic losses occurring from diminished milk production (Schroeder and Moys, 1954). The identification of specific antibodies to the virus, in a stored sample of blood collected in 1941, indicated, however, that the disease, although previously unrecognized, existed earlier (Gillespie, Lee, and Baker, 1957). While the disease in dairy cattle continued at a low incidence, in feedlot cattle of Colorado and California the incidence was very high and threatening to producers (Brown *et al.*, 1957; McKercher *et al.*, 1955; Miller, 1955). To the cattle fattening industry, viral bovine rhinotracheitis assumed greater importance than any other disease. In a survey extending from August 1954 to July 1956, more than 100,000 cattle from 64 outbreaks in Colorado were studied. In the involved herds 24.7% of all cattle were affected. While the vast majority of cases was in feedlot cattle, the acute disease with virus isolations was diagnosed and studied in range cattle of Nevada (McKercher and Straub, 1960) and Colorado (Chow, 1961). A subsequent survey indicated that in Colorado range cattle serums from most counties contained antibodies against the virus. Broader national surveys indicated that 10 to 30% of the cattle in the United States become exposed to the disease (York, 1968).

Early studies of the cause of viral bovine rhinotracheitis conclusively proved that during the febrile stage of the disease the causative agent was in nasal secretions of affected animals (McIntyre, 1954; Chow *et al.*, 1955; McKercher *et al.*, 1955). Important progress was made when the virus was isolated and cultivated on bovine embryonal kidney cells (Madin, York, McKercher, 1956). Since its discovery, the virus has been intensively studied. Structure, dimensions, and physicochemical characteristics of the virion were determined (Tousimis *et al.*, 1958; Straub, 1965; Watrach and Bahenmann, 1966; Bocciarelli *et al.*, 1966), pathogenesis within the cell was investigated (Hahnefeld and Hahnefeld, 1964; Jasty and Chang, 1969; Straub, 1965) and classification of the virus as a member of the herpes group was made (Armstrong, 1961).

As a result of its discovery and cultivation, the virus was attenuated and live vaccines were produced (Report on Bovine Respiratory Disease, 1968). Controlled field tests demonstrated that the vaccines were both safe and efficacious (Brown *et al.*, 1959). Extensive use of the vaccines reduced the incidence of the disease in feedlot cattle of the United States to manageable levels. The administration of live vaccine to pregnant cattle, however, commonly resulted in loss of fetuses through abortion, absorption, and premature births (McFeeley *et al.*, 1968).

Clinical observations followed by laboratory investigations revealed that besides respiratory infection, the virus of bovine rhinotracheitis has caused additional clinical manifestations. Recriprocal immunity studies established that the virus of bovine rhinotracheitis is the same agent that causes infectious pustular vulvovaginitis (Kendrick, Gillespie and McIntee, 1958; Gillespie, Baker and Wagner, 1958). Clinical signs of the two diseases, however, have frequently existed separately. In South Africa, viruses were isolated from the semen of bulls affected with epididymitis and from mucus of cows with vaginitis. Serum-virus neutralization tests disclosed that viral strains from 1 bull, 2 cows, and 3 heifers were identical to the virus of bovine rhinotracheitis and pustular vulvovaginitis (Mare and Von Rensburg, 1961). An additional viral complication was its effect on pregnancies. The exposure of 7 pregnant cows to virulent virus caused the loss of 6 fetuses by abortion, resorption or premature birth. Virus was recovered from fetuses (Satter, Bohl and Trapp, 1967). Experimental inoculation of 25 pregnant heifers with virulent virus resulted in a 16% abortion rate. Intervals from inoculation to abortion varied from 15 to 35 days. Pathologic changes, including necrosis and edema, were severe in fetuses and minimal in amounts in placentas (Molello *et al.*, 1966; Owens *et al.*, 1968; Kendrick and Straub, 1967). The use of attenuated live virus vaccine on 119 pregnant cows in the second trimester of gestation resulted in 20 abortions (McFeeley *et al.*, 1968). Acute conjunctivitis has been another manifestation of infection with the virus of bovine rhinotracheitis. In a herd of 125 yearling beef cattle, approximately 67% of the animals developed conjunctivitis, and even though virus was isolated from both conjunctival and nasal secretions, signs of respiratory infection were absent (Abinanti and Plumer, 1961). In another investigation, however, viral conjunctivitis was followed by slight corneal opacities that resembled keratoconjunctivitis (St. George, 1965). Encephalitis as a complication of respiratory disease was also observed in young cattle, and the virus of bovine rhinotracheitis was isolated from infected brain on monolayer cultures of bovine kidney cells (Barenfus, Delli Quadri, and McIntyre, 1963). In a study of development of encephalitis, 2 calves were inoculated intracerebrally, 2 intranasally, 2 intravaginally, and 2 orally. The animals inoculated intracerebrally developed meningoencephalitis, and the virus was recovered from brain tissue. Of the 2 cattle inoculated intravaginally, one developed rhinitis; this animal plus the 2 inoculated intranasally subsequently manifested meningoencephalitis. The route of virus movement from nose to brain was not determined (Hall *et al.*, 1966).

Several types of commercial vaccines have been developed, marketed and successfully used. Early products consisted of attenuated live virus only (Report of Panel for Symposium on Immunity to Respiratory Diseases, 1968), while others were combinations of modified bovine rhinotracheitis virus, parainfluenza-3 virus, *Leptospira pomona* bacterins, bovine viral diarrhea-mucosal disease virus (Plimpton, 1966; Kahrs and Baker, 1966). All combinations appeared to be compatible antigens and, in general, recipient animals were more healthy than their control counterparts.

Thus since 1949 phenomenal achievements were made in the study of viral bovine rhinotracheitis. The disease was identified and characterized, the cause was discovered, and a safe and efficacious vaccine was produced. As a result of these achievements, the field incidence in feedlot cattle was reduced to an insignificant level.

Occurrence. Viral bovine rhinotracheitis has been observed and confirmed in cattle only. While dairy cattle are attacked at all ages, the disease is more serious and of higher incidence in feedlot cattle. Range and pasture cattle seldom develop clinically detectable viral bovine rhinotracheitis. Frequent exposure to the virus and subclinical disease are indicated by high incidence of specific antibodies among range cattle. Experimentally, other species have been refractory to the disease. Limited evidence suggests susceptibility in deer and swine.

Geographically, the virus has been isolated from diseased cattle in the United States, Canada, New Zealand, Britain, Germany, Yugoslavia, Russia, Japan, and Australia.

In the western United States, although some cases have been observed during all months, the seasonal incidence has been significantly higher during autumn and early winter months.

Etiology and Pathogenesis. As a typical member of the herpesvirus group, the virus of viral bovine rhinotracheitis is relatively large in particle size. The cubically symmetrical virion, containing DNA and envelope, measures 120 to 180 mμ in diameter. It is sensitive to ether, ethyl alcohol and acetone and is inactivated in ½ minute by 0.5% caustic soda, in 1 minute by 5% formalin, and in 5 minutes by 1% phenol or 1% quarternary ammonium compounds, and in 21 minutes by temperature of 50° C. The virus retains viability for 50 days at 22° C and for 10 days at 37° C. When stored at −60° C at pH 6 to 9, it endures 9 months.

Outside the bovine host, the virus adapts to and grows in culture systems of embryonal bovine, porcine, ovine, caprine and monkey kidney cells and of HeLa cells. Cytopathic effects in bovine cells include plaque formation and intranuclear inclusion bodies.

Although only a single antigenic form of the virus is recognized, the disease may assume the separate or combined forms of anterior respiratory infection, conjunctivitis, metritis, genital infection and meningoencephalitis. The virus may be isolated from nasal and conjunctival secretions and from infected fetuses, genitalia and brains.

The virus of bovine rhinotracheitis escapes to the external environment from the host in nasal secretions. Although some virus contaminates feed and water and through that means may spread to susceptible cattle, the important method of spread is through infective aerosol. Violent breathing and coughing sprays secretion droplets contaminated with virus into the air and on to eyes, nostrils, muzzle and genitals of nearby susceptible animals. In addition muzzle and nostril to vulva contact among heifers and cows may transfer virus by direct contact from either of these organs. Crowding of animals, a universal practice in feedlots, provides easy opportunity for spread of the virus.

Following entrance into the upper respiratory organs, the virus penetrates epithelial cells and replicates in the nuclei. Injured primarily by the virus and secondarily by bacteria, the mucous membranes of the nose, paranasal sinuses, pharynx, larynx and anterior part of the trachea swell and produce copious exudates that accumulate on the surfaces. These tissue changes fill the cavities of the paranasal sinuses and seriously diminish dimensions of the nasal meatuses. Consequently, breathing may be difficult and through the mouth. Antibodies become identifiable at approximately the ninth day of infection. Healing is usually complete, and recovered animals are immune to subsequent attacks. Complications are common and may add to economic losses. Bronchopneumonia may result from inhalation of detached exudate. Fatalities usually come from pneumonia. Virus may spread from the nose to the brain and cause meningoencephalitis.

The method of transfer into the brain is not known, but may be along the olfactory or other nerves. In pregnant cattle, the virus may move from a primary location in the nose or genitalia by way of the blood to the uterus and placenta. Passing through the placenta the virus enters the fetus where it causes fetal septicemia, necrosis, edema, death and abortion. In some animals virus may transfer mechanically between the nose and genitalia. Frequently, however, infections of conjunctiva, nose and genitalia remain as separate individual and herd maladies.

Clinical Signs and Postmortem Lesions. Following an incubation period of 2 to 4 days, body temperature rises to 104° to 108° F. Sick cattle show anorexia and depression. Fat animals lose body weight rapidly to the extent of 200 pounds per animal. Dairy cattle show diminished milk production. Respiration is accelerated and accompanied by deep moist coughing. Dyspnea is prominent and, in severe cases, is associated with oral breathing and a double expiratory effort. Serous to mucopurulent and, in some cases, sanguineous exudate extends from the nostrils, and salivation is excessive. In approximately 10% of affected cattle, the muzzle is hyperemic and crusted. Conjunctivitis and lacrimation seldom accompany respiratory clinical signs in the same animal. In some outbreaks, however, the disease begins in a herd with conjunctivitis. Serous conjunctivitis progresses to purulent granular conjunctivitis. After a course of 5 to 10 days of the ocular form, other animals of the herd may develop the respiratory syndrome. Animals in advanced pregnancy may abort. The average morbidity is 30% but may be as high as 90%. Mortality is approximately 3% of sick cattle. A limited number of animals develop signs of meningoencephalitis.

The course of the disease within an affected animal varies from 4 to 8 days. Courses within a herd are of two types: first, the entire herd may become sick nearly simultaneously and recover following a course of 2 to 3 weeks; second, individual animals are affected sequentially and the course within the herds extends over a period of many weeks.

In the genital form, vulvovaginal membranes contain vesicles and pustules. The swollen penis and prepuce reveal similar lesions.

The hematological values are normal, and urinalysis shows no significant alterations.

At necropsy, changes are limited to the respiratory system. The muzzle is dry and may be encrusted with mucopurulent exudate. The nasal mucosa is acutely swollen and congested. The surface, especially in the ventral meatus, contains a heavy deposit of mucus which is mixed with purulent and fibrinous exudate. In case of an abnormally prolonged course, masses of dehydrated exudate may be present. Minute erosions and hemorrhages may be discernible. The mucous membrane of the paranasal sinuses is hyperemic and swollen; exudate may fill the lumens. The pharynx and larynx are swollen and may be petechiated and eroded. The mucous membrane of the trachea is affected in variable degrees. In early stages, or mild cases, the mucosa is swollen and petechiated and also contains moderate amounts of mucopurulent exudate. In severe cases, the tracheal mucosa is diptheritic. The necrotic tissue, swollen membranes and accumulated exudate significantly diminish the size of the

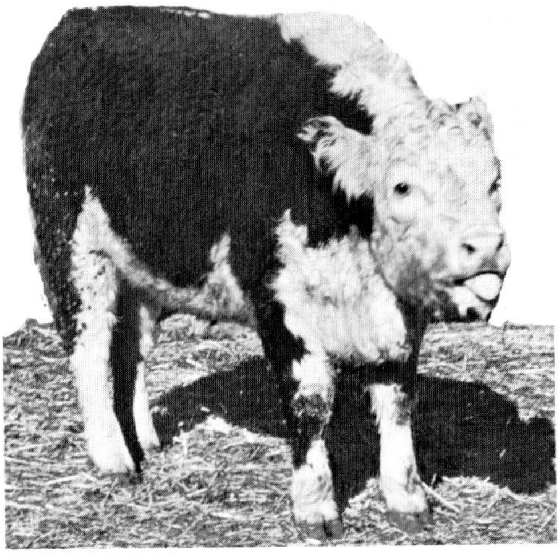

FIG. 2-1. *Feedlot animal with viral bovine rhinotracheitis.*

tracheal lumen. In fatal cases bronchopneumonia may be present.

Other disease forms reveal characteristic lesions. In the genital type, the acutely inflammed vulvovaginal, penile, and prepucial membranes contain vesicles and/or pustules. Aborted fetuses commonly are edematous and visceral organs, such as liver, have pale foci of necrosis.

Histopathologically, the mucous membranes show acute catarrhal inflammation. In animals sacrificed from 30 to 60 hours following exposure, intranuclear inclusion bodies may be found in some epithelial cells of the nose, pharynx and larynx. Since inclusion bodies disappear after a course of 4 to 7 days, they are not identifiable in most fatal cases. Swollen epithelial cells of vulvovaginal, penile, and prepucial pustules have prominent intranuclear inclusion bodies.

Diagnosis. Clinical diagnosis in an endemic area is based on signs and, if available, postmortem findings. While these are nonspecific they are reliable. If necessary, nasal or genital secretions can be submitted to a laboratory for the isolation and identification

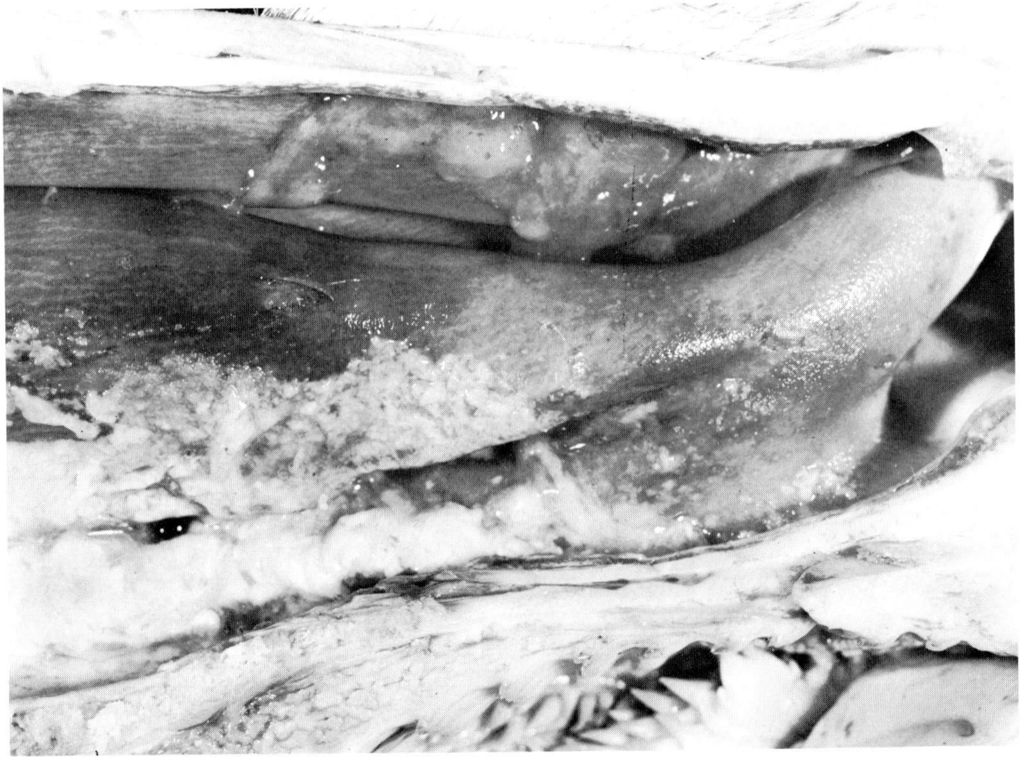

FIG. 2-2. *Anterior part of left nasal cavity from a fatal case of viral bovine rhinotracheitis.* × 0.9.

of the virus by neutralization with known antisera. Finding typical gross and histopathologic lesions on genital organs assists in the diagnosis.

Differential diagnosis requires the consideration of shipping fever and laryngeal calf diphtheria. Among feedlot cattle, shipping fever commonly develops within a few days following admission to the feedlot. Many animals show clinical signs of fibrinous pneumonia. Calf diphtheria usually occurs in a low incidence. Breathing is stertorous and laryngeal lesions can be identified by manipulation and by visual examination of the larynx. In fatal or sacrificed cases, lesions assist in establishing a diagnosis.

Prevention and Treatment. Currently, commercial vaccines are available. These are prepared from live attenuated virus and should be administered to feedlot cattle soon after arrival of animals at the feedlots. The duration of immunity from vaccination, though unknown, is of sufficient length to provide protection through the usual fattening period. Cattle remaining in the feedlot for 300 days, however, may require revaccination after the first 100 to 150 days. Extensive use of the vaccine in endemic areas has controlled the disease to a low and insignificant incidence.

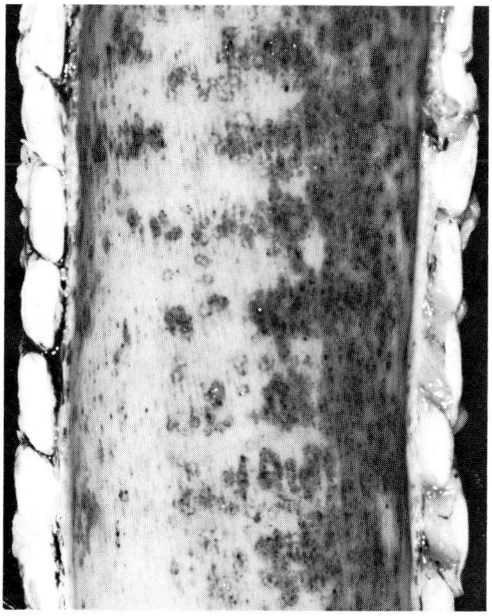

FIG. 2-3. *Trachea from animal with viral bovine rhinotracheitis.* × 1.0.

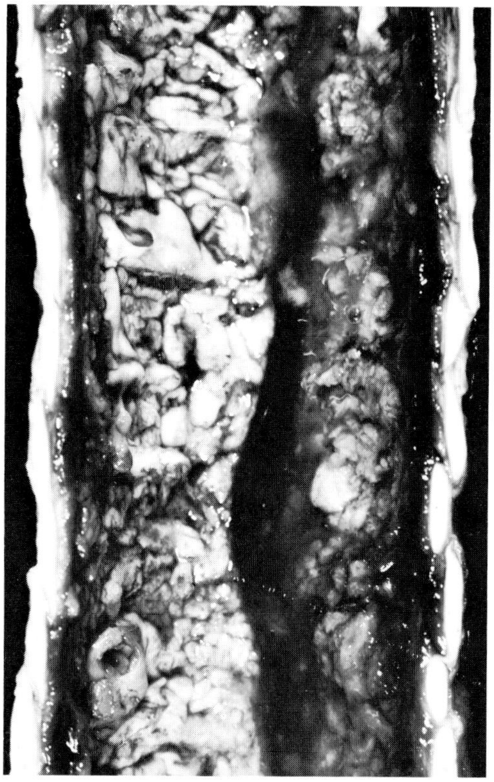

FIG. 2-4. *Exudate and necrotic tissue in mucous membrane from a steer affected with severe viral bovine rhinotracheitis.* × 0.9.

The use of antibiotics and sulfonamides is directed towards the control of secondary bacterial infection, especially bronchopneumonia. In case of diphtheritic tracheitis, the administration of a proteolytic enzyme as an intratracheal spray is helpful and shortens the course. Heavily infected herds can be treated with sulfathizole or sulfamethazine in the drinking water at the rate of 1 pound per 100 gallons for 2 to 3 days, followed by one-half the dosage for 2 to 3 more days. Another herd treatment is the inclusion of oxytetracycline or chlortetracycline in the feed at the rate of 1 mg per

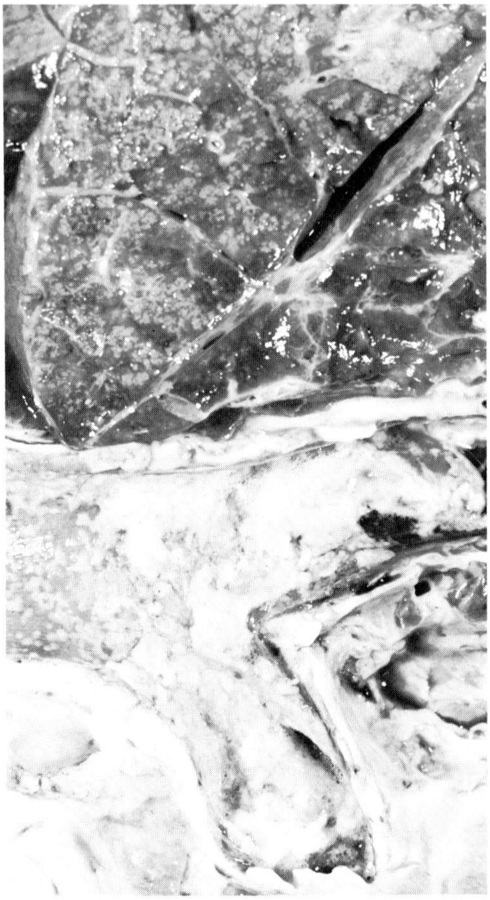

FIG. 2-5. *Bronchitis and bronchopneumonia from a fatal case of viral bovine rhinotracheitis.* × 1.6.

pound of body weight per day for 7 days, followed by one-half the dosage for 7 more days.

References

Abinati, F. R. and Plumer, G. J.: The Isolation of Infectious Bovine Rhinotracheitis Virus from Cattle Affected with Conjunctivitis—Observations on the Experimental Infection. AJVR, *22* (1961): 13–17.

Adams, O. R., Brown, W. W., Chow, T. L., Collier, J. R., Davis, R. W., Griner, L. A., Jensen, Rue, Pierson, R. E. and Wayt, L. K.: Comparison of Infectious Bovine Rhinotracheitis, Shipping Fever, and Calf Diphtheria of Cattle. JAVMA, *134* (1959): 85–89.

Armstrong, J. A., Pereira, H. G. and Andrews, C. H.: Observations on the Virus of Infectious Bovine Rhinotracheitis and its Affinity with the Herpesvirus Group. Virology, *14* (1961): 276.

Barenfus, M., Delli Quadri, C. A. and McIntyre, R. W.: Isolation of Bovine Rhinotracheitis Virus from Calves with Meningoencephalitis. JAVMA, *143* (1963): 725–728.

Bocciarelli, D. S., Orfei, Z., Mondino, G. and Persechino, A.: The Core of a Herpes Virus. Virology, *30* (1966): 58–61.

Brown, W. W. and Chow, T. L.: Field trials of Infectious Bovine Rhinotracheitis Vaccine. JAVMA, *134* (1959): 29–31.

Brown, W. W., Chow, T. L. and Jensen, Rue.: Symposium on the Mucosal Disease Complex. I. Infectious Bovine Rhinotracheitis in Feedlots of Colorado. JAVMA, *130* (1957): 379–381.

Chow, T. L.: Infectious Bovine Rhinotracheitis in Range Cattle of Colorado. JAVMA, *138* (1961): 59–60.

Chow, T. L., and Davis, R. W.: Susceptibility of Deer to Rhinotracheitis. JAVMA, *25* (1964): 518–519.

Chow, T. L., Deem, A. W. and Jensen, Rue.: Infectious Rhinotracheitis in Cattle. II. Experimental Reproduction. Proceedings, U.S.L.S.A., 59th annual meeting (1955): 168–172.

Chow, T. L., Palotay, J. L. and Deem, A. W.: Infectious Rhinotracheitis in Feedlot Cattle. III. An Epizootiological Study in a Feedlot. JAVMA, *128* (1956): 348–351.

Crandell, R. A., Cheatham, W. J. and Maurer, F. D.: Infectious Bovine Rhinotracheitis—The Occurrence of Intranuclear Inclusion Bodies in Experimentally Infected Animals. AJVR, *20* (1959): 505.

Gillespie, J. H., Baker, J. A. and Wagner, W. C.: The Relationship of Infectious Pustular Vulvovaginitis Virus to Infectious Bovine Rhinotracheitis Virus. Proceedings, U.S.L.S.A., 62nd annual meeting (1958): 119.

Gillespie, J. H., Lee, K. M. and Baker, J. A.: Infectious Bovine Rhinotracheitis. AJVR, *18* (1957): 530.

Griffin, T. P., Howells, W. V., Crandell, R. A. and Maurer, F. D.: Stability of the Virus of Infectious Bovine Rhinotracheitis. AJVR, *19* (1958): 990.

Hahnfeld, H. and Hahnfeld, E.: Nucleic Acid of Infectious Bovine Rhinotracheitis Virus and Coital Vesicular Exanthema Virus. Arch. Exp. Vet., Med., *18* (1964): 921–928.

Hall, W. T. K., Simmons, G. C., French, E. L., Snowdon, W. A. and Asdell, M.: The Pathogenesis of Encephalitis Caused by the Infectious Bovine Rhinotracheitis. Aust. Vet. J., *42* (1966): 229–237.

Jasty, V. and Chang, P. W.: Infectious Bovine Rhinotracheitis Virus in Bovine Kidney Cells: Sequence of Viral Production, Cellular Changes, and Location of Viral Nucleic Acid and Protein. AJVR, *30* (1969): 1325–1332.

Jensen, Rue, Griner, L. A., Chow, T. L. and Brown, W. W.: Infectious Rhinotracheitis in Feedlot Cattle. I. Pathology and Symptoms. Proceedings, U.S.L.S.A., 59th annual meeting (1955): 189–199.

Kahrs, R. F. and Baker, J. A.: Combined Vaccines for Dairy Cattle. Proc. 69th annual meeting. U.S.L.S.A., (1965): 177–182.

Kendrick, J. W., Gillespie, J. H. and McEntee, K.: Infectious Pustular Vulvaovaginitis of Cattle. Corn. Vet., *48* (1958): 458–495.

Kendrick, J. W. and Straub, O. C.: IBR-IPV Vulvovaginitis Virus Infection in Pregnant Cows. AJVR, *28* (1967): 1269–1282.

Madin, S. H., York, C. J. and McKercher, D. G.: Isolation of the Infectious Bovine Rhinotracheitis Virus. Science, *124* (1956): 721.

Mare, John and Von Rensburg, S. J.: The Isolation of Viruses Associated with Sterility in Cattle. A Preliminary Report. J. So. African Vet. Med. Assoc., *32* (1961): 201–210.

McFeeley, R. A., Merritt, A. M. and Stearly, E. L.: Abortion in a Dairy Herd Vaccinated for Infectious Bovine Rhinotracheitis. JAVMA, *153* (1968): 657–661.

McIntyre, R. W.: Experimental Studies of Acute Upper Respiratory Infection of Calves. JAVMA, *125* (1954): 473.

McKercher, D. G., Moulton, J. E., Kendrick, J. W. and Saito, J.: Proceedings U.S.L.S.A., 59th annual meeting (1955): 151–167.

McKercher, D. G. and Straub, O. C.: Isolation of the Virus of Infectious Bovine Rhinotracheitis from Range Cattle. JAVMA, *137* (1960): 661–664.

Miller, N. J.: Infectious Necrotic Rhinotracheitis of Cattle. JAVMA, *126* (1955): 463.

Molello, J. A., Chow, T. L., Owen, N. and Jensen, Rue.: Placental Pathology. V. Placental Lesions of Cattle Infected with IBR Virus. AJVR, *27* (1966): 907–915.

Owen, N. V., Chow, T. L. and Molello, J. A.: I. IBR: Correlation of Fetal and Placental Lesions with Viral Isolations. II. IBR: Relationship of Level of Maternal Antibody Titre to Incidence of Fetal Death and Abortion. AJVR, *29* (1968): 1959–1965; 1967–1970.

Plimpton, R. F.: Studies on Combination Vaccines for Dairy Cattle. Diss. Abst. *26* (1966): 3565–3566.

Report Panel for Symposium on Immunity to Bovine Respiratory Disease. JAVMA, *152* (1968): 713–719.

Satter, S. A., Bohl, E. H. and Trapp, A. L.: Abortion in Cattle Caused by Experimental Infection with IBR Virus. Corn. Vet., *57* (1967): 438–454.

Schroeder, R. J. and Moys, M. D.: An Acute Upper Respiratory Infection of Dairy Cattle. JAVMA, 125 (1954): 471.

St. George, T. D.: Keratoconjunctivitis Associated with IBR Infection in Victorian Cattle. Aust. Vet. J., *41* (1965): 222–223.

Straub, O. C.: Effects of Some Disinfectants on IBR-IPV Vaginitis Virus. Tierärztl. Umsch., *20* (1965): 568–570.

Tousimis, A. J., Howells, W. V., Griffin, T. P., Chaetham, R. P. and Maurer, F. D.: Biophysical Characterization of the IBR Virus. Proc. Soc. Exp. Biol. and Med., *99* (1958): 614–617.

Watrach, A. M., and Bahnemann, H.: The Structure of IBR Virus. Arch. Ges. Virusforsch., *18* (1966): 1–7.

York, C. J.: Infectious Bovine Rhinotracheitis. JAVMA, *152* (1968): 758–762.

Aujeszky's Disease

(PSEUDORABIES; MAD ITCH; INFECTIOUS BULBAR PARALYSIS)

Characterized by both severe focal itching and central nervous disturbance, bovine Aujeszky's disease is an acute, non-contagious viral infection. During its course body temperature elevates and respirations accelerate. The disease affects most domestic mammals, has scattered world-wide distribution, but is of minor economic importance to the cattle industry because herd incidence is sporadic and low. Within an affected herd, however, the morbidity incidence commonly reaches 40% and the mortality rate 90 to 100%. Economic losses result not only from the mortality of diseased cattle, but also from inpropitious marketing of herds threatened with decimation by the malady. The actual monetary losses have not been assayed or recorded.

Review of Literature. During investigations of rabies, brain tissues from suspected animals were subcutaneously inoculated into rabbits. Within 36 hours of injection rabbits inoculated with tissues from an ox and from a dog developed severe pruritus near the points of inoculation. Death occurred after an additional 12 hours. These effects on rabbits varied from the known rabid signs and led the investigator to conclude that the disease was distinct from rabies. (Aujeszky,

1902). The disease, now bearing the name of its discoverer, A. Aujeszky, has been encountered in feedlot (Anonymous, 1956) and pasture cattle (Hoyt, 1946) where the intra-herd incidence was from 40 to 50%. In addition, the presence of specific antibodies against its virus in a large number of serums from swine of the midwestern states indicated a high incidence among pigs (Shope, 1935a). Dogs, cats, sheep, horses and rats were also observed with the natural disease (Galloway, 1938).

Some biological characteristics of the virus of Aujeszky's disease have been investigated and described. Multiple passages through guinea pigs by intracerebral inoculation reduced pathogenicity of the strain by subcutaneous injection. The same passaged virus, however, was highly pathogenic when subcutaneously administered to highly susceptible rabbits (Shope, 1933). Some adapted strains of the virus grew in embryonating chicken eggs (Morrill and Graham, 1941; Skoda, 1962), in minced rabbit testes producing intranuclear inclusion bodies (Traub, 1933), and in monolayer cell cultures of swine kidney cells, chick embryo fibroblasts (Skoda and Mayer, 1961; Zuffa and Skoda, 1962), in monkey kidney cells (Tokumaru, 1957) and in HeLa cells (Sacco and Maglione, 1968). On the basis of cytopathogenic effects on monkey kidney cell cultures, two different viral strains were identified: one strain caused rounding of the cells while the other resulted in cytolytic giant cell formation (Tokumaru, 1957). The study of viruses from herpes simplex and from Aujeszky's disease demonstrated deoxyribonucleic acid in both (Ben-Porat and Kaplan, 1962).

Investigation of the pathogenesis revealed that the virus moved from the point of inoculation along afferent nerve trunks to their corresponding spinal ganglia. Inflammatory reactions were evoked along the nerves and within the ganglia. From the ganglia the virus entered the spinal cord and moved anteriorly to the medulla. Some spinal ganglionic neurons degenerated and developed intranuclear inclusion bodies (Dow and McFerran, 1962; Hurst, 1933; Dow and McFerran, 1966). Application of the fluorescent antibody technique revealed virus in Schwann cells (Rajcani and Sabo, 1969). The transection of nerves leading from the point of inoculation altered the disease course. Neuronal damage with respiratory failure was the cause of death. In addition to entering nerve tissue, the virus temporarily entered the blood but probably did not traverse the blood-brain barrier to enter the central nervous system (Hurst, 1934).

Studies of disease transmission indicated that rats consuming virus infected tissues of other rats or dead swine may acquire Aujeszky's disease and that pigs may acquire the disease from consuming infected rats (Shope, 1935a). With their nasal secretions infected swine excreted the virus and may have inoculated susceptible cattle through contact of the swine nose with bovine abraded skin (Shope, 1935).

Occurrence. All ages, breeds, and sexes of cattle are susceptible to Aujeszky's disease, but naturally it usually occurs among cattle 6 months to 4 years of age. Among feedlot and pastured cattle the disease often occurs where swine and cattle cohabitate and frequently where rat populations are abundant. In addition to cattle, the disease is encountered in swine, sheep, dogs, horses, rats, and occasionally in people.

Geographically, the disease occurs sporadically in Europe, Russia, Britain, North Africa, North America and South America. The high incidence of specific antibodies in swine serums suggests common occurrence in the mid-western region of the United States.

Etiology. The virus causing pseudorabies is a typical member of the herpesvirus group. The virion, consisting of nucleocapsid with double stranded DNA and envelope, measures 150 to 180 mμ in diameter. Sensitive to ether and heat, the virus is inactivated at temperatures of 60° C for 40 minutes, 70° C for 10 minutes, and 80° C for 3 minutes. It is destroyed by 5% phenol in 2 hours, by 1%

sodium hydroxide in a short time, and by decomposing animal tissues in 11 days.

In the laboratory the virus can be grown in small animals and cell culture systems. Rabbits are susceptible to subcutaneous inoculation and develop disease with manifestations of extreme pruritus. It grows in the chorioallantoic membrane of embryonating chicken eggs and produces pock-like lesions. The embryos usually die 3 to 5 days following inoculation. In addition the virus grows in culture systems of guinea pig testicle cells, monkey kidney cells, and HeLa cells. Cytopathic effects include enlargement and rounding of infected cells. Only a single antigenic form is known. Antibodies to the virus are common in swine sera of the midwest of the United States and much less common in the sera of cattle.

Transmission. Because the probable reservoir of virus is an infection of brown rats and swine, live rats become fatally infected from consuming virulent tissues of dead rats, swine, cattle, or other animals. Hogs may contract the disease from consuming infected dead rats or infected tissues from other dead animals and also may be inoculated either orally or intranasally. In diseased swine the virus is excreted through nasal secretions and contaminates the external surface of the snout. Cattle may be inoculated by pigs rubbing their virus infected snouts against bovine skin abrasions, or occasionally by infected swine biting or rooting recumbent cattle. Cattle may be inoculated intranasally with virus contaminated food or water.

Pathogenesis. Following inoculation, the virus moves centripetally along the afferent nerves to their respective spinal ganglia and into the dorsal horns of the spinal cord. Continually moving centrally, the virus ascends to the medulla oblongata but, in some cases, more rosterally in the brain stem. In case of inoculation around the face, the virus ascends along the afferent portions of cranial nerves, enters the ganglia, such as the semilunar ganglion of the trigeminal nerve, and goes to the brain. Since the distance traversed in reaching the brain is short, the incubation period following head inoculations is commonly shorter than the similar period for inoculations over the posterior part of the body. In some animals at least, inoculation is followed by transitory viremia. The virus is removed from the blood and deposited in secondarily infected tissues. From the new location it moves along afferent nerves to the central nervous system. Antibodies form in the blood and in swine, at least, the virus is excreted to the external environment in nasal secretions.

Tissue reactions to the virus occur throughout the infected portion of the nervous system. At the point of inoculation, an acute serous inflammation may develop, but the direct reaction to the virus is negligible. Subsequent trauma results in hemorrhage, necrosis, and severe inflammation. Along the infected nerves lymphocytes accumulate and within the infected ganglia neurons degenerate and necrose. Some neurons and some mesenchymal cells develop intranuclear inclusion bodies. Within the spinal cord and brain, foci of neuronal degeneration and inflammation develop. Neuronal injury in the ganglia results in the severe itching sensation, and most infected cattle die from neuronal injury in the medulla followed by respiratory failure.

Clinical Signs and Postmorten Lesions. Following an incubation period of 3 to 6 days, body temperature ranges between 104° and 105° F. As the disease progresses and manifests its maximum signs, the temperature rises and ranges from 105° to 107° F, and then prior to death declines to below normal levels. Simultaneous with the beginning pyrexia, itching develops at the points of virus inoculation. As the disease advances, the pruritus augments and torments. Cattle continuously lick, bite, kick and rub the affected area. Commonly these reactions result in depillation, excoriation, hemorrhage and mutilation. In extreme cases the injuries extend through the skin and into the deep subcutaneous and muscular tissues. Constant attention to the itching prevents the intake of feed or water. Salivation, rapid respiration and incoordination of movements are usually present. Sweating and grinding of the teeth are also evident. Muscular tremors and spasms are accompanied by prostration, convulsions and progressive weakness. Inconstantly, some animals become aggressive and attack with snorting noises. While most affected cattle manifest tormenting pruritus and consequential self-mutilation, some infections are accompanied by pyrexia, depression, circling, muscular tremors, aggression, stupor and prostration without pruritus.

While the morbidity rate in feedlot cattle is often low, it may reach 40 to 50% of a herd, but the mortality rate of affected animals is always high and 90 to 100% is not unusual. While the disease course usually varies from 36 to 48 hours, it may be shortened as a result of viral inoculation around the head.

At necropsy lesions are limited to the point of inoculation and the central nervous system. In the itching area the hair is absent and the skin hyperemic, hemorrhagic, and lacerated. In some animals excoriations extend through the skin into subcutaneous and muscular tissues, the affected area is swollen, and inflammatory edema and hemorrhage are prominent. The vascular system of the central nervous system is congested. In some animals the lungs are edematous and petechial hemorrhages are distributed throughout the serosal surfaces. Animals having Aujeszky's disease, but submitted for emergency slaughter, should be condemned as unsuitable for human food. The tissues should be incinerated or deeply buried in unslaked lime; contaminated instruments and floor surfaces should be chemically disinfected.

The significant histopathologic changes are found in the area of inoculation and in the affected parts of the nervous system. Acute inflammation with edema, hemorrhage, necrosis, and leukocytosis are prominent in the area of pruritus. Most of the changes are the result of traumatic injury from continuous licking, biting, kicking, and rubbing. Foci of lymphocytic infiltration of the perineurium and epineurium may be found along the affected afferent nerve. In the corresponding spinal ganglia changes are found in both epidermal and mesodermal cells. Many neurons show swelling, chromatolysis of Nissl granules, eccentric displacement of the nuclei, intranuclear inclusion bodies, and necrosis. Many capsular cells which surround the neurons contain intranuclear inclusion bodies. Lymphocytes and mononuclear macrophages may infiltrate the stroma. These changes are limited to the affected side. In the spinal cord, from the level of the affected spinal ganglion to the medulla oblongata, neuronal degeneration and necrosis are usually present. Perivascular accumulations of lymphocytes and mononuclear macrophages are discernible. In case of inoculation around the head and the movement of virus along the trigeminal nerve, similar cellular changes are found in the semilunar ganglion. In case of viral ascension along the olfactory nerve, neuronal degeneration, necrosis, and inflammation are found in the olfactory lobe.

Diagnosis. Aujeszky's disease is identified on the basis of typical clinical signs and specific laboratory findings. The febrile reaction, severe pruritus, self-mutilation, muscular tremors, and short course are evident visual signs of paramount importance. In many outbreaks these distinctive manifestations are sufficient evidence for a positive diagnosis. In cases not showing pruritus, however, Aujeszky's disease may be suspect but not diagnosed. Muscular tremors, incoordination, depression, and aggression in cattle associated with swine, but without obvious cause for these signs, may be suspect of Aujeszky's disease. Laboratory confirmation is obtained by subcutaneously inoculating infected emulsified spinal cord into rabbits. Following an incubation period of 36 to 48 hours the rabbits also develop severe pruritus and traumatize the itching area. Death usually occurs after a course of 12 to 24 hours.

Rabbits also develop the neuronal changes similar to those of affected cattle. The fluorescent antibody technique may also be used with high accuracy. In addition the virus may be isolated from infected brains in cell culture systems and identified.

The differential diagnosis requires consideration of rabies, polioencephalomalacia and poisoning. In rabies, stressed animals salivate and often become aggressive, but seldom show the severe pruritus of Aujeszky's disease. Histopathologically, Negri bodies can usually be demonstrated in neurons of the hippocampus and in Purkinje cells of the cerebellum. Subcutaneous inoculation of rabbits with tissue suspensions containing rabies virus does not produce pruritus. Polioencephalomalacia should be considered in animals showing normal body temperature, impaired vision and no pruritus. Many cattle with polioencephalomalacia recover following thiamin administration, although partial blindness persists. At necropsy focal necrosis is discernible in many areas of the cerebral cortex. Careful consideration of the animal history and chemical analysis of gastric contents assist in the diagnosis of poisonings.

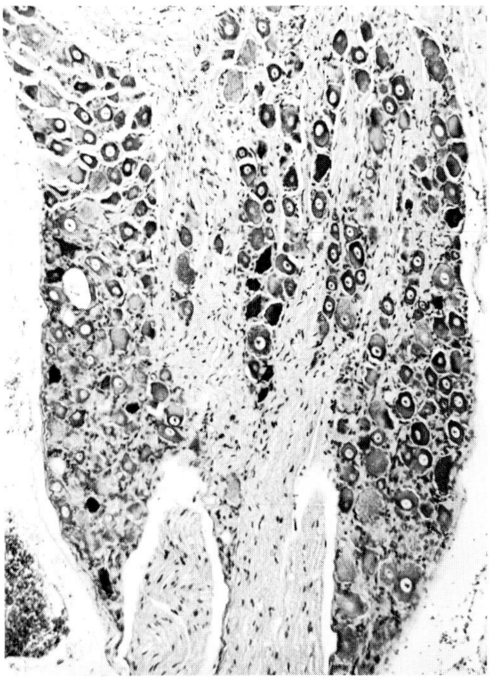

FIG. 2-6. *Necrotic neurons in a spinal ganglion from Aujeszky's disease. Nocht's stain.* × 82.

Prevention and Treatment. Many outbreaks of Aujeszky's disease in feedlot cattle can be prevented by excluding swine from the pens, feed, and water of cattle. Excessive rat populations around feedlots should be avoided by sanitation and by removing rat shelters, such as junk piles and decomposing feed. Although vaccines have been developed and used in some European countries, they have not been adopted in the United States. In case of an outbreak, affected cattle should be removed from the pen and isolated. Effective treatment against Aujeszky's disease has not been developed. The local administration of anesthetic does not relieve the itching, but the use of tranquilizers and a quiet, non-stimulating environment may increase the comfort of the animal.

References

Anonymous: Aujeszky's Disease in Cattle. JAVMA, *128* (1956): 602.

Aujeszky, A.: Uber eine Neue Infecktionskrankheit bei Haustieren. Centr. fur Bakt., Parasit., und Infekt., *32* (1902): 353–373.

Ben-Porat, T. and Kaplan, A. S.: The Chemical Composition of Herpes Simplex and Pseudorabies Viruses. Virology, *16* (1962): 261–266.

Dow, C. and McFerran, J. B.: The Pathology of Aujeszky's Disease in Cattle. J. Comp. Path., *72* (1962): 337–347.

———: Experimental Studies on Aujeszky's Disease in Cattle. J. Comp. Path., *76* (1966): 379–385.

Galloway, I. A.: Aujeszky's Disease. Vet. Rec., *50* (1938): 745–762.

Hoyt, H. H.: Aujeszky's Disease in Wisconsin, JAVMA, *108* (1946): 422–424.

Hurst, E. W.: Studies on Pseudorabies (Infectious Bulbar Paralysis, Mad Itch) I. Histology of the Disease, With a Note on Symptomatology. J. Exp. Med., *38* (1933): 415–433.

———: Studies on Pseudorabies (Infectious Bulbar Paralysis, Mad Itch) II. Routes of Infection in the Rabbit, With Remarks on the Relation of the Virus to Other Viruses Affecting the Nervous System. J. Exp. Med. *59* (1934): 729–749.

Morrill, C. C. and Graham, R.: An Outbreak of Bovine Pseudorabies, or "Mad Itch". AJVR, *2* (1941): 35–40.

Rajčáni, J. and Sabó, A.: Histological and Immunohistological Studies on the Pathogenesis of Aujeszky's Disease in Piglets. Zentbl. Vet., Med., *16B* (1969): 541–552.

Sacco, T. and Maglione, E.: Culture of Aujeszky's Disease Virus in He La Cells. Annali. Fac. Med. Vet. Torino, *17* (1968): 303–314.

Sellers, A. F., Pomeroy, B. S., Sautter, J. H., Pint, C. H. and Schrafel, C. E.: Atypical Pseudorabies and Listeriosis in Cattle. JAVMA, *114* (1949): 69–73.

Shahan, M. S., Knudson, R. L., Seibold, H. R. and Dale, C. N.: Aujeszky's Disease (Pseudorabies) A Review, with Notes on Two Strains of the Virus. North Am. Vet., *28* (1947): 441–449; 511.

Shope, R. E.: Modification of the Pathogenicity of Pseudorabies Virus by Animal Passage. J. Exp. Med., *57* (1933): 925–931.

———: Experiments on the Epidemiology of Pseudorabies. I. Mode of Transmission of the Disease in Swine and Their Possible Role in its Spread to Cattle. J. Exp. Med., *62* (1935): 85–99.

———: Experiments on the Epidemiology of Pseudorabies. II. Prevalence of the Disease Among Middle Western Swine and the Possible Role of Rats in Herd-to-Herd Infections. J. Exp. Med., *62* (1935a); 101–117.

Škoda, R.: Immunization of Calves with Modified Virus of Aujeszky's Disease. Veterinarystvi, *12* (1962): 101–102. [V. B., *32* (1962): 747]

Škoda, R., and Mayer, V.: Propogation of Aujeszky's Disease Virus in Monolayer Culture of Chick Embryo Fibroblasts. Arch. Exp. Vet. Med., *15* (1961): 391–396.

Tokumaru, Tadasu: Pseudorabies Virus in Tissue Culture: Differentiation of Two Distinct Strains of Virus by Cytopathogenic Pattern Induced. Proc. Soc. Exp. Biol. Med., *96* (1957): 55–60.

Traub, Erich: Cultivation of Pseudorabies Virus. J. Exp. Med., *58* (1933): 663–681.

Žuffa, A. and Škoda, R.: Some Biological Properties of Aujeszky Virus. Vet. Cas., *11* (1962): 155–164.

Malignant Catarrhal Fever

(MALIGNANT CATARRH; MALIGNANT HEAD CATARRH; SNOTSIEKTE)

Malignant catarrhal fever, an acute infectious but non-contagious condition of cattle, is characterized by high fever and panophthalmitis, and by inflammation of the membranes of the respiratory, digestive and urinary systems. The cause is a virus. Economically, the disease is of minor importance because of its low and sporadic incidence.

Review of Literature. While malignant catarrh was observed and recognized as an entity throughout much of the nineteenth century, productive studies of the disease began in the early twentieth century. In experiments conducted in Africa in 1923, infectivity of the disease was established when it was transmitted by the inoculation of large amounts of blood from affected to normal cattle (Mettam, 1923). In subsequent experiments many other investigators confirmed transmissibility by transferring large amounts of blood from diseased to healthy experimental animals (Blood *et al.*, 1961; Daubney and Hudson, 1936; Goetz and Leiss, 1929; Piercy, 1952; Plowright, 1953a), and by inoculation of lymph node tissue suspension from affected cattle into the lymph nodes of healthy cattle (Piercy, 1952). By inoculating blood or lymph node tissue suspension into lymph nodes of cattle, the disease was transmitted sequentially to at least 19 cattle (Blood *et al.*, 1961; Daubney and Hudson, 1936; Piercy, 1952). Many similar attempts at transmission, however, were unsuccessful, even though large amounts of blood and tissue suspensions were transferred from affected to healthy cattle (de Kock and Neitz, 1950; Doberstein *et al.*, 1928). Among laboratory animals, rabbits have proved susceptible to intracerebral inoculation of infected tissue (Daubney and Hudson, 1936; Plowright, 1953a).

In Europe it was recognized that cattle affected with malignant catarrh had been, in many cases, associated with sheep. Between 1945 and 1949, 72% of 849 Finnish cases had been associated directly or indirectly with sheep (Stenius, 1952). The implication of sheep in the epizootiology was strengthened when sheep from an infected farm were transported to a distant clean farm which contained 50 healthy cattle. Of the latter, 94% developed malignant catarrh subsequent to introduction of sheep from the infected farm (Gotze, 1930). Many studied outbreaks of the disease, however, have not been associated with sheep (Henning, 1956).

Even though proof has been lacking until recently, malignant catarrh has long been considered as a viral disease. In unsuccessful transmission experiments the causative agent could not be passed through bacteria-retaining filters (Piercy, 1952a), and plasma without cells was not infective (Mettam, 1923). As little as 0.05 ml of leukocytes from infected blood inoculated into susceptible animals produced the disease (Piercy, 1952a). This led to the conclusion that the virus is attached to leukocytes. Later, the viral nature of the causative agent was established by growing the agent on monolayer cell culture of thyroid epithelium (Plowright and Ferris, 1960; 1961). Growth of virus in cell culture systems lead to its characterization and classification as a member of the Herpesvirus group (Plowright, Macadam, and Armstrong, 1963). The cultivated virus reproduced the disease when returned by parenteral inoculation to susceptible cattle.

In East Africa, the discovery of malignant catarrh in the blue wildebeest (*Gorgon taurinus taurinus*, Burchell) led to increased understanding of the disease. The study of 181 serum samples from all ages of animals in a free-living population of wildebeest indicated that all animals over 7 months of age contained antibodies against the virus of malignant catarrh (Plowright, 1963; 1968). Large numbers of blood samples were investigated for virus, and in animals up to 3 months of age the infection rate was approximately 30%; in those 4 to 9 months, 7%; and in older animals, 2% (Plowright, 1965; 1967). Virus was isolated from a fetal spleen (Plowright, 1965) and from calves as young as 1 week of age (Plowright, 1965a; 1967). When a captive wildebeest calf was inoculated with virulent bovine blood, it became viremic from the eighth day to the thirty-first week after inoculation. Three bovine calves housed with the viremic wildebeest calf acquired infection after incubation periods of 30, 38, and 40 days (Plowright, 1965a).

Pathologic changes have been studied in natural and experimentally produced cases. Detailed investigation of 36 East African bovine cases established that the basic changes were in the lymphoid-macrophage system. During early disease stages small lymphocytes were destroyed and depleted from nodes, spleen and Peyer's patches and macrophages phagocytized the cellular debris. Lymphogenous tissue throughout the body then was intensely stimulated to produce large and medium sized lymphocytes. Undifferentiated cells accumulated around small vessels. This vascular change resulted in inadequate nutrition for surrounding cells, including epithelium of the alimentary tract; this change led to the formation of vast numbers of erosions in the mouth, pharynx, esophagus and forestomachs (Plowright, 1953; Berkman *et al.*, 1960). In addition, viral inclusion bodies have been described for cytoplasm of epithelial cells of the conjunctiva, mouth, nose and pharynx (Goss, Cole, Kissling, 1947), of neurons of the vagoglossopharyngeal nucleus (Stenius, 1952), and of reticuloendothelial cells of spleen, lymph nodes and lungs (Danskin, 1955).

Besides cattle, malignant catarrh has been observed in wild deer (Huck, Shand, and Allsop, 1961; Senior, Halnan, and Tong, 1962). The disease was transmitted experimentally from Pere Davids deer to red deer to calves and to rabbits. In deer the disease was similar to malignant catarrh of cattle. Wildebeest in Africa (Plowright, 1963) and sheep in many countries are known to be inapparent carriers (Gotze, 1930; Mettam, 1923; Stenius, 1952).

Occurrence. Both sexes and all breeds of cattle are equally susceptible to malignant catarrh. While cattle of all ages are attacked, the disease rarely occurs in animals under 4 months of age. The incidence is highest in ages 6 months to 4 years. While sheep do not develop the disease, they appear, in some cases, to carry the virus. In Africa the wildebeest may also be an inapparent carrier. Some species of deer develop the disease and manifest clinical signs which are similar to the disease in cattle. In the laboratory, rabbits are susceptible to parenteral inoculation of the virus.

Malignant catarrh occurs during all seasons, but the incidence is higher during autumn and spring. Geographically, it is worldwide in distribution.

Etiology and Pathogenesis. The virus causing malignant catarrhal fever is classified as a member of the herpesvirus group. The virion, consisting of nucleocapsid with DNA and envelope, measures 140 to 240 $m\mu$ in diameter, is sensitive to the action of ether, and is inhibited by 5-iodo-2′-deoxyuridine. Because it is sensitive to physical adversities, the virus survives only a few days in storage at 4° C. Mixed with 20 to 40% bovine serum and 10% glycerol, it maintains viability in storage at −70° C for approximately 15 months.

The virus has been cultivated in biological systems outside the mammalian body. It grows on cultures of calf thyroid cells which may be used for initial isolation; after adaptation to thyroid cells it may be transferred to calf kidney cells. Induced cytopathologic changes in cultured cells include cytoplasmic vacuolation, multinucleated syncytia, and intranuclear inclusion bodies. The virus does not grow in embryonating chicken eggs.

In the bovine host the virus is strongly associated with cells. In circulating blood, it is attached to leukocytes, especially mononuclear cells. It is also found in lymphoid tissue of nodes and spleen but not in secretions or excretions. In addition to cattle, the virus exists without clinical manifestation in sheep of America and Europe and in the blue wildebeest of East Africa. Among laboratory animals the rabbit is susceptible to parenteral inoculation of virus-containing tissues and cells.

The method of transmission of malignant catarrhal fever is not known. The virus apparently does not transfer between cattle, and for this reason cattle may be an unnatural host. In America and Europe the reservoir of virus and the source of infection in many but not all outbreaks are sheep, but in East Africa they are the blue wildebeest. Even though statistical evidence often indicates that affected cattle have recently associated with sheep, the virus has not been identified in ovine excretions or secretions. In East Africa susceptible bovine calves housed with infected wildebeest calves developed the disease, but again the means of transmission was not determined. Transmission by arthropod vectors has been considered and studied, but this method has not been demonstrated in any case.

Only fragmentary information on pathogenesis of bovine malignant catarrhal fever is available. Following close association of susceptible cattle with virus-carrying sheep, some cattle develop the disease. The anatomical points of entrance of the virus into cattle are not known. On parenteral entrance, however, the virus first attacks and replicates in lymphoid tissues, such as lymph nodes, Peyer's patches, and splenic germinal centers. Many small lymphocytes are destroyed and germinal centers depleted. As a result of these degenerative changes, the lymphoreticular centers of the entire body are stimulated to produce medium sized and large lymphocytes. Undifferentiated lymphoid cells frequently accumulate around small blood vessels, especially venules. In some vessels the walls become infiltrated. The vascular changes interfere with diffusion of nutrients from plasma into adjacent perivascular tissue and cells. In the mouth, esophagus and forestomachs, where the mucous membrane is stratified squamous epithelium, inadequate cell nutrition around vessels causes degeneration of tunica adventitia and necrosis of basal epithelial cells of the stratum germinativum. Dissolution and detachment of these cells create epithelial erosions that characterize the disease. Lymphoid cells also accumulate in stromal tissues of liver, kidneys, adrenals, lungs and heart.

In experimentally induced bovine malignant catarrhal fever, prominent changes occur in the blood. Leukocytes, especially mononuclear cells, containing virus discharge from the lymphoid tissues into the blood, and the viremia may persist from approximately the eighth day after inoculation until near death. Virus does not occur free of cells in plasma. At the time of rise in body temperatures, leukopenia develops and persists throughout the course of the disease.

The clinical course begins with nasal and ocular discharge, and these signs are followed by fever and changes in the mucous membranes. Most affected cattle die, but the few surviving cases are immune to subsequent exposures.

Clinical Signs and Postmortem Lesions. Following a highly variable but average incubation period of approximately 9 days to 9 weeks, body temperature rises to 105° to 108° F, and tends to maintain a high level. Anorexia develops early. Respiration is rapid and, in some cases, difficult and noisy because of swelling and congestion in the mucous membranes and copious exudate in the nasal meatuses and nostrils. The exudate protrudes from the nostrils in tenacious strands. At first, the exudate is translucent mucus, while later it becomes an opaque mixture of mucus and pus. Flakes of blood may be present. In early stages the muzzle is red from hyperemia, while in later stages the mucous membrane is eroded and covered with a heavy crust of dried exudate. Removal of the crust reveals an eroded, hemorrhaging surface. In early stages the mucosa of the mouth is hyperemic and cyanotic. Later, multiple small erosions develop on the buccal papillae, dental pad, hard palate, around the teeth, and especially at the junction of the skin and mucous membrane. As a result of meningitis, affected animals become aggressive and may attack attendants and inflict self-injury. Bilateral conjunctivitis and panophthalmitis result in lacrimation and photophobia. Purulent exudate accumulates in the conjunctival sacs and on the periocular skin. The corneas become opaque beginning at the limbus and progressing towards the center. During stages of corneal translucence, free moving exudate may be detectable in the anterior chambers. In advanced stages the opaque corneas may ulcerate and even perforate.

Lymph nodes are enlarged and easily palpable. Concurrent with the rise in body temperature is the development of leukopenia. The total white cell count may be reduced to 6,000 to 3,000 per cu mm and the mononuclear or non-granular cells may constitute 80 to 90% of total leukocytes. In cases with a long course, the leukocytes may rise in late stages because of secondary bacterial infection.

Many animals develop dermatitis which is characterized by erythema and eczema. Common locations are the skin around the eyes, at the base of the horns, on the neck, udder, vulva and medial surfaces of the thighs. The mucosa of the vulva may contain a diphtheritic membrane. The dermatitis and meningitis result in hypersensitivity of the skin. In a prolonged course the hooves, horns and hair may slough.

Following early stages of the disease, diarrhea develops and causes severe dehydration.

The course of the disease is highly variable. Some animals die within 1 to 2 days. Many animals, however, live 2 to 3 weeks. The morbidity rate is low and usually sporadic, while the mortality rate of affected animals is very high.

At necropsy, most gross lesions are in the eyes, skin, respiratory, digestive and urinary systems. In affected areas the skin is hyperemic and eczematous. The moist hair is erect and may be depillated. The eyes, often retracted from dehydration, are inflamed throughout the conjunctival sacs and purulent exudate may unite the eyelids. The corneas are opaque and may be ulcerated. Careful dissection of the eyes usually reveals fibrinopurulent exudate in the anterior chambers. A crust of exudate covers the muzzle and extends into the nostrils. Removal of the crust reveals extensive erosion. The nasal mucosa is swollen, hyperemic and covered with a heavy deposit of mucopurulent exudate. The swelling and exudate seriously reduce the size of the meatuses. In some cases, masses of dehydrated exudate occlude the external nares. Removal of exudate from the mucosa discloses multiple erosions. Inflammation extends also into the paranasal sinuses, larynx, and trachea. In some cases, a diphtheritic membrane extends along portions of the trachea. Bronchopneumonia is usually present in terminal stages. In the digestive system erosions up to 1 mm in diameter with some confluence extend throughout the buccal and oral membranes, pharynx, and esophagus. Occasionally, they are discernible in the forestomachs. The mucous membrane of the abomasum is swollen and hyperemic, and often contains petechial hemorrhages and erosions. The hyperemic and petechiated intestine is also eroded. The lymph nodes, especially of the head, are enlarged. The liver is usually swollen, and the stromal network may be prominent. The mucous membrane of the urinary bladder is often swollen and hemorrhagic. Some blood may escape into the urine. The ureters may show similar changes. Kidneys often contain pale foci. Meninges of the brain are slightly edematous.

Histopathologically, changes are present in most organs. These can be categorized as degenerative, proliferative and infiltrative. In the mouth, some epithelial cells degenerate and die. Detachment of the dead epithelial cells produces erosion. Rete pegs proliferate. Blood vessels of the lamina propria and submucosa are affected with considerable uniformity. In the tunica adventitia, some fibrocytes proliferate and some collagenous fibers fragment. Lymphocytes, mononuclear macrophages, eosinophils and plasma cells infiltrate the tunica adventitia and the tunica media. These changes are prominent in and around vessels of the papillae. In the skin and esophagus, changes are similar to those of the mouth. In the liver, lymphocytes and mononuclear macrophages infiltrate the interlobular stroma and Glisson's capsule. In lymph nodes small lymphocytes are depleted through degeneration. The reticuloendothelial cells are hyperplastic and macrophages accumulate in large numbers. In the kidneys, lymphocytes and mononuclear macrophages accumulate in large numbers in the intertubular stroma. In the central nervous system, the meninges are edematous. Lymphocytes infiltrate the tunica adventitia of blood vessels. In many areas of the brain the perivascular spaces of Virchow-Robin are filled with lymphocytes and mononuclear macrophages. Frequently, neurons of the vagoglossopharyngeal nucleus contain cytoplasmic inclusion bodies which are clusters of eosinophilic granules. In the eye, conjunctiva is hyperemic and eroded. Leukocytes form exudate in the sac, and they infiltrate the subepithelial tissues. The cornea may be eroded and ulcerated with leukocytes infiltrating the edematous substantia propria. Fibrin, blood and leukocytes accumulate in the anterior chamber.

Diagnosis. Clinical diagnosis is based on typical signs. Of special importance are high persisting fever, nasal discharge, muzzle erosion and encrustation, oral hyperemia and erosions, conjunctivitis with corneal opacity and leukopenia. In early stages, before typical signs and lesions have developed, diagnosis may be difficult. Following necropsy confirmation can be obtained from histopathologic studies. The non-specificity of inclusion bodies reduces their diagnostic utility.

The differential diagnosis requires consideration of bovine viral diarrhea, rinderpest, shipping fever, dermatitis and viral bovine

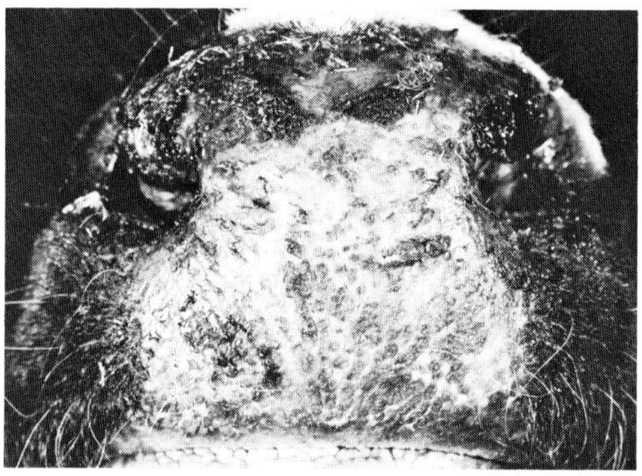

FIG. 2-7. *Eroded muzzle of a steer with malignant catarrhal fever.* × 0.5.

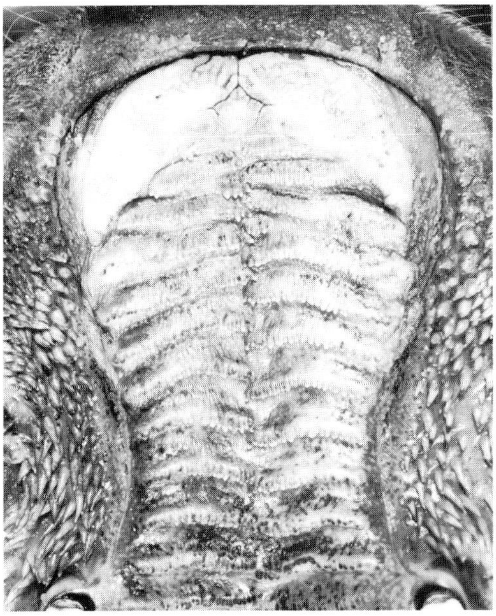

FIG. 2-8. *Eroded hard palate and buccal mucosa of a steer with malignant catarrhal fever.* × 0.5.

rhinotracheitis. Viral diarrhea, like malignant catarrh, is characterized by fever, oral erosions, diarrhea and leukopenia. Unlike malignant catarrh, viral diarrhea usually has an incidence of at least 20% within a herd, and affected animals do not develop corneal opacity. In some cases the virus from bovine viral diarrhea may be isolated in the laboratory and identified.

Rinderpest, not present in America, spreads rapidly and has a high incidence. Corneal opacity does not develop.

Because of conjunctivitis, early stages of shipping fever may be confused with malignant catarrh. Shipping fever, however, does not produce oral erosions. Pneumonia develops early and usually affects a large number of animals simultaneously.

Dermatitis from many causes may be confused with malignant catarrh. Dermatitis, however, is not associated with leukopenia, corneal opacities and oral erosions.

Prevention and Treatment. Since viral reservoirs and means of transmission are poorly understood, methods of prevention have not been developed. Some cases, however, may be prevented by avoiding association of cattle with sheep. Active cases of the disease should be isolated from other cattle. An effective vaccine against malignant catarrh has not been developed.

Treatment is non-specific and often ineffective. The course of the disease, however,

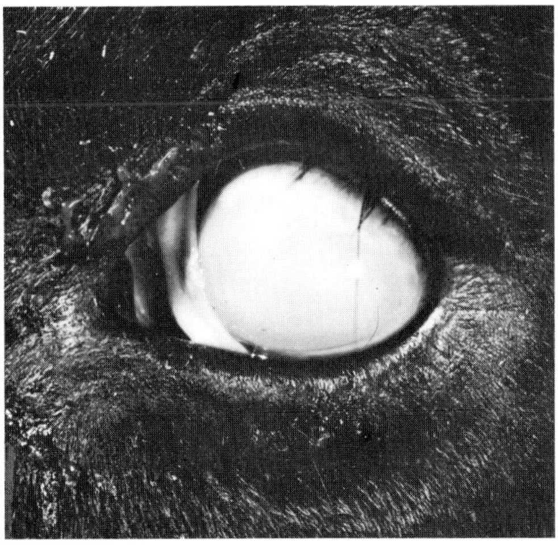

FIG. 2-9. *Keratoconjunctivitis in the eye of a heifer with malignant catarrhal fever. Opacity is due to edema of the cornea and exudate in the anterior chamber.* × 1.0.

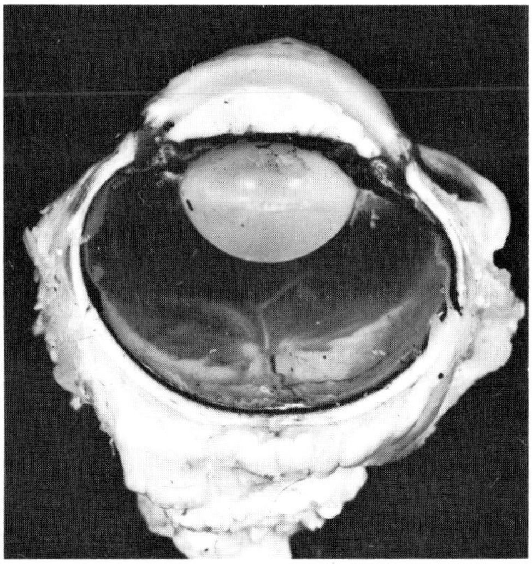

FIG. 2-10. *Same eye as in figure 2-9. The anterior chamber is filled with fibrinopurulent exudate and the cornea is edematous.* × 1.2.

may be shortened and the mortality lowered by providing good management. Because of photophobia, affected animals should be isolated in a dark stall. Excited animals should be given tranquilizers. Bacterial infections may be controlled by the use of sulfamethazine, sulfamerazine or sulfa brom methazine. Aspirin at the rate of 60 to 120 grains per day increases animal comfort. Cortical steroids may be used to reduce the severity of inflammation.

During stages of anorexia adequate water and nutriment should be force-fed and solutions of glucose in physiological salt solution should be administered intravenously. The nostrils and nasal meatuses should be cleaned to facilitate breathing and topically medicated with healing oils and antibiotics.

References

Berkman, R. N., Barner, R. D., Morrill, C. C. and Langham, R. F.: Bovine Malignant Catarrhal Fever. II. Pathology. AJVR, *21* (1960): 1015–1026.

Blood, D. C., Rowsell, H. C. and Savan, M.: An Outbreak of Bovine Malignant Catarrh in a Dairy Herd. II. Transmission Experiments. Canad. Vet. J., *2* (1961): 319–325.

Danskin, D.: Elementary Bodies in Bovine Malignant Catarrh. Nature, *176* (1955): 518.

Daubney, R. and Hudson, J. R.: Transmission Experiments with Bovine Malignant Catarrh. J. Comp. Path., *49* (1963): 63–89.

deKock, G. and Neitz, W. O.: Sheep as a Reservoir Host of Snotsiekte or Bovine Malignant Catarrhal Fever of Cattle of South Africa. So. African J. Sci., *46* (1950): 176.

Dobberstein, J. and Hemmert-Halswick, A.: Beitrage zur Pathologischen Histologie des Boesartigen Katarrhalfieber. Zeit. Infekt. Kr. Haust. *34* (1928): 160–181.

Goss, L. W., Cole, C. R. and Kissling, R. E.: The Pathology of Malignant Catarrhal Fever (Bovine epitheliosis) with Special Reference to Cytoplasmic Inclusions. Amer. J. Path., *23* (1947): 837–841.

Gotze, R. and Leiss, J.: Erfolgreiche Uebertragungsversuche des boesartigen Katarrhalfieber von Rind zu Rind. Deutsch. Tierarztl. Wschr., *37* (1929): 433–437.

Gotze, R.: Untersuchungen uber das boesartigen Katarrhalfieber des Rindes. Dtsch. Tierarztl. Wschr., *38* (1930): 487–491.

Henning, M. W.: *Animal Diseases of South Africa.* 3rd Ed. South Africa Central News Agency Ltd. (1956): 1038–1052.

Huck, R. A., Shand, A. and Allsop, P. J.: Malignant Catarrh in Deer. Vet. Rec., *73* (1961): 457–464.

Mettam, R. W. M.: 9th and 10th Reports Director Vet. Educ. and Research So. Africa, (1923): 395.

Piercy, S. E.: Studies in Bovine Malignant Catarrh. I. Experimental Infection in Cattle, Brit. Vet. J., *108* (1952): 35–47.

———: Studies on Bovine Malignant Catarrh. II. Experimental Infection of Cattle (continued) i. Infectivity of Material Other Than Glands. ii. Routes of Infection. Brit. Vet. J., *108* (1952a): 214–220.

———: Studies in Bovine Malignant Catarrh. III. The Effect of Storage and Temperature on Viability of Virus. Brit. Vet. J., *109* (1953): 59–65.

Plowright, W.: The Pathology of Infectious Bovine Malignant Catarrh in Cattle and Rabbits. XVth International Veterinary Congress. Proceedings Part I, Vol. 1, (1953): 323–328.

———: The Blood Leukocytes in Infectious Malignant Catarrh of the Ox and Rabbit. J. Comp. Path. & Therap., *63* (1953a): 318–334.

———: Studies on the Virus of Malignant Catarrhal Fever in Africa. XVII World Veterinary Congress, Hanover, *1* (1963): 519–523.

———: Malignant Catarrhal Fever in East Africa. I. Behavior of the Virus in Free-Living Populations of Blue Wildebeest (*Gorgon taurinus taurinus*, Burchell). Res. Vet. Sc., *6* (1965): 56–68.

———: Malignant Catarrhal Fever in East Africa. II. Observations on the Wildebeest Calves at the Laboratory and Contact Transmission of the Infection to Cattle. Res. Vet. Sc., *6* (1965a): 69–83.

———: Malignant Catarrhal Fever in East Africa. III. Neutralizing Antibody in Free-Living Wildebeest. Res. Vet. Sc., *8* (1967): 129–136.

———: Malignant Catarrhal Fever. JAVMA, *152* (1968): 795–804.

Plowright, W., and Ferris, R. D.: The Preparation of Bovine Thyroid Monolayers for Use in Virological Investigations. Res. Vet. Sci., *2* (1961): 149–152.

Plowright, W., Ferris, R. D. and Scott, G. R.: Blue Wildebeest and the Aetiological Agent of Bovine Malignant Catarrhal Fever. Nature, *188* (1960): 1167–1169.

Plowright, W., Macadam, R. F. and Armstrong, J. A.: Growth and Characterization of the Virus of Bovine Malignant Catarrhal Fever in East Africa. J. Gen. Micro., *39* (1963): 253–266.

Senior, M., Halnan, C. R. E. and Tong, E. H.: An Outbreak of Malignant Catarrh Among the Pere Deer. Vet. Record, *74* (1962): 932–936.

Stenius, P. I.: Bovine Malignant Catarrh. Institute of Pathology, Veterinary College, Helsinki-State Veterinary Medical Institute, Stockholm. Helsinki, (1952).

Viral Papillomatosis

(CUTANEOUS BOVINE PAPILLOMATOSIS; WARTS; ANGLEBERRY)

A chronic proliferative disease, viral papillomatosis is characterized by cutaneous warts and genital polypi. While the importance of this common infectious disease has not been economically measured, losses do result from damage to hides, unthriftiness from heavy infection over the face and neck, diminished breeding efficiency from penile and vaginal papillomas, and an occasional death. Since the disease has a prolonged course, the economic losses, although small for any one time, extend and accumulate over a long period.

Review of Literature. In addition to bovine papillomatosis, a similar disease has been observed in horses (Cook and Olson, 1951), dogs (DeMonbreun and Goodpasture, 1932), people (Ormsby, 1927), rabbits, goats (Davis and Kemperer, 1936) and deer (Tajima, Gordon and Olson, 1968). The comparison of viruses from papillomas of several species of animals indicated that the bovine virus is similar in size, shape, and structure to the papilloma virus of people, dogs and rabbits (Crawford and Crawford, 1963). In studying the cause of the disease, researchers ground cutaneous papillomas and from them made a fresh tissue suspension and a bacteria-free filtrate. When the inoculae were injected subcutaneously into 2 lots of calves, 8 animals of 11 receiving unfiltered tissue and 7 of 11 receiving the filtrate developed papillomatosis. This experiment established the viral nature of the causative agent (Creech, 1929). Injection of the virus into skin, meninges, peripheral nerve, urinary bladder, testicle, tongue, rumen and intestines of young calves caused fibroblastic tumors in those organs (Gordon, 1968). Using fluorescene labeled antiserum, researchers found the antigen in nuclei of cells in the keratohyaline and keratinized layers of hyperplastic epithelium but not in the germinal basal cells of the papilloma (Smithies and Olson, 1961). Later studies using electron microscopy identified virus particles in cell nuclei of the upper stratum granulosum (Tajima, Gordon, and Olson, 1968). When injected into guinea pigs, isolates of virus from papillomas of different cattle caused subcutaneous fibrosarcomas in 67 to 100% of the injected animals (Robl and Olson, 1968). The relationship of bovine papilloma virus to equine sarcoid has been investigated. The sera of 9 horses affected with equine sarcoid failed to neutralize the bovine cutaneous virus, and 4 other horses having equine sarcoid plus 4 normal horses reacted alike to intradermal injections of the virus. These experiments failed to demonstrate a relationship of the bovine virus to the equine disease (Ragland and Spencer, 1968).

Transmission of bovine cutaneous papillomatosis has been studied under both natural and experimental conditions. Clinical observations revealed a natural outbreak with two prominent episodes developing among 10 lots of Hereford cattle. Of the 110 animals, 12 developed the disease in the original loci. From these animals the disease spread by direct contact to 29 additional cattle and by indirect contact through fence and water tank to an additional 14 animals (Bragdonas and Olson, 1953). Papillomas often developed in anatomical areas exposed to superficial trauma of the skin (Bragdonas and Olson, 1953; Grunder, 1959). Under experimental conditions the disease has been transmitted by subcutaneous and intradermal inoculation of cattle with suspensions of papilloma tissue and bacteria-free filtrates from papilloma tissue (Bragdonas and Olson, 1953; 1954). The inoculation of 15 calves into the submucosa of the urinary bladder with bovine cutaneous papilloma tissue suspension resulted in the development of polypi of the mucosa in 13 animals. While the growth suggested malignancy, no metastases were observed (Olson, Pamukcu *et al.*, 1959). The intradermal inoculation of 12 horses with

0.01 ml each of a supernatant fluid from bovine warts produced in 5 of the animals sarcoid-like lesions. The nodular growths were visible 12 to 27 days after inoculation and attained diameters of 2 to 3 cm (Olson and Cook, 1951).

Vaccines have been produced by inactivating the virus of naturally occurring bovine cutaneous papillomas and by inactivating the virus grown in incubating chicken embryos. In one experiment, each vaccine was administered in two separate doses with a 2-week interval. Two to 3 weeks following the last administration the immunized and control animals were challenged with three strains of virus. Animals receiving the papilloma tissue vaccine showed an average of 50% susceptibility, while cattle receiving the chick embryo vaccine showed a 95% susceptibility, and were not significantly different from the unvaccinated controls (Bragdonas and Olson, 1954). In another experiment, cattle received vaccine whose strain of virus was capable of producing skin and vaginal papillomas. Challenge inoculations after vaccination indicated considerable immunity to skin papillomas but not to vaginal papillomas (Olson, Luedke and Brobst, 1962).

Bovine papillomatosis has been treated with various drugs, biological agents, and surgical excision. The drugs were totally ineffective in altering the course of the disease. The use of autogenous vaccines, given as 2 doses with an interval of 2 weeks, was in some cases highly effective (du Casse, 1961; Pearson *et al.*, 1958). In one trial involving 122 cattle, 87% of animals receiving the autogenous vaccine made rapid recovery from the cutaneous form, and 4 of 5 bulls with penile papillomas recovered following vaccination (Pearson *et al.*, 1958). While the field trials indicated a high degree of efficacy for autogenous vaccines, controlled experiments showed that the course of the disease was not shortened by the use of vaccine or by a combination of autogenous vaccine and surgical excision. Warts excised after 3 months' duration, however, tended not to recur (Olson, Segre, and Skidmore, 1954; Olson and Skidmore, 1959).

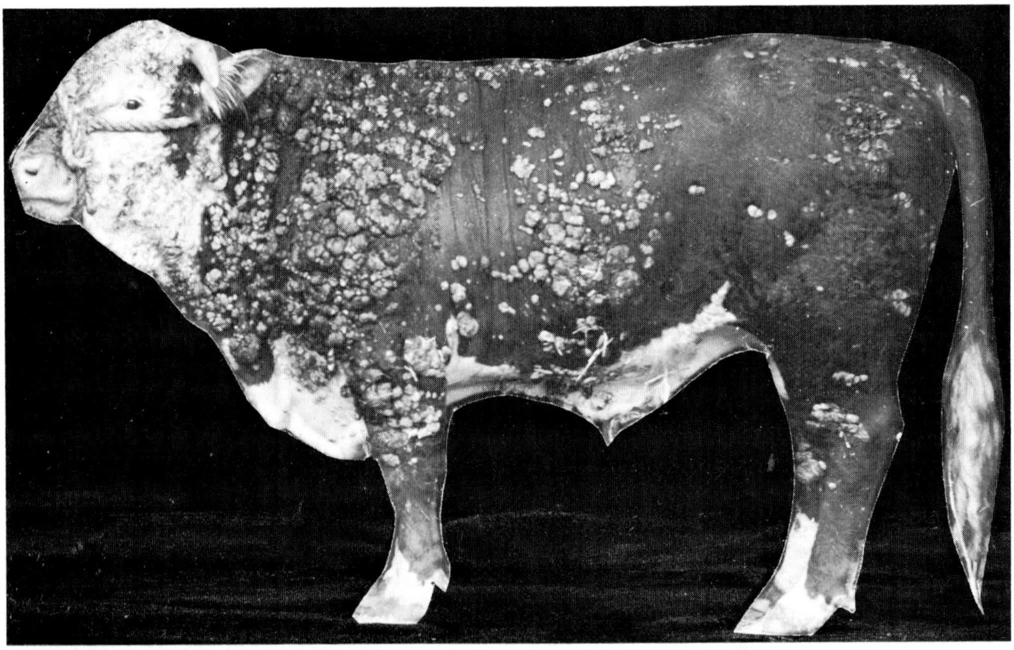

FIG. 2-11. *Generalized cutaneous papillomatosis.*

Occurrence. Occasionally found in all sexes and breeds of cattle, papillomatosis probably occurs more commonly among Hereford, Angus and Shorthorn breeds because animals of those breeds are often assembled in crowded pens where direct contacts are possible. While all ages of cattle may be susceptible, animals under 2 years of age are more commonly affected. In 998 show cattle, 228 (23%) contained warts. To reveal the age incidence the animals were divided into three age groups: group 1, age 10 to 12 months, showed an incidence of 28% papillomatosis; group 2, age 14 to 16 months, 25%; and group 3, 18 to 20 months, 19% (Olson, Leudke *et al.*, 1962). The study of hides from slaughtered cattle indicated an incidence of 15 to 25% papillomatosis in some parts of the United States (Creech, 1929).

Geographically, the disease is found in all major cattle producing countries, but some local areas and individual herds have great annual differences in incidence.

Besides cattle, papillomatosis occurs in horses, sheep, deer, dogs, rabbits and man. For each host, however, the causative virus is specific and antigenetically different.

Etiology and Pathogenesis. Bovine papilloma virus is typical of the papovavirus group of which it is a member. It is resistant to ether, moderate heat and changes in pH, but it is sensitive to ultraviolet light radiation and formalin solutions. Containing no envelope, the virion possesses DNA in the nucleocapsid. Having cubic symmetry it measures approximately 40 to 50 mμ in diameter. Mixed with 50% glycerene and stored in refrigeration, it retains viability for approximately 3 to 6 months.

The virus can be cultivated independently of the bovine host. It can be grown in several cell types in culture systems, and it has been adapted to embryonating chicken eggs and cytopathogenicity appears to be low. Following experimental inoculation, the virus grows, temporarily at least, in the skin of horses.

As a mildly contagious disease, papillomatosis is transmitted by both direct and indirect contact and presumedly its virus is inoculated into susceptible cattle through inconspicuous skin abrasions and lacerations. The rubbing between and among affected and susceptible cattle crowded in a feedlot provides ample opportunity for direct physical contact. Feeding, watering, and back rubbing equipment is used by all animals within a lot and may become contaminated with the virus. Small lacerations of the skin of the ears, chin, face and neck may occur from the virus contaminated equipment and result in inoculation. Since the incubation period is usually long, many cattle inoculated within the feedlot are marketed before the papillomas have had sufficient time to develop in either great numbers or large size. In young cattle, however, which enter the feedlot and are fattened over periods greater than 4 months, papillomatosis may develop a high incidence and to a severe degree. A small number of warts usually cause little discomfort and no adverse fattening effect. Generalized papillomatosis, however, especially over the face, neck and around the eyes and mouth may result in unthriftiness, diminished rates of gain, loss of body weight, and even death. Following the normal course of the disease most animals recover without treatment and are immune, at least temporarily. The etiological relationship of esophageal papillomas to other types of papillomas has not been determined.

Breeding animals affected with genital papillomatosis have diminished reproductive capacity. Penile papillomas frequently become large, traumatized, ulcerated and infected. Either penile or vaginal papillomas may mechanically interfere with breeding and may predispose to genital infection.

Clinical Signs and Lesions. According to anatomical location of the warts, bovine papillomatoses are classified clinically as cutaneous, genital, and/or esophageal. In the common cutaneous form, the papilloma is pedunculated, hairless, and cauliflower-shaped. The irregular surface is nodular,

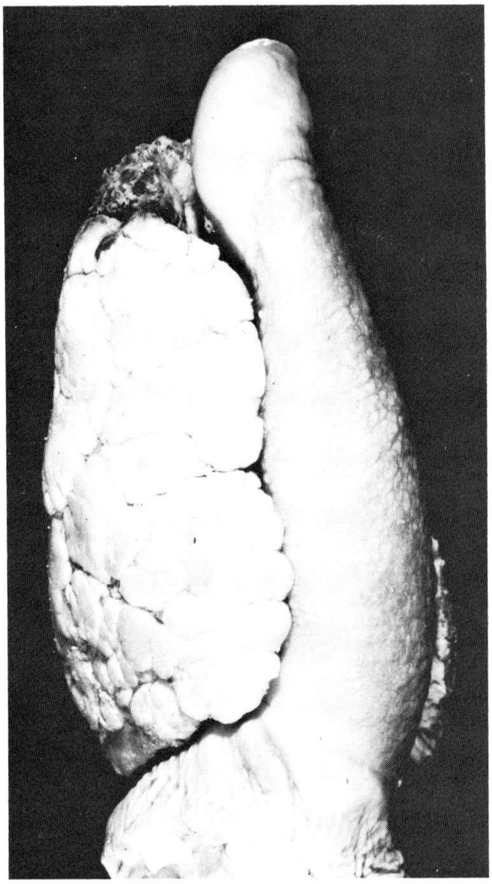

FIG. 2-12. *Penile papilloma.* × 1.0.

scaly, and sometimes spiny. The size varies from 1 to 20 cm in diameter and projects from the skin surface 1 to 10 cm. An affected animal may contain one or multiple papillomas which are commonly located on the neck, chin, face, shoulders, dewlap, ears, eyes, throat, lips and udder. The original warts are frequently located on skin wounded by abrasion, tattooing, branding and ear tagging. Large papillomas of the face and neck commonly become traumatized by rubbing against equipment and against other animals in a crowded feedlot. Repeated injury and continuous hemorrhage may result in anemia and physical weakness. Attraction of gravid screwworm and blow flies to the traumatized warts may result in ovaposition and myiasis. Severe papillomatosis results in some anorexia and diminished rates of gain in body weight. Under natural conditions the incubation period varies from $3\frac{1}{2}$ to 4 months and experimentally from 3 to 8 weeks. While the incidence within a herd often varies tremendously, 75% or more of the animals may be affected, and the course is from 1 to $5\frac{1}{2}$ months.

In the genital form of the disease, both males and females are affected. In the male a single papilloma develops on or near the glans penis, grows to dimensions as great as 8 cm in diameter and often becomes traumatized and infected. In advanced stages, a penile papilloma partially incapacitates the bull for breeding. In females the papillomas develop on the vulva and vagina and trau-

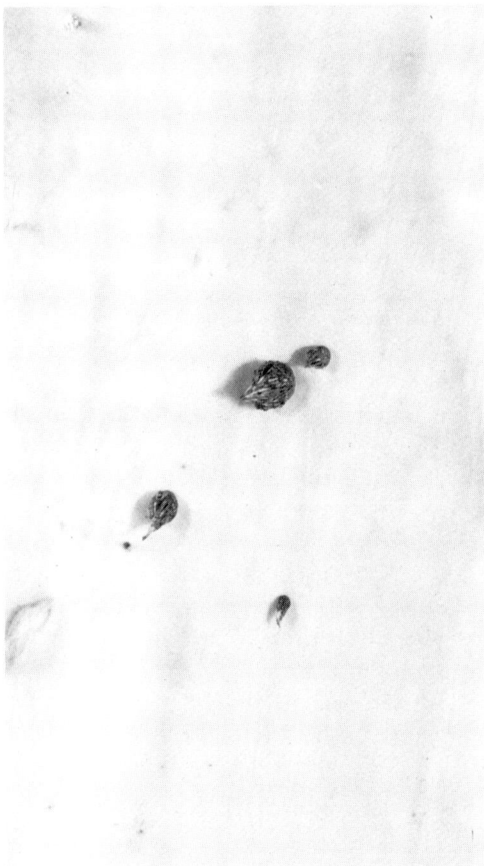

FIG. 2-13. *Small papillomas in the esophageal mucosa.* × 1.3.

matized vaginal papillomas may become infected and result in vaginitis.

Esophageal papillomatosis is the formation of single or multiple papillomas on the mucosal surface of the esophagus and occasionally the forestomachs. While small esophageal papillomas produce no clinical signs, large ones may obstruct the lumen and result in dysphagia and esophageal choke.

Diagnosis. Papillomatosis is identified by the presence of single or multiple warts on the skin, genitalia and esophagus. The skin lesions, of medium size, are conspicuous and easily identified, but the genital form requires careful examination of the glans penis, vulva, and vagina. Esophageal papillomatosis is usually diagnosed at necropsy or slaughter inspection.

The differential diagnosis requires consideration of true neoplasms usually having a single point of origin. Malignant skin tumors infiltrate surrounding tissues and commonly metastasize to other organs. Histopathologic studies are necessary to identify the specific neoplasm.

Prevention and Treatment. Since the virus of papillomatosis is usually transmitted through areas of trauma, lacerating objects such as nails, wire and wood splinters should be eliminated from feedlot equipment surfaces. Surgical instruments for tattooing and other minor operations should be kept clean and disinfected to avoid mechanical spread of the virus.

Considerable immunity can be induced by the use of a general or autogenous vaccines. Either product is prepared from viable papillomatous tissue excised from the skin, cleaned, and ground and added at the rate of 5% to a solution of equal parts glycerin and physiological saline solution.

The virus in the suspension is inactivated by adding formalin to a concentration of 0.5% of the mixture. After discarding the settled solids, the supernatant fluid as the vaccine is administered in 2 doses given subcutaneously with an interval of 2 weeks. To be effective the vaccine should be administered prior to or at the time of the animals' admission to the feedlot. Although vaccination immunity does not provide protection to all animals, the duration of protection usually extends over the standard fattening period.

While affected animals have been treated with either general commercial or autogenous vaccines, the efficacy of their administration is questionable. If vaccine is to be used prophylactically, the autogenous preparation is preferred. Drugs are not effective. In early stages of the disease, surgical excision may prolong the disease course, while in late stages excised papillomas tend not to recur.

References

Bragdonas, V. and Olson, C.: Observations on the Epizootiology of Cutaneous Papillomatosis (warts) of Cattle. JAVMA, *122* (1953): 393.

———: Observations on Immunity in Cutaneous Bovine Papillomatosis. AJVR, *15* (1954): 240–245.

Cook, R. H. and Olson, C.: Experimental Transmission of Cutaneous Papilloma of the Horse. Amer. J. Path., *27* (1951): 1087–1097.

Crawford, L. V. and Crawford, E. M.: A Comparative Study of Polyoma and Papilloma Viruses. Virology, *21* (1963): 258–263.

Creech, G. T.: Experimental Studies of the Etiology of Common Warts in Cattle. J. Ag. Res., *39* (1929): 723–737.

Davis, C. L. and Kemperer, H. E.: Common Warts in Goats. JAVMA, *88* (1936): 175–179.

DeMonbreun, W. A. and Goodpasture, E. W.: Infectious Oral Papillomatosis of Dogs. Amer. J. Path., *8* (1932): 43–55.

de Casse, F. B. W.: Bovine Papillomatosis, With Special Reference to Treatment With Tissue Vaccines. J. So. Afr. Vet. Med. Assoc., *32* (1961): 59–63.

Gordon, D. E.: The Response of Various Tissues in Neonate Calves to Bovine Papilloma Virus. Diss. Abst., *29B* (1968): 5.

Grunder, H. D.: Die Tierpapillomatosen. Deutsche Tierarzt. Wschr., *66* (1959): 219–221.

McIntee, K.: Fibropapillomas of the External Genitals of Cattle. Corn. Vet., *60* (1950): 304–312.

Olson, C. and Cook, R. H.: Cutaneous Sarcoma-like Lesions of the Horse Caused by the Agent of Bovine Papilloma. Proc. Soc. Exp. Biol. & Med., *77* (1951): 281–284.

Olson, C. Luedke, A. J. and Brobst, D. F.: Induced Immunity of Skin, Vagina, and Urinary Bladder to

Bovine Cutaneous Papilloma Agent. Cancer Res., *22* (1962): 463–468.

———: Incidence of Bovine Cutaneous Papillomatosis in Beef Cattle. JAVMA, *140* (1962a): 50–52.

Olson, C. Pamukcu, M., Brobst, D. F., Komalczyk, T., Satter, E. J. and Price, J. M.: A Urinary Bladder Tumor Induced by a Bovine Cutaneous Papilloma Agent. Cancer Res., *19* (1959): 779–782.

Olson, C., Segre, D. and Skidmore, I. V.: Cutaneous Papillomatosis (warts) of Cattle. Proc. U.S.L.S.A., (1954): 219–226.

———: Immunity to Bovine Cutaneous Papillomatosis Produced by Vaccine Homologous to the Challenge Agent. JAVMA, *135* (1959): 499–502.

———: Further Observations on Immunity to Bovine Cutaneous Papillomatosis. AJVR, *21* (1960): 233–242.

Olson, C. and Skidmore, L. V.: Therapy of Experimentally Produced Bovine Cutaneous Papillomatosis with Vaccine and Excision. JAVMA, *135* (1959): 339–343.

Ormsby, O. S.: *Disease of the Skin.* Lea & Febiger. Philadelphia. (1927): 502–510.

Pearson, J. K. L., Kerr, W. R., McCartney, W. D. J. and Steele, T. H. J.: Tissue Vaccines in the Treatment of Bovine Papilloma. Vet. Rec., *70* (1958): 971–973.

Ragland, W. L. and Spencer, G. R.: Attempts to Relate Bovine Papilloma Virus to the Cause of Equine Sarcoid. AJVR, *29* (1968): 1363–1366.

Robl, M. G. and Olson, C.: Oncogenic Action of Bovine Papilloma Virus in Hamsters. Cancer Research, *128* (1968): 1596–1604.

Smithies, L. K. and Olson, C.: Antigen of Bovine Cutaneous Papilloma Detected by Fluorescent Antibodies. Cancer Res., *21* (1961): 1557–1559.

Tajima, M., Gordon, D. E. and Olson, C.: Electron Microscopy of Bovine Papilloma and Deer Fibroma Viruses. AJVR, *29* (1968): 1185–1194.

Thomas, M., Boiron, M. and Geraldes, A.: Some Physicochemical Properties of the Virus of Bovine Papillomatosis. Séanc. Acad. Sci., Paris. *262D* (1969): 2383–2386.

Bluetongue

An acute infectious but non-contagious disease, bluetongue in cattle is characterized by inflammation of the mucous membrane of the mouth and tongue and of the skin of the feet. The causative virus is transmitted by a dipterous insect, *Culicoides variipenis.* Although the virus attacks many ruminant species, the disease is major in sheep and minor in cattle. The reason for the name of the disease is the characteristic cyanotic tongue in affected sheep.

The importance of the disease to the cattle industry has not been specifically measured. Economic loss, however, results from unthriftiness, inefficient use of feed, reduction in body weight and milk production, expensive treatment and prevention, and lower meat quality in affected cattle. In addition, the value of feedlots, pasture land and range land in disease endemic areas may be diminished. Estimates of economic losses to the sheep industry are greater than the losses to the cattle industry because the sheep disease has high incidence, great severity and significant mortality.

Review of Literature. Bluetongue probably evolved in Africa where for almost 100 years it has been endemic, and where it has great economic importance. Although the disease was recognized as early as the seventeenth century, the first formal description came as a report of serious losses among sheep imported from Europe to South Africa (Hutcheon, 1880). As a result of careful studies, many details of the disease, including its pathologic changes, geographic distribution, and the results of attempted immunization, came later (Spreull, 1905). During the same period of study the presence of the causative agent in the blood of affected sheep and its filtrability were discovered (Theiler, 1905). For a long time bluetongue was limited to Africa, but it was finally identified in Cyprus (Gambles, 1949), Turkey (Aral, 1949), Palestine (Komarov and Goldsmidt, 1951), the United States (McKercher *et al.,* 1953), Portugal (Ribeiro and Noronha, 1958), Spain (Lopez and Botija, 1958), Pakistan (Howell, 1960), and Japan (Omori, 1961).

Even though most research on bluetongue has been directed towards the disease in sheep, a significant number of studies have been in cattle. In 1932 South Africa encountered an epizootic bovine disease whose manifestations resembled foot-and-mouth disease, but the cases lacked vesicles on both the tongue and feet. All breeds of cattle were affected and economic losses were high. Eventually the bluetongue virus was isolated from affected animals (Bekker, DeKock and Quinlan, 1934). Later in South Africa bluetongue virus was isolated from some range cattle manifesting only slight clinical signs of depression, stiffness, and disinclination to eat (DeKock, DuToit and Neitz, 1937), as well as from completely healthy cattle that had been exposed to cases of natural bluetongue (Owen, DuToit and Howell, 1965). During 1959 and 1960, cattle in Japan developed a disease that was characterized by fever, leukopenia, erosions and ulcers of the mouth, difficult swallowing, conjunctivitis and lachrymation, dermatitis and lameness. Throughout the course of the disease outbreak approximately 43,500 cattle were sick, and of these animals 4,500 died or were slaughtered because of the disease. From these cattle bluetongue virus was isolated and identified (Omori, 1961; Inaba, Ishii and Omori, 1966). In the United States between 1962 and 1965, bluetongue virus was isolated from 28 cattle of many herds of 6 western states. The affected animals manifested minor amounts of combinations of erosions of the tongue, mouth, muzzle, and nostrils and muscular stiffness and lameness in all feet (Bowne, Luedke, Foster and Jochim, 1966). One cow had a history of suffering an acute illness 5 months previously. From her, bluetongue virus was isolated by inoculating her blood into bluetongue-susceptible sheep on each of two occasions at 2-month intervals. Following death of the cow, bluetongue virus was isolated from internal organs (Bowne, Luedke, Jochim and Metcalf, 1968). According to one investigation bluetongue virus appeared to transmit from feedlot cattle to sheep. During the fall months a large number of lambs were shipped to a field near the cattle feedlot. Fourteen days after arrival the lambs developed bluetongue, but the parent herd remained healthy. Bluetongue virus was isolated from the apparently healthy cattle, and the researchers concluded that the disease was transmitted from the cattle to the sheep (Bowne, Luedke, Foster and Jochim, 1966).

Cattle have been inoculated with live bluetongue virus, and in these animals the disease has been invariably mild. When sheep blood containing bluetongue virus was injected into susceptible cattle, some of the inoculated animals developed mild fever as the only sign of disease. The infected cattle, however, harbored the virus for as long as 22 days after injection (Dekock, DuToit and Neitz, 1937; Mason and Neitz, 1940). In other experiments, cattle injected with virulent bluetongue virus developed mild leukopenia and a rise in body temperature of 1 to 2° F. Some animals lost appetite and a few suffered dermatitis, and others had no perceivable reaction. Virus was intermittently detected in the cattle blood for as long as 50 days after inoculation. By using the fluorescent antibody technique, researchers identified the virus in the mucous membrane of the lips within 4 to 7 days after inoculation (Luedke, Jochim and Jones, 1969; Gleiser, Stair and McGill, 1969).

From studies emphasizing the biological and physico-chemical properties of the particle, the bluetongue virus has been tentatively classified as a member of the arbovirus group. Recent investigators using electron microscopy have indicated that the viral particle has a diameter of approximately 50 to 60 mμ, is noncapsulated, and has double-stranded RNA (Verwoerd, 1969; Els and Verwoerd, 1969; Owen and Munz, 1966; Studdert, Pangborn, and Addison, 1966). The virus was resistant to ether, chloroform and sodium deoxycholate, but sensitive to the action of trypsin, and was stable at pH 6 to 8 (Svehag *et al.*, 1966). In the laboratory the virus readily grew in cell cultures, where it produced intracytoplasmic inclusion bodies, and in embryonating chicken eggs (Howell, Verwoerd and Oellermann, 1967; Bowne and Jochim, 1967). Immunogenic studies identified 12 antigenic groups. Although some common antigens were found, the antigens were mostly type specific (Howell, 1963).

With epizootiologic evidence of vector

transmission, many dipterous insects were studied. After eliminating various species of mosquitoes, the prevalent midge, *Culicoides variipenis,* was incriminated (DuToit, 1944). Subsequently, 14 midge transmissions of virus—5 from cattle to sheep, 5 from sheep to sheep, 3 from sheep to cattle, and one between cattle—were demonstrated (Luedke, Jones and Jochim, 1967). After allowing laboratory-reared midges to feed on virus, the insects fed on bluetongue susceptible sheep. Transmission occurred after 10, 13, and 15 days of virus incubation in the midge. Feeding after incubation periods shorter than 10 days did not result in bluetongue transmission (Foster, Jones and McCrory, 1963). In further biological studies, bluetongue virus was inoculated into the thoracic hemocoel of the vector. Thirty-three days after injection, virus particles were demonstrated by electron microscopy in cells of the insect salivary glands (Bowne and Jones, 1966). Multiplication of the virus within the insect varied directly with time and size of inoculated dose. The average viral increase within the fly was of the order of 10^4 fold in 5 to 8 days (Jochim and Jones, 1966).

Investigations have been conducted to determine the susceptibility to bluetongue of wild ruminant species. Blood samples, obtained from antelope, bighorn sheep, moose and deer, were tested for bluetongue antibodies. Many individuals reacted positively. The geographic distribution of the number of reactors paralleled the number of reactors among domestic ruminants. In southern Texas 85% of the deer were positive reactors (Trainer and Jochim, 1969). In Texas a spontaneous outbreak of bluetongue occurred in a captive herd of deer, and virus was isolated from some animals (Stair, Robinson and Jones, 1968). In one controlled experiment, 9 white-tailed deer, exposed to bluetongue virus, manifested clinical signs similar to hemorrhagic disease of deer. Seven of the diseased deer died (Vosdingh, Trainer, and Easterday, 1968).

Occurrence. Bluetongue occurs in most species of ruminants, both domestic and wild. Among cattle, all breeds, sexes and ages are susceptible, but breeds native to endemic areas probably are more resistant than breeds from bluetongue-free regions. Unless immunized by passive transfer of antibodies from immune dams, calves, as well as adults, are fully vulnerable. Although most ruminants can be attacked, sheep appear to be the most susceptible, and with these animals the disease has major economic importance. Native African and Asiatic breeds, such as the Karakul and Black Head Persian, are more resistant than animals of European breeds. The susceptibility of goats to bluetongue is approximately equal to that of cattle. Among wild ruminants, deer appear to be highly susceptible, and may suffer serious losses from the disease. Antelope, bighorn sheep and moose are also susceptible, but the actual degree is unknown. Some wild rodents in Africa also harbor the virus.

The seasonal variance of bluetongue relates to availability of the vector, *Culicoides varripenis.* In America, and other parts of the temperate zone, the disease occurs during late summer and early fall months. During summers of high rainfall the disease appears early in the season. Transmission ceases following a *Culicoides*-killing frost. Altitudes of ruminant habitats do not affect the disease.

During the first half century of bluetongue history, the disease was geographically limited to Africa. On that continent the disease exists in most countries which have developed animal agriculture, and careful search and diagnoses probably will reveal a distribution in all African countries. Since 1949, the disease has been identified by virus isolation in Cyprus, Palestine, Syria, Turkey, United States, Portugal, Spain, Japan and West Pakistan. In the United States, diagnoses have been limited to the west and southwest. Except in Africa, most geographic locations contain only a few of the 12 antigenic types of virus.

Etiology and Pathogenesis. Because the bluetongue virus transmits by and replicates in the insect, *Culicoides variipenis,* it has been tentatively classified as a member of the Arbovirus group. Some features of the nucleic acid, however, resemble the Reovirus group. The virus particle, containing double stranded RNA, appears to be 50 to 60 mμ in diameter when measured by electron microscopy and 100 to 150 mμ when measured by ultracentrifugation. Probably lacking an envelop, the virus resists chloroform, ether and sodium deoxycholate, but is sensitive to the action of trypsin.

The bluetongue virus is remarkably stable. In citrated blood or properly prepared splenic tissue stored at 4° C, infectivity persists for many years. Even at room temperature, virus in citrated blood has remained viable for more than 25 years. Minimal losses in titer result from lyophilization and storage at −70° C. Values of pH favoring stability vary from 6 to 8; values below 6 rapidly inactivate the virus. At 60° C the virus is destroyed in 30 minutes.

Outside the ruminant host and the vector insect, the virus adapts to and grows in artificial systems. In chicken eggs embryonated 8 days, it grows and concentrates at 33.5° C; embryo death usually occurs 3 to 4 days after inoculation. Following intracerebral inoculation of suckling mice, the virus grows in the central nervous system. Eight to 12 hours are required for replication, and most infected mice die. Mice older than 13 days are resistant. In culture systems, the virus grows in cells of sheep kidney, bovine kidney, bovine lymph node, lamb testicle, Chang liver, HeLa clones and human amnion. Cytopathologic changes are lysis of infected cells.

Multiple antigenic types of virus have been identified. In Africa, 12 separate types exist; these, on the basis of relationship, have been arranged into 4 groups. Each type evokes antibodies which protect against the homologous, but not heterologous virus. In America, and other infected areas outside of Africa, only a few of the 12 types have been found. Under natural conditions the virus can be found in the blood of affected ruminants and in pools of *Culicoides* collected from endemic areas.

The transmission of bluetongue virus is achieved by the dipterous midge, *Culicoides varripenis.* The virus replicates by as much as 10,000 fold, but transmission, by feeding of the vector on susceptible hosts, can occur no sooner than 10 days after the insect becomes infected. Transovarian passage of the virus has not been determined. Because of nocturnal feeding habits, the midge attacks host ruminants on night pasture and in nearby open pens, such as feedlots. The insect breeds in running streams and, consequently, is abundant along stream and river valleys, especially during periods of heavy rainfall. The existence of a viral reservoir, besides cattle and sheep, has been suspected but not identified nor adequately investigated. The fact that endemic areas remain infective after prolonged periods of absence of cattle and sheep supports the possibility of a viral reservoir in some other animal species. Experimentally, the virus can be transmitted by inoculating susceptible animals with infective blood or tissue.

Although the pathogenesis of bluetongue is inadequately understood, some important points are known, and others conjectural. The transmitting midge acquires the bluetongue virus by feeding on viremic ruminants, especially sheep or cattle. After an incubation period of 10 days in the insect, the virus locates in the salivary glands, and during subsequent feedings on ruminants, the virus, along with saliva, passes from the vector into the ruminant. In the vertebrate host the virus reaches highest blood titer 48 hours after the beginning of the febrile reaction. Although the blood titer descends to a low level, viremia may persist for as long as several months. Neutralizing antibodies develop early and pass into the colostrum of dams. Feeding of a new insect vector on infective blood spreads the virus to other susceptible ruminants and completes the life cycle for the virus.

Because of an affinity for epithelium, the virus attacks cells of the Malpighian and spinose layers of the tongue, mouth, esophagus, rumen and probably skin. The epithelial cells undergo ballooning degeneration and eventually necrose. Detachment of the dead cells produces erosions and ulcers. Leukocytopoiesis is temporarily suppressed. In pregnant sheep, and possibly cattle, the virus traverses the placenta and, during the first trimester, may seriously interfere with organogenesis.

Clinical Signs and Postmortem Lesions. In cattle, bluetongue, although viremic, is usually benign and may be visually inapparent. Two clinical forms, mild and acute, are discernible. Reasons for variance in disease manifestations have not been determined.

Mild bluetongue probably is the usual form and includes most bovine cases in endemic regions. Some affected cattle and perhaps most cattle exposed to the virus, develop viremia, experience slight transitory fever and sustain mild leukopenia. Such cases casually appear normal and probably escape detection. The application of laboratory procedures are necessary for identification. A minority of cases, however, undergo viremia and leukopenia, and develop any combination of mild fever, slight stiffness, lameness, and inappetitance, and few and inconspicuous erosions of the dental pad, lips and muzzle. These latter cases also may escape detection, but observant husbandmen usually note some of the adverse reactions. By using laboratory procedures and by inoculating the bovine blood into susceptible sheep, viremia and ascending antibody titers can be detected. One possible explanation for the mild form is the passive transfer of antibodies from the dam through colostrum to the calves. During and following passive immunity, exposure to the virus may maintain a low level of antibodies which provide some, but incomplete protection.

The acute form of bovine bluetongue is uncommon, but individual cases may occur in endemic areas or as epizootic outbreaks in areas where the disease has not previously existed and where the cattle population is highly susceptible. After an incubation period of 5 to 7 days, affected cattle develop viremia and acute sickness with variable combinations of signs and lesions in any one animal. Body temperature may rise to as much as 107° F. Soon after the febrile reaction there is a short period of leukopenia. Depression and anorexia with nasal and oral discharge are apparent. Mucous membranes of the mouth and tongue are hyperemic and, unless pigmented, are reddened. The tips of papillae of the buccal mucosa may be red and cyanotic. The lips are swollen. Erosions form on the dental pad, the dorsal and ventral surface of the tongue, on the lips at the junction of skin and mucous membrane, and on the muzzle. A crust of dried mucus and necrotic cells may form on the nostrils, muzzle and lips. Muscular stiffness may impare movements, and lameness may be evident in all feet. Clipping the hair from clean non-pigmented feet may reveal hyperemia and reddening at the coronary bands and on the skin between the claws and immediately dorsal to the hooves. Focal dermatitis may form above the hooves, around bases of the horns and at the perineum. The hoof may separate from the skin. Lacrymation may be prominent for a few days and, as in Japanese cattle, swallowing may be difficult. Interruptions in weight gains and losses of body weight may occur. Morbidity rate varies from individual cases in endemic areas to as much as a few per cent of a susceptible herd. The mortality rate is low. The variable course of the disease extends from a few days to 2 weeks.

Histopathologic changes are limited largely to the epithelium and vasculature. In erosive lesions of the mouth, tongue and skin, epithelial cells of the Malpighian and spinose layers undergo ballooning degeneration and eventually necrose. Leukocytes accumulate between the enlarged epithelial cells, and erosions result from detachment of the dead cells. In affected mouths, feet and skin, the blood vessels are heavily congested and hemorrhages are present. The sensitive laminae of lame feet sustain exaggerated vascular changes.

In sheep, bluetongue is severe, often fatal, and industrially important. Affected sheep develop swelling of the lips and nostrils and subcutaneous edema of the intermandibular space. The alimentary tract contains erosions, ulcers, and hemorrhages on the lips, tongue, mouth, esophagus, forestomachs, abomasum and small intestine. Laminitis, manifested by unwillingness to stand, is severe. At necropsy hemorrhages are prominent on the heart and in skeletal muscles. Subcutaneous and intermuscular edema and muscular degeneration are generalized. Morbidity rate varies up to 20% and mortality rate of affected animals may reach 50% or more.

Diagnosis. Bovine bluetongue is diagnosed by correlating clinical signs, postmortem findings, and laboratory data. Fever, leukopenia, erosions of the dental pad, tongue, and buccal cavity, swelling of the lips, and lameness in cattle during the insect season, are highly indicative. In mild cases of bluetongue, however, clinical signs and lesions are inadequate for diagnosis, except in an area where the disease is actively occurring and already diagnosed. A positive diagnosis of isolated cases, of epizootics in nonendemic areas, and of new outbreaks in endemic areas, requires isolation and identification of the bluetongue virus. Virus isolation can be achieved by inoculating suspected bovine blood into: (1) bluetongue susceptible sheep. A linear series of inoculations may be necessary for evoking characteristic bluetongue signs in the inoculated sheep; (2) appropriate cell culture systems. This method also may require a series of subcultures for adapting and concentrating the virus; and (3) suckling mice under 13 days of age. The isolated virus may be identified by neutralization with known antiserum. Serum neutralization identifies the homologous virus type. The complement fixation test, however, may identify the group to which the virus belongs.

The differential diagnosis requires consideration of vesicular stomatitis, foot-and-mouth disease, malignant catarrhal fever, bovine viral diarrhea and photosensitization. Vesicular stomatitis, like bluetongue, occurs during insect season; but it produces vesicles on the tongue and feet, and affects both cattle and horses. Foot-and-mouth disease produces vesicles on the tongue and feet, spreads rapidly by direct and indirect contact, and does not affect horses. Vesicular stomatitis and foot-and-mouth disease can be differentiated by controlled animal inoculations and by laboratory procedures using serum neutralization tests. Malignant catarrhal fever, usually sporadic in occurrence, causes extensive erosions of the buccal cavity, tongue, hard palate and forestomachs. Severe panophthalmitis produces opacity of the cornea. Fever is high and persistent. Bovine viral diarrhea causes severe and extensive erosion of the buccal cavity, tongue, hard and soft palates, esophagus, and forestomachs, and ulcers over Peyers patches. The causative virus can be isolated and identified. Photosensitization results in dermatitis of white skin only, but may also cause lacrymation and hyperemia of non-pigmented eyes and facial skin.

Prevention and Treatment. Commercial vaccine for preventing bluetongue in sheep is available, and it contains viral antigen types known to exist in the involved region. This product could be effectively used for vaccinating cattle. In the United States, vaccination of cattle against bluetongue has not been practiced because the disease has usually been mild and of minor importance, and because immunization is expensive in labor and material. Vaccination is recommended only for protecting valuable breeding cattle against anticipated bluetongue.

Some husbandry practices can be followed to reduce the incidence of bluetongue. In endemic areas, feedlots should be constructed on high land away from streams where the vector midge breeds and feeds. Maintaining cattle under shelter and without artificial

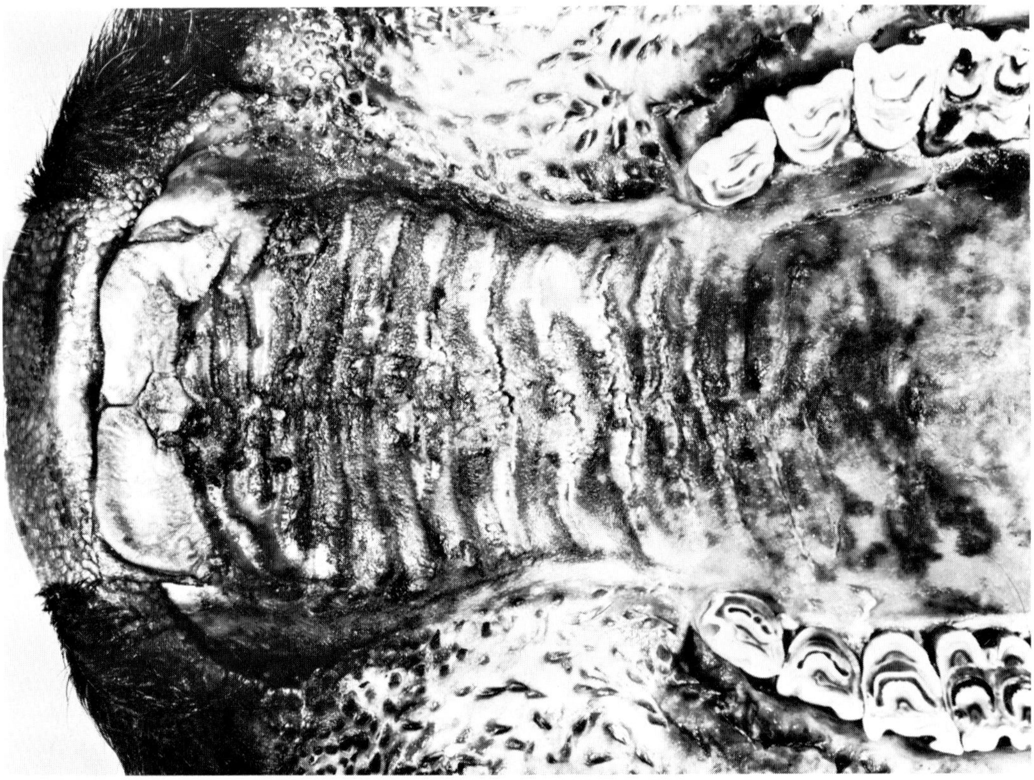

FIG. 2-14. *Stomatitis in an heifer affected with bluetongue. Note necrosis, erosions and inflammation of hard palate, lips, muzzle and buccal mucosa.* × 0.8.

light during hours of darkness may protect animals against the transmitting midge.

Specific drug treatment for bluetongue has not been developed. The administration of antibiotics and sulfonamides controls secondary bacterial infections, such as pneumonia. Good nursing should be practiced to maintain affected animals on feed and to avoid excessive loss of body weight during the course of the disease. Soreness and pain in the mouth can be mitigated with anesthetic sprays or ointments and laminitis and coronitis may be alleviated by injecting cortical steroids. Providing animal comfort helps to maintain appetite and to avoid excessive weight losses. In case of anorexia, affected cattle should be artificially fed milk replacers and fluids by use of a stomach tube. Such equipment should be sterilized before subsequent uses.

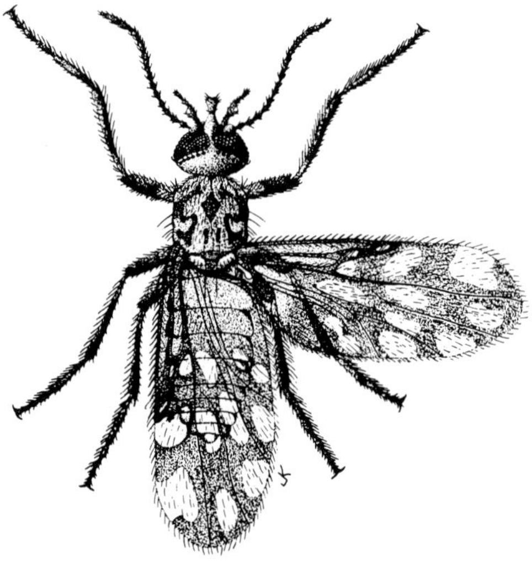

FIG. 2-15. *Culicoides.* × 32. (*Courtesy of J. H. Shaw, T. O. Thatcher, and James Kretzmeir.*)

References

Aral (See Gambles, R. M.: Bluetongue of Sheep in Cyprus. J. Comp. Path. *59* (1949): 176–189.)

Bekker, J. F., DeKock, G. W. and Quinlan, J. B.: The Occurrence and Identification of Bluetongue in Cattle—The So-called Pseudo Foot and Mouth Disease in South Africa. Onderstepoort J. Vet. Sc. and An. Ind., *2* (1934): 393–507.

Bowne, J. G. and Jochim, M. M.: Cytopathologic Changes and Development of Inclusion Bodies in Cultured Cells Infected with Bluetongue Virus. AJVR, *28* (1967): 1091–1105.

Bowne, J. G. and Jones, R. H.: Observations on Bluetongue Virus in Salivary Glands of an Insect Vector, *Culicoides varriipenis*. Virology, *30* (1966): 127–133.

Bowne, J. G., Luedke, A. J., Foster, N. M. and Jochim, M. M.: Current Aspects of Bluetongue in Cattle. JAVMA, *148* (1966): 1177–1180.

Bowne, J. G., Luedke, A. J., Jochim, M. M. and Metcalf, H. E.: Bluetongue Disease in Cattle. JAVMA, *153* (1968): 662–668.

DeKock, G. W., DuToit, R. and Neitz, W. O.: Observations on Bluetongue in Cattle and Sheep. Onderstep. J. Vet. Sc. and An. Ind., *8* (1937): 129–180.

DuToit, R. M.: The Transmission of Bluetongue and Horsesickness by *Culicoides*. Onderstep. J. Vet. Sc., *19* (1944): 7–16.

Els, H. J. and Verwoerd, D. W.: Morphology of Bluetongue Virus. Virology, *38* (1969): 213–219.

Estrella e Silva, F.: Língua Azul ou Febre Catarraldos Ovinos (Bluetongue). Rev. Ciencias Veterinarias, *5* (1956): 191–231.

Foster, N. M., Jones, R. H. and McCrory, B. R.: Preliminary Investigations on Insect Transmission of Bluetongue Virus in Sheep. AJVR, *24* (1963): 1195.

Gambles, R. M.: Bluetongue of Sheep in Cyprus. J. Comp. Path. Therap., *59* (1949): 176.

Gleiser, C. A., Stair, E. L. and McGill, L. D.: Diagnosis of Bluetongue in Cattle by Intravascular Inoculation of Chicken Embryos and Immunofluorescence. AJVR, *30* (1969): 981–999.

Howell, P. G.: A Preliminary Antigenical Classification of Strains of Bluetongue Virus. Onderstep. J. Vet. Res. *28* (1960): 357–363.

———: *Emerging Diseases of Animals*. Food and Agriculture Organization. Rome (1963): 109–176.

Howell, P. G., Vorwoerd, D. W. and Oellermann, R. A.: Plaque Formation by Bluetongue Virus, Onderstep. J. Vet. Res., *34* (1967): 317–332.

Hutcheon, D.: Fever or Epizootic Catarrh. Report of the College of Vet. Surgery, (1880): 12.

Inaba, Y., Ishii, S. and Omori, T.: Bluetongue-like Disease in Japan. Bulletin Office Internat. Epizoot., *66* (1966): 329–340.

Jochim, M. M. and Chow, T. L.: Immunodiffusion of Bluetongue Virus. AJVR, *30* (1969): 33–41.

Jochim, M. M. and Jones, R. H.: Multiplication of Bluetongue Virus in *Culicoides variipenis* Following Artificial Infection. Am. J. Epidem., *84* (1966): 241–246.

Komarov, A. and Goldsmit, L.: A Disease Similar to Bluetongue in Cattle and Sheep of Israel. Refuah Vet., *8* (1951): 96.

Lopez, A. C. and Botija, C. S.: L'epizootie de fievre catarrhale ovine en Espagne (Bluetongue) Bulletin Office Internat. Epizoot., *50* (1958): 65.

Luedke, A. J., Jochim, M. M. and Jones, R. H.: Bluetongue in Cattle: Viremia. AJVR, *30* (1969): 511–516.

Luedke, A. J., Jones, R. H. and Jochim, M. M.: Transmission of Bluetongue Between Sheep and Cattle by *Culicoides variipenis*. AJVR, *28* (1967): 457–460.

Mason, J. G. and Neitz, W. O.: The Susceptibility of Cattle to the Virus of Bluetongue. Onderstep. J. Vet. Sc. and An. Ind., *15* (1940): 149–157.

McKercher, D. G., McGowan, B., Howarth, J. A. and Saito, J. K.: A Preliminary Report on the Isolation and Identification of Bluetongue Virus from Sheep in California. JAVMA, *122* (1953): 300.

Omori, T.: Bluetongue-like Disease in Japan. Bulletin Office Internat. des Epizoot., *55* (1961): 1109–1117.

Owen, N. C., du Toit, R. M. and Howell, P. G.: Bluetongue in Cattle: Typing of Viruses Isolated from Cattle Exposed to Natural Infection. Onderstep. J. Vet. Res., *32* (1965): 3–6.

Owen, N. C. and Munz, E. K.: Observations on a Strain of Bluetongue Virus by Electron Microscopy. Onderstep. J. Vet. Res., *33* (1966): 9–14.

Ribeiro, J. M. and Noronha, F. M. O.: Fievre Catarrhale du Mouton au Portugal (Bluetongue). Bulletin Office Internat. Epizoot., *50* (1958): 46.

Spreull, J.: Malarial Catarrhal Fever (Bluetongue) of Sheep in South Africa. J. Comp. Path., *18* (1905): 321–337.

Stair, E. L., Robinson, R. M. and Jones, L. P.: Spontaneous Bluetongue in Texas White-tailed Deer. Pathologia Vet., *5* (1968): 164–173.

Studdert, M. J., Pangborn, J. and Addison, R. B.: Bluetongue Virus Structure. Virology, *29* (1966): 509–511.

Svehag, S. E., Leendertsen, L. and Gorham, J. R.: Sensitivity of Bluetongue Virus to Lipid Solvents, Trypsin and pH Changes and its Serological Relationship to Arbovirus. J. Hyg. Camb., *64* (1966): 339–346.

Theiler, A.: Bluetongue in Sheep in Transvaal. Director of Agriculture. Annual Report, (1904–05): 110–121.

Trainer, D. O. and Jochim, M. M.: Serologic Evidence of Bluetongue in Wild Ruminants of North America. AJVR, *30* (1969): 2007–2011.

Verwoerd, D. W.: Purification and Characterization of Bluetongue Virus. Virology, *38* (1969): 203–212.

Vosdingh, R. A., Trainer, D. O., and Easterday, B. C.: Experimental Bluetongue Disease in White-tailed Deer. Canad. J. Comp. Med., *32* (1968): 382–387.

Shipping Fever

(SHIPPING PNEUMONIA; HEMORRHAGIC SEPTICEMIA; PASTEURELLOSIS)

An acute infectious disease of cattle, shipping fever is characterized by acute inflammation of the nasal cavities, paranasal sinuses, larynx, pharynx, trachea and bronchi, and in advanced and fatal cases by acute fibrinous bronchopneumonia and is caused by interaction of *Pasteurella hemolytica* or *P. multocida*, Myxovirus parainfluenza-3 (SF-4), and environmental stressing agents. Because they describe, in a partial way, only some of the limited aspects of the complex syndrome of shipping fever, the various names applied to this disease are unsatisfactory. The popular, but inaccurate term, hemorrhagic septicemia, should be discarded because it erroneously implies an invasion of the blood by pathogenic organisms. When, through research, the precise etiology is determined, a more satisfactory name may be devised.

Along with viral bovine rhinotracheitis and calf diphtheria, shipping fever is a member of the triumvirate of respiratory diseases of feedlot cattle, and it causes annual economic losses which have been conservatively estimated for the United States at $20 million. The losses are due to diminished body weight, high mortality rate, expensive treatments, and delayed marketability.

Review of Literature. Throughout much of the 20th century, research on shipping fever has been sporadic. During the 1960's, however, accelerated investigations have been concentrated on bacterial, viral, and environmental stressing agents.

Repeatedly the lungs and other organs, as well as blood, from animals sacrificed and from animals fatally affected, were collected for bacteriological and pathological studies. With considerable constancy *Pasteurella hemolytica* and/or *P. multocida* were isolated from diseased lungs (Carter, 1954; 1955; Collier, Brown and Chow, 1962; Horlein and Saxena, 1961). Rarely, pasteurellas were isolated from the spleen and seldom from the blood except in terminal stages of the disease (Collier, Brown and Chow, 1962). In Canada, 26 affected cattle were studied, and *P. hemolytica* was isolated from the lungs of 15 and *P. multocida* from 10 (Carter, 1954). One year later 33 affected cattle were examined, and *P. hemolytica* was isolated from the lungs of 27 animals, while *P. multocida* was not found (Carter, 1955). In affected cattle of the midwestern and western United States, *P. hemolytica* also predominated. In one project involving the investigation of 13 epizootics, *P. hemolytica* was isolated from 12 outbreaks and *P. multocida* from one (Collier, Brown and Chow, 1962). When freshly isolated cultures of *P. hemolytica* and *P. multocida* were inoculated into healthy cattle, variable results were obtained. When the organisms in aerosol were administered into the nose a mild febrile reaction was produced (Baldwin, Marshall and Wessman, 1967; Collier, Chow, Benjamin and Deem, 1960), but essentially no reaction occurred when similar organisms were injected subcutaneously (Gale and Smith, 1958). In some attempts, however, fibrinous bronchopneumonia was produced (Collier, 1968). Normal cattle have also been studied. The tracheas, lungs and bronchial lymph nodes of 88 apparently healthy cattle contained no pasteurellas (Collier and Rossow, 1964), but *P. hemolytica* and/or *P. multocida* were isolated from the palatine tonsils of 7 of 100 healthy slaughtered cattle (Collier, 1965). A laboratory study of 98 strains of *P. hemolytica* by a modified indirect hemagglutination test established 11 different serotypes. All strains from bovine pneumonia were of type 1 (Biberstein and Gills, 1960).

Numerous failures to reproduce shipping fever with bacterial pathogens led invesitgators to postulate that the primary cause is some other agent. The possibility of a virus as a primary causative agent was investigated. The first successful effort came in 1959 when nasal secretions from 11 young cattle affected with shipping fever were studied.

From each of 2 of these animals virus was isolated and grown in embryonal bovine kidney cell cultures and classified as Myxovirus parainfluenza 3 (SF-4) (Reisinger, Heddleston and Manthei, 1959). Subsequent to the first discovery other scientists isolated this virus from the respiratory tracts of cattle affected with clinical shipping fever (Gale and King, 1961; Hamdy, 1966; Sweat, 1967; Burroughs, 1967). A similar virus was also found in horses suffering from upper respiratory disease (Ditchfield *et al.*, 1963). Additional attempts to evaluate the importance of Myxovirus parainfluenza 3 (SF-4) as a causative factor of shipping fever were made in calves 6 months of age. Antibody titers against Myxovirus parainfluenza 3 (SF-4) from the same cattle were made before and after prolonged shipment and exposure to shipping fever. Of 191 cattle studied, 131 (68.6%) made a significant rise in titer (Hoerlein, Mansfield, Abinanti and Huebner, 1959). When subjected to comparative studies, Myxovirus parainfluenza 3 (SF-4) proved to be similar, but not identical, to Myxovirus parainfluenza 3 isolated from children (Abinanti and Huebner, 1959). When inoculated intranasally as an aerosol into healthy young cattle, the newly isolated virus usually caused a febrile reaction for about 6 days, but it did not cause the entire and typical syndrome of shipping fever (Reisinger, Heddleston and Manthei, 1959; Gale and King, 1961; Baldwin, Marshall and Wessman, 1967). The exposure of healthy cattle in a close sequence to both Myxovirus parainfluenza 3 (SF-4) and *P. hemolytica* or *P. multocida* caused more severe disease than virus alone, but still did not in general reproduce the entire syndrome of shipping fever (Heddleston, Reisinger and Watko, 1962; Baldwin, Marshall and Wessman, 1967). The inclusion of a third causative factor, appropriate environmental stress, may be a requirement for full manifestation of shipping fever.

Concurrent with research on the etiology were pathological studies which have established that in outbreaks of typical and fatal shipping fever cattle suffer from bilateral fibrinous bronchopneumonia (Graham, 1953; Carter, 1954).

The efficacy of vaccines, as well as management regimen, have also been studied. Live virus modified by multiple serial passages through cell cultures was administered to 6-month-old calves 5 weeks before weaning. Twenty cattle received the vaccine intramuscularly and 20 as an intranasal aerosol. After shipment for 150 miles all animals received an intranasal challenge of virulent Myxovirus parainfluenza 3 (SF-4). Fewer of the intranasally vaccinated calves excreted virus for a shorter period and manifested milder clinical signs than did calves vaccinated intramuscularly (Gutekunst, Paton and Volenec, 1969). A few other vaccines containing variable combinations of antigens from Myxovirus parainfluenza 3 and *Pasteurella* spp. have been prepared, but more could be developed (Report of Panel on Immunity to Bovine Respiratory Disease, 1967). Their efficacy needs further clarification by field use and laboratory evaluation. In an effort to protect feedlot cattle against respiratory diseases, 1432 similar animals were randomly arranged into two groups of 712 control and 720 treated cattle. Each of the treated animals daily, for the first 28 days of the fattening period received in the ration 350 mg of chlortetracycline and/or 350 mg of sulfamethazine. The treated cattle, especially those receiving chlortetracycline, gained 12 pounds extra weight with 23% greater rate of weight gain, made 19% more efficient conversion of feed, and had 54% fewer cases of disease (Beeson, 1969).

Occurrence. Usually the disease occurs in cattle of both sexes, 6 to 24 months of age. The incidence, greatest during late autumn and winter, develops within 10 days of arrival of cattle in feedlots. High incidence occurs in cattle that receive no immunizations 6 weeks before transit and that during shipment travel long distances to feedlots, suffer hunger and thirst, encounter inclement weather, and pass through central markets and other public areas for assembling cattle. The disease exists in all major cattle producing countries.

Etiology. The complex cause of shipping fever appears to be an interaction of Myxovirus parainfluenza-3 (SF-4), *Pasteurella hemolytica* and/or *P. multocida,* and environmental stressing agents.

Since its first discovery in 1959, Myxovirus parainfluenza-3 (SF-4) has been studied extensively. The virus particle consists of coiled ribonucleoprotein inner helix surrounded by an outer spiked lipoprotein envelope. The particle diameter varies from 150 to 250 mμ, and the single strand diameter from 15 to 18 μ. Growing in many types of cell cultures, the virus causes syncytia and eosinophilic inclusion bodies in both the nucleus and cytoplasm. Erythrocyte receptors are destroyed by enzyme. Hemagglutination, hemadsorption, and hemolysis can be demonstrated. Sensitive to ethyl-ether, the outer lipoprotein membrane dissolves when exposed to this solvent and releases the fragmenting ribonucleoprotein. When exposed to temperature of 50 to 56° C, the virus rapidly inactivates, but survives freezing at $-70°$ C. The virus has been found in cattle with shipping fever and probably is carried by some apparently healthy adults. Horses affected with upper respiratory disease also contain a similar virus. Although closely related Myxovirus parainfluenza 3 of children and the bovine virus are antigenicly separable.

Pasteurella hemolytica, a non-motile, nonspore forming, encapsulated, coccoid, but pleomorphic rod, measures 0.25 to 0.4 by 0.6 to 2.6 μ in size. In staining it is gram-negative and bi-polar. On serum agar it forms round, smooth, moist colonies. The colonies of encapsulated organisms are iridescent. Freshly isolated strains hemolyze erythrocytes, but some of this capacity is lost by multiple passages in series on media. While the capacity to ferment carbohydrates varies with different strains, most organisms produce acid from raffinose, saccharose, glucose and lactose, but not from rhamnose and inulin. Litmus milk is acidified. Commonly found in pneumonic lungs of cattle affected with shipping fever, the organisms are also carried in the palatine tonsils of some apparently healthy cattle and from these animals the bacteria may spread to other cattle by direct contact and by contaminating feed and water. Strains pathogenic to cattle usually classify as serotype 1 of Biberstein and Gills.

Pasteurella multocida resembles *P. hemolytica* in cell morphology and staining characteristics. On serum agar three colony types may form: fluorescent, blue and intermediate. Fluorescent forms are white and opaque and usually pathogenic. Blue colonies are dew-drop-shaped and commonly not pathogenic. As the name suggests, intermediate forms vary in appearance between the blue and fluorescent colonies. Erythrocytes are not hemolyzed. Indole is formed, and glucose and saccharose are fermented to form acid, but not raffinose. Like *P. hemolytica,* this species commonly occurs in pneumonic lungs of cattle with shipping fever and in palatine tonsils of some healthy adult cattle. Both species of *Pasteurella* are delicate and destroyed in 10 minutes at 60° C and in 15 minutes by 0.5% phenol, but they endure for several weeks in moist soil and dead animal tissues.

Practicing and research veterinarians have often observed, but not experimentally investigated, the relationship to shipping fever of common environmental stressing agents. These include hunger, thirst, vibrations, loss of body heat, overheating, fear, fatigue and anxiety of transit and castration, dehorning, vaccination and weaning that may occur near the time of transit. Presumably combinations of these conditions depress resistance and enhance susceptibility to Myxovirus parainfluenza-3 (SF-4), *P. hemolytica* and *P. multocida,* and the three categories of pathogens combine to cause shipping fever.

Pathogenesis. While the pathogenesis of shipping fever has not been fully elucidated, considerable information on the subject has been obtained, and an additional amount can be deduced. The three causative factors, environmental stressing agents, virus, and bacteria, combine to produce the disease. Each factor separately produces adverse results on cattle, but combinations have additive effects.

Environmental stresses vary in severity and effect, and the adverse conditions during transit from pasture or range to feedlot initiate the disease process. Weaning, vehicular vibrations, crowding, cooling and overheating are among the physical factors and fear, anxiety, and noise are psychological factors. The severity of transit stresses in general vary directly with distance moved. Travel for short distance during inclement weather, however, may be more adverse than traveling long distances during mild weather. Arrival at the feedlot may present additional stresses. Minor surgical operations, such as dehorning, castration, and vaccination, often result in hemorrhage and shock, and dipping or spraying may cause chilling and mild intoxication, while change in diet may cause digestive disturbances. The combined effect of all stresses is reduction in body weight, physical and mental depression, and increased susceptibility to infections.

Opportunities for exposure to Myxovirus parainfluenza-3 (SF-4) can occur at many points as cattle move from source to feedlot. Transporting trucks and railroad cars may carry different lots of cattle in rapid succession. Unless they are disinfected between each consignment, virus in nasal secretions from carrier animals may contaminate the vehicle. Unloading, resting, and feeding cattle at public stockyards or other public assemblage facilities may expose young susceptible animals to either animals carrying and shedding the virus or live virus contaminating the pens, water and feed. On arriving at the feedlot, the new cattle may again contact live virus by comingling with virus-carrying and shedding cattle or by occupying pens contaminated with live virus. Regardless of time and point in transit of exposure, stressed and depressed cattle may receive the live virus as inhaled infective droplets or as ingested contaminant in feed and water. On entering the nasal cavities or other anatomical parts of the respiratory system, the virus particles enter the epithelial cells where they replicate. Larger numbers of particles are released to the surface of the membranes and the mucus. The movement of mucus and air assists in distributing the virus particles throughout the system from nose to bronchioles where additional epithelial cells are infected. Viral injury to the mucous membrane evokes fever and acute inflammation with the formation of voluminous mucus and lesser amounts of pus. Discharged mucus, exudate and other nasal secretions carry virus particles which contaminate the environment and transmit disease to other susceptible animals.

Simultaneously or separately with exposure of transit animals to virus may come also exposure to pathogenic *Pasteurella hemolytica* and/or *P. multocida.* The bacteria, carried and excreted by some healthy cattle, as well as by sick animals, contaminate the environment where transported cattle feed, drink and rest. As with the virus, the bacteria may be inhaled with infective droplets or ingested as contaminants in feed and water. On entering the respiratory system already infected with Myxovirus parainfluenza-3 (SF-4), the pasteurellas proliferate and distribute widely throughout the system. Some organisms are inhaled into alveoli of the lungs. A more severe inflammatory reaction than was caused by virus alone is provoked. The mucous membranes swell and blood capillaries congest. Some weakened vessels rupture and produce hemorrhage. The pathogenic pasteurellas evoke an abundant heavy fibrinous exudate which forms in the lumens of bronchi and bronchioles, in infected alveoli, and on the pleural surfaces of infected lung lobes. The fibrinous bronchopneumonia, with filling of alveoli by fibrinous exudate, results in generalized hypoxia, dyspnea, and weakness. In fatal cases, death probably results from shock and circulatory failure. In surviving cases, the fibrin in alveoli, after several days, undergoes lysis and healing occurs. If the fibrin persists excessively, it becomes organized by the proliferation into it of fibrocytes and capillaries. Organization permanently incapacitates alveoli and establishes adhesions between pleural surfaces. In addition to changes in the respiratory system, some voluntary muscles of some affected animals develop myopathy. Grossly affected muscles have pale foci which microscopically show muscle cell degeneration. The mechanism for myopathy development is unknown.

Clinical Signs and Postmortem Lesions. Following an incubation period of 2 to 5 days the body temperature rises to 104° to 108° F. In early stages of the disease the general attitude is depicted at the time of, or immediately following, the morning feed, when affected animals remain recumbent or stand isolated with the head downward. The hair coat is rough, the muzzle dry, and the appetite diminished. In early stages the lungs are fully functional. In more advanced stages the animals are profoundly affected systemically. With a mucopurulent discharge extending from the nostrils, the muzzle becomes encrusted with dehydrated exudate. Forcible removal of the crust leaves a denuded hemorrhaging surface. The eyes show profuse lacrimation and purulent conjunctivitis. Gaunt and often dehydrated from anorexia, the cattle are depressed, weak, and fatigued. Rapid respirations are accompanied by coughing and sometimes oral breathing. Auscultation reveals fibrinous pleuritis and bronchial pneumonia in the anteroventral portions of the lungs. Some animals develop mucoid diarrhea and some purulent otitis; a few show tonic clonic convulsions. In some, but not all cases, muscular weakness and severe myopathy result in flaccidity and pendulence of muscle groups. These changes are especially noticeable in the thighs. Some animals die after 2 to 3 days of illness. While morbidity varies widely, usually it does not exceed 20% of the herd. The mortality rate is 1 to 2% of affected cattle but may rise higher unless treatment is provided. Fifty to 60 days of feeding may be required to regain preshipment body weight.

At necropsy the respiratory system is severely affected. Catarrhal inflammation is general throughout the nose, paranasal sinuses, pharynx, larynx and trachea. The nasal cavities and paranasal sinuses contain a large volume of mucopurulent exudate. The mucous membranes of the bronchi are swollen and hemorrhagic. Frequently, masses of fibrin fill the lumens of bronchi. The anteroventral portions of both lungs are distended and firm because the alveoli are filled with fibrin. Emphysema, both alveolar and interstitial, is prominent at the junction of the pneumonic and normal tissue. On the cut surface of the pneumonic lung some lobules are in red and some in gray hepatization. The interlobular connective tissue is widened because of extensive edema. Occasionally, pulmonary infarcts are present. The pleural cavity contains serofibrinous exudate and strands of fibrin adhere to the pleural surfaces.

Outside of the respiratory system changes are less severe. Suprapharyngeal, mediastinal, and bronchial lymph nodes are swollen and hemorrhagic. Petechial and ecchymotic hemorrhages are abundant in the thymus, pleura, peritoneum, subepicardium and subendocardium. Occasionally they are also present in the subcutaneous tissues and muscles. Hemorrhages in the mucosa of the abomasum may progress into erosions and ulcers. The intestinal mucosa may be swollen and contain hemorrhages.

Myopathy may be found in large skeletal muscles, including the pectoralis, triceps, biceps femoris, semimembranosus, semitendonosus, and longissimus dorsi. The affected muscle tissue is pale yellow in color. With only a part of a muscle affected, the diseased tissue usually measures up to several inches in each dimension. The changes may be bilateral.

Histopathologically, acute catarrhal inflammation is present throughout the mucosa of the upper respiratory system. In the pneumonic portions of the lung, alveoli are filled

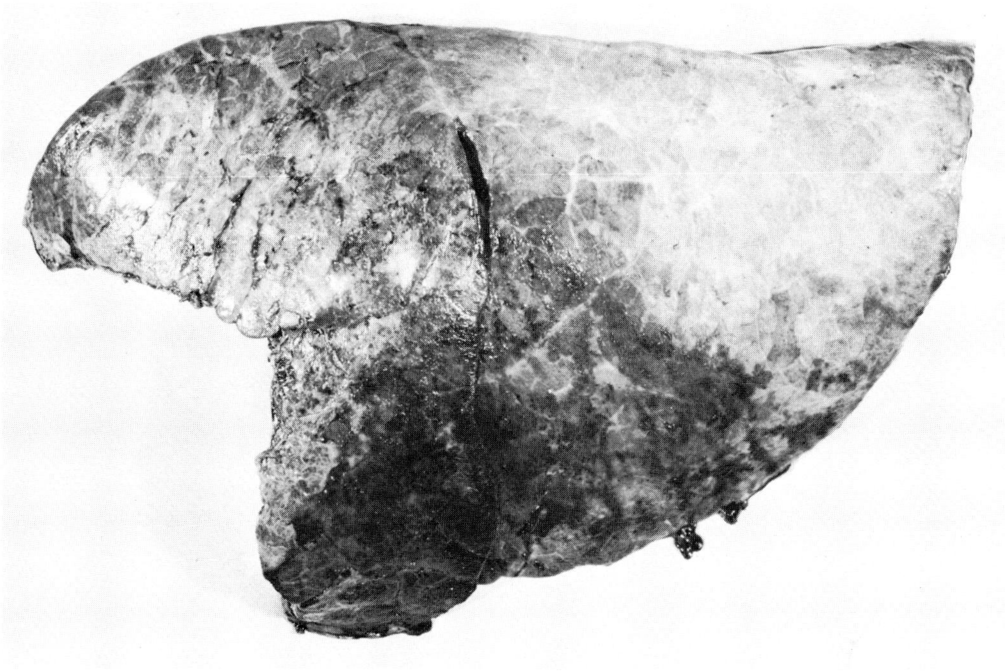

FIG. 2-16. *Lung of steer with shipping fever. The anteroventral part is pneumonic. Note the fibrinous pleuritis.* × 0.3.

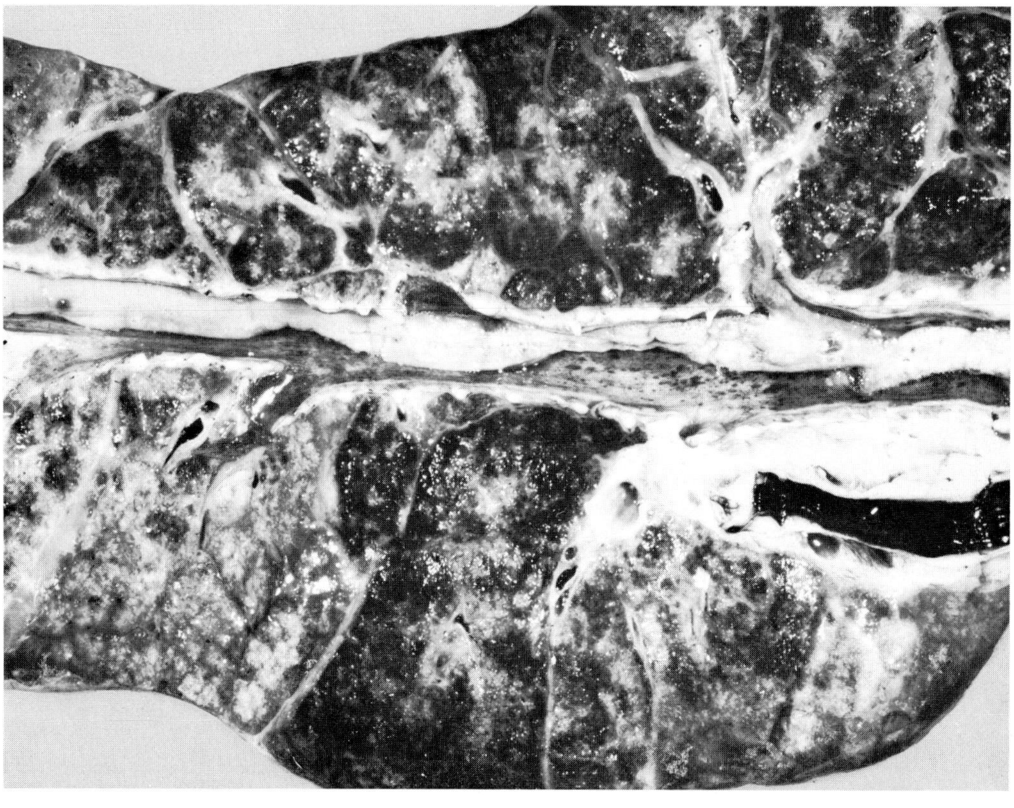

FIG. 2-17. *Cut surface of lung from steer with shipping fever. The bronchus contains fibrin.* × 1.2.

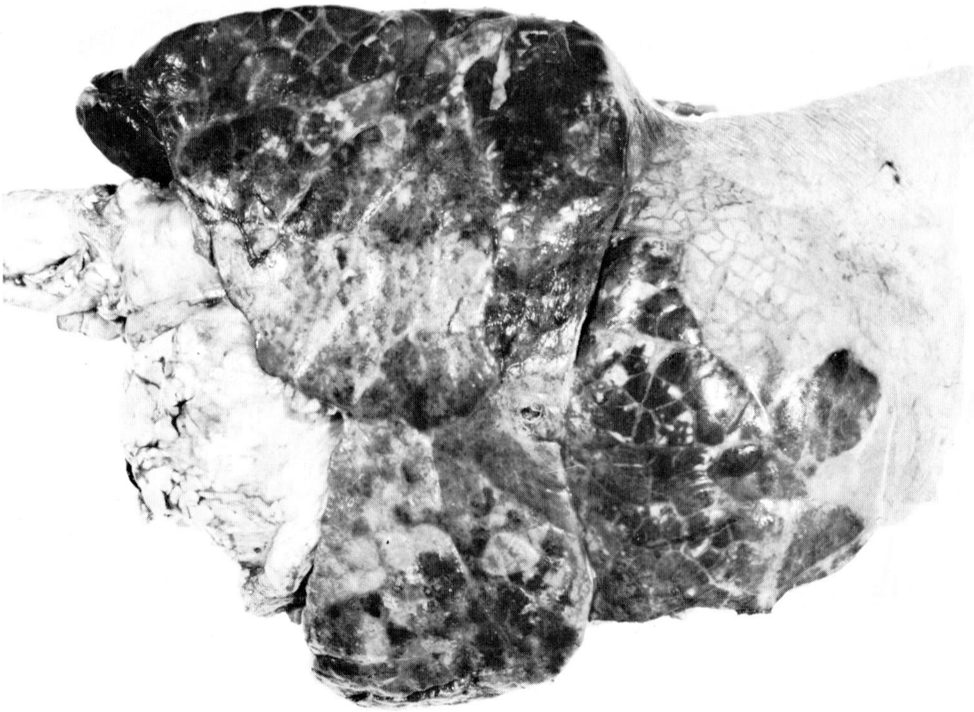

FIG. 2-18. *Pneumonic lung from an heifer with shipping fever.* × 0.3.

with fibrin. In early stages of red hepatization, the fibrin contains erythrocytes. Later, in stages of gray hepatization, leukocytes in variable stages of degeneration infiltrate the fibrin. Colonies of pasteurellas are discernible within the exudate. Many bronchioles are filled with fibrin. The interlobular connective tissue is edematous and may be infiltrated with leukocytes. Interlobular and subpleural lymphatics are distended and frequently thrombosed. The pleural surface contains serofibrinous exudate. In stages of resolution the fibrin diminishes and mononuclear macrophages accumulate within the alveoli. At the junction of the pneumonic and functional tissue many alveoli are overdistended with air, and gas bodies are discernible within the interstitial connective tissue. In diseased muscles, affected cells may be swollen and necrotic. After losing striations, the swollen cytoplasm fragments, vacuolates and undergoes lysis. Empty sarcolemmas may be discernible and mononuclear macrophages may be present.

Diagnosis. Typical signs of shipping fever are pneumonia, fever, gauntness, nasal discharge, and leukocytosis. These signs, in cattle exposed within 10 days after stressful experience, are the basis for diagnosis. Confirmation of diagnosis is dependent upon finding at necropsy of bilateral fibrinous bronchopneumonia in the anteroventral parts of the lungs and serofibrinous pleuritis. In the laboratory *P. hemolytica* and/or *P. multocida* can be isolated. Often, from some members of the herd Myxovirus parainfluenza-3 (SF-4) can be isolated in tissue culture from secretions of the respiratory system or from diseased lungs.

The differential diagnosis requires consideration of calf diphtheria and viral bovine rhinotracheitis. Calf diphtheria usually is sporadic and may develop at any time during

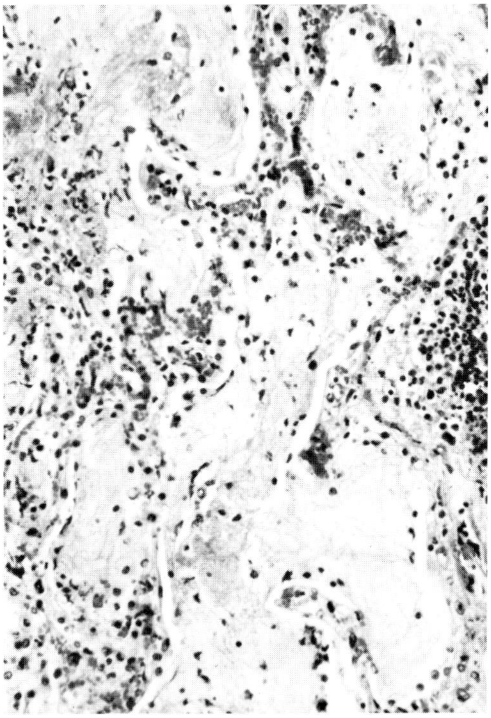

FIG. 2-19. *Lung from a steer dead from shipping fever. The alveoli are filled with fibrin and leukocytes. HE stain.* × 163.

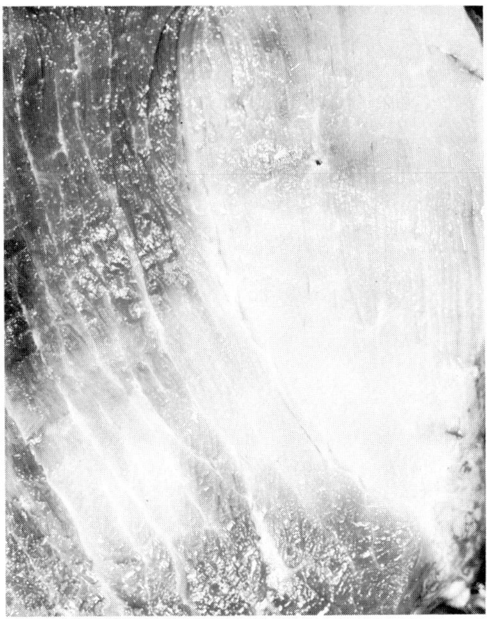

FIG. 2-20. *Myopathy of thigh muscle of a steer with shipping fever.* × 0.7.

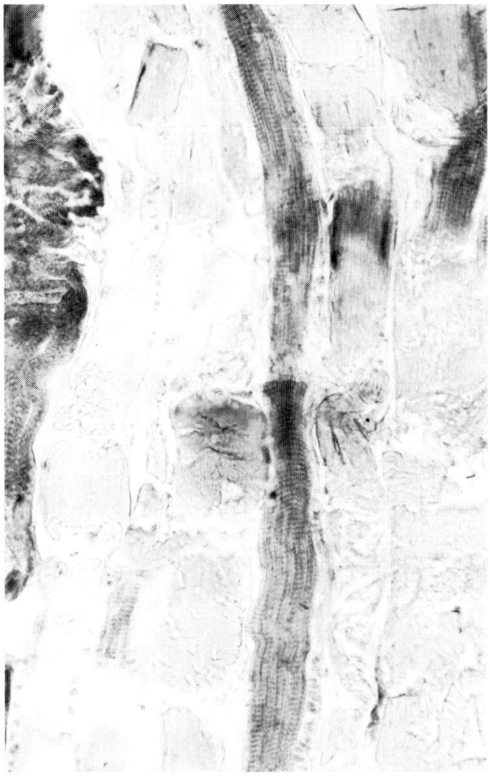

FIG. 2-21. *Muscular degeneration from a steer with shipping fever. PTAH stain.* × 383.

the fattening period. Breathing, especially during inspiration, is often stertorous, difficult, and oral. Visual examination of the larynx by means of a laryngoscope reveals the typical diphtheritic lesions of the larynx.

Viral bovine rhinotracheitis simulates and may be combined with shipping fever. Careful study usually, however, enables differentiation. Viral bovine rhinotracheitis usually develops as a herd problem several weeks following shipment into the feedlots. While many animals are febrile, most affected cattle do not manifest pneumonia or pleuritis. The virus of viral bovine rhinotracheitis can be isolated from nasal secretions, grown in bovine embryonal kidney cell cultures, and identified by means of serum neutralization with known antiserum. Following clinical recovery, specific antibodies against the virus of viral bovine rhinotracheitis manifests an ascending titer.

Prevention and Treatment. Currently two systems for preventing shipping fever are practiced: one utilizes immunizing agents; the other, drugs. Commercial vaccines are available and in use. Varying in composition, these products contain different combinations of attenuated live virus, inactivated virus and killed pasteurellas. Intranasal administration stimulates the formation of nasal secretion antibodies and may be more effective than parenteral inoculation. To be effective, any vaccine must be administered a few weeks before the vaccinated animals are exposed to the disease. In case of shipping fever, vaccine should be administered 2 to 3 weeks prior to shipment to feedlots. Some good vaccines may require 2 doses with an interval 1 to several weeks, and some may require intranasal administration a few weeks before shipment or within 36 hours after arriving at the feedlot. Unfortunately, some cattle management practices may preclude vaccination a few weeks before shipment. The use of bacterins, composed of killed pasteurellas and possibly other bacteria, alone after cattle arrive at the feedlot tends to increase the amount and severity of respiratory disease and should be avoided. If health of cattle permits, antibiotics should be avoided for 7 to 10 days after vaccination.

The shipment of cattle to feedlots during fall and winter months is followed commonly by shipping fever, and precautions should be exercised to avoid the disease. On arrival at the feedlot and continuing for 1 week, adult animals should be given grass hay, oats and bran along with adequate drinking water. Recently weaned calves can be fed rations of calf starter. Chloretetracycline, or oxytetracycline can be administered daily for 25 to 30 days in feed at the rate of 250 mg per animal per day. Sulfamethazine may be given along with the antibiotic drug at the same dosage. The combination is more effective in preventing disease than the antibiotic alone. This preventive treatment also increases the rate of gain in body weight and enhances the efficiency in utilization of feed. Following removal of antibiotic and sulfamethazine from the diet, respiratory disease may develop.

The administration of electrolytes and arsenical compounds in the drinking water appears to accelerate the rate of recovery from fatigue and to develop appetite for the new and unfamiliar diet. Medication should be continued for 7 to 10 days. During the first week large amounts of corn silage, alfalfa silage, and third or fourth cuttings of alfalfa should not be fed, especially to recently weaned calves, because of the tendency to produce diarrhea.

Fortunately, specific and effective treatment is available. When administered early in the course of the disease, sulfonamides and antibiotics are highly effective in shortening the disease course and in returning cattle to feed. Sick animals should be treated individually with chlortetracycline or oxytetracycline daily for 3 to 6 days at the rate of 5 mg per pound of body weight given intravenously. When 25% or more cattle within a pen are affected, the entire herd should be treated with sulfathiazole sodium or sulfamethazine in the drinking water at the rate of 1 pound of drug per 100 gallons of drinking water for 72 hours, followed by 1 pound of drug per 200 gallons of drinking water for an additional 48 to 72 hours. Additional individual treatment is the parenteral administration of aqueous solutions of glucose intravenously, antihistamines, expectorants and cortical steroids. Dry bedding, such as straw or wood shavings, and protection against inclement weather should be provided during periods of treatment and convalescence.

References

Abinanti, F. R. and Huebner, R. J.: Serological Relationships of Parainfluenza 3 Virus Isolated from Humans and Cattle with Respiratory Disease. Virology, 8 (1959): 391–394.

Adams, O. R., Brown, W. W., Chow, T. L., Collier, J. R., Davis, R. W., Griner, L. A., Jensen, Rue, Pierson, R. E. and Wayt, L. K.: Comparison of Infectious Bovine Rhinotracheitis, Shipping Fever, and Calf Diphtheria of Cattle. JAVMA. *134* (1959): 85–89.

Baldwin, D. E., Marshall, R. G. and Wassman, G. E.: Experimental Infection of Calves with Myxovirus Parainfluenza 3 and *Pasteurella Hemolytica*. AJVR, *28* (1967): 1773–1782.
Beeson, W. M.: How Beneficial Are Feed Additives?: JAVMA, *154* (1969): 1214–1219.
Biberstein, E. L., Gills, M. and Knight, H.: Serological Types of *Pasteurella Hemolytica*. Corn. Vet., *50* (1960): 283.
Burroughs, A. L.: Viral Respiratory Infection in Commercial Feedlot Cattle. AJVR, *28* (1967): 365–371.
Carter, G. R.: Observations on the Pathology and Bacteriology of Shipping Fever in Canada. Canad. J. Comp. Med., *18* (1954): 359–363.
———: Studies on *Pasteurella Multocida*. I. A Hemagglutination Test for Identification of Serological Types. AJVR, *16* (1955): 481–484.
Carter, G. R. and McSherry, B. J.: Further Observations on Shipping Fever in Canada. Canad. J. Comp. Med., *19* (1955): 177–181.
Collier, J. R.: Personal Communication (1965).
———: Pasteurellae in Bovine Respiratory Disease. JAVMA, *152* (1968): 824–828.
Collier, J. R., Brown, W. W., Jr. and Chow, T. L.: Microbiologic Investigations on Natural Epizootics of Shipping Fever in Cattle. JAVMA, *140* (1962): 807–810.
Collier, J. R., Chow, T. L., Benjamin, Maxine M. and Deem, A. W.: The Combined Effect of Infectious Bovine Rhinotracheitis Virus and *Pasteurella Hemolytica* on Cattle. AJVR, *21* (1960): 195–198.
Collier, J. R. and Rossow, C. F.: Microflora of Apparently Healthy Lung Tissue of Cattle. AJVR, *25* (1964): 391–393.
Ditchfield, J. and Zbitnew, A. and MacPherson, L. W.: Association of Myxovirus Parainfluenza 3 (RE 55) with Upper Respiratory Infection of Horses. Canad. Vet. J., *4* (1963): 175.
Gale, C. and King, N. B.: Isolation of a Virus from Clinical Shipping Fever in Cattle. JAVMA, *138* (1961): 235–238.
Gale, C. and Smith, H. R.: Studies on Shipping Fever of Cattle. I. Experimental Exposure of Cattle with Various Cultures of Pasteurella. AJVR, *19* (1958): 815–817.
Gossett, F. O., Gale, C., Gregory, R. P. and Matsuoka, T.: Serologic Response to a Formalized and Adjuvant Parainfluenza 3 Antigen in Calves. JAVMA, *157* (1970): 174–177.
Graham, W. R.: The Pathology of Shipping Fever in Feedlot Cattle. JAVMA, *123* (1953): 198–203.
Gutekunst, D. E., Paton, I. M. and Volenec, F. J.: Parainfluenza-3 Vaccine in Cattle: Comparative Efficacy of Intranasal and Intramuscular Routes. JAVMA, *155* (1969): 1879–1884.
Hamdy, A. H., Gale, C. and King, N. B.: Studies on Shipping Fever of Cattle. II. Isolation of Pleuropneumonia-like Organisms. AJVR, *19* (1958): 818–821.
Heddleston, K. L., Reisinger, R. C. and Watko, L. P.: Studies on the Transmission and Etiology of Bovine Shipping Fever. AJVR, *23* (1961): 548–553.
———: Studies on the Transmission and Etiology of Bovine Shipping Fever. AJVR, *23* (1962): 548–553.
Hoerlein, A. B., Mansfield, M. E., Abinanti, F. R. and Huebner, R. J.: Studies of Shipping Fever of Cattle. I. Parainfluenza 3 Virus Antibodies in Feeder Calves. JAVMA, *134* (1959): 153–160.
Hoerlein, A. B., Saxena, S. P. and Mansfield, M. E.: Studies on Shipping Fever of Cattle. II. Prevalence of Pasteurella Species in Nasal Secretions from Normal Calves and Calves with Shipping Fever. AJVR, *22* (1961): 470–472.
Losses in Agriculture. Agricultural Handbook No. 291. Agricultural Research Service. U.S.D.A. (1965).
Reisinger, R. C., Heddleston, K. L. and Manthei, C. A.: A Myxovirus (SF-4) Associated with Shipping Fever of Cattle. JAVMA, *135* (1959): 147–152.
Report of Panel for Symposium on Immunity to Bovine Respiratory Disease Complex. JAVMA, *151* (1967): 1481–1487.
Sweat, R. L.: Isolation of Myxovirus Parainfluenza 3 From Cattle with Respiratory Diseases. JAVMA, *150* (1967): 172–177.
Woods, G. T.: The Natural History of Bovine Myxovirus Parainfluenza-3. JAVMA, *152* (1968): 771–777.
Woods, G. T., Mansfield, M. E., Cmarik, G., Zinzilieta, M. and Marquis, G.: Vaccination of Beef Calves Before Weaning with a Live-Virus Bovine Myxovirus Parainfluenza-3 Vaccine. AJVR, *29* (1968a): 1349–1353.
Woods, G. T., Mansfield, M. E., Segre, D., Holper, J. C., Brandly, C. A. and Barthel, C.: The Role of Viruses in Respiratory Diseases of Cattle. III. Respiratory Disease in Beef Calves Vaccinated Before Weaning with Myxovirus Parainfluenza 3 (SF-4) Vaccine. AJVR, *23* (1962): 832–836.

Bovine Viral Diarrhea

(MUCOSAL DISEASE)

Bovine viral diarrhea, an acute, subacute or inapparent contagious disease, is characterized clinically by fever and diarrhea and pathologically by erosions of the mouth, esophagus, forestomachs, abomasum and intestines. The cause is a virus. Because of extreme variability in clinical manifestations, many cattle experience the disease without detection of illness. Although approximately 60% of cattle throughout the United States contain antibodies to the virus, only a fraction of these reacting cattle have suffered the clinically recognizable disease. Even though not measured, bovine viral diarrhea probably causes severe economic losses. Some damage comes from overt disease with marked reduction in body weight, abortions, deaths, and expensive prevention and treatment programs. Possibly greater losses accrue from subclinical infections of large numbers of cattle that become unthrifty and inefficient for variable periods.

Review of Literature. In the book *Traite des Maladies Contagieuses,* published toward the close of the nineteenth century, Galtier described an unidentified disease of cattle with clinical signs and lesions resembling bovine viral diarrhea (Provost, 1965). Modern bovine viral diarrhea, however, was first identified, described and named in New York State where it caused considerable economic losses, especially among dairy cattle. Important manifestations were diarrhea and erosions of the alimentary tract. Morbidity rate was high and mortality rate low (Olafson, MacCallum and Fox, 1946; Olafson and Rickard, 1947). Recognizing some clinical similarities between bovine viral diarrhea and rinderpest, cattle recovered from bovine viral diarrhea were inoculated with rinderpest virus and were found to be fully susceptible (Walker and Olafson, 1947). Subsequently, additional studies were conducted on similar cattle diseases of midwest areas of the United States. One such disease was observed in feedlot cattle of Iowa. Because the characteristic erosions and ulcers were limited to the mucous membranes of the alimentary tract, the disease was designated "mucosal disease." In these cattle herds, mucosal disease had low morbidity rate and high mortality rate. Early attempts to transmit the disease were unsuccessful (Ramsey and Chivers, 1953; Ramsey, 1956). In feedlot cattle of Indiana a disease similar to bovine viral diarrhea of New York State developed, but in these pens 10% of affected cattle were lame from laminitis. This malady was given the name "bovine viral diarrhea Indiana" (Pritchard, Taylor, Moses and Doyle, 1956). Although differing in some clinical features, the three bovine diseases of New York, Iowa, and Indiana possessed fundamentally similar lesions, and viruses isolated from affected cattle of each area were found to be identical (Gillespie, Baker, and McEntee, 1960; Tyler and Ramsey, 1965). Eventually the disease was identified and studied in Britain (Don, Jarrett, and McIntyre, 1956), West Germany (Kniazeff *et al.,* 1961; Bogel, 1964), France (Tournut, *et al.,* 1961), Africa (Otte and Peck, 1960), Australia (Blood, Hutchins, Jubb, Whitem and Littlejohns, 1957), and Japan (Omori *et al.,* 1967). In cattle of the United States the incidence of exposure as measured by the presence of antibodies varied greatly among herds (Mills and Lugmbuhl, 1965). The average incidence appeared to be approximately 60% (Malmquist, 1968).

Numerous strains of bovine viral diarrhea virus have been isolated and studied. Strains from affected cattle in New York and Indiana were grown in bovine kidney cells and found to be non-cytopathic (Lee and Gillespie, 1957; Gillespie and Baker, 1959). But a cytopathic strain was isolated from lymphoid tissue of cattle affected with mucosal disease and grown in bovine kidney cells (Underdahl *et al.,* 1957). Another cytopathic strain, isolated from infected calf spleen and designated "Oregon C24V," became a prototype reference for comparing other strains from many countries (Gillespie, Baker and McEntee, 1960). Eventually cultures of the other cell types, including bovine testicle, spleen and trachea, were used and some of these cultures possessed advantages over bovine kidney cells (Malmquist, 1968).

The morphology and physicochemical properties of particles of the bovine viral diarrhea virus have been investigated. The diameter of the virion has been found to be variable. Using electron microscopy following particle staining with phosphotungstic acid or uranyl acetate the particles measured 15 to 80 mμ in diameter with an average of about 40 mμ (Hafez, Petzoldt and Reczko, 1968; Hermodson and Dinter, 1962; Ritchie and Fernelius, 1969). Investigations also in-

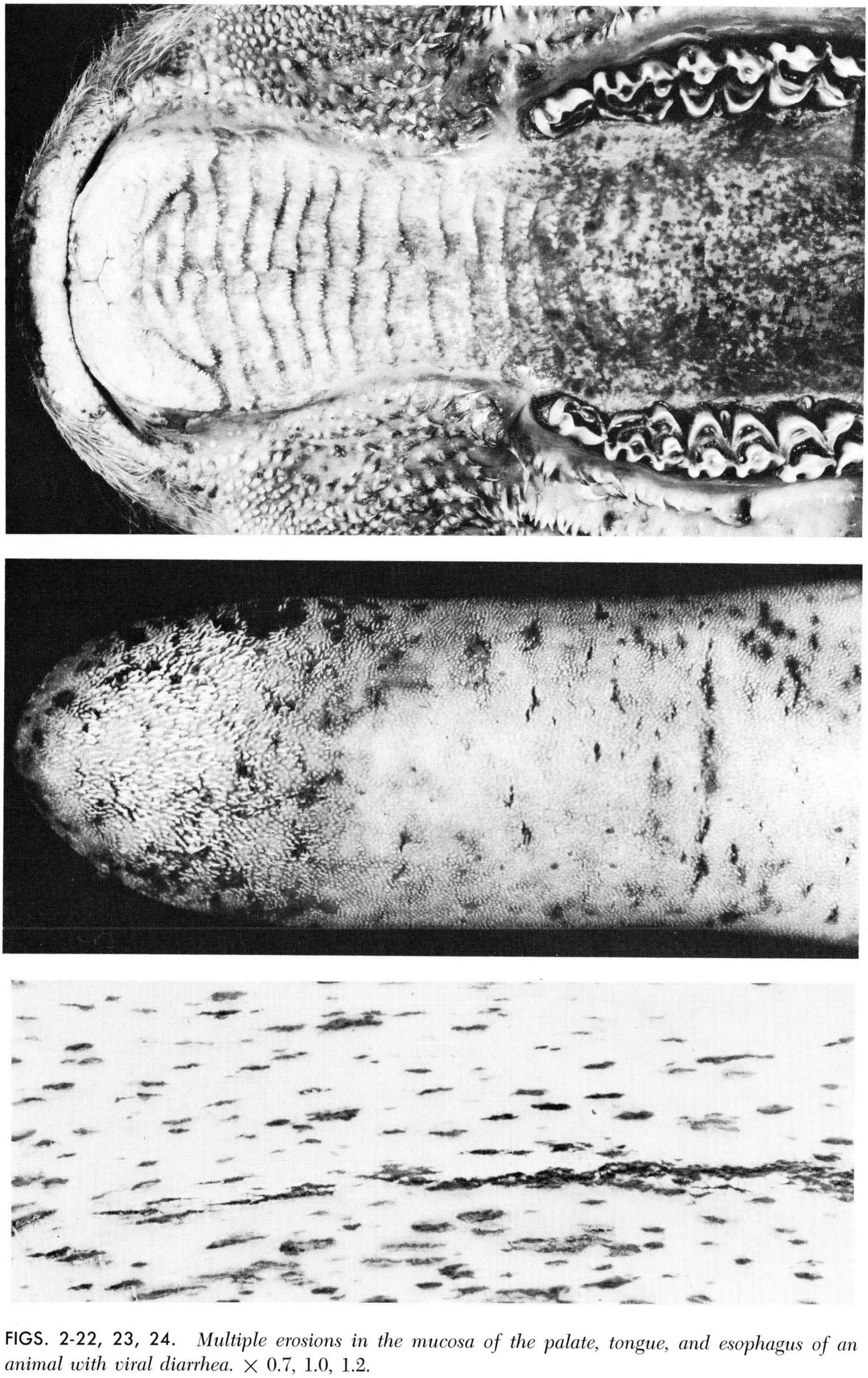

FIGS. 2-22, 23, 24. *Multiple erosions in the mucosa of the palate, tongue, and esophagus of an animal with viral diarrhea.* × 0.7, 1.0, 1.2.

dicated that the virus is sensitive to ether and chloroform and that it is not inhibited by 5-iodo-deoxypuridine (Hermodsson and Dinter, 1962).

An antigenic relationship between the causative viruses of viral bovine diarrhea and hog cholera was clearly established. In Ouchterlonyplates, a line identity was observed to form between a hog cholera system and a viral diarrhea system (Darbyshire, 1960; 1962). In a later experiment, 21 hogs inoculated with virus of bovine viral diarrhea developed immunity to hog cholera (Beckenhauer, 1961). Continued studies, however, indicated that antibodies to bovine viral diarrhea virus protect swine against hog cholera virus to a lesser extent than do antibodies evoked by hog cholera vaccine (Tamoglia *et al.*, 1965).

Systematic culturing of the virus of bovine viral diarrhea resulted in modification of the agent. After 32 serial passages, the Oregon C24V strain virus appeared to be attenuated. When inoculated into susceptible cattle no illness was detected, but the animals resisted exposure to fully virulent virus (Coggins *et al.*, 1961). This change in virus enabled the production of commercial live virus vaccine which was produced and marketed both as a single antigen and in combination with other antigens, such as virus of viral bovine rhinotracheitis, parainfluenza-3 virus, and leptospira (Report of Panel for Symposium on Bovine Respiratory Disease, 1968; Grantson and Welter, 1968). Use of the vaccine against bovine viral diarrhea resulted in a few animals developing fatal disease resembling field cases of bovine viral diarrhea (Peter, Tyler and Ramsey, 1967; McKercher *et al.*, 1968). These complications were con-

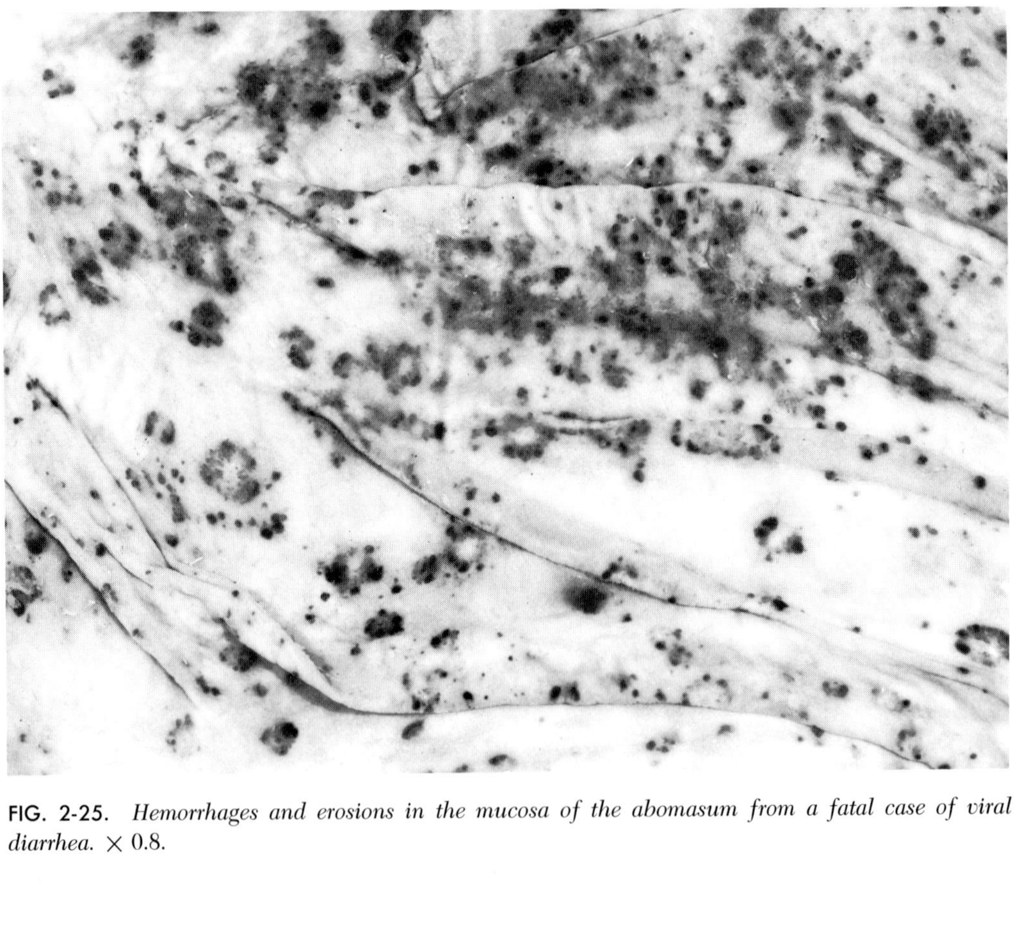

FIG. 2-25. *Hemorrhages and erosions in the mucosa of the abomasum from a fatal case of viral diarrhea.* × 0.8.

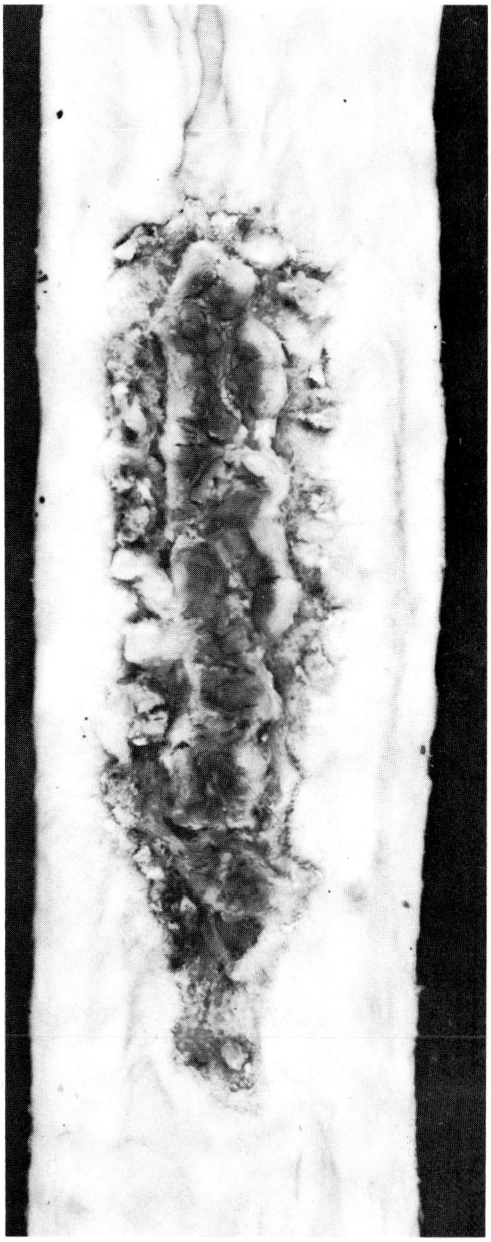

FIG: 2-26. *Necrosis and ulcer in a Peyer's patch of the small intestine from a fatal case of viral diarrhea.* × 1.4.

sidered to be due to possible failure of lymphoid tissue to produce antibodies (Malmquist, 1968) and to prevaccination exposure of animals to virulent viruses, such as bovine viral diarrhea virus and parainfluenza-3 virus (McKercher *et al.*, 1968).

In addition to cattle, clinical bovine viral diarrhea has been observed in deer from which virus was isolated and identified. Paired serum samples from affected and later recovered animals revealed an ascending titer (Romváry, 1965). While some sheep have positive blood titers (Bogel, 1964), clinical cases have not been described.

Occurrence. Borine viral diarrhea occurs during all seasons, but with higher incidence during fall and winter months. While cattle of all ages and sexes are affected, animals 6 to 24 months have been attacked more commonly. Clinical and subclinical forms of the disease are together very common. As a result of exposure to the disease approximately 60% of all young adult cattle contain antibodies against the virus. Most of the exposures cause subclinical effects. In addition to cattle some deer develop clinical bovine viral diarrhea. Some deer and some sheep contain antibodies against the virus. Clinical bovine viral diarrhea has not been observed in sheep. Geographically, the disease, in both feedlot and dairy cattle, exists in all sections of the United States, in Canada, Britain, France, Sweden, Germany, Czechoslovakia, Africa, Australia and Japan.

Etiology and Pathogenesis. Although studied extensively, the virus causing bovine viral diarrhea is not classified. The spherical virion contains RNA and measures approximately 40 mμ in diameter. It is sensitive to ether, chloroform and trypsin, and it is not stabilized by magnesium chloride. When stored for 24 hours at 26° to 37° C the titer reduces to about one-tenth the original concentration, but at 24° C little loss occurs. Lyophilized virus in blood or tissue and stored at −70° C retains viability for several years.

Outside the bovine host the virus adapts to cell culture systems. The virus grows and replicates in embryonic bovine cells from kidneys, testicles, spleen and trachea. In tissue culture some strains of virus are cytopathogenic, but many are non-cytopathogenic. The latter require special techniques for efficient and effective study. The fluorescent antibody technique is direct, simple and easy to use. It visualizes virus in its position of replication as well as in areas of relocation. Cytopathogenic strains cause cell elongation, shrinkage, vacuolization and pyknosis. Many passages of some strains cause little change in pathogenicity, but Oregon C24V strain attenuated for calves after 32 passages.

During acute febrile stages of bovine viral diarrhea, the virus can be found in and isolated from many tissues. Blood leukocytes are a good source. Virus usually disappears from the blood following the development of neutralizing antibodies. A few cases of prolonged viremia, however, have been identified. Mucous membranes of the nose, paranasal sinuses, larynx and intestine, lymphoid tissue, and some secretions and excretions are also good sources. Newborn calves from infected cows often contain virus.

Viruses isolated from cattle affected with bovine viral diarrhea appear to be antigenically homogenous. The viruses of bovine viral diarrhea and hog cholera possess an antigenic relationship. In agar gel diffusion tests a line of precipitation forms between hog cholera virus and bovine viral diarrhea antiserum. The two viruses share a common soluble antigen, but their antibodies do not completely cross neutralize the viruses. Hyperimmune hog cholera serums, however, commonly contain neutralizing antibodies against bovine viral diarrhea virus. Cattle recovered from bovine viral diarrhea appear to be immune for prolonged periods.

With virus in some secretions and excretions of affected cattle, the disease often rapidly spreads throughout a herd by both direct and indirect contact. In crowded feedlots and transport vehicles, virus-containing nasal and oral secretions easily transfer from affected cattle to the nose, face, eyes and skin of susceptible animals. Coughing and violent breathing sprays infected droplets into air breathed by susceptible cattle. Feeding and watering equipment, used jointly by all cattle within a pen, become contaminated, and transfer viable virus from diseased to susceptible cattle. Vehicles, such as trucks and tractors, and workers operating within an infected pen become contaminated and when used without decontamination in other pens or at other, even distant, feedlots may mechanically carry the virus and transmit the disease. The problems of healthy animals carrying and excreting the virus and of reservoirs of virus need additional investigations.

Even though a large amount of information is available on bovine viral diarrhea, the pathogenesis is poorly understood and extensively conjectured. Following exposure of susceptible cattle to the disease, the virus presumably enters through the respiratory and alimentary systems. Epithelial cells of the mucous membranes of the nose, paranasal sinuses, larynx, pharynx, mouth, abomasum and intestines may be attacked and invaded, and in these cells the virus replicates and concentrates. Virus then enters the blood where it associates with leukocytes. Viremia persists during febrile stages and usually terminates when neutralizing antibodies form. Virus enters lymphoid tissue either through afferent lymphatics or from the blood. In lymph nodes, spleen, and Peyer's patches, cells are destroyed and the germinal centers become depleted. Necrosis, especially in Peyer's patches, may be extensive. Granulocytes are also suppressed and generalized leukopenia temporarily develops. Strong stimulation of reticuloendothelial system results in the production of new mononuclear cells. The cells accumulate around capillaries near epithelial coverings of the mouth, pharynx, forestomachs, abomasum, intestines, nose and larynx. Consequently, some epithelial cells degenerate and necrose, and their sloughing from the membrane results in the numerous erosions that characterize bovine viral diarrhea. The virus is excreted to the external environment through secretions from the respiratory and alimentary systems. Serum neutralizing antibodies are usually demonstrable within 1 to 2 weeks after exposure to the virus and complement fixing antibodies at the beginning of the second week. Following recovery most animals are immune.

The nature of bovine viral diarrhea among cattle is highly variable. The majority of individual cattle experience a mild syndrome. Mild fever, slight leukopenia and few other clinical signs develop and subside and may escape detection. Following recovery such animals contain specific antibodies and are immune. In fatal cases tissue damage is severe and other viruses, such as the virus of bovine rhinotracheitis and parainfluenza-3, and bacteria, such as pasteurellas, complicate the disease and aggravate the injury. A few individual animals develop persistent and prolonged viremia. This complication may be due to injury to the lymphoid tissue and incapacity for producing antibodies.

Clinical Signs and Postmortem Lesions. Following an incubation period of 1 to 3 weeks, body temperature ranges from 105° to 108° F. The fever usually persists from 4 to 7 days and may have a second rise. Leukopenia develops on the fourth or fifth days after experimental inoculation and may reduce the number of leukocytes to 50% of normal. In some animals the leukopenia is followed by leukocytosis. Profuse diarrhea begins towards the end of the febrile period and continues for 3 to 5 days. The fluid feces are maloderous because of necrotic cells and tissues. Oral erosions appear 1 to 3 days following the onset of diarrhea. They are often numerous on the tongue, palate and buccal mucosa. Approximately 20% of affected cattle contain few or perhaps no erosions. Anorexia and dry coughing come early. Profuse salivation accompanied by nasal discharge and moist coughing may develop later. The roughened dry muzzle reveals erosions beneath the crust. Some cases develop conjunctivitis with a mucopurulent ocular discharge and inflamed erosions near the medial canthi, and a few eyes develop mild keratitis and corneal opacity. In some outbreaks approximately 10% of infected cattle are lame. Dermatitis, with necrosis and scab formation, is present at the junction of skin and hoof. Interdigital skin lesions may resemble changes found in foot rot. Similar skin lesions may develop at the base of the horns and occasionally at the perineum. Affected cattle lose large amounts of body weight and may not regain the lost pounds for several weeks after disease subsidence. Uncommonly, an affected animal develops central nervous signs of muscular tremors, weakness, incoordination and nystagmus. Peripheral lymph nodes may be enlarged, and pregnant cows may abort.

The morbidity, while highly variable, may be as much as 90% of a herd. Mortality of affected animals, equally variable, usually does not exceed 30% in large herds. The disease syndrome originally described for New York State and Indiana State had high morbidity rate and low mortality rate, but the mucosal disease syndrome of Iowa had low morbidity rate and high mortality rate.

At necropsy, in addition to the exhibition of specific lesions, profuse diarrhea, dehydration and loss of body weight are obvious. Most lesions are limited to the alimentary tract. Multiple erosions, usually 1 to 5 mm in diameter, are present in the mucosa of the muzzle, buccal cavity, oral cavity, tongue, pharynx, esophagus, abomasum and small intestine. In some cases, similar lesions are found in the forestomach. Commonly the muzzle is encrusted with mucus and exudate. In the oral cavity the erosions are prominent on the hard palate and around the teeth. In early stages of the disease, pre-erosions are grayish foci of necrosis. The abomasum frequently is inflamed and the mucosa contains multiple hemorrhages which may surround an erosion. In the small intestine, deep necrosis or ulcers are located in the mucous membrane of Peyer's patches. The necrosis extends into the lymphoid tissue. From such lesions hemorrhage may have occurred into the intestinal lumen. Lymph nodes draining the alimentary tract, and frequently others, are swollen.

Histopathologically, the basic change is cell degeneration. In stratified squamous epithelium, the cells adjacent to the basal layer become hydropic, swollen and finally necrotic. Persistance of these cells in normal location produces an opaque plaque, while sloughing of them creates an erosion. Changes in the abomasal mucous membrane consist of necrosis of glandular epithelial cells, hemorrhage and dilation of gland lumens. In the small intestine pathologic changes are prominent over Peyer's patches. The epithelium undergoes necrosis, and mucosal glands become cystic. Lymphoid germinal centers necrose, and mature lymphocytes become depleted. Hemorrhage may be prominent. In many tissues edematous fluid accumulates at junctions of epithelium and lamina propria; this change results in erosion and ulcer

Diagnosis. The clinical diagnosis of bovine viral diarrhea is based on evidence of typical signs and postmortem lesions. Of special significance are early leukopenia, oral erosions and diarrhea in cattle affected with a febrile disease that spreads through the herd. Laboratory confirmation can be obtained by isolating and identifying the virus. During the febrile stage virus can be isolated from blood leukocytes, spleen, lymphoid tissue and mucous membranes of the herd and small intestine. Isolations commonly are made in culture systems of bovine embryonic kidney, spleen and testicle cells. The cultivated virus can be identified by neutralizing with known antibodies or by visualizing with fluorescenes conjugated to bovine viral diarrhea antibodies. A herd diagnosis can be made serologically using paired serum samples and the complement fixation test. Complement fixing antibodies begin to form approximately 1 week after exposure of the animal to the virus.

The differential diagnosis requires consideration of malignant catarrhal fever, viral bovine rhinotracheitis, Johne's disease and rinderpest. Malignant catarrh has a low sporadic incidence, high persistent fever, respiratory involvement and ophthalmitis. The causative virus can be cultivated in rabbits. Viral bovine rhinotracheitis has high incidence, respiratory signs and dyspnea without oral, esophageal and intestinal erosions. The virus can be isolated from nasal secretions, cultured in cell culture systems and identified with known neutralizing antibodies. Johne's disease, a chronic bacterial infection, has recurring periods of diarrhea. The causative organism, *Mycobacterium paratuberculosis*, can be identified in the mucous membrane of the large intestine. Rinderpest, a disease exotic to the United States, spreads rapidly because of high contagiousness and has a very high mortality rate.

Prevention and Treatment. Since bovine viral diarrhea is a contagious disease, the application of hygienic principles of isolation to an infected herd should help to limit spread of the disease to other susceptible cattle. Commercial vaccines against bovine viral diarrhea are readily available. These products contain attenuated but live virus that may be separate or combined with antigens against viral bovine rhinotracheitis and leptospirosis. The use of vaccine containing live virus of viral bovine diarrhea, however, has caused disease resembling bovine viral diarrhea in a few animals of some herds. Because of these complications, vaccine should not be used, except in those cattle where heavy losses from the natural disease are expected. If on arrival at feedlot some animals show clinical signs of the disease, the cattle shipment should be vaccinated promptly. Otherwise vaccination, if necessary, should be done 3 to 4 weeks after arrival.

Diseased animals are treated symptomatically to prevent or control secondary bacterial infections and to avoid excessive loss of body weight. The diet should be changed from corn, barley, milo and silage to prairie hay, oats, bran and protein concentrate.

References

Bechenhauer, W. H., Lidolph, A. A. and Norden, C. J.: Immunization of Swine Against Hog Cholera with a Bovine Enterovirus. Vet. Med., *56* (1961): 108–112.

Blood, D. C., Hutchins, D. R., Jubb, K. V., Whitem, J. H. and Littlejohns, I.: Mucosal Disease in Cattle in Australia. Aust. Vet. J., *33* (1957): 75.

Bogel, K.: Spread of a Virus of Mucosal Disease Group in Sheep Flocks in Southern Germany. Zentbl. Vet. Med., *11B* (1964): 687–692.

Bogel, K. and Voss, H. J.: Serological Study of the Incidence of Mucosal Disease Virus in Cattle in North Germany. Zentbl. Vet. Med., *11B* (1964): 181–189.

Coggins, L., Gillespie, J. H., Robson, D. S., Thompson, J. D., Phillips, W. V., Wagner, W. C. and Baker, J. A.: Attenuation of Virus Diarrhea Virus (Strain Oregon C24V) for Vaccine Purposes. Cornell Vet., *51* (1961): 539–545.

Darbyshire, J. H.: A Serological Relationship Between Swine Fever and Mucosal Disease of Cattle. Vet. Record, *72* (1960): 331.

———: Agar Gel Diffusion Studies with a Mucosal Disease of Cattle. I. Preliminary Results with a Technique. Res. in Vet. Sci., *3* (1962b): 118.

———: Agar Gel Diffusion Studies with a Mucosal Disease of Cattle. II. Serological Relationship Between a Mucosal Disease and Swine Fever. Res. in Vet. Sci., *3* (1962c): 125.

Don, C., Jarrett, W. F. H. and MacIntyre, W. I. M.: A Disease of Cattle in Britain Resembling Virus Diarrhea-Mucosal Disease Complex. Vet. Record, *68* (1956): 620.

Gillespie, J. H. and Baker, J. A.: Studies on Virus Diarrhea. Corn. Vet., *49* (1959): 439.

Gillespie, J. H., Baker, J. A. and McEntee, K: A Cytopathogenic Strain of Virus Diarrhea Virus. Cornell Vet., *50* (1960): 73.

Gillespie, J. H., Coggins, L., Thompson, J. and Baker, J. A.: Comparison by Neutralization Tests of Strains of Virus Isolated from Virus Diarrhea and Mucosal Disease. Cornell Vet., *51* (1961): 155–159.

Grantson, A. E. and Welter, C. J.: Preliminary Evaluation of a Trivalent Bovine Vaccine. Vet. Med. Sm. Am. Clinic, *63* (1968): 58–63.

Hafez, S. M., Petzoldt, K. and Reczko, E.: Morphology of Bovine Viral Diarrhea Virus. Acta. Virol. *12* (1968): 471–473.

Hermodsson, S. and Dinter, Z.: Properties of Bovine Viral Diarrhea Virus. Nature, *194* (1962): 893–894.

Kniazeff, A. A. *et al.*: Antigenic Relationship of Some Bovine Viral Diarrhea-Mucosal Disease Viruses From the U. S., Great Britain, and West Germany. Vet. Record, *73* (1961): 768–769.

Lee, K. M. and Gillespie, J. H.: Propogation of Virus Diarrhea Virus in Tissue Culture. AJVR, *18* (1957): 952.

Malmquist, W. A.: Bovine Viral Diarrhea-Mucosal Disease: Etiology, Pathogenesis, and Applied Immunity. JAVMA, *152* (1968): 763–768.

McKercher, D. G., Saito, J. K., Crenshaw, G. L. and Bushnell, R. B.: Complications in Cattle Following Vaccination with Combined Viral Bovine Diarrhea and Infectious Bovine Rhinotracheitis Vaccine. JAVMA, *152* (1968): 1621–1624.

Mills, J. H. L. and Lugmbuhl, R. E.: Incidence of Bovine Mucosal Disease in Connecticut. Cornell Vet., *55* (1965): 583–590.

Olafson, P., MacCallum, A. D. and Fox, F. H.: An Apparently Transmissible Disease of Cattle. Cornell Vet., *36* (1946): 205.

Olafson, P. and Rickard, C. G.: Further Observations on the Virus Diarrhea (New Transmissible Disease) of Cattle. Cornell Vet., *37* (1947): 104.

Omori, T., Inaba, Y., Moremoto, T., Tanaka, Y., Kurogi, H. and Matumoto, M.: Bovine Viral Diarrhea Virus. I. Isolation of Non-cytopathogenic Strains Detectable by END Method. Jap. J. Microbiol., *11* (1967): 133–142.

Otte, E. and Peck, E. F.: A Note on a Rinderpest-like Disease of Cattle in Ethiopia. Bull. Epiz. Dis. Africa, *8* (1960): 203–216.

Peter, C. P., Tyler, D. E. and Ramsey, F. K.: A Condition Following Vaccination With Bovine Viral Diarrhea Vaccine. JAVMA, *150* (1967): 46–52.

Pritchard, W. R., Taylor, D. B., Moses, H. E. and Doyle, L. P.: A Transmissible Disease Affecting the Mucosae of Cattle. JAVMA, *128* (1956): 1–5.

Provost, A.: A Historical Note on Mucosal Disease. Bull. Soc. Vet. Prat. Fr., *49* (1965): 123–124.

Ramsey, F. K.: Pathology of a Mucosal Disease of Cattle. A Dissertation. Iowa State College, Ames, Iowa (1956).

Ramsey, F. K. and Chivers, W. H.: Mucosal Disease of Cattle. North Am. Vet., *34* (1953): 629–633.

Report Panel for Symposium on Immunity to Bovine Respiratory Disease Complex. JAVMA, *152* (1968): 713–719.

Ritchie, A. E. and Fernelius, A. L.: Characterization of Bovine Viral Diarrhea Viruses. V. Morphology of Characteristic Particles Studies by Electron Microscopy. Arch. Ges. Virusforsch., *28* (1969): 369–389.

Romvary, J.: Incidence of Virus Diarrhea Among Roes. Acta. Vet. Hung. *15* (1965): 451–455.

Tamoglia, T. W., Tellejohn, A. L., Phillips, C. E. and Wilkenson, F. B.: Further Evaluation of Hog Cholera Immunizing Agents: Bovine Virus Diarrhea and Hog Cholera Vaccine. Proc. 69th Ann. Meet. U.S.L.S.A. (1965): 385–389.

Tournut, J., Lacaze, B., Redon, P. and Laporte, J.: Identification of Bovine Mucosal Disease in Southwest France. Rev. Med. Vet., *112* (1961): 81–90.

Tyler, D. E. and Ramsey, F. K.: Comparative Pathologic, Immunologic, and Clinical Responses Produced by Selected Agents by the Bovine Viral Diarrhea-Mucosal Disease Complex. AJVR, *26* (1965): 903–913.

Underdahl, N. R., Grace, O. D. and Hoerlein, A. B.: Cultivation in Tissue Culture of Cytopathogenic Agent From Bovine Mucosal Disease. Proc. Soc. Exp. Biol. and Med., *94* (1957): 795–797.
Walker, R. V. L. and Olafson, P.: Failure of Virus Diarrhea of Cattle to Immunize Against Rinderpest. Cornell Vet., *37* (1947): 107.

Rabies

(HYDROPHOBIA; TOLLWUT; LE RAGE; LYSSA)

An acute viral infection of the central nervous system and salivary glands, rabies is characterized by a syndrome of excitation, depression, paralysis, coma and death. The disease occurs in all species of warm blooded animals, but especially in mammals, and is widely distributed throughout the world. Even though state and federal control of the incidence of rabies has recently diminished its economic importance in the United States, the diagnosis of 10,743 bovine cases was confirmed in the laboratory in the period 1953–1970. Economic losses accrue not only from the deaths of affected cattle, but from the costs of protective cattle vaccination and from the operation of rabies control programs involving the protection against rabies exposure of all animals, including people. Total annual monetary loss to the cattle industry has been estimated at $27,000. Additional economic loss results from the public health significance of rabies. During 1953 through 1970, 72 fatal cases occurred in people and large numbers of individuals received prophylactic treatment following bites from rabid animals.

Review of Literature. In ancient Greek literature both Democritus (460 B.C.) and Aristotle (384–322 B.C.) referred to rabies, and other writers observed the disease throughout subsequent periods of civilization. Continuous interest and sporadic investigations have resulted in the accumulation of information. While often observed in diverse species of mammals and other warm blooded animals (Tierkel, 1959), the disease has been more common among dogs, cats, and cattle (Camargo, 1955; Schroeder, 1952; Tierkel, 1959) of the domestic animals and in foxes, skunks, coyotes, and wolves of the wild animals (Ballantyne and O'Donoghue, 1954; Kleckner, 1958). A survey in southeastern United States of randomly trapped wild animals indicated a rabies incidence of 2.2% in foxes and 1% in skunks (Kleckner, 1958). In South and Central America (1956) where the incidence of rabies in cattle has been high, estimates indicated the losses of 100,000 livestock animals or of 80 million dollars (Tierkel, 1959). Some herds in Mexico suffered an incidence and mortality of 50 to 80% (Camargo, 1955). In the area from northern Argentina and further northward through Mexico the virus of rabies has been found in vampire bats which feed on the blood of cattle and other animals (Camargo, 1955; Schroeder, 1952). Transmission studies in Brazil (Johnson, 1959), indicated that some bats, without evincing the disease, contain rabies virus in the saliva for several months (Queiroz Lima, 1934).

While the rabies virus always occurs in the nervous central system of animals affected with the disease, it is also present in the saliva of some cases other than the vampire bat. In one study the saliva from 50% of 34 cattle, 87% of 150 foxes, and 75% of 28 dogs affected with rabies contained the virus (Starr *et al.*, 1954). The virus in the saliva of human rabies cases was demonstrated by experimentally producing canine rabies by inoculation of the animals with saliva from an affected person (Magendie and Breschet, 1910). Although some strains have been difficult to cultivate outside the animal body, others have been propagated in chicken embryos (Kligler and Bernkopf, 1938), baby chicks (Johnson, 1959) and in cultures of hamster kidney cells (Kissling, 1958). Histopathologic studies revealed neuronal cytoplasmic inclusion bodies which bear, from their discoverer (Negri, 1903), the name of Negri bodies. The attachment of specific fluorescent antibodies to the Negri bodies indicated the presence of virus (Goldwasser and Kissling, 1958).

While artificial immunization against rabies has been practiced in people and pet animals since the historic demonstrations by Pasteur, the immunization of cattle was not done extensively until the Flury strain virus was avianized and an easily administered vaccine was developed (Johnson, 1959). Originating from a human case of rabies, the Flury strain was passed serially through day-old chicks and then through embryonating chicken eggs. Viable vaccine prepared from the fortieth to the fiftieth egg passage was experimentally administered to cattle with some adverse effect (Gomez, Black and Koprowski, 1955). Live virus vaccine prepared from the one hundred and eighty-fifth egg passage was innocuous but immunogenic to cattle. In Mexico this vaccine was used over 3.5 years to immunize approximately 2.3 million cattle (Comargo, 1955). Losses from rabies among the vaccinated cattle was low, while deaths among non-vaccinated animals continued at a high level. In vaccinated cattle the development of an antibody titer was closely correlated to the resistance to challenge with Street virus (Koprowski and Black, 1954). The vaccine has been used to protect cattle and partially control rabies in Canada (Ballantyne and O'Donoghue, 1954), Mexico (Comargo, 1955), and Brazil (Carneiro, Black and Koprowski, 1955).

Occurrence. Among domestic animals, cattle are highly susceptible. While all bovine breeds and both sexes are susceptible, cattle 6 months of age and older are more commonly affected. In the older animals, adult curiosity motivates interest in and possible exposure to rabid dogs, cats, skunks, and foxes. In general the incidence in feedlot cattle is low but may be high in individual herds because of accidental entrance of a rabid biting animal into a crowded feedlot. In South and Central America the incidence in cattle may be 50 to 80% because of attack by transmitting vampire bats. As shown in table 3, the annual incidence of bovine rabies in the United States declined gradually during the 17 years beginning with 1953. The decline perhaps was due to more effective control of the disease in transmitting animals. In addition to cattle, the disease occurs commonly in dogs, cats, skunks, and foxes, and while other animal species are susceptible, the rabies incidence among them is lower. In the same period, the incidence of rabies

TABLE 3 *Incidence of rabies in the United States*

Year	*Cattle*	*Dogs*	*Cats*	*Skunks*	*Foxes*	*Man*
1953	1,012	5,688	538	319	1,033	14
1954	930	4,083	464	547	1,028	8
1955	835	2,657	343	580	1,223	5
1956	700	2,592	371	631	1,281	10
1957	654	1,758	382	775	1,021	6
1958	660	1,643	353	1,005	845	6
1959	700	1,119	292	789	920	6
1960	563	697	277	725	915	2
1961	435	594	217	1,254	614	3
1962	547	565	232	1,449	594	2
1963	459	573	217	1,462	622	1
1964	529	409	220	1,909	1,061	1
1965	536	412	289	1,582	1,038	1
1966	519	412	256	1,522	864	1
1967	612	412	293	1,568	979	2
1968	365	296	157	1,400	801	1
1969	359	256	165	1,156	888	1
1970	328	182	131	1,195	761	2

in the United States declined in dogs, cats, and foxes, but increased in skunks.

Although occurring in cattle in all seasons, the incidence often rises during spring and early summer when dogs, cats, skunks, and foxes are mobile and active during the spring breeding season.

Geographically, rabies occurs universally but Australia, Britain, and Scandinavia have been free of the disease for prolonged periods. Within the United States in a geographic zone extending northeast from Texas towards New York State, the disease incidence has been higher than in other zones.

Etiology. Even though the virus causing rabies has not been classified, it possesses some morphologic features of the rhabdovirus group. Containing RNA and lipid material, the virions vary in morphology. As shown by electron microscopy, the rounded elongated, and bullet-shaped particles measure 100 to 150 $\times$ 250 to 1,000 mμ. Electron microscopy reveals an external membrane containing radial surface projections. Because of apparent lack of hemagglutinins, however, the virus differs from typical myxoviruses.

In media with which it is usually associated, rabies virus is sensitive to environmental adversities. In a fluid medium at 70° C it is killed in 15 minutes, but when dried it withstands 100° C for 2 to 3 minutes. Contact exposure to acids, bases, phenol, mercuric chloride, formalin and ultraviolet light rapidly destroy the virus. Ether inactivates, but at an inconstant rate. Storage in 50% glycerol or in the lyophilized state maintains viability for approximately 1 year.

Rabies virus can be cultivated in cell culture systems and in living laboratory animals. Cell cultures from mouse embryo, chick embryo and baby hamster kidney, support virus growth. Cytopathogenic effects include cytoplasmic fibrils early in the growth process and mature virus particles by the end of 24 hours. Following intracerebral inoculation of mice and rabbits, the virus grows, produces Negri bodies, and causes disease.

Even though the virus occurs as a single antigenic form, "street" virus and "fixed" virus demonstrate biological differences. Street virus is the pathogenic form in field outbreaks of rabies, and fixed virus is a laboratory form adapted to a specific host, such as mice or rabbits. Both forms are lethal and found in tissues of the central nervous system and in the salivary glands of some affected animals. In cattle, street virus usually causes furious clinical manifestations.

Transmission. In cattle, rabies is transmitted exclusively from the bite of saliva infected rabid animals. Rabid dogs, cats, foxes and skunks are the usual vectors in the United States and, when infected, these animals wander widely and often fearlessly enter cattle feedlots. Being curious animals, the cattle closely approach, smell the intruding rabid animal, and frequently are bitten on the muzzle or other parts of the face. Less commonly bites are inflicted on the limbs.

In South and Central America hematophagous vampire bats often are infected and transmit the disease to cattle; consequently, the incidence of bovine rabies from bat transmission has been high and costly. The common vampire bat, *Desmodus rotundus*, and the hairy-legged vampire bat, *Diphyalla ecaudata*, are transmitters, and as night feeders they attack cattle and other large animals. Inflicting tooth incisions in the skin of the head, neck and back, the bat laps the exuding blood. In the process of biting and lapping, virus-infected saliva may contaminate the wound and inoculate the host animal. The bat saliva may contain virus several months before onset of the disease. In the United States, rabies virus has been isolated from the saliva of insectivorous bats. While no cases have been proved, rabid insectivorous bats theoretically could attack, bite, and inoculate large mammals, including cattle.

Pathogenesis. Following viral inoculation of cattle with saliva from an infected dog, cat, fox, skunk or bat, the virus remains temporarily localized but eventually it multiplies and moves centripetally along peripheral nerves into the central nervous system. Since most bovine cases result from inoculation near the face, the virus usually ascends the cranial nerves. Within the brain the virus attacks and injures neurons and commonly produces cytoplasmic Negri bodies in neurons of the hippocampus and Purkinje cells of the cerebellum. In some affected animals, neurons throughout much of the brain contain Negri bodies. A mild encephalitis is produced especially along the brain stem. In approximately 50% of affected cattle, the virus moves centrifugally along the peripheral nerves to the salivary glands and enters the saliva.

The high variability of the incubation period appears to depend upon virulence of the virus, the amount of virus inoculated, and the anatomical location of the point of inoculation. Large amounts of highly pathogenic virus inoculated on the face often results in a short incubation period. All affected cattle die.

Clinical Signs and Postmortem Lesions. The course of rabies is divisible into three phases: prodromal, excitative, and paralytic. Following an incubation period of 10 days to several months, with an average of 3 weeks, the prodromal phase is initiated, and in cattle it is short and inconspicuous. The affected animal is depressed and usually prefers isolation from other cattle. Unless the animal has a history of exposure to rabies these signs are of little diagnostic importance. This transitory phase endures from a few to 48 hours. The virus may be present in the saliva. In contrast with the prodromal phase, the excitative, or furious phase, is prominent and attracts the attention of animal owners and practicing veterinarians. Even though isolated from other cattle, the animal becomes nervous and irritable, often alternating its standing and reclining positions. Butting with the head and stamping with the feet are apparent, and the infuriated animal may attack attending persons. Because of dysphagia, saliva drips and prehended feed may be held in the mouth for a prolonged period. Little or no water is consumed and the animal becomes dehydrated and gaunt. Straining is common and often rectal prolapse results. Both males and females may exhibit sexual excitement. A characteristic bellowing with a low-pitched voice occurs sporadically, or more or less continuously in some cattle. Throughout the second phase the animal is alert to visual and auditory stimuli, and the ears are erect and the eyes staring. Sudden strong stimuli may cause violent reactions and sudden loud noises may cause falling and convulsions. Moving objects may provoke attacks or retreats. After one to two days the animal becomes prostrated, and the third phase begins. During the paralytic phase the limbs, usually first the posterior, become paralyzed. Coma supervenes and death occurs after 1 to 2 days.

At necropsy organic changes are minimal and are of little diagnostic importance. The dehydrated carcass may be traumatized from violence during the clinical course of the disease. The central nervous system is congested and in some cattle edematous. Microscopically, neurons of many parts of the brain, especially the brain stem, are swollen, degenerated, and occasionally necrotic. Specific Negri bodies are usually present in neurons of the hippocampus and in Purkinje cells of the cerebellum. Inflammation and neuronophagia may be found along the brain stem and in the semilunar ganglion of the trigeminal nerve. Negri bodies are absent in approximately 12% of fatal cases and in many animals destroyed before natural termination.

Diagnosis. Bovine rabies is diagnosed on case history, clinical manifestations, and laboratory findings. The history of exposure to the bite of animals or residence in an endemic area is important. Typical clinical signs during the excitative and paralytic phases direct attention to rabies. Of great significance are the excitement, dysphagia, characteristic raucous bellowing, and subsequent paralysis.

Following natural termination of the disease, the head should be removed, refrigerated and shipped promptly to a diagnostic laboratory for further studies. In the laboratory, smears and/or sections of the hippocampus and cerebellum are examined for specific evidence of the rabies virus. The fluorescent antibody technique possesses high accuracy and has frequent use. In this method, fluorescene dye conjugated with antibodies to rabies virus is applied to brain tissue smears and sections. As a specific reaction, the conjugation fixes to rabies virus infected cells and produces a recognizable and diagnostic fluorescence. Other methods differentiate Negri bodies with agents such as Seller's stain. The identification of Negri bodies is conclusive evidence of the disease. In the absence of Negri bodies, 3 to 5 young adult Swiss mice are inoculated intracerebrally with 0.03 ml of suspected brain suspension. If rabies virus is present, the inoculated mice usually die within 7 to 10 days following inoculation. A positive diagnosis requires the identification of Negri bodies in the mouse brain or neutralization of the virus with known antibodies.

The differential diagnosis requires consideration of listeriosis, esophageal choke and nervous acetonemia. Cattle affected with listerosis seldom are aggressive and often exhibit unilateral facial paralysis. Frequently the course is prolonged and in the laboratory *Listeria monocytogenes* can be isolated from the brain stem and identified. Choke results in dysphagia and salivation. The affected animal may bloat and the choking object, if located in the neck, can be detected by palpation and with a probe if located within the thorax. Animals affected with nervous acetonemia are usually not aggressive and acetone bodies are detectable in the urine.

Prevention. Feedlot cattle can be protected against rabies by management practices and immunization programs. Since feedlots are usually limited to relatively small dimensions, most rabid animals, especially dogs, can be excluded by the use of proper fencing. Rabid cats, rats and possibly some other animals cannot economically be mechanically excluded.

In rabies endemic areas where the probability of exposure is high, immunization of cattle at the time of admission into feedlots should be practiced. This procedure usually provides adequate time for immunization before actual exposure. Available immunizing agents include killed virus vaccines and attenuated but living virus vaccines. The Flury strain virus has been attenuated by serial passage through 136 day old chicks, and later through a series of 175 serial passages in chicken embryos. Virus passed through a series of 45 to 50 embryonating chicken eggs is sufficiently attenuated for canine vaccine, but passage through a series of 175 embryonating chicken eggs is necessary for bovine vaccine. Vaccine prepared in this manner is safe and efficacious for immunizing cattle. A single dose of approximately 15 ml administered intramuscularly produces protective immunization for at least 9 months. The low cost of materials and labor makes immunization economically feasible.

Until recent years rabies vaccines for cattle contained phenol or chloroform killed virus. Both efficacy and safety were questionable. At least 2 doses of 30 to 50 ml were administered intramuscularly with a 5-day interval. Abscesses often developed at the point of inoculation and allergic reactions sometimes occurred. Killed vaccines require 20 to 30 days to produce effective immunity and consequently are not usable in cattle after exposure to the virus. The cost of materials, labor, and excessive manipulation of cattle made the process economically prohibitive except under conditions of high probability of repeated rabies exposure.

A preferred method of prevention is the application of regional programs for control of the disease in all animals. The programs should be administered by a veterinarian in a state or county government. Dogs should be licensed, immunized periodically, and prevented from free-roaming. If foxes and skunks of an area are infected their numbers should be reduced by systematic trapping. In the United States the application of control programs has resulted in eradicating the disease in a few areas and in reducing the incidence to low levels in other localized ones.

References

Ballantyne, E. E. and O'Donoghue, J. G.: Rabies Control in Alberta. JAVMA, *125* (1954): 316–326.

Camargo, F.: The Derriengue Problem in Mexico. Proc. 59th Annual Meeting. U.S.L.S.A. (1955): 313–318.

Carneiro, V., Black, J., and Koprowski, H.: Rabies in Cattle. V. Immunization of Cattle in Brazil Against Exposure to Street Virus of Vampire Bat Origin. JAVMA, *127* (1955): 366–369.

Communicable Disease Center, Zoonoses Surveillance: U. S. Dept. of Health, Education, and Welfare. Annual Rabies Summary, 1953–1969.

Fagan, R.: Rabies, an Epidemiological Analysis. Proc. 89th Annual Meeting, AVMA, *89* (1952): 394–407.

Goldwasser, R. A. and Kissling, R. E.: Fluorescent Antibody Staining of Street and Fixed Rabies Virus Antigens. Proc. Soc. Exp. Biol. & Med., *98* (1958): 219–223.

Gomez, C., Black, J. and Koprowski, H.: Rabies in Cattle. III. Comparative Studies on Vaccination of Cattle in Colombia with Flury Virus and Chloroform Inactivated Vaccine. JAVMA, *127* (1955): 360–363.

Johnson, H. N.: Rabies. (In Rivers, T. M. and Horsfall, F. L.: *Viral and Rickettsial Infections of Man*. 3rd ed. J. B. Lippincott Co. Philadelphia. 1959. pp. 405–431).

Kleckner, M. D.: Sylvatic Rabies Investigations in the Southeast. Proc. of CDC Conference for Teachers of Veterinary Public Health. June 1958. pp. 204–212.

Kligler, I. J. and Bernkopf, H.: Cultivation of Rabies Virus in the Allantois of the Developing Chick Embryo. Proc. Soc. Exp. Biol. & Med., *39* (1938): 212–214.

Koprowski, H. and Black, J.: Studies on Chick-Embryo-Adapted Rabies Virus. VII. Immunological Responses of Animals to Vaccination with High Egg Passage Flury Strain. Jour. Immunology, *72* (1954): 503–510.

Koprowski, H., Black, J. and Johnson, W. P.: Rabies in Cattle. IV. Vaccination of Cattle with High Egg-passage Chicken-Embryo-Adapted Rabies Virus. JAVMA, *127* (1955): 363–366.

Losses in Agriculture. Agricultural Research Service. U.S.D.A. Agricultural Handbook no. 291 (1965).

Magendie, F. and Breschet, G.: J. Physiol. Exptl., *1* (1821): 42. (From Stimson, A. M. Facts and Problems of Rabies. Hyg. Lab. Bull. U. S. Public Health Service, No. 65 (1910): 1–90.

Negri, A.: Beitrag zum Stadium der Aetiology der Tollwut. Zeit. Hyg. Infektionskrankheit, *43* (1903): 507–528.

Queiroz Lima, E. De: A Transmissao da Ravia bovina pelo morcego hematophago *Desmodus rotundus*. Brazil Med., *48* (1934): 38–40.

Schroeder, C. R.: Rabies in Central and South America. Proc. 89th Annual Meeting AVMA, *89* (1952): 411–412.

Starr, L. E., Clower, T. B., Bromley, C. L. and Routh, C. F.: Antirabic Immunization of Cattle in Georgia Using Living Virus Vaccine of Chick Embryo Origin. Vet. Med., *49* (1954): 366–370.

Tierkel, E. S.: Rabies. Advances in Vet. Science, *5* (1959): 183–226.

Van Houweling, C. D.: Report of Committee on Rabies. Annual Report U.S.L.S.A. (1955): pp. 319–327.

Vesicular Stomatitis

(SORE MOUTH; SORE NOSE)

An acute infectious and mildly contagious disease, vesicular stomatitis is characterized by oral, pedal, and mammary maculae and/or vesicles. A disease of the western hemisphere, vesicular stomatitis occurs in horses, cattle, swine, some species of wild animals and man, and is caused by a filtrable virus. The herd incidence is discontinuous within an affected region and feedlot cattle are less suceptible than pastured animals; vesicular stomatitis, therefore, has moderate economic importance to the American cattle fattening industry. While not precisely measured, some monetary losses result from reduction of live body weight, prolonged fattening periods, restricted trade movements from quarantine, expensive treatments, and meticulous attention and labor in establishing accurate diagnoses. The susceptibility of people and the development of systemic reactions among laboratory personnel, veterinarians, and farmers give additional importance and also public health significance to the disease.

Review of Literature. While vesicular stomatitis has primarily been a disease of the western hemisphere (Hanson, 1964), it has occurred but apparently has failed to become established in Africa (Theiler, 1901) and in Europe (McNutt, 1963) where it developed as a result of transporting infected American horses to France for use in World War I. In the western hemisphere the disease has been encountered in North, South, and Central America with both epizootic and enzootic areas (Hanson, 1964). Along the coastal plains of Georgia, South Carolina and Florida the disease is enzootic. Reports from these states indicated that in healthy animals from 11 farms, the serums from 100% of 10 horses, 57% of 59 pigs, and 50% of 116 cattle, contained antibodies specific for the vesicular stomatitis virus (Hanson and Karstadt, 1956). Wild deer of the area also contained antibodies and susceptibility of the species was confirmed by deer inoculations (Hanson and Karstadt, 1958).

While occurring annually in enzootic areas, the epizootic regions of the North Central and Western states have suffered less frequent outbreaks. Major epizootics occurred in 1906, 1916, 1926, 1936–37, 1942–43, 1964, and 1965 (Hanson, 1952; Heiney, 1945; Sudia, Fields, Fields and Calisher, 1967). In 1942, 200 Colorado farms were infected with 50% of 4,000 cattle contracting the disease; in 1943 40% of 5,000 cattle on 250 premises, mostly ranches, were affected (Heiney, 1945). The personnel in research and diagnostic laboratories where the vesicular stomatitis virus was manipulated (Patterson, Mott and Jenney, 1958; Laserna, 1968), the farmers on infected farms, and also veterinarians contracted an influenza-like disease and subsequently manifested rising antibody titers (Brandley, Hanson and Chow, 1951).

Studied morphologically and functionally, the virus of vesicular stomatitis is well known. Filtrability of the causative agent, and its viral nature, were established early (Cotton, 1926). Viral particles in infected cells of avian chorioallantoic membranes (Patterson, Mott and Jenney, 1958), in supernatant fluids following centrifuging and purification (Chow, Chow and Hanson, 1954), and in ultrathin sections of cultured L cells were visualized with the electron microscope and measured. Most particles were cylindrical and dimensioned approximately 68 $\times$ 178 mμ. One investigation disclosed a cavity at one end of the cylinder and numerous filamentous surface projections (Howaton and Whitmore, 1962). Both serologic types of virus have been adapted and grown in cells of the avian chorioallantoic membranes (Chow, Chow and Hanson, 1954; Reczko, 1961). Optimum growth occurred in embryos incubated 7 days in cultures of bovine kidney cells, monkey kidney cells, He La cells, L cells, and chick fibroblasts (McClain and Hackett, 1958). Both types of virus grew rapidly with the highest virus yield in monolayer cultures of chick fibroblasts; in the latter system 62 to 75% of cells released virus at a nearly constant rate (Cooper, 1957). When the virus was grown in P_{32}-containing medium, the isotope was metabolized into the virus. Following precipitation and purification, the labeled virus was injected intravenously into mice and autoradiographs were prepared. Both types of virus were removed from the blood by the reticuloendothelial cells (Brunner, Hurex, McCluskey and Bonacerraf, 1960). Resistance to disinfecting chemicals and inimical physical factors were variable. When subjected to action of a chemical for a standard 15 minutes, the virus endured 3, 2, and 1% lye solutions, but was inactivated by 1% formalin, 1% cresylic acid-soap solution and 0.1% solution of calcium hypochlorite (Patterson, Holbrook, Hopkins, and Songer, 1958). It was made non-infective to guinea pigs by heating at 55° C for 30 minutes, by incubation at 37.5° C for 5 to 8 days, and by crystal violet dye in 2 to 3 days (Shahan, 1946). Under conventional refrigeration the virus survived 11 to 23 days.

By studying the pathogenesis of oral lesions, the infection was found to begin in the stratum spinosum and to spread towards the surface and deeper basal layer. The cellular changes were shrinkage of cytoplasm, prominence of intercellular bridges, and pyknosis; the changes occurred within 24 hours of infection (Ribelin, 1958).

Until recently vesicular stomatitis was

considered to be typically manifested by oral vesication with an occasional atypical case failing to vesicate. This concept was questioned when oral examination of 11 infected herds failed to disclose any vesicles (Brandley, Hanson and Chow, 1951). In a controlled experiment the tongues of 20 steers were inoculated with viable virus and sacrificed on the second, third, and fourth subsequent days. Vesicles developed in less than 30% of the tongues and were present within 24 hours. Histopathologically, the lesions were characterized by intercellular edema, epithelial necrosis, and leukocytic infiltration (Seibold and Sharp, 1960).

Even though the means of transmission are not fully understood, some investigations suggest insects as vectors. In Panama where the disease is endemic, serum samples from people, domestic animals and wild animals were collected and tested for antibodies. People and domestic animals possessed high antibody rates for both New Jersey and Indiana virus types, while arboreal and semi-arboreal animals contained antibodies to the Indiana type, and bats, carnivors and rodents had antibodies to the New Jersey type (Tesh, Peralta and Johnson, 1969). In the same geographic area, phlebotomus sandflies were collected from the rainforest; from these insects 4 strains of vesicular stomatitis Indiana virus were isolated. Of 497 serum samples from people of a nearby village, 26% contained antibodies to the same virus type (Shelokov and Peralta, 1967), and in an endemic area of Georgia, 30% of the people contained antibodies to the New Jersey virus (Johnson, Tesh and Peralta, 1969). During an epizootic of vesicular stomatitis in cattle and horses of Colorado and New Mexico, a mosquito pool from the area was collected; from these insects and from cattle and horses of the area vesicular stomatitis Indiana virus was isolated (Sudia, Fields and Calisher, 1967).

Occurrence. Although vesicular stomatitis is found in all breeds and sexes of cattle, field animals under one year of age are generally resistant. Under laboratory conditions, calves are susceptible to viral inoculation and develop typical lesions at points of injection. Usually cattle on pasture and in open pens develop a higher incidence than stabled animals. In addition to cattle, vesicular stomatitis occurs in horses, swine and people; in deer, raccoons and bobcats it is inapparent. Guinea pigs, ferrets, embryonating chicken eggs, chickens, mice, rats and chinchillas are susceptible to viral inoculation in the laboratory. Young mice and ferrets develop encephalitis from intranasal inoculations.

Geographically a disease of the western hemisphere, vesicular stomatitis may be enzootic or epizootic in character. In enzootic areas, susceptible indigenous species commonly contain specific antibodies, while in epizootic regions susceptible species show antibodies only after an epizootic exposure. Enzootic areas include the United States coastal plains of Georgia, South Carolina, and Florida; eastern coastal Mexico; Venezuela; Colombia, Panama, and Costa Rica. Epizootic areas are Manitoba, Canada; Minnesota, Wisconsin, Utah, Montana, Colorado, Arizona, New Mexico, Texas, Maryland, West Virginia, North Carolina, Georgia, and California of the United States; Peru and Ecuador of South America.

Possibly because of arthropod vectors the disease occurs during warm months and ceases during months of environmental freezing temperatures. In the United States, cases often begin in May or June and stop in September or October with a peak incidence in August. Within an enzootic or epizootic area, herd outbreaks are spatially discontinuous without evidence of direct or indirect contact.

Etiology and Pathogenesis. Although versatile and enigmatic, the virus causing vesicular stomatitis is officially unclassified. The bullet-shaped virion contains a rounded end and a flattened end and measures 65 by 175 mμ. The inner part of the cylindrical particle contains a helical spiral of ribonucleic acid surrounded by a membrane with surface projections 10 mμ in length. This morphologic feature characterizes the rhabdovirus group of microorganisms. The group contains both animal viruses, such as rabies virus, and plant viruses, such as wheat striate mosaic virus. When exposed to adverse physical agents the vesicular stomatitis virus reacts variably. It is stable at pH 4 to 5, endures 0.5% phenol for 23 days, 3% lye solution for 15 minutes, and retains viability for prolonged periods when stored at low temperatures. But it is inactivated by ether, 0.05% crystal violet solution, 1% formalin, 1% cresylic acid, 0.1% hypochlorite and exposure to temperature of 58° C for 30 minutes.

In addition to several natural animal hosts, the virus readily adapts to live cell culture systems. It grows in the chorioallantoic membrane of embryonated chicken eggs and causes necrosis and frequently death of the embryo within 1 to 2 days. In live mosquitos and fruit flies it appears to grow and replicate, and it adapts to live cell cultures from humans, subhuman primates, cattle, mice, hamsters, birds, reptiles, fish and insects. In cultures it causes necrosis of cells and plaque formations.

Two antigenic forms, New Jersey and Indiana, have been identified. The two types can be separated from each other and from foot-and-mouth disease virus by serum neutralization and complement fixation tests.

In addition to saliva of cattle, horses and swine, the natural hosts, the virus is found in man, deer and raccoon. Experimentally it also infects sheep, goats, guinea pigs and rabbits.

Transmission. During active stages of the disease, saliva containing virus is emitted from the mouth and may contaminate feed, water and feedlot equipment. While in cattle the disease is not known to be contagious, the opportunity for contact transmission is maximal in crowded feedlots. Abrasions of the mouth, feet, or teats facilitate successful establishment and growth of inoculated virus. Foot rot lesions and oral lacerations from coarse fibrous feed or from foreign bodies in the feed can be points of inoculation.

The low rate of contact spread, warm season occurrence, identification of the virus in mosquitos and sandflies, and geographically discontinuous development within an infected region support the concept of spread by highly mobile arthropod vectors. The annual occurrence in enzootic areas, and less frequent outbreaks in epizootic areas, indicate active reservoirs where the virus is maintained during cold months and during years without disease incidence. To date neither vector nor reservoir have been discovered and proven.

Pathogenesis. Following inoculation or exposure to the disease, the virus, through abrasions in oral mucosa, pedal skin or teat skin, enters the stratum spinosum, attacks the epithelial cells and grows rapidly. Within a few hours many cells are injured and viral particles are released. The virus invades cells toward the deeper basal layer and toward the superficial stratum granulosum. Intercellular edema causes extension and rupture of many intercellular bridges, spatial separation of cells and the formation of maculae. In approximately 30% of cattle, the necrosis of cells and confluence of adjacent intercellular spaces produce fluid-filled spaces or vesicles which rupture, discharge virus to the surface and heal. The remaining cases retain the maculae which lose fluid by seepage, collapse and erode. The course is short and healing rapid except for cases with secondary bacterial infection which may create deeply infected ulcers and prolong the course. During early stages, virus may temporarily enter the blood. After clinical recovery humoral antibodies increase and the animal is immune to the specific viral type for 2 to 3 months.

Clinical Signs and Lesions. After an incubation period of 12 to 24 hours, the oral, pedal, or mammary lesions develop, and body temperature rises to a range of 105° to 107° F.

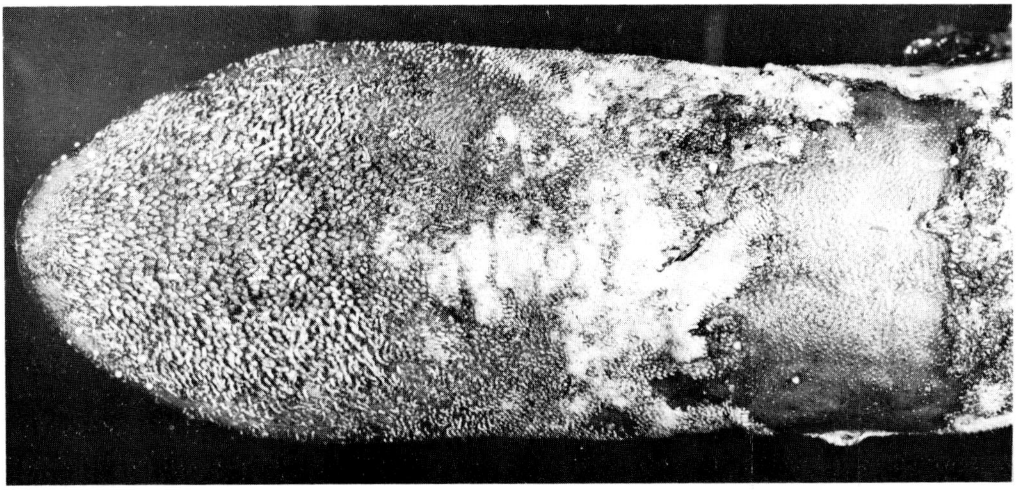

FIG. 2-27. *Bovine tongue showing ruptured vesicles and flaps of necrotic mucosa from vesicular stomatitis.* × 0.9.

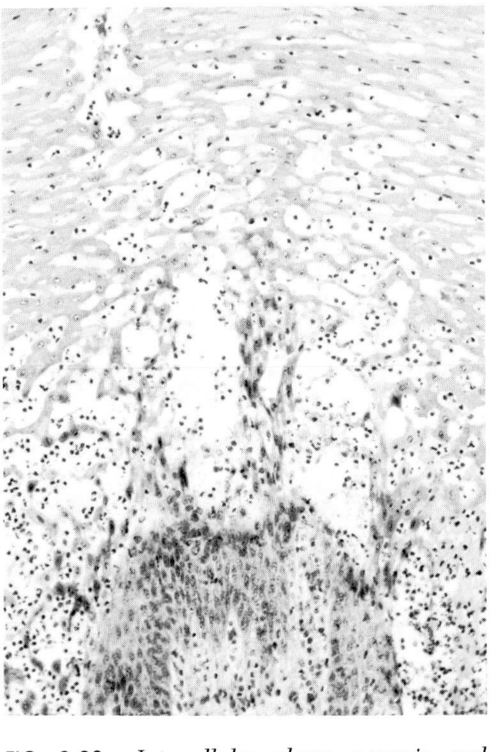

FIG. 2-28. *Intercellular edema, necrosis, and leukocytic infiltration in a macula of bovine tongue affected with vesicular stomatitis. HE stain.* × 105.

Most affected cattle show depression, local soreness, and general discomfort. Because of oral lesions, food is declined 2 to 3 days and gauntness develops; water, however, is consumed. Strands of saliva drip from the mouth. With the tip of the tongue projecting slightly from the mouth, a smacking sucking noise is emitted. The muzzle is hyperemic, and a serous fluid escapes from the nose.

Foot lesions may affect from one to all feet of the same animal. Lameness is usually manifested and becomes exaggerated with secondary bacterial infection from manure. The standing position is maintained much of the time. In feedlot cattle teat lesions are rare. In dairy animals, however, the skin of affected teats is vesicated and later ulcerated and encrusted. The adjacent udder skin is hyperemic and tender.

In cattle the morbidity rate is highly variable. Usually 30 to 50% of the animals in a herd become infected. Occasionally, however, a single case may develop. Mortality does not occur from uncomplicated vesicular stomatitis. Rarely deep secondary bacterial infection of the tongue, coffin joint, or udder may result in death or prolonged incapacitation, and eventually euthanasia. The course is 7 to 14 days for healing.

The lesions of vesicular stomatitis in cattle and especially feedlot animals show propensity, in any single outbreak, for one anatomical area. Usually either oral lesions only or pedal lesions only occur. In the mouth the dorsum of the tongue, hard palate, dental pad, and buccal mucosa are affected and these tissues may be observed clinically in any stage of lesion development. Early changes are maculae which are elevated foci with smooth surfaces from 2 to 20 mm in diameter. All infected mouths contain maculae. After 24 hours approximately 30% of infected mouths develop vesicles or blisters which are elevated and each contains a fluid-filled cavity. The latter may have ruptured leaving a raw reddened surface and flaps of necrotic mucosa. After 48 hours the nonvesicating maculae have dehydrated, collapsed, and eroded.

In foot infections vesicles are located at the coronary bands of the abaxial hoof surfaces and in the interdigital tissues. The proximal skin is hyperemic and tender. After 24 hours many of the vesicles have ruptured, leaving the opened cavity and flaps of necrotic skin. The floor of the vesicle is red and may be filled with exudate from secondary bacterial infection. In some cattle the latter progresses laterally from the interdigital tissue into the coffin joint and persists for several months.

Teat lesions, like those of the feet, consist of yellow-gray vesicles in early stages and ruptured cavities with eroded surfaces in later stages. Following rupture of vesicles the healing surface forms a dry fissured crust. In some animals mastitis from entrance of the virus into the teat canal is present.

Histopathologically, the lesions, regardless of location, show intercellular edema, epithelial necrosis, and leukocytic infiltration. Only 30% of the oral, but most foot and mammary lesions, contain vesicles. The remaining oral lesions fail to develop cavities and heal from the macular stage. The submucosa and derma are hyperemic and slightly edematous. Lesions complicated with secondary bacterial infections show colonies of microorganisms, necrosis and abundance of exudate.

Diagnosis. The clinical diagnosis of vesicular stomatitis is based on the occurrence of typical oral, pedal or mammary lesions in adult cattle and horses during warm months within a known enzootic or epizootic area. For new cases within a confirmed outbreak, a clinical diagnosis may be adequate. A mistaken diagnosis may permit an extensive invasion of the devastating foot-and-mouth disease. Within the United States, the clinical diagnosis must be confirmed by reliable laboratory procedures in order to differentiate vesicular stomatitis from clinically and pathologically similar foot-and-mouth disease which does not normally occur in North America. Usually vesicular fluid is submitted to a federal laboratory. The complement fixation test and viral neutralization with known antibodies are accurate diagnostic methods in an experienced laboratory. Cell cultures, embryonating chicken eggs, guinea pigs and baby mice are useful testing systems. Cattle and horses, having no previous exposure to the vesicular diseases, can be inoculated at the infected premises. Virus is obtained from oral vesicles and is inoculated as follows:

Animal	*Inoculation*	*Foot-and-mouth disease*	*Vesicular Stomatitis*
horse	lingual	−	+
bovine	lingual	+	+
bovine	intramuscular	+	−
guinea pigs	foot pad	+	+

Prevention and Treatment. While vesicular stomatitis is not highly contagious, the exposure of susceptible to infected animals should be avoided. Infected animals should be isolated and separate equipment used for

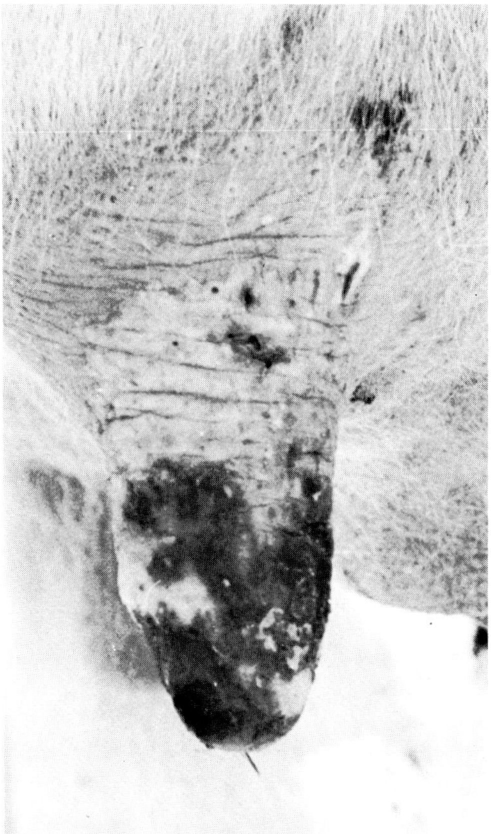

FIG. 2-29. *Bovine teat containing crusts, vesicles, and hyperemic adjacent skin from vesicular stomatitis.* × 1.0.

their care and treatment. Even though strict quarantine is seldom applied, owners of diseased cattle should avoid direct or indirect exposure of other feedlots or farms. Feedlot insects should be controlled.

The treatment of cattle affected with mild and uncomplicated vesicular stomatitis is seldom necessary. In case of severe oral, pedal, or mammary lesions, the local application of topical anesthetic ointment containing antibiotics or sulfonamides helps to relieve pain and maintain appetite. Cortical steroids with antibiotics of sulfonamides reduce inflammation and hasten recovery. Lesions with secondary bacterial infection may require systemic treatment with antibiotics and/or sulfonamides. Adequate fresh water and non-fibrous feed should be readily available, and gruels and fluids can be given by means of a stomach tube to animals with diminished appetites.

References

Brandley, C. A., Hanson, R. P. and Chow, T. L.: Vesicular Stomatitis With Particular Reference to the 1949 Wisconsin Epizootic. Proc. Book. Meeting AVMA, *88* (1951): 61–67.

Brunner, K. T., Hurez, D., McCluskey, R. T. and Bonacerraf, B.: Blood Clearance of P_{32}-labeled Vesicular Stomatitis and New Castle Viruses by the Reticuloendothelial System in Mice. J. Immun., *85* (1960): 99–105.

Chow, T. L., Chow, Fu-Ho and Hansen, R. P.: Morphology of Vesicular Stomatitis Virus. J. Bact., *68* (1954): 724–725.

Cooper, P. D.: Some Characteristics of Vesicular Stomatitis Virus Growth Curves in Tissue Culture. J. Gen. Microbiol., *17* (1957): 327–334.

Cotton, W. E.: The Causal Agent of Vesicular Stomatitis Proved to be a Filter-Passing Virus. JAVMA, *70* (1926): 168–184.

Griesemer, R. A. and Cole, C. R.: Bovine Papular Stomatitis. JAVMA, *137* (1960): 404–409.

Hanson, R. P.: The Natural History of Vesicular Stomatitis. Bact. Rev., *16* (1952): 179–204.

———: Vesicular Stomatitis. *Diseases of Swine.* 2nd Ed. Iowa State University Press. Ames, Iowa. (1964): 235–249.

Hanson, R. P. and Karstad, L.: Enzootic Vesicular Stomatitis. Proc. U.S.L.S.A., (1956): 288–292.

———: Further Studies on Enzootic Vesicular Stomatitis. Proc. U.S.L.S.A., (1958): 300.

Heiny, E.: Vesicular Stomatitis in Cattle and Horses in Colorado, North Am. Vet., *26* (1945): 726–730.

Holbrook, A. A. and Geleta, J. N.: Vesicular Stomatitis. Immunization With Inactivated Vaccines of Chicken Embryo Origin. Proc. U.S.L.S.A., (1957): 308–315.

Howaton, A. F. and Whitmore, G. F.: The Development and Structure of Vesicular Stomatitis Virus. Virology, *16* (1962): 466–478.

Johnson, K. M., Tesh, R. B. and Peralta, P. H.: Epidemiology of Vesicular Stomatitis Virus: Some New Data and a Hypothesis of Transmission of the Indiana Serotype. JAVMA, *155* (1969): 2133–2140.

Laserna, Z. B.: Infection of Laboratory Personnel With Vesicular Stomatitis Virus. Vet. Colombia, *2* (1968): 209–213.

McClain, M. E. and Hackett, A. J.: A Comparative Study of the Growth of Vesicular Stomatitis Virus in Five Tissue Culture Systems. J. Immun., *80* (1958): 356–361.

McNutt, S. H.: Vesicular Stomatitis. *Diseases of Cattle.* 2nd Ed. Am. Vet. Pub., Inc. Wheaton, Ill. (1963): 509–516.

Patterson, W. C., Holbrook, A. A., Hopkins, S. R. and Songer, J. R.: The Effects of Chemical and Physical Agents on the Viruses of Vesicular Stomatitis and Vesicular Exanthema. Proc. U.S.L.S.A., (1958): 294.

Patterson, W. C., Mott, L. O. and Jenney, E. W.: A Study of Vesicular Stomatitis in Man. JAVMA, *133* (1958): 57–62.

Reczko, E.: Electron Microscopy of the Virus of Vesicular Stomatitis. Arch. Ges. Virusforsch., *10* (1961): 588–605.

Ribelin, W. E.: The Cytopathogenesis of Vesicular Stomatitis in Cattle. AJVR, *19* (1958): 66–73.

Seibold, H. R. and Sharp, J. B.: A Revised Concept of the Pathologic Changes of the Tongue in Cattle With Vesicular Stomatitis. AJVR, *21* (1960): 35–51.

Shahan, M. S.: Effects of Temperature, Phenol, and Crystal Violet on Vesicular Stomatitis Virus. AJVR, *7* (1946): 27–31.

Shelokov, A. and Peralta, P. H.: Vesicular Stomatitis Indiana Type: An Arbovirus Infection of Tropical Sandflies and Humans. Am. J. Epidem., *86* (1967): 149–157.

Stone, S. S. and DeLay, P. D.: A Rapid Complement Fixation Test for Identification of Vesicular Stomatitis Virus in Cattle. AJVR, *24* (1963): 1060–1062.

Sudia, W. D., Fields, B. N. and Calisher, C. H.: Isolation of Vesicular Stomatitis Virus (Indiana Strain) and Other Viruses From Mosquitos in New Mexico. Am. J. Epidem., *86* (1967): 598–602.

Tesh, R. B., Peralta, P. H. and Johnson, K. M.: Ecological Studies of Vesicular Stomatitis Virus. I. Prevalence of Infection Among Animals and Humans Living in an Area of Endemic VSV Activity. Am. J. Epidem., *90* (1969): 255–261.

Theiler, A.: Eine Contagiose Stomatitis des Pferdes in Sud-Africa. Deutsche Tierarztl. Wchnschr., *9* (1901): 131–132.

3

Diseases caused by rickettsia and chlamydia

Anaplasmosis

(GALL SICKNESS; GALSIEKTE)

An acutely infectious but non-contagious disease, anaplasmosis is clinically characterized by fever, anemia, icterus and physical weakness and pathologically marked by complex intraerythrocytic parasitism. The causative agent, *Anaplasma marginale,* has disputed classification between rickettsiae and protozoa and is transmitted by either or both biological and mechanical vectors. Although continentally distributed, anaplasmosis occurs more commonly in pastured than in feedlot cattle. Economic losses from the disease accumulate from bovine mortality, diminished gains in body weight, reduced rates of growth, lowered milk production, inefficient feed conversion in cattle specifically and also from expensive treatment, extensive research and costly eradication programs. In the United States, the annual loss estimates to the cattle industry extend to 50 million dollars (Oglesby, 1962) and 50,000 fatal cases (Riemenschneider, 1962).

Review of Literature. Apparently *Anaplasma marginale* was first observed in the United States as a mixed bovine infection with *Babesia bigeminum* (Smith and Kilborne, 1893). In an experimental study of piroplasmosis, *A. marginale* was observed in erythrocytes, described as "coccus-like or marginal bodies" and considered as one morphologic form in the life history of *B. bigeminum.* In South Africa the organism was studied in stained blood smears and a new genus, *Anaplasma,* was described. Because it frequently located in the periphery of the erythrocyte researchers applied the name *Anaplasma marginale,* and classified it as a protozoan (Theiler, 1910). The first uncomplicated case of American anaplasmosis was observed and described in cattle in Kansas (Darlington, 1926).

While many taxonomists have continued to label the organism a protozoan, recently acquired morphologic (Albritten and Parker, 1962; Ristic, 1960) and physiologic (Pilcher, Wu and Muth, 1961) evidence suggested a closer and more vital relationship to the order Rickettsiales, and the utilization of special techniques indicated the morphologic complexity of the organism. Three of these techniques, light microscopy with Wright's-Giemsa stained blood films and Toisson's stained blood films (Espana, Espana and Gonzalez, 1959; Espana and Espana, 1962; Kreier and Ristic, 1963), phase microscopy with hemolyzed infected erythrocytes, and ultraviolet light microscopy with fluorescein-labeled antibody stained blood films (Kreier and Ristic, 1963; Ristic, White and Saunders, 1957) gave evidence of three morphologic types: (1) tailed and dumbbell forms, (2) bipolar disc-shaped forms, and (3) the classical globular inclusion bodies. The globular marginal bodies predominated and were common to all cases of anaplasmosis (Espana, Espana and Gonzalez, 1959), but the tailed, dumbbell, and bipolar disc-shaped forms were present in some cases of anaplasmosis (Kreier and Ristic, 1963; Espana and Espana, 1962; Pilcher, Wu and Muth, 1961). When infected bovine blood containing a mixture of the morphologic forms was passed through susceptible sheep, only the globular marginal morphologic form survived. The two-way process of staining the parasites with fluorescein-labeled antibody from cattle recovering from infection with the pure marginal body type of infection, and from cattle recovering from infection with the tailed, dumbbell, and bipolar-disc type of morphology, indicated that the globular marginal morphologic type was immunogenically distinct from the other morphologic types (Kreier and Ristic, 1963). From these intricate data investigators concluded that the tailed dumbbell, and bipolar disc-shaped types are different species of parasites. They proposed the names *Paranplasma caudata* for the tailed forms and *Paranplasma discoides* for the bipolar disc forms (Kreier and Ristic, 1963a). Electron microscopy of the classical marginal bodies within the red cells provided additional morphologic details: a marginal body consisted of submicroscopic units designated as initial bodies (Ristic, 1960) or elementary bodies (DeRoberts and Epstein, 1951). The round initial bodies were dispersed throughout the erythrocyte and in the plasma. As a component of the marginal body, they were arranged singly, in pairs, or in aggregates. Measuring 0.3 to 0.4 μ in diameter, the initial bodies were abundant in blood from cases of bovine anaplasmosis and in 5 to 10% of erythrocytes of cattle in the carrier-state of anaplasmosis (Ristic, 1960). The initial body possessed a peripheral membrane, had erythrocyte penetrating capability (Ristic and Watrach, 1961), and divided by fission (Ristic and Watrach, 1963). Following disruption of *A. marginale* infected erythrocytes, the organism was filtrable. After passing through a millipore filter having average pore diameters of 0.65 μ, the initial bodies penetrated normal bovine cells and produced clinical anaplasmosis in susceptible calves (Ristic, 1960). Viable initial bodies also passed through filters with an average pore diameter of 0.30 μ but were retained by filters having an average pore diameter of 0.22 μ (Albritten and Parker, 1962).

When *A. marginale* was removed from the host, glycerinized, and stored at $-70°$ C, it remained infective 1 to 2.5 years (Barnett, 1964; Summers, 1968).

From their attempts at accurate diagnosis through laboratory procedures scientists of the U. S. Department of Agriculture developed a complement-fixation test (Gates *et al.*, 1954). The use of the test on the blood of cattle having had anaplasmosis, or free of the disease, indicated a 97.9% accuracy. Use of the complement fixation test under field conditions evinced a high degree of accuracy and feasibility (Riff, Breen, and Thomas, 1964). The search for additional tests, however, continued. When adapted to *A. marginale*, the fluorescein-labeled antibody technique became highly accurate and useful in experimentation, but its cost and complexity rendered the test unfeasible for routine diagnosis (Ristic, White and Sanders, 1957). In their search for a simplified means of diagnosis, scientists developed a capillary tube agglutination test (Ristic, 1962). A comparison of the complement fixation and the capillary agglutination test on the same serum samples of known anaplasmosis revealed both the accuracy and agreement of the two tests (Merriman *et al.*, 1964). Further simplification and efficiency in herd testing came with development of a rapid card agglutination test. Consisting of washed and stained *A.*

marginale organisms, the antigen was standardized to amount per dose (Brock, Kliewer and Pearson, 1965). When tested against 22 sera known to be positive, 19 were in agreement (Amerault and Roby, 1968).

In the quest for effective and specific treatments, many drugs were screened for anaplasmacidal properties. In one study of acute cases of anaplasmosis, chlortetracycline (Aureomycin) was administered daily at the rate of 5 mg per pound of body weight; of 32 treated cattle, 100% recovered, while in 24 untreated controls, only 20% recovered (Miller *et al.*, 1952). The treatment of cattle recovered from anaplasmosis with chlortetracycline administered orally and daily at the rate of 5 mg per pound of body weight for 30 to 60 days destroyed the anaplasma and freed animals from the carrier state (Brock, Pearson and Kliewer, 1958; Twiehaus, 1962).

While studying other aspects of anaplasmosis, means for preventing the disease were also investigated. The first commercial vaccine was developed in Oklahoma. The antigen consisted of *A. marginale* organisms. After release from infected erythrocytes, they were washed, concentrated and freeze-dried. Immediately preceding injection the antigen, administered in two doses at 6-week intervals, was suspended in adjuvant. When vaccinated animals were challenged by injecting infective blood or by field exposure, some protection was demonstrated. Approximately 1% of erythrocytes, however, became infected with viable *A. marginale* (Brock, Kliewer and Pearson, 1965).

Recognizing the need for a strong antigen, another vaccine containing attenuated but viable *A. marginale* was prepared. Virulent *A. marginale* organisms were exposed to 60,000 r per minute for 45 minutes, and passed in series through splenectomized deer and sheep. These adversities attenuated the organism for cattle. In preparing the vaccine, live, but attenuated, organisms were released from infected erythrocytes and concentrated into an antigen. Safety and efficacy were tested on 900 cattle and found to be satisfactory (Ristic, Sibinovic and Welter, 1968). Efficacy was reaffirmed by additional field tests (Lora and Koechlin, 1969; Welter and Woods, 1968).

Occurrence. Anaplasmosis occurs in all bovine breeds and sexes, but susceptibility varies directly with age, and the highly specialized beef breeds, especially Herefords, Angus and Shorthorns, are fully susceptible. Previously unexposed bulls placed with herds of anaplasmosis carriers are commonly and fatally attacked. While calves under 6 months of age are highly resistant, steers and heifers 1 to 2 years of age, are sufficiently susceptible to develop a high disease incidence and to suffer a mortality of 50% or more. Old cattle are highly susceptible and calves can be rendered susceptible to experimental infection by splenectomy. In feedlot cattle, the incidence may be high because of rapid disease spread by mechanically transmitting insects. The stress from long shipment, excessive fasting, and shipping fever may cause carrier cattle to relapse into acute anaplasmosis soon after arrival at a feedlot. In addition to cattle *A. marginale* lives naturally in Columbian black-tailed deer and can be maintained in sheep.

Because anaplasmosis is transmitted by vectors, the incidence is high during spring, summer, and autumn when arthropods are active and low during late autumn, winter, and early spring when inactive. The disease may occur during any season in situations where surgical instruments are used in rapid succession on both carrier and susceptible cattle. Instruments required for venipuncturing, dehorning, and castrating and used without disinfection may transmit the disease at any time.

Geographically, anaplasmosis occurs where cattle production is an important industry in tropical, subtropical and temperate zones. In the United States the disease is endemic in central coastal California, in coastal areas northward and westward from Florida, and in the northern Rocky Mountain states. Surrounding endemic areas are zones of medium and slight incidence. (See table

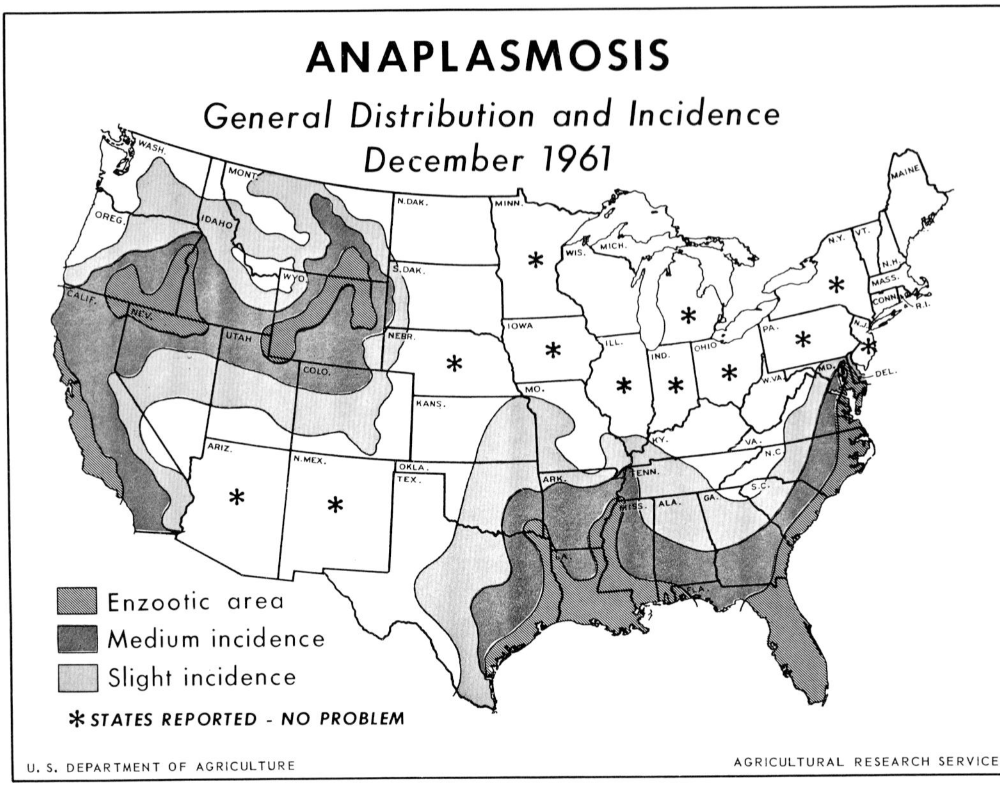

FIG. 3-1. *Geographic distribution of anaplasmosis within the United States (Courtesy of U. S. Dept. of Agriculture).*

for record of occurrence.) Outside the United States the disease has been reported in Central America, South America, Africa, Asia, Asia Minor, the Philippines and the USSR.

Etiology. While *Anaplasma marginale* has been classified as a protozoan, the recent discovery that *A. marginale* infected erythrocytes consume oxygen at approximately twice the rate of normal erythrocytes and a small fraction of the rate of oxygen consumption of malaria infected cells gives support to the classification of *A. marginale* in the order *Rickettsiales.* A dense, round, globular mass staining nearly uniformly basic with Giemsa or Wright's stains and measuring 0.3 to 1.0 μ in diameter, *A. marginale* contains no discernible cytoplasm and is usually located within the marginal part of the erythrocyte. Under laboratory conditions, but outside the bovine tissues, the infectivity of *A. marginale* is destroyed in 50 minutes but not in 15 to 30 minutes when heated to 60° C, and endures 1 to 2 years when stored in glycerinized whole blood at −70° C. Infected erythrocytes usually contain one or two and seldom more marginal bodies per cell.

As revealed by electron microscopy, a marginal body consists of 1 to 8 initial bodies or subunits, which are commonly contiguous or partially fused and arranged singly or in pairs within the marginal body. Each body, measuring 0.2 to 0.4 μ in diameter and surrounded by a membrane is globular, grows in size, divides by fission, and probably is the dynamic infecting unit of the disease and carrier-states. Initial bodies are also dispersed within individual erythrocytes, and extracellularly within the plasma. In clinical anaplasmosis as many as 90% of erythrocytes contain at least one initial body, while in the carrier state 5 to 10% of erythrocytes may contain one or more.

After hemolysis of infected erythrocytes, these initial bodies traverse filters with average pore diameters of 0.3 μ. Although known by researchers to consume oxygen and parasitize cells, *A. marginale* has not been isolated nor grown in artificial media, cell culture systems or laboratory animals. Viability of the organism, however, has been maintained in sheep without attenuation for cattle, and *A. centrale,* a bovine parasite, and *A. ovis,* an ovine parasite have been described as related species.

Transmission. Among susceptible cattle anaplasmosis is communicated by inadvertent surgical contamination and by either or both mechanical or biological vectors. The latter are ticks in which *A. marginale* persists for prolonged periods and undergoes life-cyclical changes. At least twenty species of ticks are recognized anaplasma vectors, and in the United States these seven are important: *Argas persicus, Dermacentor variabilis, D. andorsoni, D. occidentalis, D. albapictas, Rhipicephalus sanguineus* and *Ixodes scapularis.*

Mechanical vectors are hematophagous insects whose piercing mouth parts become contaminated while feeding on clinically sick or carrier cattle. During the activities of feeding, rising, flying, alighting and feeding again and again, the contaminated vector meets susceptible bovine hosts and through continued feeding inoculates *A. marginale* into other new hosts. Many species of horse flies (*Tabanus* spp.) are known mechanical vectors and in the beef fattening lots feed freely on many hosts.

During minor but rapid sequential surgical operations such as vaccinations, venipuncture, dehorning and castration, both carrier and susceptible cattle may be included and small quantities of infected blood may be inoculated into susceptible animals from the instruments contaminated from carrier cattle. To avoid this type of accidental transmission, many instruments, especially hypodermic needles for vaccination, should be used and each thoroughly cleaned and chemically sterilized between successive uses.

Pathogenesis. In the process of anaplasma inoculation, viable initial bodies, transferred from the sick or carrier animals to susceptible cattle, penetrate normal bovine erythrocytes, increase in size, and divide by fission into two to eight other initial bodies and clusters of these form marginal bodies. Eventually the initial bodies are liberated from the parasitized erythrocyte, and the cycle of cell penetration and parasite reproduction is repeated. After approximately 1% of erythrocytes are visibly infected with marginal bodies, the percentage of infected erythrocytes doubles daily for 8 to 13 days when 60 to 80% of erythrocytes are infected, and in this stage anemia begins. Growth of the anaplasma is accompanied by reduction in the amount of phospholipid within the erythrocyte stroma and by development of erythrocyte fragility. Erythrocyte fragility is inversely proportional to the phospholipid content of the stroma. While fragility and anemia acquire peaks at approximately the same time, hemolysis does not occur within the plasma. Gradually the parasitized and injured erythrocytes are removed from circulation through erythrophagia by the reticuloendothelial cells in the bone marrow, spleen, liver and lymph nodes. The erythrocyte count may decline from a normal number of 7 million per cu mm to 2 to $1\frac{1}{2}$ millions per cu mm, and the hemoglobin values may decline from the normal 12 to 3 gm per 100 ml of blood. Many clinical signs and death result from hypoxia. In recovering animals, polychromasia of erythrocytes appears in the peripheral blood and the number of discernible anaplasma rapidly declines. Recovered cattle are permanent carriers of the disease. In carrier animals an acute exacerbation of anaplasmosis can be induced by splenectomy.

Clinical Signs and Postmortem Lesions. The clinical disease course of anaplasmosis, varying directly with the natural resistance of cattle, may be mild or severe. In young calves with natural resistance, the disease is mild and commonly characterized by inappetence, moderate depression, and slight fever. Because of mild symptoms such cases are frequently unnoticed and undiagnosed, but small numbers of anaplasma infected erythrocytes may be found by microscopic examination of stained blood films.

The more severe form occurs in cattle 1 year of age and older. Following an incubation period of 17 to 45 days, body temperature ranges from 104° to 107° F. The animal's muzzle is dry, and its appetite and rumination are reduced. As a result of anemia affected animals are physically weak and mentally depressed. When the packed red cell volume is reduced to a range 40 to 50% of normal, pallor and icterus are discernible in mucous membranes of the sclera, mouth, vulva and prepuce, and also in nonpigmented skin. The urine is normal in amount, content and color. The pulse and respiration rates are accelerated. While diarrhea may occur, constipation is more common, and body weight may diminish 7% in 10 to 12 days of sickness. Muscular tremors, abortion, and suppressed libido are apparent. Hematologic examinations reveal the anaplasma infected erythrocytes.

Disease statistics show high variability. Morbidity rate varies from single isolated cases to 75 to 80% of a herd, and the mortality rate of affected cattle varies from 5 to 80%. The disease course varies from 3 to 14 days and is followed in non-fatal cases by a prolonged convalescence of 5 to 10 weeks.

At necropsy, some tick vectors may be attached to the skin, but most organ changes relate to anemia. The animal body may be emaciated and the organs dehydrated. The blood is thin and most tissues are pale and icteric. Small amounts of transudate may be found in the body cavities and in subcutaneous tissues of the lower planes of the neck, thorax and abdomen. Abundant petechiae may be found in the subepicardium, subendocardium and other serous membranes. The spleen and occasionally lymph nodes are enlarged. The hyperplastic bone marrow is transformed to the red type. Because of hyperventilation the lungs may be emphysematous. The gallbladder is distended with grumous bile, and the liver is pale.

Histopathologically, the erythrocytes are numerically reduced; many cells contain one or more marginal bodies; and after critical anemia, polychromasia of many erythrocytes is common. Reticuloendothelial cells of the spleen, bone marrow, liver and lymph nodes evince erythrophagia of damaged and parasitized cells. Hepatic cells of the central zone of liver lobules and tubular epithelial cells of the kidneys manifest fatty metamorphosis. Animals with anaplasmosis when submitted for slaughter are condemned because of fever, dehydration and beginning emaciation.

Diagnosis. A clinical diagnosis of anaplasmosis depends upon observation of typical clinical signs and postmortem lesions, and laboratory findings. Fever, anemia, icterus, clear and sometimes foamy urine and exposure to potential vectors are significant signs. In the laboratory, blood smears stained with Giemsa or Wright's solutions disclose the presence of single or multiple marginal bodies in some erythrocytes, and detection of infection in at least 0.5% of erythrocytes is usually required for a positive diagnosis. A more accurate indicator of anaplasma than classical staining is fluorescent-antibody staining which relies on the fact that a fluorescein dye, conjugated with plasma globulin from anaplasmosis recovered cattle, attaches to the marginal bodies in blood smears and fluoresces microscopically under ultraviolet illumination. Generally fluorescent antibody staining is too complex and costly for routine diagnosis, but is used in experimentation and special cases.

The bovine carrier state has epizootic and disease control importance, and can be identified by use of either the complement fixation or the capillary tube agglutination test. The former is commonly used within the United States, has an accuracy of approximately 97% and is officially performed by many state and federal diagnostic laboratories. The capillary tube agglutination test, while apparently simple and accurate, is not commonly used. The rapid card agglutination test, similar to the brucellosis card agglutination test, may be used to detect carrier animals in herds. Speed of the method allows collection and test of the blood while the animal undergoes one restraint. The entire process requires approximately 5 minutes.

The differential diagnosis requires consideration of convalescent leptospirosis, bacillary hemoglobinuria and piroplasmosis. During acute stages, the three diseases each cause hemoglobinuria, a sign not present in anaplasmosis. Animals recovering from leptospirosis show an ascending agglutination titer against leptospiras. Very few cases of bacillary hemoglobinuria recover. While bovine piroplasmosis does not occur in the United States, the possibility of the disease should not be ignored. Animals recovering from anaplasmosis possess a positive complement fixation titer against anaplasma antigen, while the other three diseases are negative to complement fixation tests, unless previously premunized by anaplasmosis or by inoculation of infected blood.

Prevention and Treatment. The incidence of anaplasmosis in feedlot cattle is reduced by the control of vectors, and the standard procedure of dipping cattle on entrance to the feedlot for ticks and other ectoparasites usually prevents its transmission. While biting flies, such as horse flies, can be numerically reduced by eliminating aquatic breeding places, they cannot be eliminated. Horse flies travel long distances, attack feedlot cattle in rapid succession, and by feeding activities commonly transmit anaplasmosis. When performing minor surgical operations on a series of cattle, all instruments should be cleaned and disinfected before use on each animal.

In some countries, but not the United States, high mortality in susceptible cattle introduced into endemic areas is avoided by premunizing with *A. centrale* or *A. marginale.* In some African countries where the virulent *A. marginale* and the relatively nonpathogenic *A. centrale* coexist, animals susceptible to *A. marginale* are inoculated with 5 ml of fresh defibrinated blood infected with pure *A. centrale.* Following a mild reaction 3 to 6 weeks after inoculation, the cattle are sufficiently resistant to avoid mortality from natural infection with *A. marginale.* Premunization with virulent *A. marginale* is feasible with and limited to young naturally resistant cattle, preferably calves. In the immunizing process, a few milliliters of infected blood from a carrier are, during winter months, inoculated into susceptible cattle. Usually a non-fatal reaction occurs 17 to 48 days after inoculation and following recovery the animals are resistant carriers.

During recent years commercial vaccines for protecting cattle against anaplasmosis have become available. Consisting of inactivated organisms, one vaccine, *e.g.,* "Anaplaz," provides some protection against field exposure to *A. marginale.* The vaccine requires two injections with an interval of 6 to 12 weeks and an annual booster injection for reinforcement of the immunity. Another vaccine, attenuated but viable, may become available when secure evidence is obtained

FIG. 3-2. *Typical marginal bodies of A. marginale in erythrocytes of a steer affected with anaplasmosis. Giemsa stain.* × 1113.

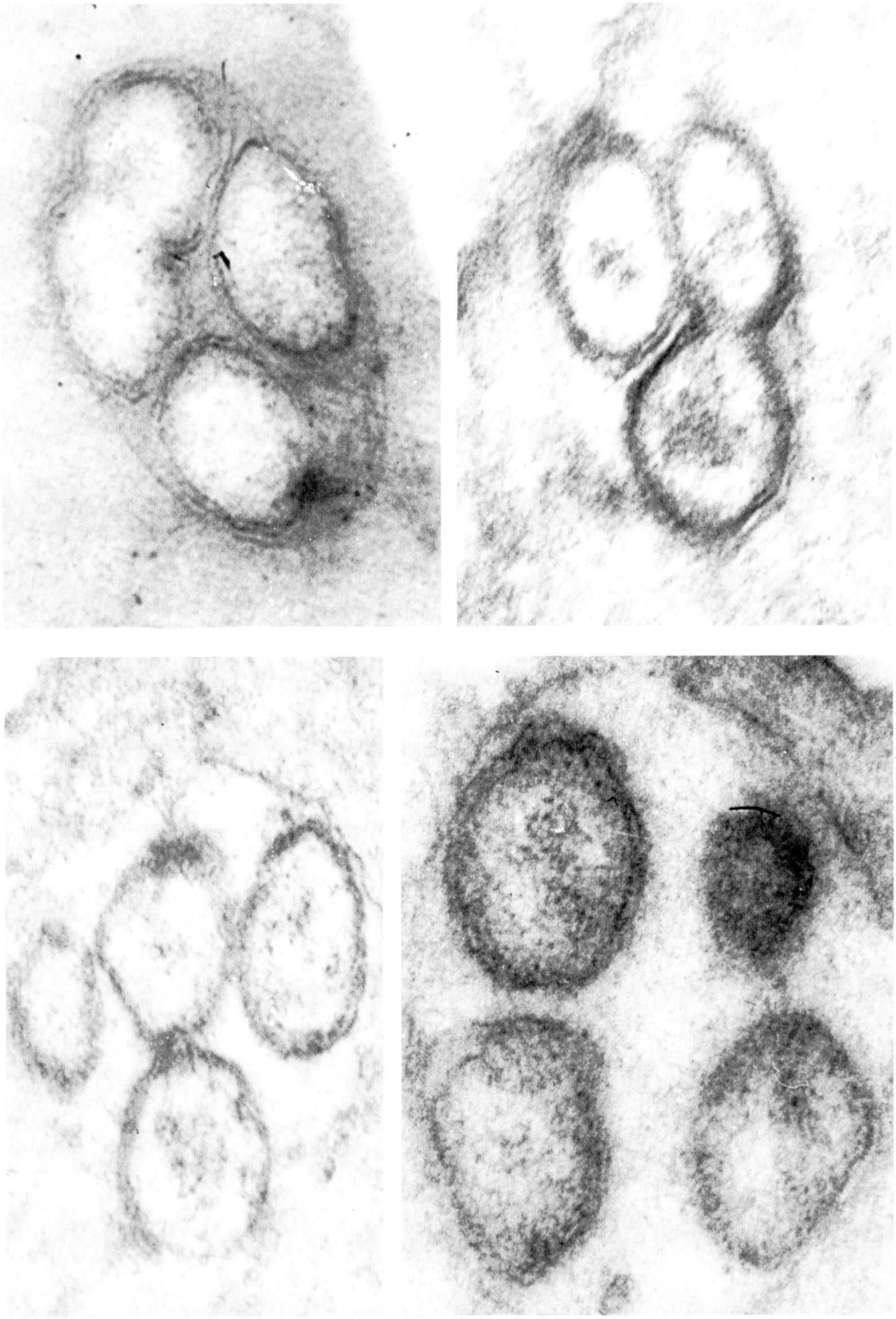

FIG. 3-3. *Electron micrographs of initial bodies dividing by fission in erythrocytes of a bovine affected with anaplasmosis.* × 78,000. (*Courtesy Dr. Miodrag Ristic, College of Veterinary Medicine, University of Illinois.*)

that the organism in the vaccine will not revert to its original pathogenicity. Because the vaccine premunizes, cattle on which it is used may carry the attenuated organism and react to the test. Immunity, however, should be strong.

The removal of sources of infection would effectively prevent anaplasmosis and in the future may become a feasible practice. Carrier cattle can be identified by appropriate blood tests and either slaughtered or given prolonged daily treatment. Chlortetracycline or oxytetracycline administered orally and daily at the rate of 5 mg per pound of body weight for 30 to 60 days destroys the infection in the carrier animal. The existence of carrier deer would complicate eradication as a means of prevention.

Animals with clinical anaplasmosis should be isolated from the herd, kept in cool pens, given adequate appetizing feed and water and sprayed daily with fly repellents. Chlortetracycline (Aureomycin) or oxytetracyclene (Terramycin) are anaplasmacidal and should be daily administered at the rate of 5 mg per pound of body weight. Anemic animals should be given 1 to 1.5 gallons of healthy blood by transfusion. Administration should be slow to avoid shock. If the large single transfusion is not feasible, 1 liter daily can be given for 4 to 6 days. Chloroquine hydrochloride (Aralen by Winthrop Laboratories) may be given intramuscularly at the rate of 250 to 500 mg daily for 5 days. An obsolescent treatment is the intramuscular or subcutaneous administration of sodium cacodylate at the rate of 200 grains per 1000 pounds of body weight at 3 to 5 day intervals.

Weak and anxious cases should not be subjected to aggravating restraint.

Since the lives of feedlot cattle are short, the carrier state in this category is temporary, of minor importance and, consequently, is not treated. In valuable breeding cattle, however, the anaplasma carrier state can be destroyed by the daily oral administration of chlortetracycline at the rate of 5 mg per pound of body weight for 30 to 60 days.

References

Allbritton, A. R. and Parker, L. T.: Filtration of the Infective Agent of Bovine Anaplasmosis. AJVR, *23* (1962): 809–812.

Amerault, T. E. and Roby, T. O.: A Rapid Card Agglutination Test for Bovine Anaplasmosis. JAVMA, *153* (1968): 1828–1834.

Barnett, S. F.: The Preservation of *Babesia bigemina*, *Anaplasma centrale* and *Anaplasma marginale* by Deep Freezing. Vet. Rec., *76* (1964): 4–8.

Breed, R. S., Murray, E. G. D. and Hitchens, A. P.: Bergey's Manual of Determinative Bacteriology. 6th Ed. The Williams and Wilkins Co. Baltimore (1948): 1100.

Brock, W. E., Pearson, C. C. and Kliewer, I. O.: Anaplasmosis Control by Test and Subsequent Treatment with Chlortetracycline. Proc. U.S.L.S.A., (1958): 66–70.

Brock, W. E., Kliewer, I. O. and Pearson, C. C.: A Vaccine for Anaplasmosis. JAVMA, *147* (1965): 948–951.

Christensen, J. F., Osebold, J. W., Harrold, J. B. and Rosen, M. N.: Persistence of Latent *Anaplasma marginale* Infection in Deer. JAVMA, *136* (1960): 426–427.

Darlington, P. B.: Anaplasmosis in Cattle (Galziekte) Found to Exist in Kansas. North Am. Vet., *7* (1926): 39–41.

DeRoberts, E., and Epstein, B.: Electron Microscope Study of Anaplasmosis in Bovine Red Blood Cells. Soc. Exp. Biol. and Med., *77* (1951): 254–258.

Espana, C., Espana, E. M. and Gonzalez, D.: *Anaplasma marginale*. I. Studies with Phase Contrast and Electron Microscopy. AJVR, *20* (1959): 795–805.

Espana, C. and Espana, E. M.: Further Studies on the Morphology of *Anaplasma marginale* with the Phase Contrast and Light Microscopy. Proc. Fourth National Anaplasmosis Conference, Reno, Nevada. (1962): 17–21.

Gates, D. W., Mohler, W. M., Mott, L. O., Poelma, L. J. and Price, K. E.: A Comparison of Antigen Production Methods and Complement-Fixation Procedures for Diagnosing Bovine Anaplasmosis. Proc. U.S.L.S.A., (1954): 105–114.

Kreier, J. P.: Tailed Forms in Anaplasmosis and Their Relationship to *Anaplasma marginale*. Proc. Fourth National Anaplasmosis Conference. Reno, Nev. (1962): 24–25.

Kreier, J. P. and Ristic, M.: Anaplasmosis. X. Morphologic Characteristics of the Parasites Present in the Blood of Calves Infected With the Oregon Strain of *Anaplasma marginale*. AJVR, *24* (1963): 676–686.

———: Anaplasmosis. XII. The Growth and Survival in Deer and Sheep of the Parasites Present in the Blood of Calves Infected with the Oregon Strain of *Anaplasma marginale.* AJVR, *24* (1963a): 697–702.

Lora, C. A. and Koechlin, A.: An Attenuated *Anaplasma marginale* Vaccine in Peru. AJVR, *30* (1969): 1993–1998.

Merriman, G. M., Owens, L. Karolee and Chung, P. K.: Complement-Fixation and Capillary-Agglutination Tests in Anaplasmosis-Infected Herd of Cattle. JAVMA, *145* (1964): 258–262.

Miller, J. G., Levy, H. E., Torbert, B. J. and Oglesby, W. T.: A Method of Screening Drugs to be Used in Treatment of Anaplasmosis—Results of Testing With Aureomycin and Terramycin. Proc. Book. Am. Vet. M. Assoc. (1952): 160–167.

Oglesby, W. T.: Financial Losses from Anaplasmosis. Proc. Fourth National Anaplasmosis Conference. Reno, Nevada (1962): 1–2.

Pilcher, K. S., Wu, W. G. and Muth, O. H.: Studies on the Morphology and Respiration of *Anaplasma marginale.* AJVR, *22* (1961): 298–307.

Riemenschneider, M. N.: Report of Committee on Anaplasmosis. JAVMA, *141* (1962): 1461.

Ristic, M.: Structural Characterization of *Anaplasma marginale* in Acute and Carrier Infections. JAVMA, *136* (1960): 417–425.

———: A Capillary Tube-Agglutination Test for Anaplasmosis—A Preliminary Report. JAVMA, *141* (1962): 588–594.

Ristic, M., Sibinovic, S. and Welter, C. J.: An Attempted *Anaplasma marginale* Vaccine. Proc. 72nd Ann. Meet. U. S. Livestock Sanit. Assoc. (1968): 56–69.

Ristic, M. and Watrach, A. M.: Studies in Anaplasmosis. II. Electron Microscopy of *Anaplasma marginale* in Deer. AJVR, *22* (1961): 109–116.

———: Anaplasmosis. VI. Studies and a Hypothesis Concerning the Cycle of Development of the Causative Agent. AJVR, *24* (1963): 267–276.

Ristic, M., White, F. H. and Sanders, D. A.: Detection of *Anaplasma marginale* by Means of Fluorescein-Labeled Antibody. AJVR, *18* (1957): 924–928.

Ryff, J. F., Breen, Harold and Thomas, George M.: Control of Anaplasmosis Under Wyoming Conditions. JAVMA, *145* (1964): 43–46.

Smith, T. and Kilborne, F. L.: Investigations into the Nature, Causation, and Prevention of Texas or Southern Cattle Fever. U. S. Dept. of Agri. Bur. Animal Industry Bulletin, *1* (1893): 1–301.

Summers, W. A.: Preservation of Infectivity of *Anaplasma marginale.* AJVR, *29* (1968): 1489–1490.

Theiler, A.: Gall Sickness of South Africa (Anaplasmosis of Cattle). J. Comp. Path. & Therap., *23* (1910): 98–115.

Welter, C. J. and Woods, R. D.: Preliminary Evaluation of an Attenuated *Anaplasma marginale* Vaccine in Cattle. Vet. Med. Small Animal Clinic, *63* (1968): 798–802.

Sporadic Bovine Encephalomyelitis

(BUSS DISEASE)

An acute generalized infectious disease, sporadic bovine encephalomyelitis is characterized clinically by fever, weakness and incoordination, and pathologically by peritonitis, pleuritis, pericarditis and encephalomyelitis. The disease occurs in cattle and is caused by a Chlamydial microorganism.

Because the natural disease is sporadic and has an apparently low incidence, its economic importance to the cattle industry is generally slight. Losses result from reduced body weight, interrupted feed consumption, and low mortality rate in affected animals; however, some individual herds may suffer severe economic losses. The susceptibility of people to sporadic bovine encephalomyelitis lends public health significance to the disease and adds to its total economic importance.

Review of Literature. Since the first report (McNutt, 1940) many aspects of sporadic bovine encephalomyelitis have been investigated. The etiologic agent has been recognized and described as a Chlamydial organism (Tustin, Mare, and Van Heerden, 1961; Wenner *et al.,* 1953), and also has been cultivated in embryonating chicken eggs (Bannister *et al.,* 1962; McNutt, 1940; Tustin *et al.,* 1961; Wenner *et al.,* 1953; Harshfield, 1970). The disease has been reproduced experimentally by subcutaneous inoculation of susceptible cattle with infected bovine tissue and infected chick embryo tissue suspensions (McNutt, 1940; Tustin *et al.,* 1961; Wenner *et al.,* 1954), and with bacteria-free infected tissue (Sterns and McNutt, 1942). Recent published reports indicated a wide but sporadic distribution of the disease. Within the United States it has been identified in nine states (Menges *et al.,* 1953), with most cases being in the midwestern region of the country. In addition, it has been found in

Canada (Bannister *et al.*, 1962), Japan (Omori *et al.*, 1953), Australia, and South Africa (Tustin *et al.*, 1961). While numerous pathological investigations indicated that the virus affects cattle, serologic methods suggested that sheep, pigeons (Bannister *et al.*, 1962), and people (Enright, Sadler and Robinson, 1959) may also be affected. Among laboratory animals guinea pigs are highly susceptible and when infected manifest peritonitis and pleuritis, features of the disease in cattle (Harshfield, 1957; McNutt, 1940; Menges *et al.*, 1953). Experimentally the virus has produced encephalitis but not peritonitis in rats, hamsters and monkeys (Harshfield, 1957).

During 1946 to 1970 numerous aspects of the disease were studied in 38 naturally infected herds and experimentally induced cases. Clinical signs, pathologic changes and epizootologic features were intensively investigated (Harshfield, 1970).

Occurrence. Sporadic bovine encephalomyelitis occurs in all breeds and sexes, and while the disease may be found in adult cattle, animals under 2 years of age are more susceptible. In South Dakota in an age incidence study involving 1,774 cattle from 21 affected herds, 269 animals or 28% were affected. Among the 482 adults and 400 yearlings, 5% of each were affected, while of the 892 calves, 25% were attacked. Although the disease may occur during all seasons, most cases were encountered during the summer and autumn months. Geographically, sporadic bovine encephalomyelitis has been diagnosed in California, Idaho, Indiana, Iowa, Maryland, Minnesota, Missouri, South Dakota and Texas of the United States, and also in Canada, Japan, South Africa and Australia.

Etiology and Pathogenesis. One of the Chlamydial organisms causes sporadic bovine encephalomyelitis. As an intracytoplasmic parasite, the spherical shaped organism varies in particle diameter from 200 to 1000 mμ. The elementary body possesses a cell wall and both DNA and RNA types of nucleic acid. Inside the parasitized cell, clumps of particles contribute to the formation of cytoplasmic inclusion bodies each with a diameter up to 12 μ. The staining affinity is mildly gram-negative, but with Giemsa's stain the particles are purple, with Macchievello's red, and with Castenada's blue. The small sized organisms possess a dense center and the large ones a light center and occupy a cytoplasmic vesicle.

Outside the bovine host, the organism can be readily cultured. Through intraperitoneal inoculation, guinea pigs support growth in abdominal viscera and in fluid of the peritoneal cavity. Following intracerebral inoculation, mice, rats, hamsters and monkeys also support growth. Chicken embryos incubated approximately 7 days sustain good growth and develop high concentration of the organism in the membrane of the yolk sac.

The Chlamydial agent is sensitive to the action of many physical factors. At temperature 56° C it inactivates in 10 minutes, but it maintains viability for 1 year when stored at −60° C. Standard disinfecting compounds kill it in a short time. The organism is destroyed in 5 minutes when exposed to either 2% sodium hydroxide, 5% cresol, or 0.3% quarternary ammonium compounds. Because of lipid material in the cell wall, the organism is inactivated by ether and some other fat solvents. It is also sensitive, *in vitro* at least, to several antibiotics.

The mature Chlamydial organism contains several antigens. As with bacteria these compounds commonly reside in the cell wall. The animal Chlamydia possess an antigen common to the group that is heat stable at 100° C for 30 minutes. Other more specific antigens are less stable to heat, and this difference is used for separating the two antigens. In affected cattle the organism can be found in peritoneal fluids and exudate, liver, kidney, brain and spinal cord. Some sick cattle excrete the organism in feces, urine and conjunctival secretions.

Because the means of transmission are

inadequately known, the pathogenesis of sporadic bovine encephalomyelitis is poorly understood. Since outbreaks of the disease, however, tend to remain localized to the herd where the outbreak originates, transmission by either direct contact or by a potential vector having low mobility seems reasonable, and crowding in feedlots provides ample opportunity for both methods. Regardless of the method, the Chlamydial inoculation of susceptible cattle is followed by wide dissemination throughout the body cavities, the central nervous system, spleen, liver and other organs, and probably takes place through the blood. The spread and growth of the organism results in a generalized systemic infection, but it is on the overt manifestation of lesions produced in the central nervous system that the affliction derives its name. Generalized inflammation in the body cavities and in the other viscera causes death of many infected animals, but cattle recovering from the disease are permanently immune. Some sick cattle excrete viable organisms in conjunctival secretions, feces and urine. This source of Chlamydia may account for spread of the disease to susceptible animals by direct and indirect contact.

Clinical Signs and Postmortem Lesions. Under natural conditions, the incubation period in feedlot cattle is uncertain in length, but observations indicate that it varies from 4 to 27 days. Experimentally, following inoculation of the Chlamydia, the incubation period is more precise but varies according to route of inoculation: 12 to 14 days following oral, 5 to 7 days following subcutaneous, and 2 to 4 days following intravenous and intracerebral inoculation. An early detectable sign is a sudden rise in body temperature ranging from 105° to 107° F. The pyrexia persists for 7 to 10 days and during the first few days of fever, the animal continues to eat but then loses appetite and becomes dehydrated. Salivation and coughing are apparent. Body weight and physical strength diminish rapidly and the animal walks with stiff incoordinated movements and, because of weakness, involuntarily flexes the fetlock joints. The stifle and hock joints may be swollen and tender. Movements may be circular, and affected cattle may show hyperexcitability and a tendency to push with the head against solid objects. Some animals develop a nasal discharge and some a diarrhea. The physical weakness results in prostration and profound depression. Some cases show oposthotonis and convulsions during terminal stages.

Morbidity and mortality rates are highly variable. Morbidity rate, however, averages 12% and mortality rate 30%. The course varies from 3 to 5 weeks.

At necropsy the animal is usually dehydrated and may be emaciated. Pathologic changes are widespread because of the generalized infection, and inflammation of the peritoneal, pleural and pericardial cavities is prominent. In early stages of the disease, the cavities contain a serous exudate, but after a course of 5 to 10 days, films of fibrinous exudate extend over the serous surfaces and may unite adjacent viscera. Plaques of fibrin may fill depressions of some surfaces. The spleen and lymph nodes commonly are enlarged. The blood vessels of the meninges and central nervous system are congested.

Histopathologically, the serous membranes of the body cavities and many organs show focal or general inflammatory reactions. Serous surfaces of the peritoneal, pleural and pericardial cavities contain deposits of serofibrinous exudate with some leukocytes distributed among the strands of fibrin. In the liver lymphocytes and some mononuclear macrophages accumulate in foci in the stroma, especially around portal trinities. The central nervous system contains inflammatory foci throughout the entire brain, cord, and meninges, but the inflammatory reactions are more numerous in the brain stem and cerebellum than in the cerebral cortex. The meninges are infiltrated, especially around blood vessels, with lymphocytes and mononuclear macrophages. Foci of cephalic and spinal infection are characterized by neuronal degeneration, necrosis of glial cells, limited liquefaction of tracts, and

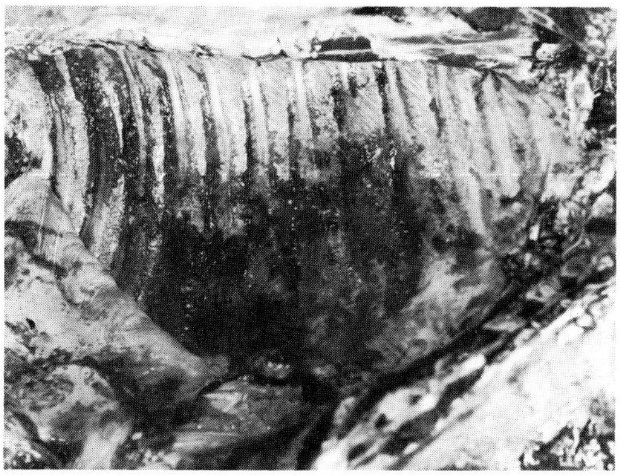

FIG. 3-4. *Fibrinous pleuritis in a bovine affected with sporadic bovine encephalomyelitis. (Courtesy Dr. G. S. Harshfield.)*

infiltration of lymphocytes, mononuclear macrophages, gitter cells, and neutrophils. Many blood vessels contain a perivascular accumulations of lymphocytes and mononuclear macrophages. In the spinal cord grey matter is more commonly affected than the myelinated tracts.

Elementary Chlamydial bodies, while not abundant, are discernible in the cytoplasm of some mononuclear macrophages of the inflammatory exudate of body cavities or of the central nervous system and when differentiated by using Machiavello's or Giemsa stain they appear as minute granules. While most of them are intracytoplasmic, some may be free and intercellular in the exudate. The elementary bodies are more easily differentiated and identified in stained smears of exudate than in stained tissue sections.

Diagnosis. Sporadic bovine encephalomyelitis is diagnosed on the basis of clinical, necropsy, and laboratory findings. While the clinical signs are non-specific, fever, physical weakness, stiffness and depression, accompanied by circling and head-pushing movements suggest this disease. At necropsy, peritonitis, pleuritis and pericarditis are important additional manifestations and in an enzootic area are sufficient evidence for a positive diagnosis. In the laboratory, paired serum samples from cattle affected with a prolonged course may show an ascending complement fixation titer with antigen prepared from the yolk sac of infected chicken embryos. Histopathologic lesions, especially with the demonstration of elementary bodies is confirming evidence. Young guinea pigs and embryonating chicken eggs may be inoculated. Young male guinea pigs, injected intraperitoneally with infected exudate or tissues, usually do not die from the infection, but when sacrificed after a few days show generalized peritonitis, and elementary bodies can be demonstrated in stained smears of the exudate. Chicken embryos, previously incubated 6 days, die in 4 to 7 days following inoculation and show characteristic elementary bodies in the yolk sac.

The differential diagnosis requires consideration of listeriosis, shipping fever, viral bovine rhinotracheitis and viral diarrhea. Listeriosis is clinically characterized by unilateral facial paralysis, and at necropsy in-

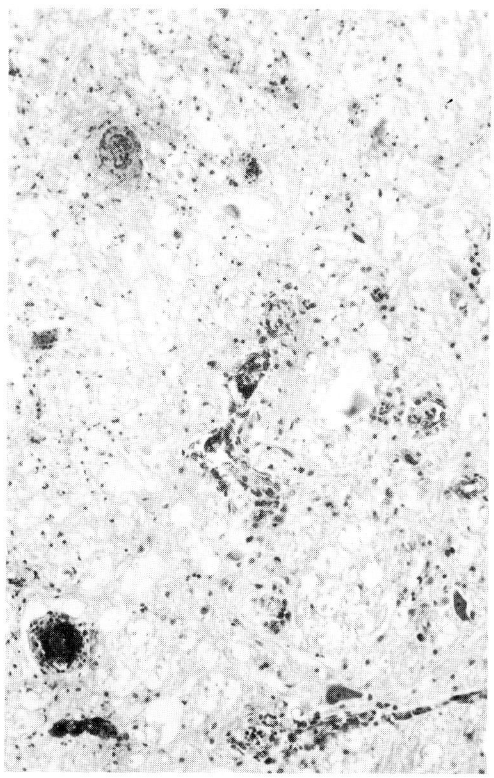

FIG. 3-5. *A focus of encephalitis. Nocht's stain.* × 100.

flammation of the body cavities is usually absent. In shipping fever, respiratory infection, including pneumonia and pleuritis, is prominent and detectable by auscultation. The disease usually follows shipment, dehorning, branding, castration, or some other stressful influence. At necropsy, pleuritis and fibrinous pneumonia are common but peritonitis and pericarditis are rare.

Viral bovine rhinotracheitis commonly affects many cattle simultaneously and produces prominent respiratory signs. While encephalitis has been reported in cattle infected with the virus of viral bovine rhinotracheitis, signs of central nervous infection are uncommon. The virus can be isolated from nasal secretions during febrile stages of the disease. At necropsy, peritonitis, pleuritis and pericarditis are absent.

In viral diarrhea, the development of oral erosions follows the beginning of fever and diarrhea. At necropsy, additional erosions are found in the esophagus and abomasum. Inflammation of the body cavities is absent.

Prevention and Treatment. Since the means of transmission are insufficiently understood, valid principles for preventing sporadic bovine encephalomyelitis have not been developed. A vaccine is not available. Because viable organisms are excreted in feces, urine and conjunctival secretions, cattle known to be infected should be removed from the feedlot and as early in the course of the disease as possible and isolated from other cattle.

Sick cattle should be treated individually by daily intramuscular administration of chlortetracycline or oxytetracycline at the rate of 5 mg per pound of body weight for 5 days or of erythromycin at the rate of 4 mg per pound of body weight for 5 days. Nutritious attractive feed and ample fresh water should be available. In case many animals are sick or exposed, the entire herd may be treated with chlortetracycline or oxytetracycline administered daily for 7 to 10 days in the feed or water at the rate of 1 mg per pound of body weight, followed by one-half the dosage for an additional week.

References

Bannister, G. L., Boulanger, P., Chapman, C. H., Avery, R. J. and Corner, A. H.: Sporadic Bovine Encephalomyelitis in Canada. Cana. J. Comp. Med. & Vet. Sci., *26* (1962): 25–32.

Enright, J. B., Sadler, W. W. and Robinson, E. A.: Sporadic Bovine Encephalomyelitis in California. U.S.L.S.A. (1959): 127–135.

Harshfield, G. S.: Sporadic Bovine Encephalomyelitis. South Dakota Agri. Expt. Sta. Tech., Bull. 18, 1957.

———: Sporadic Bovine Encephalomyelitis, JAVMA, *156* (1970): 466–477.

McNutt, S. H.: Preliminary Report on Infectious Encephalomyelitis of Cattle. Vet. Med., *35* (1940): 228–230.

Menges, R. W., Harshfield, G. S. and Wenner, H. A.: Sporadic Bovine Encephalomyelitis. Studies on Pathogenesis and Etiology of the Disease. JAVMA, *122* (1952): 294–299.

———: Sporadic Bovine Encephalomyelitis. I. The Natural History of the Disease in Cattle. Amer. Hygiene *57* (1953): 1–14.

———: Sporadic Bovine Encephalomyelitis: Etiologic Studies, Epizootiologic and Epidemologic Implications. Vet. Med., *68* (1953a): 301–305.

Omori, T., Kawakami, Y., Ishii, S., Ishitani, R. and Harada, K.: Studies on the Disease of Cattle by a Psittacosis-lymphogranuloma group Virus. IV. Identification of a Virus (Shizuoka Strain) as a Causative Agent of Bovine Encephalomyelitis, Jap. J. Exp. Med., *24* (1953): 257–273.

Sterns, T. W. and McNutt, S. H.: Sporadic Bovine Encephalomyelitis: Filtration of the Causal Agent. AJVR, *3* (1942): 253–257.

Tustin, R. C., Mare, J. and Van Heerden, A.: A Disease of Calves Resembling Sporadic Bovine Encephalomyelitis. J. So. Afr. Vet. Med. Assoc., *32* (1961): 117–123.

Wenner, H. A., Harshfield, G. S., Chang, Te Wen and Menges, R. W.: Spradic Bovine Encephalomyelitis. II. Studies on the Etiology of the Disease. Isolation of Nine Strains of an Infectious Agent from Naturally Infected Cattle. Amer. J. Hygiene, *57* (1953): 15–29.

Wenner, H. A., Menges, R. W. and Harshfield, G. S.: Sporadic Bovine Encephalomyelitis. III. Reproduction of the Disease, with Particular Reference to the Role of Poliomyelitis Viruses in Experimental Infection in Calves. J. Infect. Dis., *94* (1954): 284–296.

4

Diseases caused by bacteria

Listeriosis

(LISTERELLOSIS; CIRCLING DISEASE)

Listeriosis, an acute infectious disease, is characterized by encephalitis, septicemia and abortion, occurs in cattle, in most other species of domestic animals and man, and is caused by *Listeria monocytogenes.* On the basis of clinical manifestations the disease is usually classified as three forms: (1) encephalitis or neurolisteriosis with clinical signs of disturbance in the central nervous system, (2) gastrointestinal septicemia with lesions in many visceral organs, including liver, spleen and lungs, and (3) placentitis with abortion commonly occurring during the second half of gestation. Among feedlot cattle, encephalitis is the common form, the type referred to by the unqualified disease name. Listeriosis causes economic losses from a high mortality rate of affected cattle, loss of body weight during the prolonged disease course and expensive handling and treatment of sick animals. The possibility of transmission to man adds public health significance to the disease in cattle.

Review of Literature. The disease and the causative agent, *Listeria monocytogenes,* were first discovered in an epizootic disease of domestic rabbits in a laboratory colony (Murray, Webb, and Swann, 1926). In 1949 *Listeria monocytogenes* was isolated from grass silage which sheep had eaten, and consequently they had developed the disease (Palsson, 1963). In another experiment, the organisms of the same serotype were isolated from corn silage and from the brains of sheep fed on the silage (Gray, 1960). In addition the organisms have been isolated from milk (Dykstra, 1966), and from nasal secretion and manure (Darie, 1969). By studying the antigenic structure of 54 strains from animals and man, four serotypes were identified (Paterson, 1940). In a large number of isolants from cattle, including 179 from encephalitic brains and 370 aborted foeti, types I and IV predominated (Dykstra, 1966).

The occurrence of listeriosis in host animals has been extensively investigated. Large numbers of individual human cases are now on record (Gray, 1963; Graham, 1943). Of the domestic animals, cattle (Jones and Little, 1934), sheep (Gill, 1931), swine (Biester and Schwarte, 1940) and poultry (Seastone, 1935) are frequently infected. Occasionally, some wild species including birds and rodents have been found to be infected (Pirie, 1927). After feeding on infected cattle, ticks, *Rhipicepha-*

lus bursa and *Hyalomma ssp* and *Boophilus spp.*, harbored the bacteria for several months (Ganiev and Mamedova, 1962; Petrov, 1966). Infected farms have been investigated for recurrence of the disease. Of 20 feedlots where infected animals occupied pens during winter months only, 9 experienced recurrence of the disease in new animals during the following year (Jensen and Mackey, 1949).

Although recognizing various forms of the disease, veterinarians have tried to determine pathogenesis of the disease. In mice and goats septicemia and placentitis have been produced experimentally, but with inconsistent results, by feeding virulent cultures (Asahi, 1963) and by intravenous inoculations of *L. monocytogenes* (Molello and Jensen, 1964). Animals in these experiments developed severe placentitis with abortion and focal infection in liver, spleen and lungs. The distribution of lesions, however, in listeric encephalitis could not be satisfactorily explained by septicemia. Using serial sections of infected animal brains and tracing the inflammatory reaction from the brain stem into the trigeminal nerve, a Japanese scientist suspected movement of the bacteria from peripheral tissues along nerve trunks into the brain stem. When by minute needle punctures the mucosa and skin of the lips of mice were wounded and viable culture of *L. monocytogenes* was applied to the injured surfaces, the inoculated organisms were found in the trigeminal nerve trunk within 3 days and in the medulla oblongata within 4 days. Clinical signs of listeric encephalitis were noted 6 to 7 days after inoculation. Similar techniques produced trigeminal neuritis, brain stem infection and clinical signs in 4 of 11 inoculated young goats. Clinical signs appeared 17 to 28 days after inoculation. The trigeminal nerves were dissected from each of 8 naturally affected sheep, and all animals contained histopathologic evidence of neuritis from the nerve endings through the trunk into the medulla. From these astute observations and ingenious experiments, the investigators postulated that in listeric encephalitis the causative bacteria enter the brain stem by way of trigeminal nerve (Asahi, 1963).

The possibility of artificial immunization against listeriosis has also been investigated. In one project *L. monocytogenes* was grown in a successive series on media containing sublethal concentrations of acriflavine. By this procedure, the bacteria became attenuated and were injected parenterally into mice. When challenged with virulent bacteria by the lip inoculation method, the animals were protected. In a similar manner, 13 young goats were given the attenuated bacteria. When these animals were challenged with virulent organisms injected into the lip, none developed the disease, while all 5 nonimmunized goats inoculated in the same manner and with the same virulent culture contracted listeriosis (Asahi, 1963a). *L. monocytogenes,* grown on solid media, separated into rough and smooth colonies. Laboratory mice were injected parenterally with viable nonpathogenic rough colonies. When challenged by injection of virulent organisms, the mice were protected (Potel, 1963).

Occurrence. In cattle listeriosis occurs only in confined or semi-confined animals. Commonly, the disease develops in animals being fed silage. Cattle 6 to 24 months of age and occasionally older animals and animals of both sexes are affected. Other species of domestic animals as well as man are susceptible. The disease occurs in all major cattle producing countries. In the United States, it occurs commonly in feedlot cattle of western and mid-western states, but it does not necessarily recur in the same feedlot on successive seasons or years.

Etiology and Pathogenesis. *Listeria monocytogenes,* the bacterium causing listeriosis, is a rod-shaped organism that measures 0.4 to 0.5 μ by 0.2 to 2.0 μ and has rounded ends with straight or slightly curved sides. Some individual cells resemble coccobacilli. Staining gram-positive, it is nonspore forming and nonencapsulated. When grown at 20° C the organism is motile with peritrichous flagella. Cultures on enriched media are optimum at 37° C. On blood agar, the small, smooth, circular, flat and opaque colonies hemolyze erythrocytes in a narrow zone surrounding the colony. Isolations from infected brain tissue may require prior storage of the ground brain stem at 4° C for a few days to several weeks. The organism readily produces acid but not gas from glucose, salicin and trehalose and slowly and inconsistently from maltose, lactose and sucrose. On the basis of H and O antigens the bacteria have been classified in 4 serotypes. *L. monocytogenes* may be found in the brain stem of cattle and other animals affected with listeric encephalitis; in liver, spleen and lungs from animals suffering from septicemia; and in placentas of cattle and sheep contracting the uterine form of the disease. In addition, the organism may be encountered in silage, milk from infected cows, nasal secretions and water.

Available information now indicates that encephalitis, the important and common form of listeriosis in feedlot cattle, develops as a local infection. Susceptible cattle are exposed to the organism in contaminated feed, especially silage, contaminated water and possibly infected secretions and excretions from diseased cattle. Feeding on diets containing grass and grain awns and fragments of metal, such as wire and nails, results in abrasions and small puncture wounds of the mucosa of the mouth and lips and of skin of the lips, muzzle and nose. These anatomical areas may also be injured by infectious agents, such as vesicating viruses, by caustic irritants and by photosensitization. Through areas of injury in the mouth, lips and face, the causative bacteria, especially in the feed, penetrate tissues innervated by the trigeminal nerve. The organisms enter branches of the trigeminal nerve, grow and move along lymphatics of the trunk and enter the brain stem where they grow and spread throughout much of the medulla and pons. Throughout the infected nerve and brain stem an inflammatory reaction is provoked, and neurons and fibers are damaged or destroyed. Clinical signs vary according to function of damaged neurons. In severe cases death probably comes from respiratory failure. Non-fatal cases recover slowly. During the course of the disease the causative bacteria may be excreted in nasal secretions.

Septecemic listeriosis probably develops from ingestion or possibly inhalation of the bacteria. From the alimentary system, the bacteria penetrate tissues and enter the blood. Focal infections form in liver, spleen, lungs, mammary gland and kidneys. Organisms may be discharged to the external environment in feces, milk, and urine.

Clinical Signs and Postmortem Lesions. Following an incubation period of 2 to 3 weeks, affected cattle are distressed, disoriented, and mildly febrile. The head inclines laterally and shows unilaterial facial paralysis. On the paralyzed side the ear is pendulous, the eye partly closed, and the nostril immobilized. The paralyzed side is opposite the direction of flexion of the head. Saliva may discharge from the mouth and nasal secretions from the nose. Walking tends to be in a circular direction and often follows the fence of a pen. In a course of 10 to 14 days the animal may become prostrated and comatose, and finally die. During recumbency, even in coma, the affected animal lies constantly on the same side. When forcibly changed to the opposite side, resumption of the original position is attempted. Laboratory examination of cerebrospinal fluid reveals an increased volume, some turbidity and an increase in leukocytes and globulin content. Pregnant cows may abort.

At necropsy of fatal feedlot cases, gross changes usually are not discernible. Occasionally, the cut surface of the medulla and the pons are hyperemic. Histopathologically, the changes are in the brain stem, usually concentrated in the medulla and pons, and the trigeminal nerves. The brain stem exhibits multiple foci of infection. In each focus neutrophils, mononuclear macrophages, and lymphocytes are usually present. In some foci, however, neutrophils are scarce or absent. Neurons within a focus may be necrotic and occasionally bacilli are discernible. Blood vessels of the region disclose perivascular accumulations of lymphocytes and mononuclear macrophages. A meningitis with infiltration of lymphocytes and mononuclear macrophages is also present. The morbidity rate commonly approximates 5%, but in some outbreaks it may reach 10%. The mortality rate of affected animals is high.

Diagnosis. Circling movements, lateral inclination of the head, unilateral facial paralysis, followed by prostration, are highly characteristic clinical signs. The signs are especially indicative if more than one animal is affected. In fatal cases *Listeria monocytogenes* can usually be isolated from the brain stem. Isolations from ground infected brain stem may require prior storage of the tissue at 4° C for several days to weeks. Sections prepared from the pons and medulla exhibit characteristic histopathologic changes. While an agglutination test has been developed, it has a very limited application. The bacteria may be isolated from feed, especially silage.

Differential diagnosis requires consideration of other diseases of the central nervous system: these include sporadic bovine encephalomyelitis, rabies, brain abscesses, infectious embolic meningo-encephalitis, polioencephalomalacia, middle ear infections, and traumatic facial paralysis. Sporadic bovine encephalomyelitis is a febrile disease characterized by depression, occasionally circling, and fibrinous peritonitis and pleuritis. Rabies in cattle causes aggressiveness and characteristic changes in voice; virus can be identified following necropsy. Depending on anatomical location, abscesses of the brain may cause symptoms similar to listeriosis. This disease, however, affects usually a single animal only, and the course of the disease is long. Infectious embolic meningo-encephalitis usually produces irritation and convulsions, with prostration and coma rapidly following. Polioencephalomalacia, a non-febrile disease, is characterized by depression, blindness and often prostration and

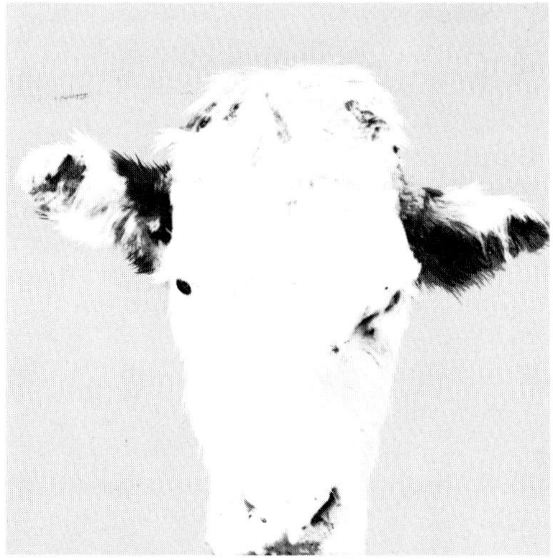

FIG. 4-1. *Left facial paralysis in a steer with listeriosis. The left ear is pendulous, the left eye is partly closed, and the left nostril is immobilized.*

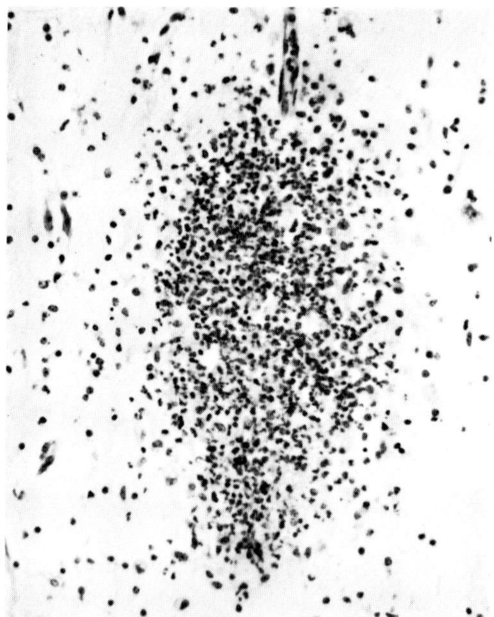

FIG. 4-2. *A focus of infection in the medulla of a steer with listeriosis. Cresyl ect violet stain.* × 222.

coma. Middle ear infection causes drooping of the affected ear. Other muscles of the face are not paralyzed. Exudate exudes from the ear canal. Facial nerve paralysis from trauma is nonfebrile. The locomotor abnormalities of listeriosis are not manifested.

Prevention and Treatment. As of 1970 no effective vaccine is available for immunizing cattle against listeriosis. Some cases may be prevented by avoiding exposure of susceptible cattle to infected herds. In some outbreaks, further spread of the disease can be prevented by changing feed, such as silage to grain, and sometimes by relocating the animals in new clean pens. Affected animals may be treated in the early stages with sulfonamides and/or antibiotics. Specific treatment requires the use of drugs which penetrate the blood-brain membranes and form high concentrations in the cerebrospinal fluid. Sulfamerazine and sulfabrommethazine administered at the rate of 1 to 1.5 grains per pound of body weight per day give good results. Supportive therapy should include daily intravenous administrations of aqueous solutions of glucose and daily intragastric administration of adequate amounts of water and protein concentrates, as milk and eggs, until self-feeding is resumed.

References

Asahi, O.: Pathogenesis of Listeric Encephalitis: Invasion of Nerve Fibers by *Listeria Monocytogenes.* Chapter in *Second Symposium on Listeric Infection.* Artcraft Printers, Bozeman, Mont., (1963): 99–108.

———: Present Situation of *Listeria* Vaccine for Animal Use. Chapter in *Second Symposium on Listeric Infection.* Artcraft Printers, Bozeman, Mont., (1963a): 74–84.

Biester, H. E. and Schwarte, L. H.: *Listerella* Infection in Swine. JAVMA, *96* (1940): 339–342.

Darie, P.: Presence of *Listeria Monocytogenes* in Excretions and Secretions from Sheep in Listeriosis Outbreaks. Vet. Bull., *39* (1969): 324.

Dumont, J. and Cotoni, L.: Bacille semblable au bacille du roughet du porc recontre dans le liquide cephalo-rachidien d'un meningitique. Inst. Past. Paris Ann., *35* (1921): 625–633.

Dykstra, R. G.: Listeriosis in Cattle. Vet. Bull., *36* (1966): 68–69.

Ganiev, T. L. and Mamedova, D. G.: The Question of Location of Listeriosis in Agricultural Animals. Veterinariya, *39* (1962): August: 22.

Gill, D. A.: "Circling Disease" of Sheep in New Zealand. Vet. J., *87* (1931): 60–74.

Graham, R., Levine, N. D. and Morrill, C. C.: Listerellosis in Domestic Animals. Bull. 499, Univ. of Ill. Agri. Exp. Sta. (1943).

Gray, M. L.: Isolation of *Listeria Monocytogenes* from Oat Silage. Science, *132* (1960): 1767–1768.

———: Listeric Infections in Man in the United States. Chapter in *Second Symposium on Listeric Infections.* Artcraft Printers, Bozeman, Mont. (1963): 290–292.

Jensen, Rue and Mackey, D. R.: Listerellosis in Cattle and Sheep. JAVMA, *64* (1949): 420–424.

Jones, F. S. and Little, R. B.: Sporadic Encephalitis in Cows. Arch Path., *18* (1934): 580–581.

Julianello, L. A. and Pons, C. A.: Identification of *Listeria Monocytogenes.* Proc. Soc. Exp. Biol. and Med., *40* (1939): 362–363.

Khalimbekov, M. M.: Epidemiological Significance of Carriers in Listeriosis of Sheep and Goats. Veterinariya, Moscow, *34* (1957): No. 6, 17–20.

Mollelo, J. A. and Jensen, R.: Placental Pathology. IV. Placental Lesions of Sheep Experimentally Infected with *Listeria Monocytogenes.* AJVR, *25* (1964): 441–449.

Murray, E. G. D., Webb, R. A. and Swann, M. B. R.: A Disease of Rabbits Characterized by a Large Mononuclear Leucocytosis, Caused by a Hitherto Undescribed Bacillus *Bacterium Monocytogenes.* J. Path. and Bact., *29* (1926): 407–439.

Olafson, P.: Listeria Encephalitis (Circling Disease of Sheep, Cattle, and Goats) Corn. Vet., *30* (1940): 141–150.

Palsson, P. A.: Relation of Silage Feeding to Listeric Infection in Sheep. Chapter in *Second Symposium on Listeric Infection.* Artcraft Printers, Bozeman, Mont. (1963): 74–84.

Paterson, S. J.: The Antigenic Structure of Organisms of the Genus *Listeria.* J. Path. and Bact., *51* (1940): 427–436.

Petrov, D.: The Tick *Rhipicephalus bursa* as a Carrier of *Listeria Monocytogenes.* Vet. Med. Nauki, Sofi, *3* (1966): 737–741.

Pirie, H. H. H.: A New Disease of Veld Rodents, "Tiger River Disease." South Afr. Inst. Med. Res. Pub., *3* (1927): 163–186.

Potel, J.: Active Immunization Against Listeriosis with Avirulent *Listeria Monocytogenes.* Chapter in *Second Symposium on Listeric Infection.* Artcraft Printers, Bozeman, Mont. (1963): 57–59.

Seastone, C. V.: Pathogenic Organisms of the Genus *Listerella.* J. Exp. Med., *62* (1935): 203–212.

Young, Stuart and Firehammer, B. C.: Abortion Attributed to *Listeria Monocytogenes* Infection in a Range Herd of Beef Cattle. JAVMA, *132* (1958): 434–438.

Yoorkov, G. G.: Epizoology of Listeriosis of Agricultural Animals in Luganskov Oblast. Veterinarii, *37* (1960): No. 11, 48.

Salmonellosis

(PARATYPHOID)

An acute contagious disease, salmonellosis is characterized by moderate fever and profuse hemorrhagic diarrhea, occurs in cattle of all ages, and is caused by *Salmonella typhimurium* and S. *dublin.* The disease results in economic losses from marked reduction in body weight, both temporary and permanent incapacity to gain weight, and limited mortality. The apparent association of the disease with the feeding of freshly chopped corn and freshly chopped alfalfa reduces the utility of those feeds.

Review of Literature. In America the original observation and study of salmonellosis in adult cattle was in 1902 (Mohler and Buckley, 1902). Since that time sporadic outbreaks have been studied in the United States (Edwards, Bruner and Moran, 1948; Edwards and Bruner, 1948; Scheal, 1962), Canada (Schofield, 1946), and Britain (Field, 1949). The disease, however, has been observed more commonly in calves (Edwards, Bruner and Moran, 1948; Edwards and Bruner, 1948). Salmonellae have been isolated from calves and adult cattle.

One extensive study was made of cultures of Salmonellae isolated from many species of mammals, birds, and reptiles. A total of 7,365 outbreaks of disease were reported. Of these, 1,896 (25.7%) were caused by S. *typhimurium.* Of the latter number, 39 outbreaks were in ruminants. S. *typhimurium* and S. *dublin* were the more common species in cattle. In outbreaks in the United States, S. *typhimurium* predominated (Edwards, Bruner and Moran, 1948).

While salmonellosis may occur during any month, the incidence has been significantly higher during May through October (Field, 1949; Scheel, 1962; Stableforth and Galloway, 1959).

Since S. *typhimurium* and S. *dublin* are occasional causes of food poisoning in people, the epizootiology of salmonellosis in cattle has been investigated. By use of the agglutination test healthy carriers of the organisms have been identified (Bythell, 1946; Stableforth and Galloway, 1959). Salmonellae also have been isolated from the bile and mesenteric lymph nodes of carrier animals.

Occurrence. Salmonellosis may develop in feedlot cattle any time during the fattening period, but the disease occurs also in adult dairy cows and, still more frequently, in calves. While the disease may occur during any month of the year, the incidence is much higher from June through October. Geographically, the disease has been observed in feedlot cattle of the western region of the United States. In addition, it has been found in adult dairy cattle and calves throughout the United States, and in Canada, Britain, Europe and other areas.

Etiology and Pathogenesis. *Salmonella typhimurium* is the usual cause of salmonellosis in feedlot cattle. In some regions, however, S. *dublin* may be the causative species. Being non-host specific, S. *typhimurium* affects, in addition to cattle, many other species of domestic mammals, including man, domestic birds, and reptiles. In contrast, S. *dublin* manifests considerable host specificity for cattle. S. *typhimurium,* a gram-negative, non-sporeforming, motile rod produces acid and gas in arabinose, inositol, maltose, trehalose and zylose; it also produces H_2S. The bacterium measures approximately 2 to 3 microns in length by 0.5 micron in width. At a temperature of 60° C it is killed in 20 minutes; but in moist soil it may endure 12 months or more.

Most outbreaks in feedlot cattle occur during months when green chopped alfalfa or green chopped corn is being fed free choice. Consequently, this type of feed has been suggested as an accessory causative factor.

The route of infection in cattle is through the alimentary tract. In the intestines the organism proliferates and causes severe injury to the mucosa. Necrosis of epithelial cells and opening of blood vessels causes hemorrhage into the intestinal lumen. Irritation to the intestine provokes diarrhea early in the course of the disease. Some organisms may penetrate the blood vessels to produce a septicemia and foci of infection in the liver, spleen, and lymph nodes. After a short course death may result from dehydration, hemorrhage, intoxication and septicemia. In surviving cattle, the infection may localize in the gallbladder and in hepatic and mesenteric lymph nodes. The localization and survival of the organisms produce carriers. Such carrier animals may excrete the organism in the feces. Demonstrable antibodies are evoked in carriers after a few weeks of infection. In clinically recovered cattle, permanent injury to the intestinal mucosa may be sufficient to deter normal digestion and render the animal incapable of efficient utilization of feeds and of normal growth in body weight.

Transmission. Salmonellosis is transmitted by direct exposure of susceptible cattle: (1) to other cattle affected with the active disease, (2) to carrier cattle excreting the causative agent, (3) to infected feces and soil, and (4) to water and feed contaminated with feces and tissues from infected rodents.

The same organism may cause food poisoning in people through heavy contamination of human food. In feedlots, *Salmonellas* from infected cattle discharge into manure. Fluid runoff containing the bacteria may enter and contaminate streams and rivers, and create a public health hazard to human consumers of the untreated water.

Clinical Signs and Postmortem Lesions. After a sudden onset, affected cattle exhibit semifluidity of stools which is followed by a short period of profuse diarrhea with varying amounts of blood and mucus in the feces after 24 to 48 hours. In some cases hemorrhage is profuse and may cause anemia. Fecal material becomes black and may contain blood clots. Early in the disease, body temperature ranges from 103° to 106° F. Exhaustion develops rapidly and may be followed by prostration and death. In some lots of cattle, morbidity rate may be as high as 30% with a mortality rate among affected animals of 1 to 3%. The course is from 3 to 7 days. Approximately 10% of clinically recovered cattle fail to make normal rates of gain in body weight.

At necropsy, most lesions are limited to the alimentary system. Severe inflammation of the mucosa is diffuse throughout the colon and cecum with less severe changes in the small intestine and abomasum. The fecal content is fluid and may contain blood. In case of severe intestinal hemorrhage, anemia is present. The spleen and mesenteric lymph nodes may be swollen. All animal tissues may be dehydrated.

Diagnosis. Clinical diagnosis is based on the presence of typical signs. Profuse diarrhea with blood in the feces is highly significant. Failure of cattle to benefit from treatment for coccidiosis should generate suspicion of salmonellosis. In a laboratory, confirmation can be obtained by isolation and identification of a species of Salmonella from feces and, less commonly, from blood and organs collected at necropsy.

Differential diagnosis requires consideration of coccidiosis and pasteurellosis. The former produces hemorrhagic diarrhea but less profuse than salmonellosis, and oocysts can be identified in significant numbers in the feces. Pasteurellosis, although capable of causing diarrhea, usually affects primarily the respiratory system and causes pneumonia.

Prevention and Treatment. Prevention of salmonellosis may be achieved through avoiding exposure of susceptible animals to

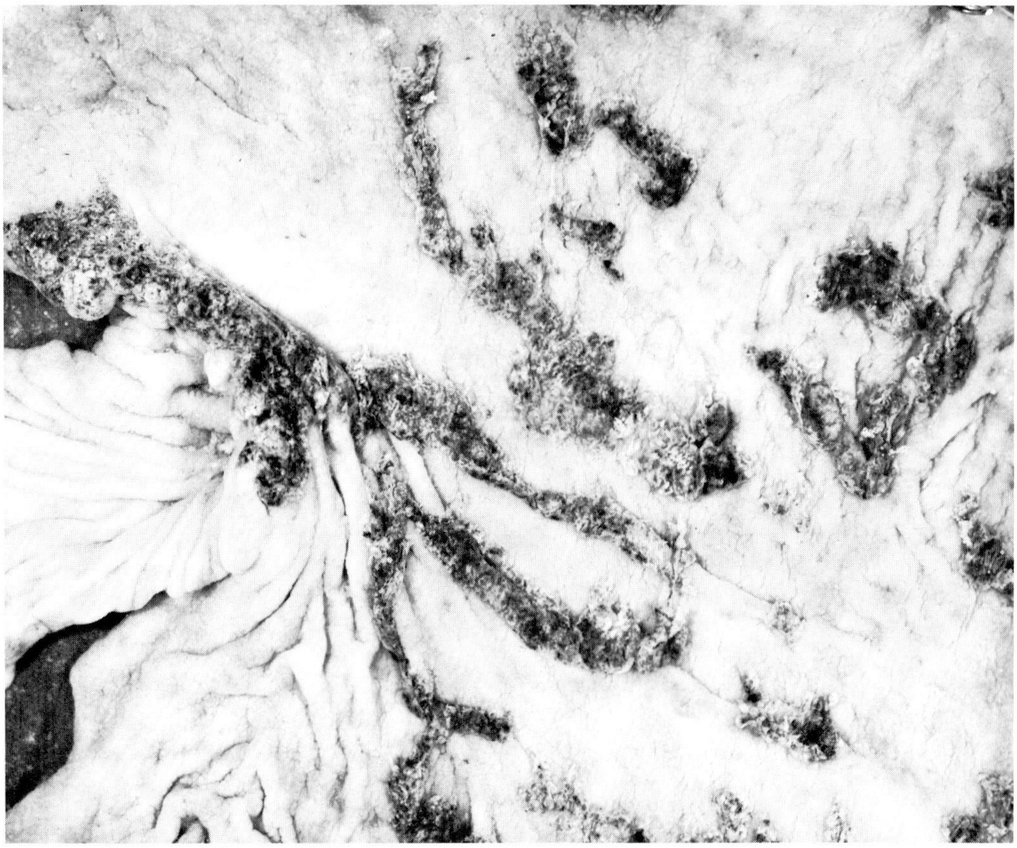

FIG. 4-3. *Cecum and ileocaecal valve from a steer affected with salmonellosis. The mucosa contains foci of necrosis.* × 0.8.

sources containing the causative agent. Active cases should be isolated. Contaminated lots or stalls should be cleaned thoroughly and disinfected chemically. Non-occupancy of pens and exposure of them to sunshine are additional means of prevention. Carrier cattle may be identified by the agglutination test and eliminated from the herd. Feed and water should be protected against contamination by rodents. In some cases discontinuing or limiting chopped green feed as a part of the diet may avoid outbreaks of the disease. While bacterins have been used, their efficacy lacks verification.

Treatment consists in the use of neomycin at the rate of 4 mg per pound of body weight per day for 3 to 5 days. Administration may be for individual animals in the form of oral tablets or for infected pens as a solution added to drinking water. Nitrofurans, such as furadantin, may be used especially for individual treatment at the rate of 2 mg per pound of body weight per day. Supportive treatment with quaternary ammonium preparations in the drinking water at the rate of 2 gm per animal per day for 7 to 10 days and with mucosal protectants such as salol, bismuth and pectins is indicated.

References

Bythell, D. W. P.: Two Outbreaks of *Salmonella dublin* Infection in Adult Cattle. Vet. Rec., *58* (1946): 425–426.

Edwards, P. R., Bruner, D. W. and Moran, A. B.: Further Studies on the Occurrence and Distribution of Salmonella Types in the United States. J. Inf. Dis., *83* (1948): 220–231.

Edwards, P. R. and Bruner, D. W.: The Genus Salmonella: Its Occurrence and Distribution in the United States. Kentucky Agri. Experiment Sta. Bull. 525, 1948.
Field, H. I.: Salmonella Infection in Cattle. Vet. Rec., *61* (1949): 109–112.
Mohler, J. R. and Buckley, J. S.: Report on an Enzootic Among Cattle Caused by a Bacillus of the Enteritidis Groups. U.S.D.A., B.A.I., 19th Report, 1902, p. 297.
Scheel, H. E.: Personal Communications. 1962.
Schofield, F. W.: *Salmonella typhimurium*. A Case of Acute Fatal Enteritis Among Cattle. Canadian J. Comp. Med., *10* (1946): 271–273.
Stableforth, A. W. and Galloway, I. A.: Infectious Diseases of Animals. *Diseases due to Bacteria*. Vol. 2. Academic Press, Inc., New York, 1959. pp. 481–556.

Actinobacillosis

(WOODEN TONGUE; BIG HEAD)

Actinobacillosis, a chronic infectious but noncontagious disease, is characterized by purulent granulomas in soft tissue of the head and elsewhere, and is caused by *Actinobacillus lignieresi*. Commonly a sporadic disease, actinobacillosis occasionally occurs in high incidence. Extensive economic loss results from reduced capacity of affected animals to gain weight, from condemnation of entire carcasses or affected parts at the time of slaughter, and from occasional mortality.

Review of Literature. Since *A. lignieresi* was first discovered in Argentina (Lignieres and Spitz, 1902), actinobacillosis has been observed in most major cattle producing countries of the world (Farquharson, 1937; Phillips, 1961; Stableforth and Galloway, 1959). In addition to cattle, the disease has been studied in sheep (Davis and Stiles, 1939; Marsh and Wilkins, 1939; Tunnicliff, 1941) and in other animals, including horses and people (Pathak and Ristic, 1962; Stableforth and Galloway, 1959).

The incidence of actinobacillosis is higher in cattle than in other species of livestock. During the period 1967 through 1969, approximately 29 million adult cattle were slaughtered annually in the United States under federal inspection. Of these, 0.7% were affected with either actinobacillosis or actinomycosis. Approximately 800 carcasses were condemned annually; in the other animals, affected parts were condemned (Federal Meat Inspection, 1967–1969). In one experiment designed to measure the relative incidence of actinobacillosis and actinomycosis, 72 cattle affected with a granulomatous disease were selected at random from different lots of western cattle. Different ages and breeds were in the sample. Differential diagnosis was made on the basis of bacteriologic and histopathologic findings. Of the 72 affected, a ratio of 6 cases of actinobacillosis to 1 case of actinomycosis was found (Shahan and Davis, 1942).

In the laboratory, strains of *A. lignieresi* isolated from people and animals have been studied. Human strains and bovine strains were morphologically and biochemically similar (Pathak and Ristic, 1962; Stableforth and Galloway, 1959). From 218 strains of organism isolated from bovine and ovine lesions and investigated for relationships by the slide and tube agglutination tests, six antigenic types were identified. The majority of cattle strains belonged to type 1 and most sheep strains to types 2, 3, and 4 (Phillips, 1967). While seeking sources of infection, *A. lignieresi* was isolated commonly from the contents of the mouth and the contents of the rumens from cattle not affected with actinobacillosis (Frost, 1940; Phillips, 1961). These findings led the investigators to postulate that the organism is commonly present on mucous membranes and skin, and that it may cause lesions by penetration through wounds or other discontinuities of the covering tissue. Regional lymph nodes of primary sites of infection were infected commonly, and occasionally wide dissemination occurred through the blood. Consequently, infection has been observed in brain, meninges, liver, kidneys, stomachs, muscle, testes and bone marrow (Mawditt, 1962; Stableforth and Galloway, 1959). Usually *A. lignieresi* affected soft tissues, but in one study of 64 cases of bovine actinobacillosis, the bone was affected in one animal (Shahan and Davis, 1942).

The search for satisfactory means of treatment has been continuous. The use of sodium iodide, administered intravenously, proved highly effective in experimental and field cases (Farquharson, 1937). Consequently, this treatment has gained wide and popular use. However, studies of many strains of *A. lignieresi in vitro* indicated that growth of the organism is inhibited by sulfathiazole and sulfamethazine (Smith, 1951) and by chloromycetin, aueromycin and terramycin (Ristic *et al.*, 1956), but slightly or not at all by potassium iodide (Smith, 1951).

Occurrence. Both sexes and all breeds of cattle are susceptible. Though more common in old cattle, the disease appears in all ages of animals, including calves. In addition to cattle, the disease occurs in sheep, horses and dogs. Experimentally, guinea pigs and rabbits are slightly susceptible. In cattle the disease occurs during all seasons and in most countries of the world.

Etiology and Pathogenesis. The causative agent, A. *lignieresi*, is a pleomorphic, nonmotile, non-spore-forming, gram-negative rod. In cultures, coccoid and rod forms, measuring 0.4 μ in width and 1 to 15 μ in length, may occur. Although aerobic, the organism grows best in an atmosphere of 10% carbon dioxide. In infected tissues the bacteria form rosettes. The latter are compact bosselated colonies of organisms measuring less than 1 mm in diameter. Small club-shaped projections radiate from the surface of the rosette. In a stained smear of crushed rosette, gram-negative organisms can be demonstrated.

Probably A. *lignieresi* is widely distributed in soil and manure. In many healthy cattle it is present on the mucous membranes of the mouth, forestomachs, abomasum, intestines, nose and larynx, as well as on the skin. Presumably the organism, unable to invade healthy intact mucosa or skin, penetrates tissue through points of injury from grass awns and other foreign bodies and enters the gums at the time of tooth expulsion. In the deep noncovering tissues the organism produces a chronic inflammatory reaction which is known as an infectious granuloma. Usually infection develops at multiple points within an area. Exudate accumulates and fibrous connective tissue proliferates around the locus of infection. Sinus tracts often discharge exudate intermittently to the surface. Often the infection spreads through lymph vessels to regional lymph nodes where secondary foci of infection are established. From here, spread may continue through the lymphatic chain and eventually enter the blood. Hematogenous dissemination establishes infection in the lungs and many other organs. Usually, however, bony tissue is not affected. The infection is progressive and often fatal unless properly treated.

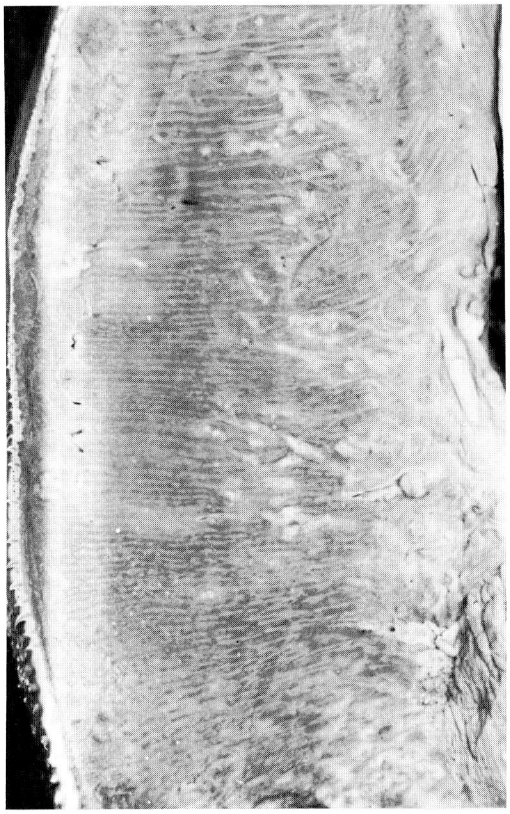

FIG. 4-4. *Actinobacillosis in tongue of a steer.* × 0.7.

Clinical Signs and Postmortem Lesions. Actinobacillosis develops insidiously in soft tissues. Specific clinical signs depend on anatomical location and stage of disease development. The granulomatous lesions, regardless of location, result in enlargement of the part and often encroachment on adjacent tubular or cavernous structures. In the head and neck, the tongue, lymph nodes and mucous membranes are commonly involved. Infected mandibular, parotid and anterior cervical nodes usually cause subcutaneous induration and surface bulging. Infection of the mucous membranes of the nose, pharynx, larynx, trachea and mouth cause localized indurated enlargements which project into the nasal, pharyngeal, laryngeal, tracheal or oral cavities. In the respiratory system the encroachment results in noisy, difficult breathing. The infected tongue, commonly known as wooden tongue, becomes enlarged, protruded and immobile. This in turn produces interference to prehension, mastication and swallowing of food. Saliva drips from the mouth.

In advanced stages, the lesion discharges tenacious pus to a surface through a sinus. The sinus opening may heal with scar tissue and re-open later at the same or different location. An infected mucous membrane, especially of the tongue, nose and larynx, commonly becomes ulcerated.

In other areas of the body, lesions of actinobacillosis are uncommonly found. Disfiguring subcutaneous lesions bulge onto the surface and at intervals discharge pus.

At necropsy, indurated granulomas of variable size and shape are located in soft tissues. Frequently, the surface of the lesion is ulcerated and contains a sinus tract. Incision of the lesion reveals single or multiple confluent cavities and tracts containing viscous bluish-yellow pus. The exudate is surrounded by a mass of firm granulation tissue.

Commonly, the lesions are located anatomically in soft tissues of the head and anterior part of the neck. The subcutis and mandibular, parotid, suprapharyngeal, and anterior cervical lymph nodes may be affected. Very often the infected tongue is enlarged, distorted, nodulated, and ulcerated.

Less commonly, granulomas are located in the lips and submucosa of the nose, pharynx, larynx and trachea. The lungs may be infected as a result of the organisms moving along lymphatics into the venous blood which conveys them into the lungs. Infected lungs are firm, nodular and variegated in color. Infection may also be found in the subcutis of the limbs and body and in many internal organs including the peritoneum, heart, liver, spleen, kidneys, testes, ovaries, brain, joints and bone marrow.

Histopathologically, the granuloma consists of rosettes of *A. lignieresi* and the surrounding reactive tissues. The rosette is located near the center and is surrounded successively by a zone of neutrophils, a zone of epithelioid cells, and a zone of fibrous connective tissue. Lymphocytes may be distributed throughout the connective tissue. Multiple granulomas may fuse to form a large infected mass. Growth of the granuloma may cause destruction of adjacent normal tissue.

At the time of slaughter, disposition of the carcass depends, in general, on the extent of infection. Infected organs or parts are unfit for food. In case of infections limited to the mandibular and/or parotid lymph nodes, the head, following excision of the nodes, is edible. Lesions in the tongue, regional lymph nodes and other soft tissues render the entire head unfit for food. Extensive infection of the lungs and other viscera, accompanied by cachexia, makes the entire carcass unsatisfactory for human food.

Diagnosis. The diagnosis is made from the presence of indurated purulent granulomas in soft tissues, especially of the head and neck. Confirmation of the diagnosis can be obtained by demonstrating the presence of rosettes in the pus and gram-negative rod-shaped bacteria in the rosettes.

In the differential diagnosis the following diseases are considered: actinomycosis, tuberculosis, pyogenic bacterial abscesses and neoplasms. Actinomycosis commonly infects a bone, especially the mandible, of cattle. Similar purulent, indurated granulomas are formed. Rosettes in the copious pus contain filamentous, branching, gram-positive organisms which can be demonstrated in stained smears of crushed rosettes. Tuberculosis may cause enlargement of lymph nodes. Usually, however, the infected node contains caseative necrotic tissue without pus. Affected animals are positive to the tuberculin test. Pyogenic bacteria, such as *Corynebacterium pyogenes*, streptococci, and staphylococci may cause abscesses in lymph nodes. These infections usually are not surrounded by the large mass of granulation tissue and the pus does not contain rosettes. The bacteria can be cultured and identified in the laboratory. Neoplasms may evoke enlargements with disfigurement in the head and elsewhere in cattle. Lymph nodes may be affected primarily or from metastatic foci. Usually a neoplasm does not contain purulent exudate. A biopsy can provide a diagnosis of the neoplasm.

Prevention and Treatment. Actinobacillosis may be partially prevented by minimizing the opportunity for either large or small traumatic injuries, especially in the mouth. The inclusion of numerous seed awns in the feed should be avoided. Protruding nails and pieces of wood should be removed from fences and other objects against which cattle rub. Continuous feeding in the diet of organic iodide compounds at the rate of 60 to 120 mg per animal per day reduces the disease incidence.

In the early stages the disease can be treated successfully by surgical drainage of lesions and with dihydrostreptomycin administered at the rate of 1 gram per 100 pounds of body weight daily for 7 to 10 days. Solutions of sodium iodide may be injected intravenously at the rate of 0.75 gr of drug per 100 pounds of body weight with several treatments at 5-day intervals. Following administration of streptomycin, the affected animal should not be slaughtered for human food for at least 30 days after the last treatment. An infected herd of cattle can be treated with organic iodide compound by the same method as is described for actinomycosis.

References

Cohrs, P.: Nieberle und Cohrs. *Lehrbuch der Speziellen Patholgischen Anatomie der Haustiere.* Vierte Auflage. Gustav Fischer Verlag. Stuttgart. 1962.

Davis, C. L. and Stiles, G. W.: Actinobacillosis of Rams. JAVMA, *95* (1939): 754–756.

Farquharson, J.: Intravenous Use of Sodium Iodide in Actinomycosis. JAVMA, *91* (1937): 551–554.

Federal Meat Inspection. Statistical Summary. USDA (1967–1969).

Frost, B. A.: Thesis. Cornell University Library. Ithaca, 1940.

Key, J. B. and Loffer, L. F.: Management of an Actinomycosis Outbreak in Feeder Cattle. A Case Report. Vet. Med., *51* (1956): 337–338.

Lignieres, J. and Spitz, G.: L'Actinobacillose. Bulletin Soc. Cent. Med. Vet., *20* (1902): 487–535.

Marsh, H. and Wilkins, H. W.: Actinobacillosis in Sheep. JAVMA, *94* (1939): 363–364.

Mawditt, A. L. and Greenham, L. W.: A Case of Subcutaneous Bovine Actinobacillosis. Vet. Rec., *74* (1962): 290–292.

Palotay, J. L.: Actinobacillosis in Cattle. Vet. Med., *46* (1951): 52–54.

Pathak, R. C. and Ristic, M.: Detection of Antibodies to *Actinobacillus lignieresi* in Infected Human Beings and the Antigenic Characterization of Isolates of Human and Bovine Origin. AJVR, *23* (1962): 310–313.

Phillips, J. E.: The Commensal Role of *Actinobacillus lignieresi.* J. Path. & Bact., *82* (1961): 205–207.

———: Antigenic Structure and Serological Typing of *Actinobacillus lignieresi.* J. Path. and Bact. *93* (1967): 463–475.

Ristic, M., Herzberg, M., Sanders, D. A. and Williams, J. W.: Actinobacillosis. I. An Evaluation of Cultural Characteristics of Selected Strains of *Actinobacillus* lignieresi. AJVR, *17* (1956): 555-562.

Sanders, D. A. and Ristic, M.: Actinobacillosis of Cattle, JAVMA, *129* (1956): 478–481.

Shahan, M. S. and Davis, C. L.: The Diagnosis of Actinomycosis and Actinobacillosis. AJVR, *3* (1942): 321–328.

Smith, H. W.: A Laboratory Consideration of the Treatment of *Actinobacillus lignieresi* Infection. Vet. Record, *63* (1951): 674–675.

Stableforth, A. W. and Galloway, I. A.: *Infectious Diseases of Animals.* Vol. 1. Academic Press, Inc. New York 1959, pp. 1–15.

Tunnicliff, E. A.: A Study of *Actinobacillus lignieresi* from Sheep Affected With Actinobacillosis. J. Inf. Dis., *69* (1941): 52–58.

Brucellosis

(BANG'S DISEASE; CONTAGIOUS ABORTION)

An acute or chronic contagious disease, often characterized by placentitis and abortion, brucellosis in cattle is caused by *Brucella abortus*. The generic term brucellosis generally refers to all diseases of mammals caused by the various species of *Brucella*, but when referring to cattle the term applies specifically to the disease caused by *Br. abortus*.

To the cattle industry, brucellosis is a disease of major economic importance. According to a survey conducted in 1954, the disease resulted in an approximate annual monetary loss of 87 million dollars. Since 1954 the incidence and, presumably the related economic loss, have as a result of brucellosis eradication programs diminished in the United States. Some losses continue, however, from the necessary maintenance of a vigilance program for detecting and eliminating new disease outbreaks and for protecting the cattle industry against new sources of infection. The development of brucellosis in other species of domestic animals and also in man further enhances the total importance of the disease.

Review of Literature. While contagious abortion in cattle was recognized during the 18th century, the specific causative organism, now known as *Br. abortus*, was discovered in Denmark (Bang, 1897). Since then the disease has been diagnosed and studied in most cattle producing countries of the world (Huddleson, 1943; Stableforth and Galloway, 1959) and eradication or reduction to a very low incidence has been achieved in some countries through systematic control programs. In infected cattle the organisms concentrated in the chorion and in allantoic and amnionic fluids (Smith, Keppie, Pearce, Fuller and Williams, 1961). The numerical disclosure that 60 to 85% of the organisms were in the fetal cotyledons was determined by separating bacteria from the constituent parts of the infected gravid uterus. Lower concentrations of bacteria were found in the mammary gland, lymph nodes, liver, spleen and muscle (Doyle, 1935; Huddleson, 1943; McCullough, *et al.*, 1951; Saddler, 1960), and in milk (Morgan and McDiarmid, 1960).

At the time of abortion the expelled fetus, membranes and exudates were heavily infected with *Br. abortus*. Systematic investigation indicated that the organisms maintain viability and presumably infectivity for variable periods under different conditions, as follows: $4\frac{1}{2}$ hours exposed to direct sunlight; 5 days in burlap in an ordinary room; 30 days in burlap in an unheated cellar; 37 days in slowly drying soil; 4 days in bovine urine; 120 days in bovine feces drying in a dark cupboard; and 75 days in an aborted fetus during cool weather (Smith *et al.*, 1949).

Intensive studies of cattle and laboratory animals have yielded significant facts about the pathogenesis of brucellosis. Susceptible pregnant cattle, inoculated either subcutaneously or intra-conjunctivally with virulent cells of *Br. abortus*, developed a bacteremia (Manthei and Carter, 1950; Payne, 1959). In guinea pigs, the duration of bacteremia varied directly with virulence of the bacteria. Organisms of low virulence, as Strain 19, produced bacteremia for 1 week, while organisms of virulent strains remained in the blood from 3 to 4 weeks (Cruickshank, 1957). In addition the organisms localized in regional lymph nodes in the area of inoculation. The infection resulted in lymphoid hyperplasia and infiltration with neutrophils and eosinophils. During pregnancy the organisms were transported by way of the blood to the gravid uterus where endometritis and placentitis developed (Payne, 1959). The organisms concentrated numerically in the chorion and allantoic and amnionic fluids (Smith *et al.*, 1961). The marked predilection for chorionic cells and for fetal fluids was shown to be due to the compound erythritol (CH_2OH CHOH CH_2OH-mesoform) in both normal and diseased placentas (Pearce *et al.*, 1962; Williams *et al.*, 1962). Following abortion, foci of infection were established in the mammary glands, supramammary lymph nodes, and other lymph nodes (Doyle, 1935; McCullough *et al.*, 1951; Saddler, 1960). Most infected mammary glands excreted viable organisms in the milk (Morgan and McDiarmid, 1960). Antibodies were evoked and demonstrable in plasma, milk and cervical mucus (Fleischhaur, 1937; Manthei and Carter, 1950; McClure and Fyvie, 1956).

Since its discovery in 1942, Strain 19, which possesses low pathogenicity and high immunogenicity, has been used extensively throughout the world as a live vaccine (Cotton, 1932). When the vaccine was administered to cattle 4 to 8 months of age, the post-vaccination titer in most animals descended to a low level by breeding age. In animals vaccinated at older ages, the post-vaccination titer in most animals persisted at higher levels beyond sexual maturity. The application of vaccine at the age of either 4 or 8 months gave equally good protection against challenge infection (Gilman and Wagner, 1959; Lambert *et al.*, 1961). The immunity from a single application of vaccine during calfhood did not diminish throughout the productive life of the cows (Goode *et al.*, 1956; McDiarmid, 1957). In beef herds the use of vaccine diminished the percentage of non-pregnant cows from 22.4% in non-vaccinated cows to 14.2% in vaccinated cattle (Blunt, 1959). As a part of a cooperative state-federal brucellosis eradication program, the extensive use of the vaccine reduced the incidence of brucellosis to a low level in the United States.

Recovery from brucellosis was indicated when most reactor cattle maintained in isolation lost their positive titers in 3 to 5 years (Grachev and Galusyan, 1957).

Occurrence. The natural geographic distribution of bovine brucellosis has been observed in most major cattle producing countries of the world. Through the application of eradication programs, the disease has been either reduced to low incidence or eradicated in countries as Norway, Denmark, Holland, Japan and the United States. While the disease may occur in all ages, calves are resistant but adult cattle are highly susceptible. Some surveys have indicated a higher incidence among cows than bulls. Besides cattle, the disease occurs in other species of domestic animals, some wild species and man.

The main reservoir for *Br. melitensis* is in sheep and goats; for *Br. suis* in swine, and for *Br. ovis* in sheep.

Etiology and Pathogenesis. The causative agent, *Br. abortus*, is bacillary to coccoid in morphology and measures 0.6 to 1.0 x 0.3 to 0.5 μ. In tissues and exudate the bacteria are coccoid but after subculturing, bacillary in shape. Staining lightly with most analine dyes, they are gram-negative. In addition they are nonsporogenous, nonmotile, but encapsulated. Although an aerobic bacterium, *Br. abortus* requires an increased carbon dioxide tension for isolation and often for some subcultures. Colonies on solid media are round, smooth and hemispherical. *Br. abortus* ferments glucose, inositol, mannose and rhamnose, but not maltose or trehalose. Although disclosing considerable similarity in morphology and metabolism, the species of *Brucella* can be differentiated as indicated in table 4.

Studies on pathogenesis have revealed that transmission of *Br. abortus* occurs naturally through ingestion and probably through inhalation of viable bacteria. Occasionally, however, pathogenic organisms may penetrate either the intact of abraded skin and the conjunctivae. In addition, the disease may be transmitted as a venereal infection from contaminated semen to susceptible cows. Experimentally, the disease can be transmitted by parenteral or conjuctival inoculation.

Following inoculation, the regional lymph nodes become infected. A low grade bacteremia develops and occurs intermittently for many months and, in some cases, as long as 2 years. As chronicity develops, a transitory bacteremia may develop at subsequent parturitions.

TABLE 4 *Growth in media containing*

	Crystal Violet 1:50,000	Basic Fuchsin 1:50,000	Thionin 1:100,000	CO_2 required	H_2S produced
Br. abortus	−	+	−	+	+
Br. melitensis	+	+	+	−	−
Br. suis	−	−	+	−	+
Br. ovis	−	±	+	+	−

As a result of the bacteremia, *Br. abortus* localizes in many tissues but especially in the placenta, mammary gland and supramammary lymph nodes. Predilection for the placental tissue may be due to the presence of erythritol in the chorionic epithelial cells. In the placentomes, bacteria penetrate the cytoplasm of chorionic epithelial cells where they multiply. The parasitized epithelial cells may necrose and detach from the basement membrane of villi. Some organisms penetrate further into the villi and enter the placental blood vessels and are carried into the fetus. Amnionic fluid also becomes infected and the organisms are swallowed by the fetus. As a result of infection, placentitis is progressive. Leukocytes accumulate in and between endometrial septa and chorionic villi. Necrosis, like inflammation, may be focal. Edema develops in the chorion.

As placentitis, necrosis and edema develop, abortion may occur. The placental changes may interfere with transmembrane exchange of nutrients and excretory metabolites. Following abortion, *Br. abortus* is excreted to the environment with the membranes, fetus and uterine discharges. Infection of the uterine discharge usually persists for a week but may continue for several months. For a few weeks following parturition, excretion of bacteria also occurs through the milk in most animals, but in some, throughout the whole period of lactation.

In bulls the bacteremia results in localized infection of the seminal vesicles, ampulae, testes and epididymi. During early stages of infection, inflammatory exudate and bacteria contaminate the semen and may be transmitted to susceptible cows through copulation or artificial insemination. In many bulls the infection becomes chronic. Testicular parenchyma undergoes progressive destruction. Adhesions form between the tunica vaginalis and tunica albiginia.

Clinical Signs and Postmortem Lesions. The incubation period, the interval from inoculation to a positive blood titer and the number of abortions tend to vary inversely with the number of organisms inoculated. In case of inoculation with infected semen, the period

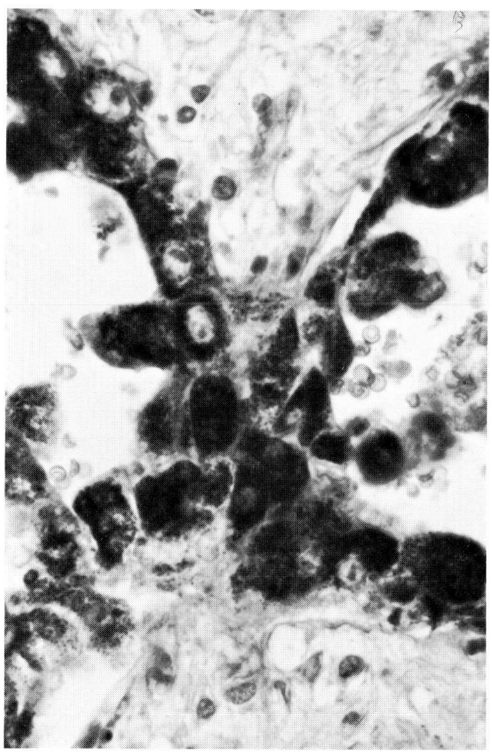

FIG. 4-5. *Brucella bacteria in chorionic epithelium. Giemsa stain.* × 620.

from breeding to abortion is approximately 225 days. Experimentally, however, inoculation with a large dose of virulent bacteria shortens the incubation period.

The main clinical sign of bovine brucellosis is abortion which is often preceded by signs of approaching parturition. While abortion may occur at any stage, the highest incidence in the natural disease is during the sixth to eighth months of gestation. For a few days preceding and for 1 to 2 weeks following abortion, an opaque uterine discharge is commonly expelled. After abortion in late gestation period, retention of the placenta is common.

Following the introduction of brucellosis into a susceptible herd, infection spreads gradually. The abortion rate increases usually to a maximum of 30 % and is then followed by a decline. In some herds, however, the maximum abortion rate may go much higher. Introduced heifers and other non-infected herd additions are fully susceptible. Recovery from the disease, as evidenced by loss of positive agglutination titer and relief from abortion, occurs after a course of 3 to 5 years in 4 to 28% of infected cows.

Signs of genital infection in bulls vary with duration of the disease. In early stages, a febrile reaction may accompany an acute painful swelling of one or both testes and seminal vesicles. After several weeks the acuteness subsides. The infected testis is enlarged and firm. The semen may contain inflammatory exudate and viable bacteria.

In cattle the lesions are limited largely to the genital system. In advanced stages of the disease, when abortion is imminent, the allanto-chorion, as observed from the amnionic surface, is heavily and uniformly edematous. The placentomes are swollen. Opaque exudate and necrotic tissue are discernible in the periplacentomal tissue as well as over the placentome. In the excised infected uterus, the cotyledon frequently separates easily from the caruncle. The separated cotyledon, instead of exhibiting a normal pink tissue coloring, is gray to yellow, especially in the periplacentomal tissue. The discoloration is due to exudate and necrosis. The uterine wall, especially at the lesser curvature of the pregnant horn, may be edematous. The placenta expelled during or following abortion discloses swelling, edema, and grayish-yellow discoloration of the infected cotyledon and pericotyledonary tissue. In some cows, arthritis and synovitis develop. In bulls, infected seminal vesicles are indurated and enlarged. Orchitis and epididymitis may be unilateral or bilateral. The infected testis is enlarged, firm and often adheres to the tunica vaginalis. The infected testis and epididymis contain single or multiple foci of inflammation and necrosis. Exudate may be abundant. In the severely infected fetus, the umbilical cord and subcutaneous tissues of the abdomen and perineum are edematous. Serous exudate may be found in the body cavities.

At slaughter of reactor cattle, the uterus and contents, udder, supra-mammary lymph nodes, testes and seminal vesicles are discarded.

Histopathologically, tissue changes vary according to the stages of disease development. In early and advanced stages, the chorion discloses focal or occasionally general inflammation and edema. In many foci, chorionic epithelial cells are filled with bacteria which may distend the cytoplasm and obscure the nuclei. Some cells may be desquamated. In foci, bacteria, inflammatory exudate and necrotic tissue accumulate between chorionic villi and endometrial septa. Frequently, bacteria enter connective tissue of the chorion and the fetal blood vessels where some organisms are found in the cytoplasm of endothelial cells.

In the periplacentome, inflammatory exudate may infiltrate the endometrium and fill lumens of endometrial glands. The space between the endometrium and the chorion may contain considerable exudate, bacteria, and desquamated chorionic cells. In a similar manner, affected testes disclose areas of necrosis of seminiferous tubules and the accumulation of inflammatory exudate and colonies of bacteria. In advanced stages, most or all seminiferous tubules may be destroyed through necrosis or non-functional from atrophy. Seminal vesicles disclose chronic inflammation with fibroplasia, focal necrosis, inflammation and destruction of some acini. Small cysts may be present.

Diagnosis. While brucellosis may be suspected clinically as the cause of abortion, a positive diagnosis of the disease depends upon the analysis of results from bacteriological or serological procedures:

1. *Bacteriological cultures.* The isolation and identification of *Br. abortus* provide the most reliability for a diagnosis of brucellosis. Bacteriological cultures can be made from: (*a*) infected uterine exudate which occurs immediately prior to, during, and usually 1 to 2 weeks following abortion; (*b*) infected aborted feti; (*c*) infected fetal membrane; and (*d*) milk from infected udders. Cultures may be made directly on artificial media or through inoculation of suspected tissues, excretions or secretions into guinea pigs and subsequent isolation on artificial media.

2. *Serology.* Because of simplicity of operation and high reliability of results, serological tests have been used extensively throughout the world for the diagnosis of brucellosis: (*a*) agglutination test. This is a procedure for the identification of specific Brucella antibodies in serum, milk, and cervical mucus. Using serum, the tube method and the rapid plate method may be utilized. Standard serum dilutions are 1:50, 1:100, and 1:200. The interpretation of the test varies among vaccinated and non-vaccinated cattle and is shown in table 5.

The milk ring test consists of mixing whole milk with stained Brucella antigen. In case of specific Brucella antibodies in the milk, the antigen is clumped and carried by fat droplets to the surface to produce a ring of clumps of stained antigen over the milk. This test is used extensively on composite samples of milk to survey herds suspected of low incidence of brucellosis. Herds positive to the milk ring test are commonly subjected to individual serological agglutination tests.

(*b*) Complement fixation test. While the complement fixation test possesses high accuracy, the complexity of the precedure has relegated it to limited application to special problems.

The differential diagnosis requires consideration of other abortifacients and infertility diseases, especially trichomoniasis, vibriosis and viral bovine rhinotracheitis. Trichomoniasis, an infectious venereal disease, is associated with infertility and occasionally with abortion during the first 5 months of gestation and, uncommonly, with pyometra. While a record of herd infertility indicates possible trichomoniasis, a positive diagnosis depends on identification of the causative protozoan, *Trichomonas fetus,* in vaginal and uterine exudate, aborted fetuses or prepucial secretions. Motile *T. fetus* can be demonstrated by microscopic examination of infected material.

TABLE 5

Vaccinates				*Others*			
1:50	*1:100*	*1:200*	*Interpretation*	*1:50*	*1:100*	*1:200*	*Interpretation*
−	−	−	negative	−	−	−	negative
±	−	−	negative	±	−	−	suspect
+	−	−	negative	+	−	−	suspect
+	±	−	suspect	+	±	−	suspect
+	+	−	suspect	+	+	−	positive
+	+	±	suspect	+	+	±	positive
+	+	+	positive	+	+	+	positive

Vibriosis, also a venereal infection, causes infertility in newly infected herds and in heifers and in susceptible cows added to long infected herds. Abortion, with a rate varying from 4 to 20%, may occur at any stage of gestation, but the highest incidence is during the fourth to seventh months. A positive diagnosis is obtained by culturing and identifying pathogenic *V. fetus* from the vaginal mucus, aborted fetus, or prepucial secretions.

Viral bovine rhinotracheitis may cause abortion 3 to 4 weeks following the disease. The virus may be isolated from the placenta and fetus.

Prevention. Brucellosis may be avoided through immunization and by reducing or preventing exposure to the disease. The vaccine, composed of viable bacterial cells of Strain 19, is administered to calves, preferably 4 to 8 months, an age range of natural resistance to brucellosis. Most calves immunized during that range lose the vaccination titer by the time of sexual maturity. The immunization evoked through calfhood vaccination endures for the life of the animal. While adult cattle may be immunized, vaccination titer persists and cannot be differentiated from the titer from natural brucellosis.

Brucellosis eradication programs have been initiated in many countries. In the United States, the procedure is a state-federal plan which utilizes calfhood vaccination together with the identification by test followed by slaughter of reactors. The plan is based on individual herd and area participation. The certified brucellosis-free herd is obtained through official participation in the eradication program. A herd may obtain the certification by passing two negative blood tests with an interval of 12 to 18 months. Additional blood tests may be conducted if the owner or certifying agencies so desire. Herd certification may also be obtained by passing three consecutive milk ring tests within 90 days and followed by a negative herd blood test within an additional 90 days of the last milk ring test.

Through cooperation of cattle herd owners, brucellosis may be eradicated from an area by application of: (1) the modified certified brucellosis area plan followed by (2) the certified brucellosis-free area plan. The modified certified brucellosis area status may be acquired by having: (1) not more than 1% positive reactors to the blood test in all cattle of the area; and (2) a herd infection rate not to exceed 5%. Infected herds are quarantined until they pass one negative blood test at least 30 days following removal of reactor cattle. Certification is for 3 years. Recertification may be obtained by blood testing all herds which contained infection on the previous test and 20% of other representative herds and by demonstrating that not more than 1% of the cattle and 5% of the herds are infected.

The certified brucellosis-free area status is obtained through complete elimination of the disease in cattle of the area as indicated by negative reactions to the blood test.

References

Bang, B.: Die Aetiologie des Seuchenhoften Verwerfens. Zeitschr. Tiermedzin, *1* (1897): 241–278.

Blunt, M. H.: The Conception Rates of Beef Cattle in the Gisborne District in Relation to Strain 19 Inoculation. New Zealand Vet. J., *7* (1959): 151–154.

Cotton, W. E.: Efficacy of Different Strains of *Brucella abortus* as an Immunizing Agent against Contagious Abortion. J. Agri. Res., *45* (1932): 705.

Cruickshank, J. C.: The Duration of Bacteremia in Relation to the Virulence of Brucella Strains. J. Hygiene, *55* (1957): 140–147.

Doyle, T. M.: The Distribution of *Br. abortus* in the System of "Carrier" Cows. J. Comp. Path., *48* (1935): 192–217.

Fleischhaur, G.: Die Abortus-Bang Ring-probe (ABR) Zur Festellung von bangverdachtigen Vollmilch proben, *53* (1937): 527–528.

Freeman, B. A., Kross, Damon, J. and Circo, R.: Host-Parasite Relationships in Brucellosis. J. Inf. Dis., *108* (1961): 333–338.

Gilman, H. L. and Wagner, W. C.: The Evaluation of Brucellosis Vaccination at 4 and 8 Months of Age. Cornell Vet., *49* (1959): 399–408.

Goode, E. R., Jr., Manthei, C. A. and Amerault, T. E.: Further Studies on Duration of Immunity to Brucellosis Induced in Calf-Vaccinated Cattle with

Strain 19 Vaccine. U. S. Livestock Sanitary Assoc. Proceed., 1956, pp. 89–96.

Grachev, I. I. and Galusyan, R. A.: Experiment in Recovery of Cattle From Brucellosis Isolation. Veterinariya, *34* (1957): No. 2, pp. 20–21.

Huddleson, I. Forest: *Brucellosis in Man and Animals.* The Commonwealth Fund. New York. 1943.

Lambert, G., Amerault, T. E., Manthei, C. A. and Goode, E. R.: Immunogenic Response of Calves Vaccinated at Different Ages with *Brucella abortus* Strain 19, U. S. Livestock Sanitary Assoc. Proceed., 1961, pp. 93–99.

Losses in Agriculture. U.S.D.A. Agri. Research Service. June, 1954. ARS-20-1. pp. 129.

Manthei, C. A. and Carter, R. W.: Persistence of *Brucella abortus* Infection in Cattle. AJVR, *11* (1950): 173–180.

McClure, T. J. and Fyvie, A. A.: Vaginal Mucus and Serum *Brucella abortus* Antibody Titres. New Zealand Vet. J., *4* (1956): 170.

McCullough, N. B., Eisele, C. W. and Byrne, A. F.: Incidence and Distribution of *Br. abortus* in Slaughtered Bangs Reactor Cattle. Public Health Rep. *66* (1951): 341–345.

McDiarmid, A.: The Degree and Duration of Immunity in Cattle Resulting from Vaccination with S 19 *Br. abortus* Vaccine and its Implication in the Future Control and Eventual Eradication of Brucellosis. Vet. Rec., *69* (1957): 877–879.

Morgan, W. J. B. and McDiarmid, A.: The Excretion of *Brucella abortus* in Milk of Experimentally Infected Cattle. Res. Vet. Sc., *1* (1960): 53–56.

Payne, J. M.: The Pathogenesis of Experimental Brucellosis in the Pregnant Cow. J. Path. & Bact., *78* (1959): 447–463.

Pearce, J. H., Williams, A. E., Harris-Smith, Patricia W., Fitzgeorge, R. B. and Smith, H.: The Chemical Basis of the Virulence of *Brucella abortus.* II. Erythritol, a Constituent of Bovine Foetal Fluids which Stimulates the Growth of *Br. abortus* in Bovine Phagocytes. Brit. Jour. Exp. Path., *43* (1962): 31–37.

Pomales-Lebron, A. and Stinebring, W. R.: Intracellular Multiplication of *Brucella abortus* in Normal and Immune Mononuclear Phagocytes. Soc. Exp. Biol. & Med. Proc., *94* (1957): 78–82.

Prohaszka, L.: A Live Vaccine Against Bovine Brucellosis. Mag. Allator. Lapja, *14* (1959): 380–382.

Richardson, M.: Parasitization *in vitro* of Bovine Cells by *Brucella abortus.* J. Bact., *78* (1959): 769–777.

Sadler, W. W.: Present Evidence on the Role of Meat in the Epidemiology of Human Brucellosis. Am. J. Public Health, *50* (1960): 504–514.

Smith, H., Keppie, J., Pearce, J. H., Fuller, R. and Williams, A. E.: The Chemical Basis of the Virulence of *Brucella abortus.* I. Isolation of *Br. abortus* from Bovine Foetal Tissues. Brit. J. Exp. Path., *42* (1961): 631-637.

Smith, R. W., Birth, R. R., Bishop, C. P., Donham, C. R. and West, R. L.: What is known about Brucellosis. U. S. Livestock Sanitary Assoc., 1949.

Stableforth, A. W. and Galloway, I. A.: *Infectious Diseases of Animals.* Diseases Due to Bacteria. Vol. 1. Academic Press, Inc. New York, 1959.

Williams, A. E., Keppie, J. and Smith, H.: Chemical Basis of Virulence of *Brucella abortus.* III. Foetal Erythritol a Cause of Localization of *Br. abortus* in Pregnant Cows. Brit. J. Exp. Path., *43* (1962): 530.

The Rumenitis-Liver Abscess Complex

(**HEPATIC NECROBACILLOSIS; LIVER ABSCESSES**)

Inflammation of the forestomachs and focal infection in the liver constitute a complex in which rumenitis is primary and hepatic necrobacillosis is secondary. Two forms are recognized: (1) chronic liver abscesses, a very prevalent condition; and (2) acute hepatic necrobacillosis, an uncommon malady. High economic loss from the disease results from liver and rumen condemnations at slaughter, limited mortality, and diminished efficiency in feed utilization. If each liver is worth $6.00, condemnations cause an annual loss to the national industry of more than $17 million. Although low in incidence, deaths from acute necrobacillosis and from ruptured liver abscesses add to the loss. Damages from reduced feed-use efficiency, even though real, have not been measured. While abscessed liver is usually asymptomatic, acute hepatic necrobacillosis causes profound illness.

Review of Literature. National surveys have indicated that approximately 10% of cattle slaughtered in the United States have abscessed livers and that, in most affected animals, abscesses are limited to the liver and only rarely occur in other organs (Federal Meat Inspection, 1967–1969). Two careful and extensive investigations revealed that *Spherophorus necrophorus* is present in pure infection in 85% of liver abscesses, that an additional 10% contain S. *necrophorus*, plus some other bacteria, and that the remaining 5% contain such bacteria as Streptococci, Staphylococci, and Corynebacteria (Newson, 1938; Madin, 1949). S. *necrophorus*, present in the stomachs of most healthy or diseased cattle, is probably ubiquitous in manure and soil (Robinson, Jasper and Gilbert, 1951). Experimental inoculation of viable S. *necrophorus* into ruminal branches of the portal vein produced abscesses in the livers of cattle (Jensen, Flint and Griner, 1954). Serial slaughter of cattle being fattened revealed that telangiectasis develops first and is followed by "sawdust" and abscesses. This sequence of developments suggested that telangiectasis predisposes to abscesses (Jensen, Frey, Cross and Connell, 1947).

Since S. *necrophorus* produces abscesses in healthy livers, is present normally in the contents of the stomach, and is unable to penetrate healthy skin and mucous membrane, the problem was how S. *necrophorus*, present in the contents of the rumen, penetrates the veins in the ruminal wall. To obtain a solution, extensive surveys were made of slaughtered cattle from which the rumens and livers were studied. The rumens were examined for evidence of inflammation and the livers for abscesses. Statistically, a positive correlation was found for the occurrence of rumenitis and liver abscesses in the same animal. Ruminal lesions were classified as acute and chronic. Grossly observed, acute rumenitis exhibited necrosis, edema and hemorrhage in the mucosa. Microscopically, S. *necrophorus* was observed in subepithelial

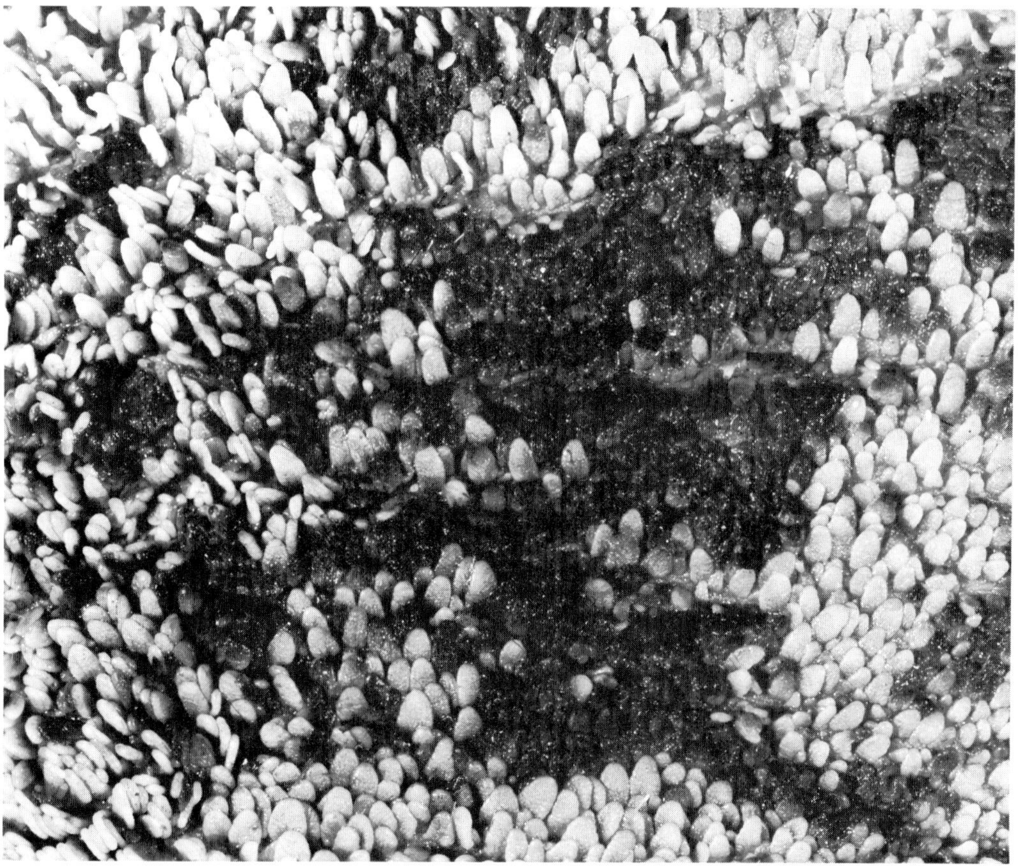

FIG. 4-6. *Acute rumenitis with necrosis of papillae.* × 1.0.

tissue where it had access to branches of the portal vein. Chronic rumenitis, viewed grossly, evinced depapillation, often depigmentation, ulcers, ulcer scars, epithelial nodules and granulation tissue nodules. *S. necrophorus* was not observed microscopically in chronic lesions (Jensen, Deane, Cooper, Miller and Graham, 1954; Smith, 1944).

The specific causes of rumenitis are multiple. In one study of the stomachs from 2,042 cattle having abscessed livers, 33% contained foreign metallic bodies in the contents. These bodies were responsible for considerable injury to the mucous membrane (Fredrick, 1943). Experimentation demonstrated that two factors contributed to rumenitis: a rapid rate of change from a ration of roughage to a ration with a high percentage of concentrate and fattening on a ration containing a 4:1 (or more) ratio of concentrate to roughage (Jensen, Connell and Deem, 1954). In Scotland where young cattle are fattened on diets containing up to 90% barley, extensive rumen lesions were found and investigated. After 2 or more weeks on the barley diet, ruminal papillae were clumped and loosely held together by ingested animal hairs, plant fibers and decomposing feed (Fell, Kay and Walker, 1967). The ruminal changes were epithelial acanthosis, hyperkeratosis and parakeratosis. Commonly, animal hairs and barley rachilla fibers had penetrated the mucous membrane and inoculated bacteria from the ruminal contents into the lamina propria. These lesions resulted in variable amounts of rumenitis (Fell, Kay, Whitelaw and Boyne, 1968).

Attempts to develop and institute rumenitis-preventive programs have had some success. In Scotland, the inclusion of 7.5% sodium bicarbonate in a diet of 82.5% barley reduced ruminal lesions to a negligible amount. The protection was interpreted as resulting from avoiding excessively low pH values in ruminal contents (Kay, Fell and Boyne, 1969). Experimentation over 2 years, involving nearly 2,000 cattle, indicated that continuous feeding of chlortetracycline in the feed at the rate of 70 to 75 mg per animal per day significantly reduced, but did not eliminate, liver abscesses (Flint and Jensen, 1958).

Occurrence. Liver abscesses are commonly observed in heavily fattened cattle. While as many as 95% of the animals within some lots contain liver abscesses, these lesions occur in and cause condemnation of approximately 10% of livers of all cattle slaughtered in the United States. Usually the abscesses begin to develop after 60 days of fattening. Incidence of the disease is high in fattened cattle of either sex and of ages 10 to 24 months. The liver lesions are reproducible by intraportal inoculation of viable *S. necrophorus* into cattle, sheep, rabbits and guinea pigs. Swine are refractory. Geographically, the disease is nationwide but of consistently higher incidence in cattle of the western United States. Areas such as the Provinces of Canada as well as Scotland and Italy where cattle are fattened have a high incidence of the disease. Acute hepatic necrobacillosis, even though uncommon, occurs sporadically at any time during fattening.

Etiology and Pathogenesis. Rumenitis and liver abscesses, each distinct entities, have specific causes, but the two lesions are related because rumenitis predisposes to liver abscesses.

Factors causing rumenitis include: (1) rapid rate of change from a diet of roughage to one high in concentrate, (2) fattening with a diet containing more than 25% concentrate, (3) foreign body penetration of the wall, and (4) miscellaneous agents. Cattle entering the feedlot from range or pasture are fully adjusted to digesting a diet of roughage. Changing the diet to concentrate commonly occurs over a period varying from a few to 10 days. Under these circumstances, ruminal microorganisms produce excessive amounts of lactic acid and probably other unidentified irritating substances. The prolonged or repeated low pH values evoke the formation of epithelial acanthosis, hyperkeratosis and

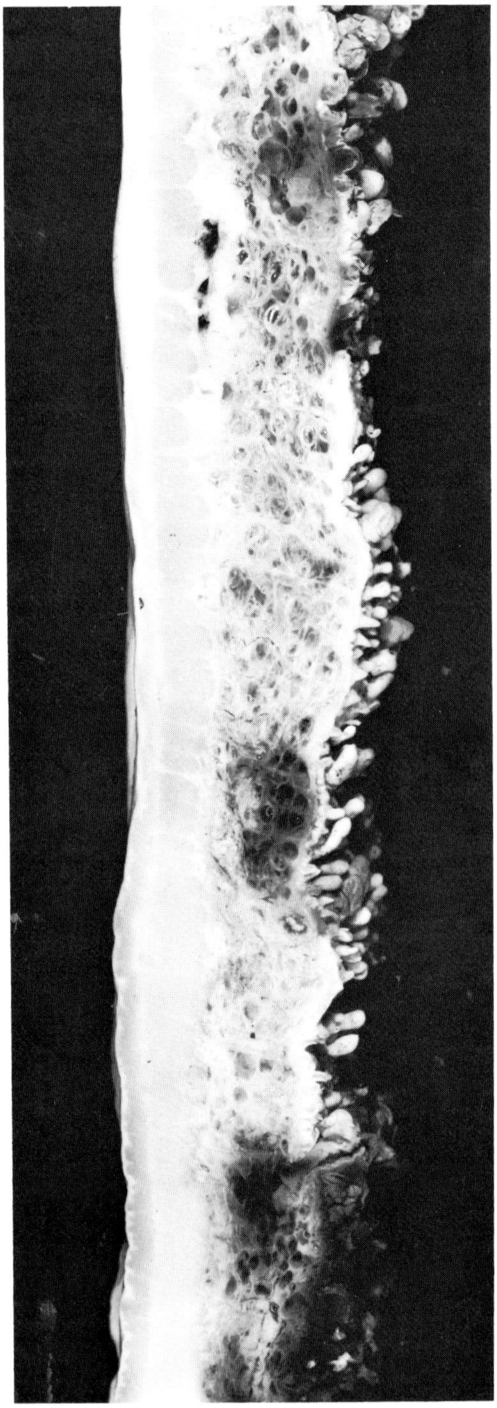

FIG. 4-7. *Cross section of ruminal wall with acute inflammation. The mucosa and submucosa are edematous, gaseous, and necrotic.* × 1.8.

parakeratosis. The mucous membrane, including papillae, become thickened and hardened. The unidentified irritants cause necrosis of epithelium and, in some cases, of the lamina propria. Hemorrhage into the necrotic tissue is common and affected papillae may slough. Affected areas are usually located in the anterior ventral sac of the rumen. Fattening cattle on rations having more than 25% concentrate is a common practice because economy of the enterprise requires fattening in the minimum time. In some feedlots the diets may be as much as 90% concentrate. The fermentation of such feed by ruminal microorganisms also causes prolonged or repeated low pH values followed possibly by acanthosis, hyperkeratosis and parakeratosis with clumping of papillae and thickening and hardening of the mucous membrane. Penetrating foreign bodies include pieces of wire, nails and other metal fragments, and animal hairs and plant fibers. The wire and nails contaminate feed, either alfalfa or grain, and are ingested along with the feed. Ruminal movements and abnormal animal positions may cause some of the metal pieces to abrade and penetrate the mucous membrane. Because of small amounts of roughage in the diet, many cattle develop abnormal appetites and consequently chew wood from fences, pull and ingest hair from their coats. Plant fibers, especially from seed awns and rachillae from barley and wheat, are ingested in large amounts. Some of the animal hairs and plant fibers accumulate between clumped papillae and in folds of hyperkeratotic epithelium. As with metals, ruminal movements cause the hairs and fibers to gradually penetrate the epithelium and enter the lamina propria. Bacteria, including S. *necrophorus* mechanically carried by the foreign bodies, contribute to the cause of rumenitis. Miscellaneous factors include vesicating viruses and ingested poisons. Occasionally these agents cause rumenitis.

The direct cause of most bovine liver abscesses is *Spherophorus necrophorus.* Widely distributed in feedlot manure and

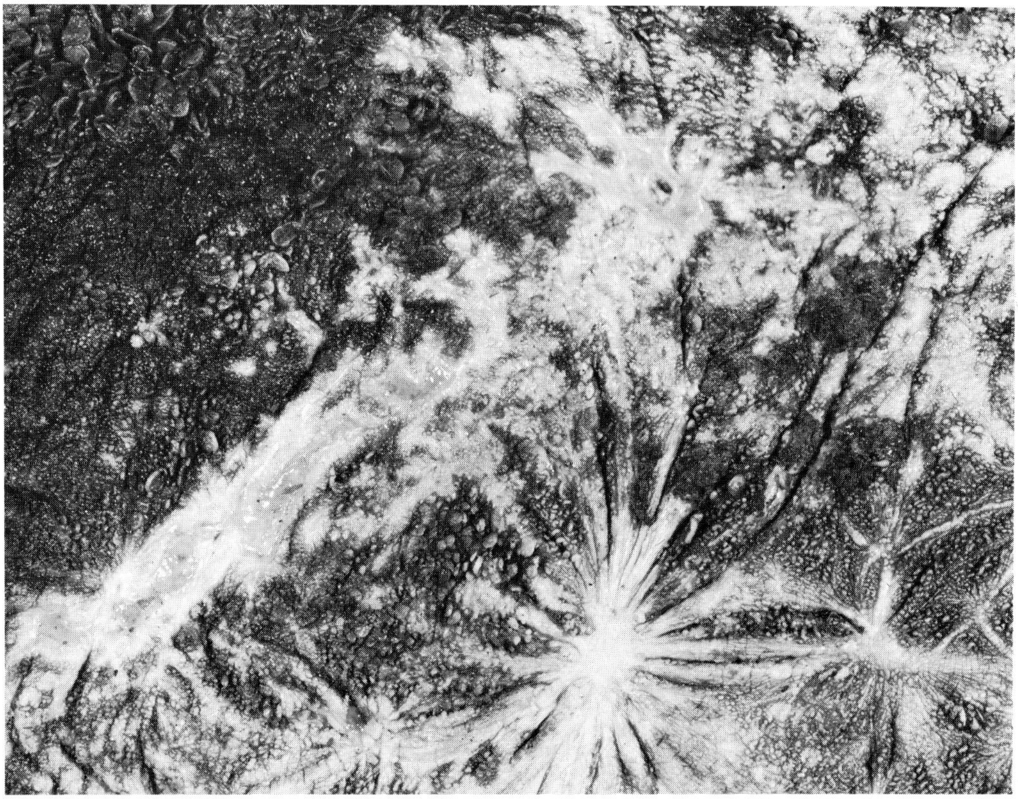

FIG. 4-8. *Chronic rumenitis. The mucosa is ulcerated, scarred, depigmented and depapillated.* × 1.0.

soil, this species of bacteria inhabits the alimentary tract, especially the rumen, of healthy and diseased cattle. In addition to liver abscesses, it is commonly found in lesions of foot rot and calf diphtheria as well as contaminated wounds. The organism has no ability to penetrate healthy and intact skin and mucous membrane. When inoculated into non-covering tissue, however, it becomes pathogenic and causes extensive necrosis, a characteristic from which it acquired its specific name. Highly pleomorphic, S. *necrophorus* in young active lesions and in new growing cultures is filamentous, non-branching, granular, variable in width and gram-negative in staining; while in old lesions and old cultures it becomes coccoid and rod-shaped. Although not easily cultured on artificial media, the organism does grow under strictly anaerobic conditions on solid

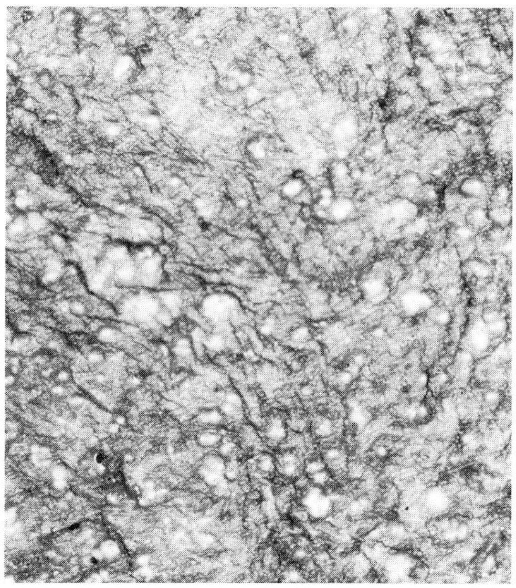

FIG. 4-9. *Chronic rumenitis with nodules of granulation tissue on surface.* × 0.9.

media, such as blood agar, and in liquid media, such as Roseneous' brain broth with a pH between 7.0 and 8.4. It produces acid and gas by fermenting glucose, maltose and glycerol, but does not ferment xylose, rhamnose, mannose, raffinose, inulin, dulcitol, dextrin, erythritol, sorbitol or inositol. The endotoxins of the organism probably contribute to the cause of necrosis. Being highly susceptible to many adverse factors, the organism is killed in 15 minutes by temperature of 55° C, and it is easily killed by most standard disinfectants.

Most aspects in the pathogenesis of liver abscesses are understood. S. *necrophorus* always present in ruminal contents, penetrates the covering epithelium through points of injury, discontinuity and necrosis. The organism may also be carried mechanically through the epithelium by penetrating foreign bodies, such as sharp metals, animal hairs and plant fibers. Once introduced beneath the epithelium, the organism proliferates, produces endotoxins and causes extensive necrosis of tissue, and these changes contribute to the cause of rumenitis. In the tissue the bacteria grow into branches of the portal vein, enter the blood and are propelled by current into the liver. Inoculation of the liver by way of the portal blood with a small number of relatively less virulent S. *necrophorus* results in single or few foci of infection. Following localization, the bacteria proliferate and produce necrosis of hepatic tissue. Each focus of necrosis commonly reaches a diameter of 15 to 20 mm. After a course of a few days, leukocytes accumulate around the focus of infection and stop further growth. After approximately 5 days from the time of inoculation, fibroplasia begins at the periphery of the lesion to form a wall of fibrous connective tissue. The abscesses endure as long as 180 days but eventually heal and form scars. Single or few liver abscesses produce little or no functional disturbance and no clinical signs. Occasionally, however, fatality results from either large numbers of abscesses and hepatic insufficiency or from rupture of an abscess followed by peritonitis.

Rarely some bacteria pass through the liver and are carried by the blood into the lungs. In this organ they localize and may produce abscesses. The aerobic conditions in the lungs, however, are unfavorable to S. *necrophorus*.

Heavy inoculation of the liver with large numbers of highly virulent S. *necrophorus* results in acute necrobacillosis. Multiple foci of infection are initiated nearly simultaneously. As many as 50 foci, many confluent, may be present. Growth of the localized organisms causes coagulative necrosis of hepatic tissue. The area of infection and necrosis expands to reach a diameter in each focus to as much as several centimeters. Some foci of infection extend through the liver capsule and into the peritoneal cavity where generalized peritonitis develops. Toxic metabolites from the liver infection and from the peritonitis are absorbed into the systemic circulation resulting in fever, profound depression, and often death. Some organisms may pass through the liver and enter the lungs where similar lesions may be produced.

The hypothesis that the etiologic organisms of this disease are inoculated into the animal through the lesions of calf diphtheria and foot rot is not tenable. Inoculation of the veins in any anatomical peripheral area of the systemic circulation, as has been shown experimentally, produces lung abscesses and, by organisms passing through the lungs, abscesses in all other organs. Extra-hepatic lesions seldom are encountered. Inoculation of the liver through the hepatic circulation logically explains the type of infection and the nature and distribution of lesions as observed in fattened cattle.

Clinical Signs and Postmortem Lesions. In the rumen, acute or chronic inflammation is discernible commonly in the antero-ventral sac. Foreign-body injuries often are in the reticulum. Grossly, foci of acute rumenitis exhibit necrosis, swelling, edema and hemorrhage. Sometimes gas bodies and edema are found in the wall. Microscopically, S. *necrophorus* can be observed in the injured tissue. Chronic rumenitis, grossly observed, manifests depapillation, depigmentation, ulcers, nodules of granulation tissue, epithelial nodules and scars. Microscopically, S. *necrophorus* is not discernible. The floor of an ulcer consists of granulation tissue. The epithelial nodule is a mass of squamous epithelium. The cleaning of affected rumens, as for the preparation of tripe, is difficult and often uneconomical.

Liver abscesses, except in rare cases, are asymptomatic. At slaughter or necropsy the liver contains single or multiple abscesses. Usually the abscess consists of a central mass of necrotic liver surrounded by pus and a wall of connective tissue. Healed abscesses leave scars. In case of rupture of an abscess, masses of pus extend onto the surface of the liver, and peritonitis is present. At slaughter most livers affected with abscesses are condemned for human food.

The acute necrobacillosis is characterized by profound intoxication and depression. Body temperature ranges from normal to 105° F. Icterus is often discernible in the sclera and other mucous membranes. The abdomen is tense from peritonitis. Diarrhea, with yellowish discoloration of fluid feces, is also common. In some animals the posterior limbs are swollen. Reluctant movements may be accompanied by grunting and by forward knuckling at the posterior fetlock joints. At necropsy, the liver discloses multiple foci of necrosis and acute peritonitis. The pale, brown, and firm foci of necrosis are readily palpable throughout the organ. Where the necrosis extends through the liver capsule, fibrinous exudate is deposited. Serofibrinous exudate is distributed throughout the peritoneal cavity. Occasionally, some organisms have passed through the liver into the lungs and there have produced additional foci of necrosis. Histopathologically, both viable and dead colonies of S. *necrophorus* are widely distributed throughout the

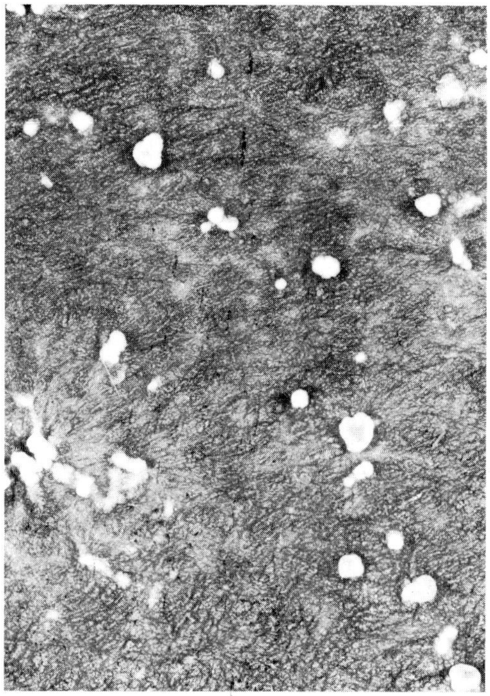

FIG. 4-10. *Chronic rumenitis with epithelial nodules in the mucosa.* × 1.0.

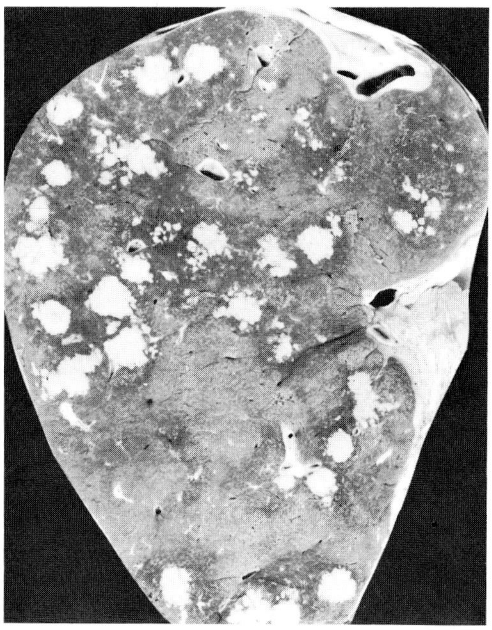

FIG. 4-11. *Cross section of liver with acute necrobacillosis.* × 0.5.

necrotic tissue. Highly viable organisms are discernible at the junction of necrotic and viable liver tissue.

Diagnosis. Liver abscesses are seldom diagnosed clinically. At slaughter or necropsy the abscesses are readily identified. Ruminal lesions are also detectable after the organ has been emptied and cleaned.

Acute necrobacillosis with peritonitis is diagnosed clinically on the basis of typical signs. Fever, grunting, icterus, reluctance to move and abdominal tenseness are of significant importance. The differential diagnosis requires consideration of traumatic reticulitis. In the latter disease, the affected animal usually is constipated and discloses a high degree of sensitivity to pressure over the xyphoid cartilage. Swelling of the posterior limbs is absent.

Prevention and Treatment. The incidence of rumenitis, and consequently liver abscesses, can be reduced by avoiding the contamination of feed with penetrating objects, such as nails, pieces of wire and glass, and by a gradual transfer of animals from a ration of roughage to a ration of concentrate over a period of 2 to 3 weeks. Fattening on a diet containing less than 75% concentrate helps to prevent rumenitis. In addition, avoiding low pH values in the rumen contents may reduce rumenitis. Protection against high acidity, especially important during early stages of fattening, can be achieved by including in the diet sodium bicarbonate at the rate of 7.5% of the concentrate. The inci-

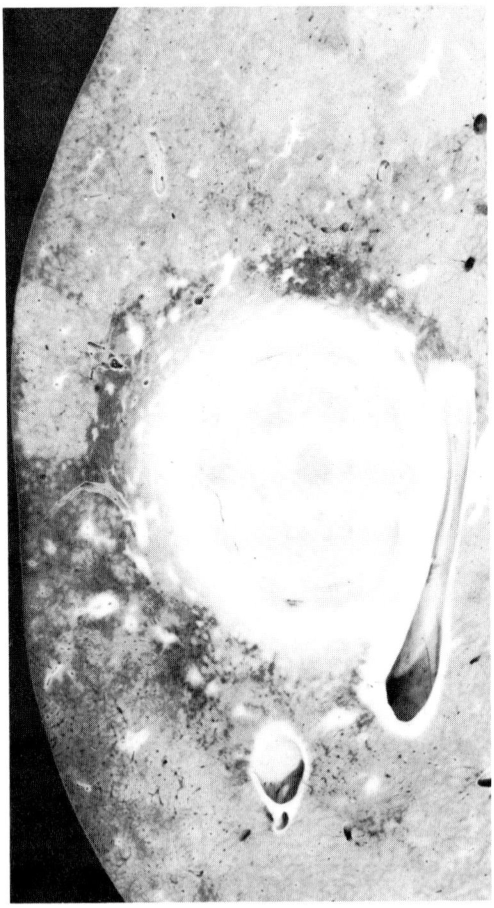

FIG. 4-12. *Cross section of liver abscess.* × 1.3.

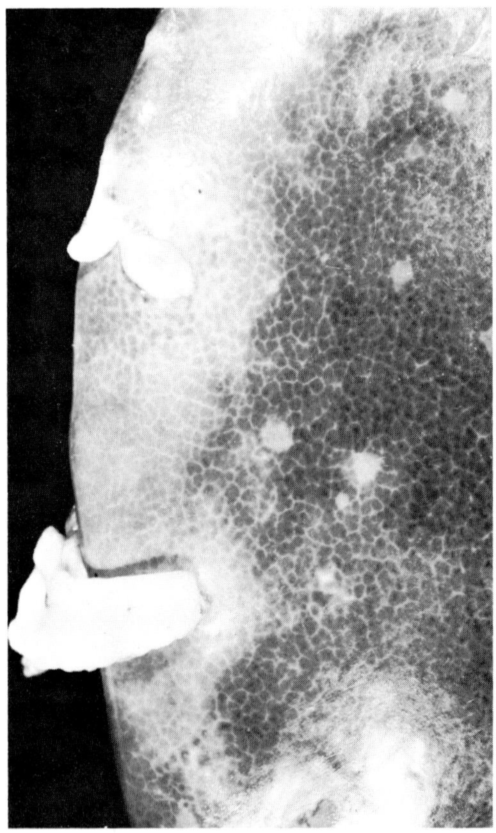

FIG. 4-13. *A liver abscess ruptured into the peritoneal cavity.* × 1.0.

dence of liver abscesses can be reduced, but not eliminated, by continuous feeding during the fattening process of chlortetracycline in the diet at the rate of 70 mg per animal per day.

References

Baker, J. A., McEntee, K. and Gillespie, J. H.: Effects of IBR-IPV Virus on New-born Calves. Cornell Vet., *50* (1960): 156.

Federal Meat Inspection. Statistical Summary. Consumer Marketing Service, USDA (1967–1969).

Fell, B. F., Kay, M. and Walker, J. T.: Ruminal Lesions in Cattle Fed on Barley. Vet. Rec., *81* (1967): 715–716.

Fell, B. F., Kay M., Whitelaw, F. G. and Boyne, R.: Observations on the Development of Ruminal Lesions in Calves Fed on Barley. Res. Vet. Sc., *9* (1968): 458–466.

Flint, J. C. and Jensen, Rue: The Effect of Chlortetracycline, Fed Continuously During Fattening, on the Incidence of Liver Abscesses in Beef Cattle. AJVR, *19* (1958): 830–832.

Frederick, L. D.: The Economic and Nutritional Importance of Bovine Hepatic Disturbances. JAVMA, *102* (1943): 338–345.

Jensen, Rue, Frey, Paul R., Cross, Floyd and Connell, W. E.: Telangiectasis, "Sawdust", and Abscesses in the Livers of Cattle. JAVMA, *110* (1947): 256–261.

Jensen, Rue, Deane, Harold M., Cooper, L. John, Miller, V. A. and Graham, W. R.: The Rumenitis-Liver Abscess Complex in Beef Cattle. AJVR, *15* (1954): 202–216.

Jensen, Rue, Flint, J. C. and Griner, L. A.: Experimental Hepatic Necrobacillosis in Beef Cattle. AJVR, *15* (1954): 5–14.

Jensen, Rue, Connell, W. E. and Deem, A. W.: Rumenitis and its Relation to Rate of Change of Ration and the Proportion of Concentrate in the Ration of Cattle. AJVR, *15* (1954): 425–428.

Kay, M., Fell, B. F. and Boyne, R.: The Relationship Between Acidity of the Rumen Contents and Rumenitis in Calves Fed on Barley. Res. Vet. Sc., *10* (1969): 181–187.

Madin, S. H.: A Bacteriologic Study of Bovine Liver Abscesses. Vet. Med., *44* (1949): 248–251.

Newsom, I. E.: A Bacteriologic Study of Liver Abscesses in Cattle. J. Inf. Dis. *63* (1938): 232–233.

Robinson, T. J., Jasper, D. E. and Guilbert, H. R.: The Isolation of *Spherophorus necrophorus* From the Rumen, Together With Some Feedlot Data on Abscesses and Telangiectasis. J. An. Sci., *10* (1951): 733–741.

Smith, H. A.: Ulcerative Lesions of the Bovine Rumen and Their Possible Relation to Hepatic Abscesses. AJVR, *5* (1944): 234–243.

Calf Diphtheria

(NECROTIC LARYNGITIS)

Calf diphtheria, an acute or chronic infectious but non-contagious disease, is characterized by bilateral necrosis of the mucous membrane of the larynx, occurs in cattle as well as in other species of animals and is caused, in part, by *Spherophorus necrophorus.* The imprecisely measured losses are high because affected cattle lose weight, delay finishing, require extra labor and medicine for treatment and occasionally die. Bovine diphtheria has no relationship to the human disease.

Review of Literature. First described in 1876, this disease was considered closely related to human diphtheria (Dammenn, 1876). Detailed bacteriological and pathological studies of infected tissues revealed the presence of a filamentous gram-negative organism (Loeffler, 1884). This organism, observed in large numbers in necrotic tissues (Davis, 1952; Kitt, 1895; Scrivner and Lee, 1934), and identified as S. *necrophorus,* is the same bacterium found in liver abscesses and foot rot of cattle. Observations led to full agreement among investigators that diphtheria of cattle was distinct and also unrelated to diphtheria of people (Mohler and Morse, 1905). Attempts to reproduce the disease experimentally by placing infected laryngeal tissue in the larynx of normal cattle and by the application of pure recently isolated cultures of S. *necrophorus* to the larynx of normal cattle were generally unsuccessful (Dammenn, 1876; Davis, 1952). However, limited success was obtained by repeated daily topical application of a culture of S. *necrophorus* to the larynx and by a laryngeal spray of *Pasteurella multocida* followed by topical application to the larynx of S. *necrophorus.* Inoculation of viable S. *necrophorus* into the thyrolaryngeal artery produced extensive necrosis, but the lesions did not resemble diphtheria. (Davis, 1952). Transmission failures led to the postulation of predisposing causes such as inclement weather, widely fluctuating diurnal temperatures and viral infections (Farquharson, 1940; Mohler and Morse, 1905; Scrivner and Lee, 1934). An epizootiological study in a large feedlot (1955–1960) failed to show a relationship between viral bovine rhinotracheitis and diphtheria. From 1955 through 1958, viral bovine rhinotracheitis showed a high incidence; in 1959 and 1960, when vaccination against viral bovine rhinotracheitis was highly effective, the incidence of calf diphtheria remained reasonably uniform. Similarity of incidence during the pre-vaccination period and the post-vaccination period suggested that infection with the virus of viral bovine rhinotracheitis is not a predisposing factor in the cause of calf diphtheria (Scheel, 1960). The effectiveness of treatment with sulfapyridine was demonstrated experimentally and through extensive field utilization (Farquharson, 1940).

Occurrence. Diphtheria occurs equally in both sexes in animals 1 to 24 months of age. The incidence is approximately 0.2% of cattle as indicated in Table 6. In addition to cattle, the disease has been reported in sheep, swine and rabbits. Seasonally, it is more common during the months of November through February. Geographically, it is found in all major cattle producing countries.

Etiology and Pathogenesis. Probably the primary cause of diphtheria is an unknown agent which produces inflammation or injury to the mucous membrane of the rima glottidis of the larynx. The injury may be slight and of little importance in itself. Table 6 indicates that the control of viral bovine rhinotracheitis by vaccination did not reduce the incidence of calf diphtheria and, consequently, that the virus of viral bovine rhinotracheitis is not a primary cause of calf diphtheria. Other viruses, bacteria, manure dust and ambient temperature variations may be contributing primary factors. The secondary cause, S. *necrophorus*, is widely distributed in feedlot manure and soil, and in the mouths, rumens, stomachs and intestines of both healthy and diseased cattle. In addition to calf diphtheria, the organism is the secondary cause of foot rot and liver abscesses. The organism has no ability to attack or penetrate healthy intact mucous membrane or skin. However, it readily grows through injured mucous membrane and penetrates the submucosa and other non-covering tissues where it becomes pathogenic and causes extensive necrosis. Highly pleomorphic, S. *necrophorus* in young active lesions and in new growing cultures is filamentous, non-branching, non-sporforming, granular, variable in width and gram-negative in staining, while in old lesions and in old cultures it becomes coccoid and rod-shaped. Although not easily cultured on artificial media, the organism grows under strictly anerobic conditions on solid media, such as blood agar, and in liquid media, such as Roseneau's brain broth with a pH value of 7.0 to 8.4. It produces acid and gas by fermenting glucose, maltose and glycerol, but does not ferment xylose, rhamnose, mannose, raffinose, inulin, dulcitol, dextrin, erythritol, sorbitol or inositol. Endotoxins probably contribute to the cause of necrosis in non-covering tissue. Being highly susceptible to many adverse factors, the organism is killed in 15 minutes by temperature of 55° C, and it is easily killed by most standard disinfectants.

In the larynx S. *necrophorus* attacks the surface of the injured mucosa at two anatomical points: (1) the dorsal angle of the larynx and (2) over the vocal process of the arytenoid cartilage. Entering the submucosa, the organism grows and penetrates along the perichondrium, especially of the arytenoid cartilage, and often extends into the crico-arytenoid dorsalis muscle. In the cartilage, muscle and connective tissue, the infection causes extensive necrosis. most necrotic lesions are bilateral. The larynx becomes swollen and exudate accumulates on the mucous membrane over the points of infection. The swelling and exudate diminish the size of the lumen. Because of paralysis of the infected cricoartenoideus dorsalis muscle, the larynx fails to dilate fully during inspiration. This results in severe dyspnea and stertorous breathing.

During inspiration or expiration the violent rush of air through the larynx may detach clumps of infected exudate. If detachment occurs during inhalation, the exudate enters the lungs as an infected foreign body and often results in fatal gangrene and pneumonia. Small foci of non-fatal gangrene may be converted to pulmonary abscesses.

Healing may occur during any stage of the acute process by interruption of spread of infection. Death, however, may occur as a result of hypoxia, intoxication, pneumonia and pulmonary gangrene.

In some animals the disease becomes chronic. The infection localizes along the perichondrium of the arytenoid cartilage. The latter becomes sequestered and is attached at the muscular process only. A sinus may drain exudate to the surface near the vocal cord. In some cases a portion of the necrotic arytenoid cartilage projects through the sinus into the lumen of the larynx. Occasionally, a mass of granulation tissue forms on the surface and projects into the lumen. Any mass, necrotic cartilage or granulation tissue, projecting into the lumen of the larynx causes chronic respiratory roaring. Healing cannot take place until the necrotic cartilage is removed.

Clinical Signs and Postmortem Lesions. Following a sudden onset, the body temperature rises to 105° F, anorexia develops, and body weight diminishes rapidly. Coughing is prominent. Breathing is difficult and noisy, especially during inspiration. Because of dyspnea the head is extended, often with mouth breathing. Digital compression of the larynx or of the trachea usually evokes coughing and exaggerates dyspnea. Bronchopneumonia or pulmonary abscesses may develop. The course of the acute form varies from 7 to 10 days.

In chronic cases, appetite returns but the regaining of body weight is slow. Because of the projection of a portion of the arytenoid cartilage into the lumen, respiratory roaring persists and the course is prolonged. The lesions of acute or chronic diphtheria can be visualized and evaluated clinically by means of a laryngoscope.

At necropsy, lesions are limited to the respiratory system. The larynx shows generalized swelling with bilateral lesions over the vocal cords and/or at the dorsal angle. The lesions consist of inflammatory exudate on the surface and of necrosis which extends through the mucosa and submucosa. In some cases, necrosis extends around the arytenoid cartilage and into the cricoarytenoideus muscle. The lumen of the larynx may be occluded by swelling, exudate and adduction. Most fatal cases show bronchopneumonia and occasionally pulmonary gangrene and/or abscesses. In chronic cases, a portion of one or both arytenoid cartilages project through a sinus into the lumen of the larynx.

At slaughter of animals with chronic diphtheria, the carcass is acceptable for food if the physical condition, except for the larynx, is good.

Histopathologically, necrosis is extensive. Colonies of filamentous S. *necrophorus,* as well as other bacteria, are discernible

TABLE 6 *Incidence of calf diptheria and viral bovine rhinotracheitis in a large feedlot*

	1955–56	*1956–57*	*1957–58*	*1958–59*	*1959–60*
Cattle	55,000	60,000	65,000	70,000	77,000
Viral bovine rhinotracheitis %	3.6	4.2	1.8*	0.25	0.03
Diphtheria %	0.17	0.29	0.33	0.23	0.5

*Vaccination began fall 1958.

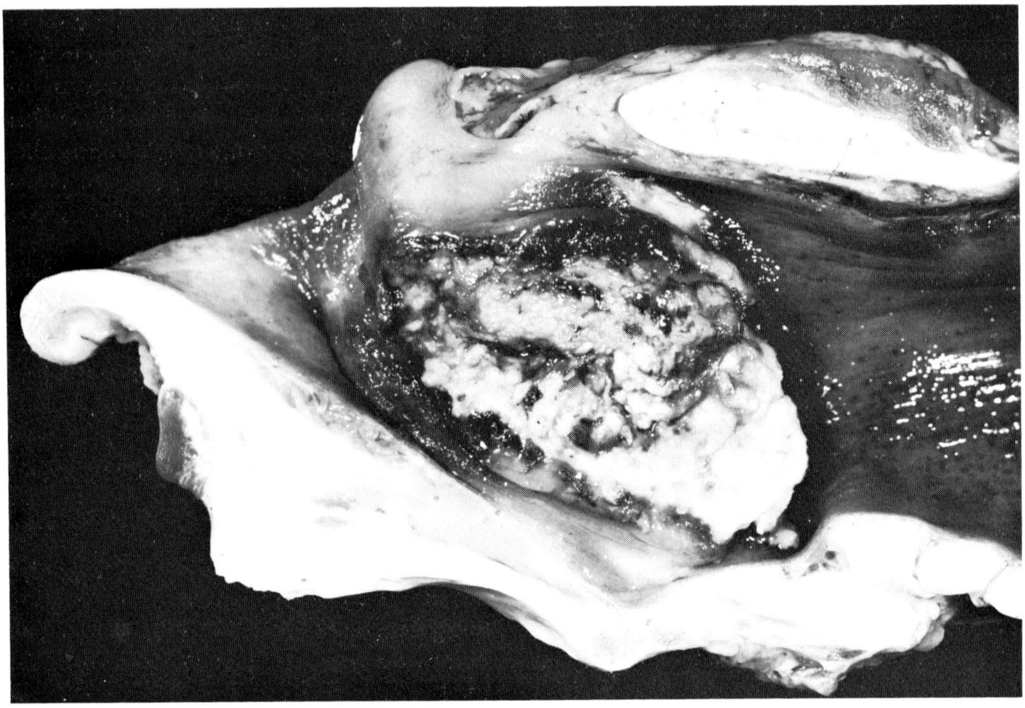

FIG. 4-14. *Necrosis and exudate over the vocal cord of the right half of the larynx from an animal with acute diphtheria.* × 1.2.

throughout the lesion. Inflammation is acute in early stages and chronic in prolonged cases.

Diagnosis. Clinically, the disease is diagnosed by typical clinical signs. Highly important are the dyspnea, roaring sounds emanating from the larynx, extension of the head and oral breathing. Visual examination of the larynx with a laryngoscope reveals the necrosis and some paralysis of the larynx in acute stages and, in chronic cases, the projection of cartilage or granulation tissue into the lumen. Differential diagnosis requires consideration of shipping fever, viral bovine rhinotracheitis, and nasal obstructions from granulomas, deformities of the turbinates, and hypoplasia of the nasal cavities in the Angus breed. Careful examination of the larynx, both externally and orally, should enable accurate differentiation.

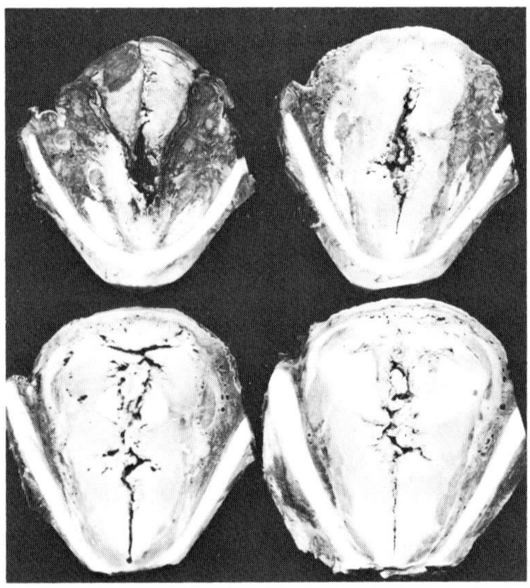

FIG. 4-15. *Serial cross sections of the larynx from an animal with acute diphtheria. Necrosis extends through mucosa and submucosa and into the muscularis. The lumen is nearly occluded.* × 0.6. (*Courtesy Dr. R. W. Davis.*)

Prevention and Treatment. Since the primary cause of calf diphtheria is not known,

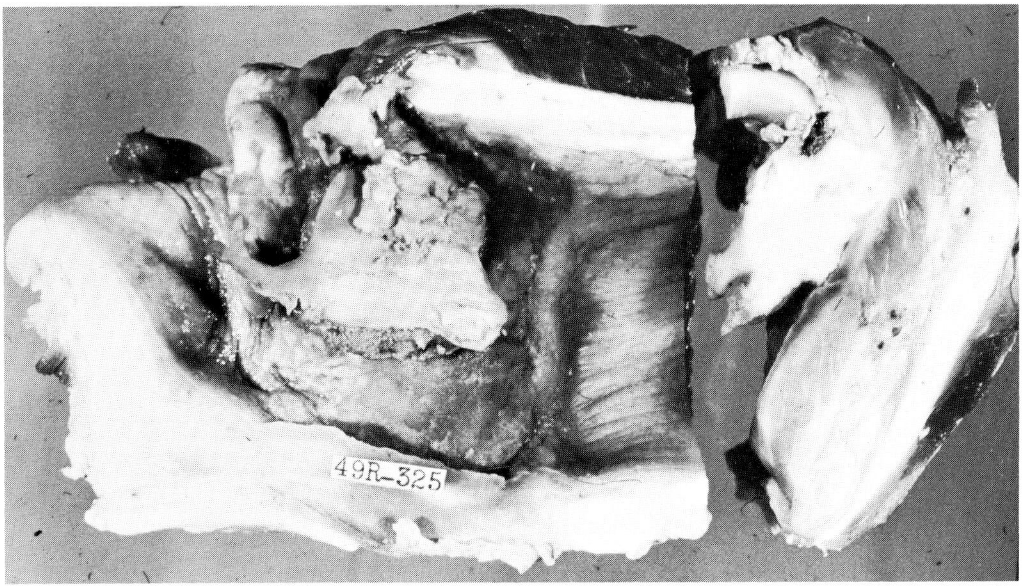

FIG. 4-16. *Chronic diphtheria in the right half of a larynx. The necrotic arytenoid cartilage projects into the lumen. At right is a cross section of the left half of the same larynx.* × 1.0. (*Courtesy Dr. R. W. Davis.*)

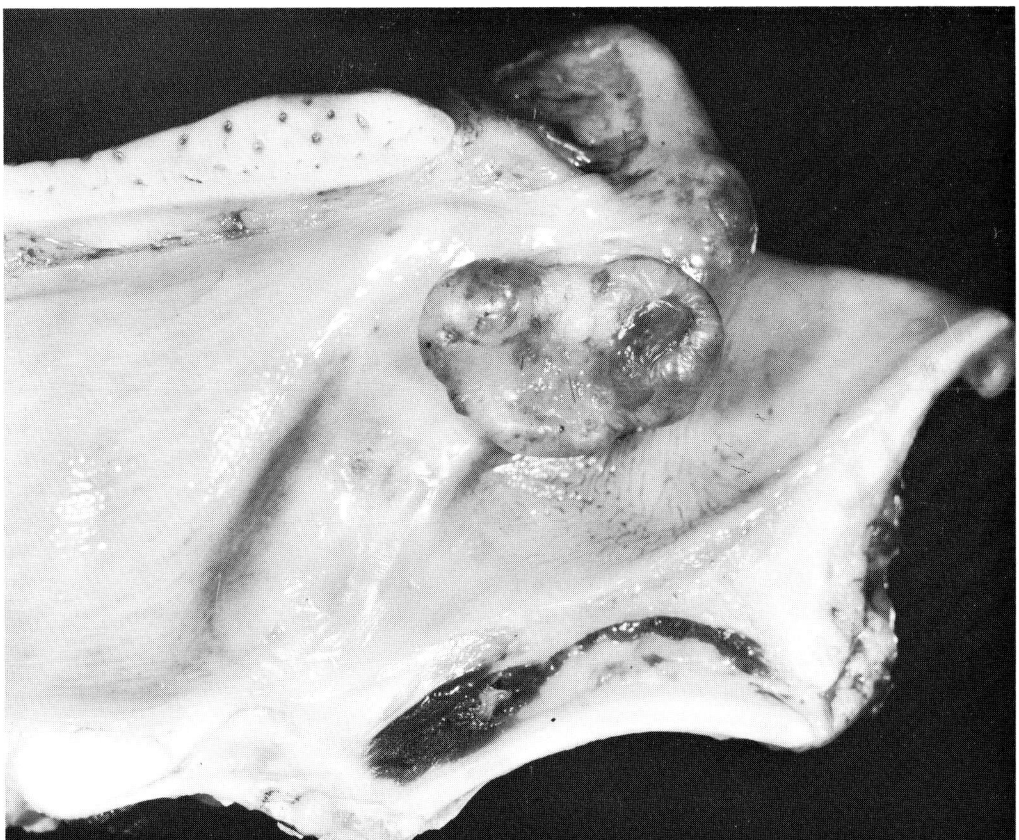

FIG. 4-17. *Left half of the larynx from an animal with chronic diphtheria. Papillary granulation tissue projects into the lumen.* × 1.4.

means of its prevention are not understood. Effective treatment of acute cases varies among animals and feedlots according to the mixture and resistance of bacterial pathogens. An effective drug is selected empirically from the following: sulfapyridine given intravenously at the rate of 1 grain per pound of body weight per day; oxytetracycline, tetracycline, chlorotetracycline, or chloromycetin given intravenously at the rate of 5 mg per pound of body weight per day. Topical administration of a proteolytic enzyme for removal of necrotic tissue is indicated. Swelling in the larynx and pharynx contraindicates the administration of drugs in boluses. In severe cases, where hypoxia has developed, a tracheal tube should be inserted. In case of chronic diphtheria with prolonged respiratory roaring, the necrotic cartilage must be excised surgically before healing can occur.

References

Adams, O. R., *et al.*: Comparison of Infectious Bovine Rhinotracheitis, Shipping Fever, and Calf Diphtheria of Cattle, JAVMA, *134* (1959): 85–89.

Dammenn, Carl: Die Diphtherie der Kalber eine neue, auf den Menschen ubertraglare Zoonose. Deutsch Zeitschrift fur Thier medcin und Vergleichende Pathologie, *3* (1876): 1–27.

Davis, R. W.: 1952. Pathology of Spontaneous and Experimental Necrotic Laryngitis in the Bovine. M.S. Thesis. Colorado State University Library, Fort Collins, Colorado.

Farquharson, J.: Sulfapyridine in the Treatment of Calf Diphtheria. JAVMA, *97* (1940): 431–436.

Kitt, T.: Diphtherischeerrkraukungen bei Schweinen und Kalbern. Dtsch. Zeitschrift fur Thiermedizen, *18* (1895) 81–88.

Loeffler, F.: Die Diphtheria beim Kalbe. Kaiserlichen gesundheitsamte Mittheilungen, *2* (1884): 489–499.

Mohler, J. R. and Morse, G. B.: *Bacillus necrophorus* and its economic Importance. (In U.S. Bureau of Animal Industry, 21st annual report, 1904. Washington Govt. Print. Off., 1905, pp. 76–116.)

Orcutt, M. L.: A Study of *Bacillus necrophorus* obtained from Cows. J. Bact., *20* (1930): 343–360.

Scrivner, L. H. and Lee, A. M.: The Morphology, Culture, Isolation, and Immunity Studies of *Actinomyces necrophorus* in Calf Diphtheria. JAVMA, *83* (1934): 360–378.

Schmorl, G.: Ueber ein Pathogenes Fadenbacterium (*Streptothrix curriculi*). Dtsch. Zeitschrift fur Thiermedizin, *17* (1891): 375–408.

Scheel, E. H. Personal communications. 1960.

Necrotic Posthitis

An acute infectious and possibly contagious disease, necrotic posthitis is characterized by evertive swelling, edema and necrosis in the prepuce of feedlot steers and bulls. The cause of the primary change, swelling and edema, is unknown, but the cause of the secondary necrosis is *Spherophorus necrophorus.* Although the economic importance of the disease has not been measured, it is assumed to be a significant cost to the industry. Losses result from reduction of body weight, delayed marketing, expensive treatments, and additional labor and care during convalescent periods. Losses can be minimized, however, by early diagnosis and treatment that prevent the development of extensive and prolonged complications. Formal research is seriously needed to determine the primary cause of the condition, and until new information is obtained, no rational preventive program is possible.

Occurrence. Necrotic posthitis occurs in feedlot steers and bulls. While the disease usually attacks cattle that have been fattened for 100 or more days, it may be encountered in animals with fewer days in the feedlot. The highest incidence is during spring and fall months and coincides with periods of rainfall and the development of muddy and unsanitary pens. Feedlots located in low-lying and insufficiently drained areas predispose animals to the disease. The geographic distribution is throughout the high plains, midwest and other cattle fattening areas where annual rainfall is seasonal and 15 or more inches in amount. Feedlots in arid areas, such as the southwestern part of the United States, are protected from serious attack because pens are drier and therefore more sanitary. Occasional outbreaks of necrotic posthitis may occur simultaneously with herd episodes of foot rot, a disease also caused by *S. necrophorus.*

Etiology and Pathogenesis. The cause of the primary swelling and edema of the preputial mucosa is not known. According to one hypothesis, moist manure, with multiple species of pathogenic and saprophytic bacteria, contaminates the preputial cavity; the irritating foreign material may actually cause swelling and edema. Another possible primary cause is the virus of bovine rhinotracheitis, a microorganism known to attack and cause primary lesions on the mucous membrane of the prepuce, penis and vulva. Necrotic posthitis, however, has not been associated with outbreaks of viral bovine rhinotracheitis, and its occurrence in animals immunized against viral bovine rhinotracheitis has not been ascertained.

The cause of secondary necrosis of the preputial mucous membrane is *Spherophorus necrophorus.* Widespread and universally present in feedlot manure, this species of bacteria inhabits the alimentary tract, feet and skin surface of healthy and diseased cattle. It probably is present also at the preputial orifice and cavity of most male cattle. The organism has no ability to penetrate healthy and intact skin and mucous membrane. After gaining access to noncovering tissue through epithelial lesions, such as degenerations and interruptions, however, it becomes pathogenic and causes extensive necrosis, a characteristic by which it acquired its name. Highly pleomorphic, *S. necrophorus* in young active lesions and in new growing cultures is filamentous, nonbranching, granular, variable in width, and gram-negative in staining; in old lesions and old cultures it becomes coccoid and rod-shaped. Although not easily cultured on artificial media, the organism does, under strictly anaerobic conditions, grow on solid media, such as blood agar, and in liquid media, such as Roseneau's brain broth with a pH between 7.0 and 8.4. It produces acid and gas by fermenting glucose, maltose and glycerol, but does not ferment xylose, rhamnose, mannose, raffinose, inulin, dulcitol, dextrin, erythritol, sorbitol or inositol. Endotoxins of the organism probably contribute to the cause of necrosis. Highly sensitive to many adverse factors, the organism is killed in 15 minutes by temperature of 55° C, and is also easily killed by most standard disinfectants.

Because the primary cause of preputial swelling and edema is not known, the pathogenesis is only conjectural. As a result of acute inflammation edematous fluid tends to accumulate in the preputial mucosa because the prepuce is located at the dependent part of the abdomen and has no muscular contractions to help propel the fluid along through afferent channels. Crowded in the preputial cavity, the mucous membrane may evert through the aperature to the exterior. During recumbency of the animal, semifluid manure, along with *S. necrophorus*, contaminates the everted membrane and also enters the cavity through the dilated orifice. The bacterium, *S. necrophorus,* attacks and penetrates the membrane damaged by inadequate circulation and acute swelling. The growing organism causes extensive and severe necrosis of the mucous membrane, including the submucosa. The infection evokes additional inflammation and edema and if untreated may spread into the penis, urethra and surrounding skin. As healing occurs, granulation tissue may form at the glans penis and at the preputial orifice. Maturation and contraction of the scar tissue may interfere with micturation.

Clinical Signs and Postmortem Lesions. Clinical signs of the disease are localized to the prepuce. During early stages the body temperature may temporarily elevate a few degrees. The prepuce is swollen, firm and tender. Nonpigmented skin, especially at the orifice, is reddened, and the mucous membrane may be everted. Edema and necrosis may extend through much of the membrane, both externally and internally. Urine and fragments of necrotic tissue drain from the cavity. Urination appears to be painful and

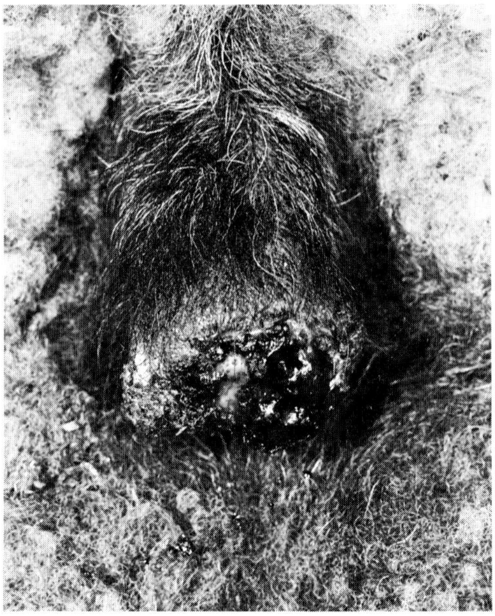

FIG. 4-18. *Necrosis of the prepuce.* × 0.5.

is accompanied by interruptions, flexings of the rear limbs and kicking at the prepuce. In advanced stages of untreated cases, necrosis is generalized throughout the preputial cavity and swelling, infection and necrosis extend into surrounding skin of the abdomen. Urine may drain through one or more skin sinuses to the exterior. A sequel to healing may be stricture of the orifice which in bulls may interfere with breeding. At necropsy early lesions are swelling and edema of parts or all of the membrane lining the preputial cavity. Some of the thickened mucosa may protrude through the orifice to the exterior. Foci of necrosis may be present, especially near the orifice. Urine and manure may contaminate the cavity. In advanced lesions, swelling, edema and necrosis are generalized throughout the cavity and may extend into the penis, up the urethra and into surrounding subcutaneous tissue. Urine may infiltrate the skin and drain to the exterior through sinus tracts. Malodors of necrotic tissue, urine and manure emanate from the affected tissues.

Histopathologic changes include extensive inflammation with edema and necrosis. At the periphery of the dead tissue masses of filimentous S. *necrophorus* are discernible. Colonies of other species of bacteria may also be present. In advanced lesions granulation tissue may be forming, especially at the preputial opening.

The morbidity rate varies from individual cases to as many as 25% of a pen. Even when untreated the mortality rate of affected animals is less than 1%. The disease course varies from 5 to 7 days, but generalized infection in the surrounding skin may, in some cases, extend the time to 2 to 3 weeks. Some animals in affected pens may develop foot rot.

Diagnosis. The clinical diagnosis is based on the presence of typical signs and on information obtained from physical examination of the animal. Painful urination, swelling and reddening of the prepuce, with eversion of edematous preputial mucous membrane, are important suggestive evidence. Confirmation can be obtained by detecting extensive necrosis through careful digital palpation or through examination of the preputial cavity with an appropriate speculum.

The differential diagnosis requires careful consideration of urinary calculosis. In this disease, the distressed animal frequently attempts urination and pulsates the urethra over the ischial arch. Rectal palpation reveals a distended urinary bladder, unless rupture has occurred; in this case, the abdomen is distended with urine which can be removed by needle centesis and identified. In animals in which the urethra has ruptured proximal to the point of calculus occlusion, urine infiltrates the abdominal subcutaneous tissue and discharges through sinus tracts to the surface. The preputial cavity of such cases is near normal.

Prevention and Treatment. The incidence of necrotic posthitis can be reduced by maintaining good pen sanitation. Adequate drainage of runoff liquids into retention basins during times of heavy rainfall, mounding or storage of manure, and provision of bedding, prevent the accumulation of excessive amounts of liquid manure and avoid conditions that frequently lead to necrotic posthitis.

Advanced cases with abdominal skin infection can be successfully treated with the same sulfonamides and antibiotics and at the same dosages as are recommended for treating foot rot. In addition, the preputial cavity should be irrigated with oil suspensions of sulfonamides and/or solutions of drying agents, such as brilliant green, methylene blue or gentian violet. Affected cattle should be kept in dry, bedded stalls or pens to avoid further contamination of the prepuce.

Infectious Thromboembolic Meningoencephalitis

(TEM)

Infectious thromboembolic meningoencephalitis, an acute and febrile disease of feedlot cattle, is characterized clinically by blindness, incoordination of movements, lameness and paresis, and pathologically by multiple infarction of the brain, arthritis and tendenosynovitis of major joints and tendon sheaths. The cause is a *Haemophilus*-like bacterium. Because of augmented incidence since 1962, thromboembolic meningoencephalitis along with polioencephalomalacia are the two prevalent neurologic diseases of feedlot cattle. Annual losses are high and result from mortality and from expensive and frequently unsuccessful treatment programs. The monetary extent of loss has not been measured.

Review of Literature. First reported in feedlot cattle of Colorado (Griner, Jensen and Brown, 1956), the disease was later diagnosed in California (Kennedy, Biberstein, Howarth, Frazier and Dungworth, 1960), in Kansas (Weide, Hibbs and Anthony, 1964), in Illinois (Case, Raudabaugh and Finnel, 1965), in Iowa (Howard and Fawcett, 1966), in Oklahoma and Texas (Panciera, Dahlgren and Rinker, 1968), and in Minnesota (Little and Sorensen, 1969). Pathological studies of natural cases revealed meningitis and a random distribution of focal lesions in the brain (Griner *et al.*, 1956; Kennedy *et al.*, 1960). An increase in volume, pressure, and neutrophils for the cerebrospinal fluid was demonstrated and used as an aid in differentiating the disease from polioencephalomalacia (Howard and Fawcett, 1966). Major joints of limbs and neck as well as many tendon sheaths contained excessive amounts of discolored synovium, and the surfaces of lungs and peritoneum in some cases disclosed fibrinous deposits. The basic change was interpreted as a generalized vasculitis (Panciera, 1968). Investigations of the specific cause led to the isolation of a *Haemophilus*-like bacterium from brain and blood of affected cattle. Injection of infected brain tissue and cultures of the *Haemophilus*-like organism inconsistently induced the disease (Kennedy, Biberstein, Howarth and Frazier, 1960). Subsequently, investigators of other states isolated the same kind of bacteria.

Classification of the *Haemophilus*-like bacterium has been only tentatively determined. Following additional morphological and physiological studies of the organism, some investigators categorized it as *Actinobacillus actinoides*-like (Bailie, Anthony and Weide, 1966; Gossling, 1966). Other researchers made detailed comparative investigations of isolations from affected cattle of Colorado and California and of *Haemophilus agni, Moraxilla bovis, Haemophilus parainfluenza, Actinobacillus actinoides* and *Bordetella bronchiseptica.* Antisera prepared against the Colorado strain and against the California strain each cross-agglutinated with the heterologous strain. The two antisera agglutinated low dilution antigen of *Haemophilus agni,* but they did not react with antigens from *Actinobacillus actinoides.* The researchers concluded that the organism from cattle affected with thromboembolic meningoencephalitis resembled *Haemophilus* more than other organisms studied (Shigidi and Hoerlein, 1970).

Occurrence. This disease frequently occurs in feedlot cattle but rarely in pastured animals, and it has been highly prevalent since 1960. However, the fall-winter seasons from 1965 to 1968 in the west and mid-west experienced higher incidence than did the 1969–70 season. The disease occurs in all breeds and sexes of animals 1 to 2 years of age. Seasonally, it is more common during fall and winter months. Usually affected cattle weigh 750 to 1,100 pounds and have resided in a feedlot 40 to 110 days. Limited to the United States, thromboembolic meningoencephalitis has been reported from Colorado, California, Illinois, Iowa, Kansas, Minnesota, Oklahoma and Texas, but states adjacent to these probably are also involved.

Etiology and Pathogenesis. The *Haemophilus*-like bacterium, the apparent cause of thromboembolic meninoencephalitis, is pleomorphic and measures 0.3 to 0.5 x 0.8 to 4.0 μ. Coccoid, bacillary and short chain forms exist. Non-motile, non-spore forming and non-capsulated, the organism stains with analine dyes and is gram-negative. The bacterium is readily isolated from brain lesions, synovial fluid, blood, spleen and kidneys of infected cattle on cystine heart blood yeast agar or on plain blood agar. As media enrichment bovine blood is superior to other sources; incubation is favorable at 37° C in an atmosphere partially replaced with carbon dioxide. Grown under these special conditions, the raised, round, smooth and

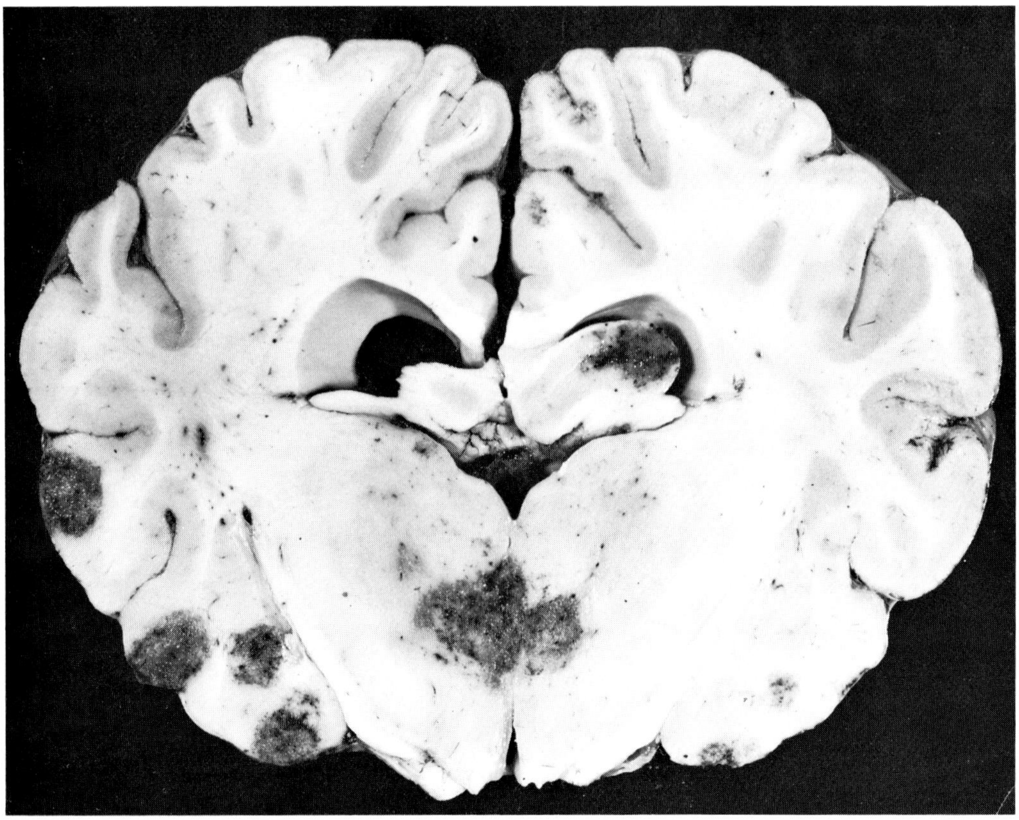

FIG. 4-19. *Multiple foci of infection in the brain of a steer with infectious embolic meningoencephalitis.* × 1.3.

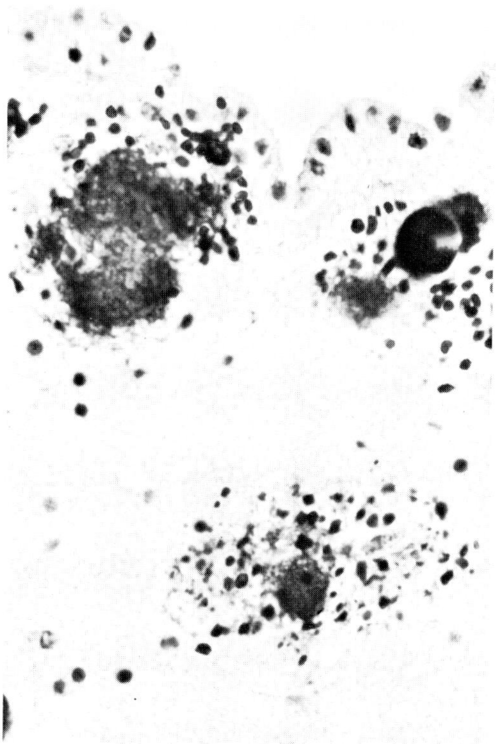

FIG. 4-20. *Bacterial colonies in inflamed vessels of the brain of a heifer with infectious embolic meningoencephalitis. Nocht's stain.* × 496.

transparent colonies do not hemolyze erythrocytes. After a series of transplants, they grow on other media not suitable for initial isolation. The organisms also grow in embryonating chicken eggs which may facilitate initial isolations.

Attempts to reproduce the disease by inoculating healthy cattle usually produce inconsistent results. Inoculations with tissue from brain lesions are more successful than inoculations with cultures of the organism. Some failures may result from bacterial attenuation on artificial media.

As determined by cross-agglutination, the isolants are antigenetically homologous.

As a disease only recently recognized, little information on pathogenesis is available. Sources of the *Haemophilus*-like organism, such as reservoir and carriers, are unknown. The means of transmission and the anatomical points of entrance into susceptible bovine tissues by the causative agent have been neither researched nor determined. Following transmission, however, septicemia develops. Vasculitis forms in vessels of brain, joint capsules and tendon sheaths, and possibly other organs. In areas of lesions, some brain capillaries and venules become occluded by masses of bacteria. Injury to the vessel walls and the presence of bacteria initiate thrombosis and result in brain infarctions. Meningeal and choroid plexus vasculitis and extension of infarcted tissue to brain surface and to the surface of the ventrical system accelerates the formation of cerebrospinal fluid and augments pressure. Leukocytes, especially neutrophils, and bacteria enter the cerebrospinal fluid. Most cattle developing neurologic signs and brain lesions die.

The random distribution of brain lesions can be explained by (1) random formation of foci of vasculitis and thrombosis, or (2) showering the brain vascular system with clumps of bacteria, as infective emboli. At points of lodgment of emboli, thrombi form and infarcts develop.

In the major joint capsules and tendon sheaths a similar mechanism for lesion development probably operates. Following vasculitis of small vessels thrombi form, and neutrophils and bacteria infiltrate tissue and synovial fluid. Pain in affected joints and tendons evokes stiffness and lameness.

Although the disease is clinically recognized by the neurologic signs and at necropsy is frequently diagnosed from characteristic brain lesions, theoretically many other cases without brain involvement may exist in an affected herd. Some infected animals may develop septicemia and mild fever. Vasculitis with or without thrombosis may form in the vessels outside the brain, and such non-encephalitic cases may escape detection, elude diagnosis, and recover. If this interpretation is correct, the infection rate is higher than the mortality rate.

Clinical Signs and Postmortem Lesions. In early stages of the disease only a few animals are simultaneously affected. Some cases are first noticed when animals are recumbent with opisthotonis, weakness and coma. Death usually follows after a few to 24 hours. As the disease continues in the herd, larger numbers of cattle become affected. These animals collectively, but not necessarily all in one animal, show febrile reaction with body temperature commonly near 107° C. Muscular weakness, knuckling at the posterior fetlock joints, stiffness, lameness with swollen joints and anorexia are evident. These signs are followed by excitement, incoordinated movements, blindness, prostration, paresis, opisthotonis, coma and convulsions. The clinical morbidity rate usually approximates 5%. Most animals showing neurologic signs die, but those individuals not developing encephalitis may have temporary fever and prolonged lameness.

At necropsy of fatal cases, lesions are found in many organs. The brain usually contains single or multiple infarctions which are randomly distributed throughout the brain stem, mid-brain, thalamus, basal nuclei and cerebrum. Both gray and white matter are affected. Brownish red in color, the discrete, circular infarctions measure 1 to 15 mm in diameter. Some extend to the cerebral surface and are visible through the meninges. Cerebrospinal fluid is increased in volume and commonly turbid. Firm fixation of the brain in 10% formalin renders the lesions, especially on the cut surface, more conspicuous. Histopathologically, the predominating change is vasculitis. In infarcted tissue some capillaries and venules may be occluded with masses of bacteria. Thrombi containing clumps of bacteria and numerous neutrophils may have formed. The affected vessel walls are infiltrated with leukocytes. Adjacent nerve tissue is necrotic and contains extravascated erthrocytes, neutrophils and some bacteria. In meninges affected vessels reveal similar changes.

The major limb and neck joints and some tendon sheaths are usually distended by excessive synovium. The fluid may be turbid or contain blood and clumps of fibrin. In early stages joint capsules and tendon sheaths are hyperemic and sometimes edematous; after prolonged course the tissues are thickened. In microscopic sections vascular changes similar to those of the brain may be observed. Inflamed walls of capillaries and venules thrombose and neutrophils infiltrate the walls and surrounding tissue.

In other organs hemorrhages are common. Ecchymotic and petechial in size, hemorrhages may form in the subepicardium, subendocardium, subpleura, subperitoneum of abdominal viscera and in muscles. The mucosa of the abomasum and intestines may also contain hemorrhages.

Diagnosis. Infectious thromboembolic meningoencephalitis is diagnosed from clinical signs, necropsy findings, and laboratory studies. Important signs include sudden onset and early deaths, fever, incoordinated movements, muscular weakness, swollen joints, lameness, blindness, prostration, opisthotonis, nystagmus, convulsions and coma. Although the cerebrospinal fluid may be clear, usually it is turbid and contains more than 200 cells per cu mm. At necropsy of fatal cases, the finding of multiple brownish-red infarcts throughout the brain, supplemented with typical clinical signs, is conclusive evidence for a diagnosis. Changes in joints and tendon sheaths are also indicative. Final confirmation can be obtained by laboratory isolation of the *Haemophilus*-like bacterium from brain lesions, blood or joints.

The differential diagnosis requires consideration of polioencephalomalacia and lead poisoning. Polioencephalomalacia, a noninfectious disease, like thromboembolic meningoencephalitis, occurs sporadically in feedlot cattle. Clinically non-febrile, it responds favorably to treatment with thiamin. The cerebrospinal fluid has no increase in leukocytes and at necropsy of fatal cases, the brain contains multiple foci of necrosis in the cerebral cortex. Lead poisoning may cause gastrointestinal disturbance with diarrhea.

Chemical analysis of blood, liver, kidneys or feed may reveal a toxic level of the lead.

Prevention and Treatment. The paucity of information on this disease provides no means for prevention. Affected animals, if identified during early febrile stages, can be treated with considerable success with antibiotics. Occasionally complete change of diet and pens is beneficial. In late stages when prostration and coma have supervened, treatment is usually unsuccessful.

References

Bailie, W. E., Anthony, H. D. and Weide, K. D.: Infectious Thromboembolic Meningoencephalomyelitis (Sleeper Syndrome) in Feedlot Cattle. JAVMA, *148* (1966): 162–166.

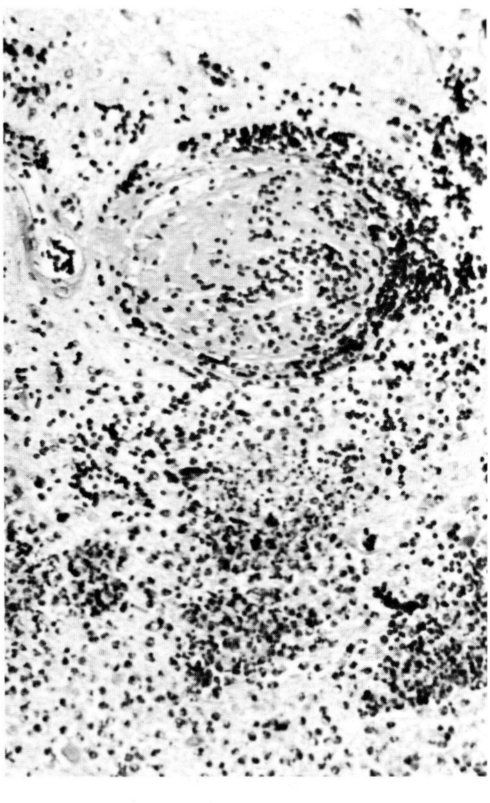

FIG. 4-21. *Thrombosed vein and surrounding inflammation in the brain of a heifer with infectious embolic meningoencephalitis. Nocht's stain.* × 204.

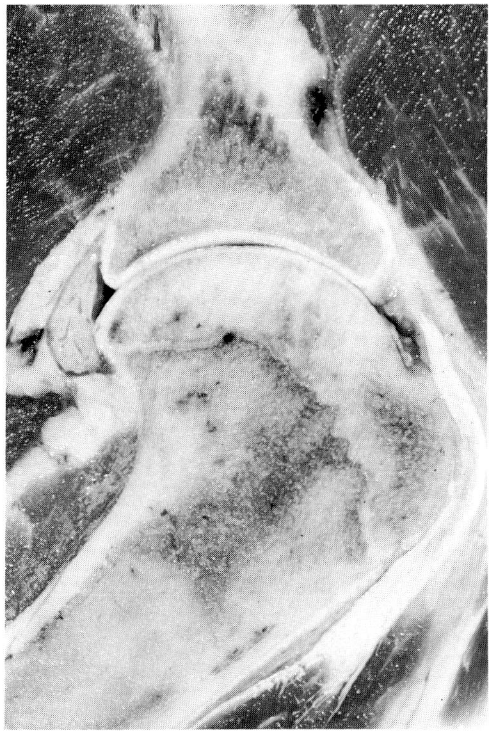

FIG. 4-22. *Acute arthritis in shoulder joint affected with infectious thromboembolic meningoencephalitis. Note exudate in joint capsule at each end of the articular surface.* × 0.9.

Case, M. T., Raudabaugh, W. G. and Finnell, J. H.: Report of Embolic Meningoencephalitis in Illinois. Illinois Vet., *8* (Spring 1965): 31–32.

Gossling, J.: The Bacteria Isolated from Lesions of Embolic Meningoencephalitis of Cattle. Illinois Vet., *9* (1966): 14–18.

Griner, L. A., Jensen, R. and Brown, W. W.: Infectious Embolic Meningo-Encephalitis in Cattle. JAVMA, *129* (1956): 417–421.

Howard, J. and Fawcett, K.: Practical Differential Diagnosis of Polioencephalomalacia and Thromboembolic Meningoencephalitis. Iowa State University Vet., *28* (1966): 101–105.

Kennedy, P. C., Biberstein, E. L., Howarth, J. A., Frazier, L. M. and Dungworth, D. L.: Infectious Meningo-Encephalitis in Cattle Caused by a *Haemophilus*-like Organism. AJVR, *21* (1960): 403–409.

Little, P. B. and Sorensen, D. K.: Bovine Polioencephalomalacia, Infectious Embolic Meningoencephalitis, and Acute Lead Poisoning. JAVMA, *155* (1969): 1892–1903.

Panciera, R. J., Dahlgren, R. R. and Rinker, H. B.: Observations on Septicemia of Cattle Caused by a *Haemophilus*-like Organism. Path. Vet., *5* (1968): 212–226.

Shigidi, M. A. and Hoerlein, A. B.: Characterization of the *Haemophilus*-like Organism of Infectious Thromboembolic Meningoencephalitis of Cattle. AJVR, *31* (1970): 1017–1022.

Weide, K. D., Hibbs, C. M. and Anthony, H. D.: Diagnosis of Bovine Feedlot Encephalitides. Proceedings Meeting of U. S. Livestock Sanit. Assoc. (1964): 469–478.

Infectious Bovine Keratoconjunctivitis

(PINKEYE; SPECIFIC OPHTHALMITIS; INFECTIOUS CONJUNCTIVITIS; INFECTIOUS KERATITIS)

An acute contagious disease, infectious bovine keratoconjunctivitis is characterized by lacrymation, seropurulent discharge, corneal opacity and ulceration, and photophobia. The complex cause is a combination of a physical factor and biological agent. Because of high herd and individual incidence, even though seasonal and of wide geographic distribution, the disease has significant economic importance. Losses result from reduced feed consumption, diminished growth rate, loss of body weight, occasional deaths and expensive treatments. Although not precisely measured, total losses to the national cattle industry are probably large.

Review of Literature. Since an early description (Billings, 1889) infectious bovine keratoconjunctivitis has been observed and studied in many regions of the United States (Baldwin, 1945; Henson and Grumbles, 1960; Sykes, Dmochowski and Grey, 1962), Europe (Cooper, 1960; Dimic *et al.*, 1960), South Africa (Coles, 1936), and Russia (Gromov, *et al.*, 1963). During the last five decades research has been directed towards its etiology. Transmissibility was established by passing swabs saturated with exudate and tears from infected eyes to the conjunctival sacs of healthy animals and thus experimentally reproducing the disease (Allen, 1918; Dimic *et al.*, 1960). The bacterial organism, *Moraxella bovis,* a short, gram-negative rod, was observed in smears from infected eyes, and was isolated and grown in pure cultures on artificial media (Baldwin, 1945; Cooper, 1960; Henson and Grumbles, 1960; Jones and Little, 1923). The same organism was isolated from nasal secretions of infected cattle. Bacterial studies of the eyes of 20 healthy cattle produced no isolations of *M. bovis*, while 82% of 90 infected eyes from 13 herds contained *M. bovis* (Baldwin, 1945). Intermittently investigators were able to reproduce the disease by instilling a small amount of viable pure culture of *M. bovis* into the conjunctival sacs of healthy cattle (Baldwin, 1945; Cooper, 1960; Henson and Grumbles, 1960a). By this method, in one investigation, 43 of 59 inoculated eyes developed lesions typical of infectious bovine keratoconjunctivitis (Henson and Grumbles, 1960). Although many investigators succeeded in reproducing the disease, others were unsuccessful; in one study involving several strains of pure cultures of *M. bovis*, 34 healthy cattle inoculated into the conjunctival sacs with viable inoculae failed to contract the disease (Farley *et al.*, 1950).

Using facilities that provided strict control of variables, the interaction of the bacterium, *Moraxella bovis*, and ultraviolet light irradiation as the cause of the disease was studied. The experimental cattle were raised in isolation and were disease-free. Ultraviolet irradiation was from a sunlamp whose emissions included wavelengths of 2,800 to 3,100 Å and simulated natural irradiation (Hughes, Pugh and McDonald, 1965; 1968). Strains of *M. bovis* were isolated from eyes naturally affected with the disease. On culture media, the organism produced two types of progeny, one hemolytic and the other non-hemolytic (Pugh and Hughes, 1968). Exposure of bovine eyes to ultraviolet light irradiation in 1 period of 20 minutes or in 2 periods of 10 minutes with a 24-hour interval caused little or no visible injury. Exposure of eyes to viable cultures of hemolytic *M. bovis* inconsistently produced slight keratoconjunctivitis.

Exposure of eyes, however, to both ultraviolet light irradiation and to viable cultures of hemolytic *M. bovis* consistently provoked the clinicopathologic signs and lesions that occur in the natural disease (Hughes, Pugh and McDonald, 1965; 1968a; Pugh and Hughes, 1968). Over a 5-year period, investigations of the disease in a field herd of cattle indicated a positive correlation between intensity of natural ultraviolet light irradiation, number of isolations of *M. bovis* and the number of natural cases of disease (Hughes and Pugh, 1970). In the search for possible non-bacterial causes, rickettsiae observed in the cytoplasm of stained smears of conjunctival epithelial cells were assumed to be pathogens (Coles, 1936; Gromov *et al.*, 1963). More recently an unclassified virus isolated from infected bovine eyes and grown on monolayer cultures of embryonic bovine lung cells produced cytopathogenic effects in 72 to 96 hours. The cytopathogenic effects included margination of chromatin and increased fluorescence of the nuclei. Some nuclei showed evidence of increased DNA. While unaffected by ethyl ether through contact for 1 hour at 38° C, the virus was inactivated in 30 minutes at 56° C. The virus was not neutralized by the antiserum from bovine viral diarrhea, mucosal disease, viral bovine rhinotracheitis or parainfluenza-3, but was neutralized by antisera from cattle recovered from contagious keratoconjunctivitis. When inoculated into the conjunctival sacs of 6 healthy calves and 12 1-year-old heifers, 3 of the calves and 5 of the heifers developed clinical signs in 4 days. The antibody titers rose from a preinoculation level of zero to a postinoculation level ranging from 1:40 to 1:320. Electron microscopy divulged the presence of the virus particles in the nucleus and cytoplasm of infected cells (Sykes, Dmochowski, Grey and Russell, 1962).

While the virus of bovine rhinotracheitis has also produced acute conjunctivitis in some outbreaks of the disease, the inflammation did not progress to ulceration and dense opacity as often occurs in bovine contagious keratoconjunctivitis (Abinanti and Plumer, 1961; Hughes, Olander and Wada, 1964). In other outbreaks of the disease where scientists were not able consistently to isolate *M. bovis* from affected eyes, other viruses were found (Wilcox, 1969; and Dyml, 1965).

Although house flies, stable flies, and face flies are suspect in the transmission of contagious bovine keratoconjunctivitis, controlled experiments did not incriminate insects as vectors (Jones and Little, 1924).

The investigation of treatment efficacy has involved many types of drugs. In early stages of the disease, when applied to infected eyes, oxytetracycline, chlortetracycline, chloramphenicol and penicillin were equally effective (Cooper, 1960). *In vitro* studies of pure cultures revealed that *M. bovis* was sensitive to penicillin, erythromycin, tetracycline, chloramphenicol and chlortetracycline. In the same investigation sulfapyridine and sulfathiazole were more efficacious than were sulfadiazine, sulfamerazine or sulfanilamide (Kliewer and Gee, 1960).

Occurrence. While infectious bovine keratoconjunctivitis occurs in both sexes, in all breeds and ages of cattle, animals with non-pigmented eyes and under 3 years of age appear to have a higher incidence with more severe reactions. Because of their non-pigmented faces, Hereford steers and heifers commonly are affected. In western feedlots and ranges the non-pigmented eyes of Shorthorns and Holsteins also are severely affected. Within congested feedlots, outbreaks develop an incidence of 60% or more. In addition to cattle a similar disease occurs in sheep, horses, swine and deer. In each species the causative agent is host specific. Seasonally, the disease commonly begins during the spring, acquires maximal incidence during late spring and early summer, and continues, but diminishes, during the late months of summer and autumn. A limited number of cases may occur during winter. Although widely distributed throughout the United States, the disease is very common in both feedlot and range cattle of the semi-arid western and south western states where altitude is high and ultraviolet light irradiation intense. Specifically reported from Canada, Britain, Europe, Russia and Africa, the disease probably occurs in all countries where the cattle industry has been developed.

Etiology. The cause of infectious bovine keratoconjunctivitis now appears to be an interaction of solar ultraviolet radiation and a bacterium, *Moraxella bovis.* These two factors have been studied both independently and in combination.

Solar radiation consists of electromagnetic emissions of different wavelengths. Wavelengths are commonly measured in Angstroms (Å) and 1 Å = 10^{-8}CM. The visible parts of the light spectrum include wavelengths in the range 4,000 to 7,500 Å. The blue and violet light is at the short and red at the long wavelengths of the range. Infrared light has wavelengths longer and ultraviolet light has wavelengths shorter than visible light. Ultraviolet light includes wavelengths from 20 to 4,000 Å. Within this range is the biologically effective sunlight having wavelengths 2,800 to 3,132 Å. Bovine eyes are damaged by exposure to excessive amounts of biologically effective sunlight and predisposed to the action of *Moraxella bovis.*

Even though the solar emission of ultraviolet light is nearly constant, the amount intercepted per unit of earth surface varies with atmospheric conditions, and seasons, clouds, dust, water and pollutants reflect solar rays. During winter at north latitudes the greater inclination of the ecliptic to the celestial equator results in a smaller amount of solar emission intercepted per unit of earth surface. Consequently, ultraviolet light irradiation is of highest intensity during clear weather of May, June, July and August and of low concentration during cloudy weather of winter months. Seasonal differences in ultraviolet light irradiation explain the high summer incidence of infectious bovine keratoconjunctivitis.

The bacterium, *M. bovis,* formerly classified in the genus *Haemophilus,* is commonly found in the conjunctival sac and nasal secretions of cattle affected with infectious bovine keratoconjunctivitis. Measuring approximately 0.5 to 1.0 x 1.5 to 2.0 μ, this rod-shaped organism is capsulated, nonmotile, non-spore bearing and gram-negative in staining affinity. Although commonly growing in pairs, it may also be found in short chains. Old cultures become pleomorphic. The organism does not ferment any common sugars. Nitrates are not reduced to nitrites and indole is not formed.

Growing on blood agar at pH 7.2 to 7.5 the organism produces round, translucent, gray colonies. Two types of progeny colony, hemolytic and non-hemolytic, are formed. The hemolytic form is pathogenic and the non-hemolytic type is nonpathogenic to bovine eyes. In addition to bovine eyes, the organism grows in the conjunctival sac of sheep and mice. In mice the ocular lesions resemble the ones in bovine eyes affected with infectious bovine keratoconjunctivitis.

In the eyes of cattle, ultraviolet irradiation in moderate amounts alone or *M. bovis* alone, usually cause little or no reaction. Occasionally, a single factor may cause limited corneal opacity and lacrymation. Exposure to ultraviolet solar irradiation of intensity commonly found during summer months followed by exposure to hemolytic *M. bovis* produces the severe ocular lesions of natural infectious bovine keratoconjunctivitis. Lesions probably are exaggerated by wind, dust, flies and trauma.

Transmission. While easily transmitted by mechanical transfer of exudates and secretions from infected to susceptible eyes, the natural means of transmission of infectious bovine keratoconjunctivitis are in dispute. Some healthy adult cattle probably carry the organism through the winter season. During spring and summer seasons, face flies, house flies and stable flies may mechanically transmit the organism by feeding on secretions and exudates of infected eyes and then moving to susceptible eyes for continued feeding. Rapid succession of flies to host cattle increases the probability of disease spread. In addition transmission may be through nasal secretions. Bacteria, secretions and exudate drain from the conjunctival sac through the nasolacrymal duct into the nasal cavities. Infective aerosols may be sprayed by violent breathing, blowing and coughing into the air and into the eyes of nearby cattle. Under crowded conditions of feedlots, the infective droplets may easily enter susceptible eyes. Rubbing and butting between diseased and susceptible cattle may also transfer infection. The common use of feeding and watering equipment facilitates indirect contact and disease transmission between animals. Viable *M. bovis* persists in ocular and nasal secretion for many months following clinical recovery. The introduction of infected or carrier cattle into susceptible herds is a common method of initiating the disease within a herd.

Pathogenesis. During clear weather days of late spring and early summer all unsheltered cattle become exposed to damaging amounts of ultraviolet light irradiation. Even though the injury may be slight, it predisposes the conjunctiva and cornea to the action of *M. bovis*. On entrance of *M. bovis* into the conjunctival sac, the epithelium is injured and the entire sac becomes acutely inflamed. Swelling and congestion at the corneoscleral junction may result in circulatory disturbances of the eye. At the filtration angle the compressed canal of Schlemm may fail to absorb fluids at the normal rate and result in increase of intraocular pressure. The inflamed cornea becomes edematous, infiltrated with leukocytes, and vascularized from the periphery, and these changes result in thickening, clouding and opacity. Three to 5 days after the beginning infection, erosion, approximately 1 mm in diameter, develops towards the center of the corneal surface. Continued action of primary and secondary pathogens increases the conjunctival exudate and often deepens the corneal erosion into an ulcer which penetrates the layers of cornea to variable degrees. Often the epithelium, Bowman's membrane and substantia propria are penetrated. In some eyes all corneal layers are perforated and infection enters the anterior chamber and leads to a generalized ophthalmitis. Aqueous humor and lens may be extruded and the infection may progress into the optic nerve and follow the subarachnoid space into the brain. In most infected eyes, however, the disease is arrested before corneal perforation, and healing occurs. Healed eyes commonly contain a small persisting opaque corneal scar. The recovered animal resists reinfection. Recovery with restoration of most vision usually follows even after corneal perforation. Deep corneal ulceration allegedly predisposes the eye to squamous cell carcinoma.

Clinical Signs and Lesions. Following an incubation period of 3 to 5 days, the disease is initiated in one or both eyes. Swelling is prominent in the conjunctivae, eyelids and nictitating membranes. Because of photophobia and pain, the infected eye is kept closed. Copious exudate and lacrimal secretion escape at the medial canthus and flood the face. The eyelashes and face hair below the eyes are soiled and adherent. Vision is impaired, the appetite reduced and the animal seeks darkened, cool areas for rest. Because of diminished food and water intake body weight reduces. Forcible opening of the swollen eyelids reveals the acute inflammatory reaction. The conjunctivae of the eyelids and the nictitating membranes are congested and edematous. Petechial hemorrhages may be present and apparent over the sclera. Purulent exudate and tears fill the conjunctival sac. In early stages the translucent cornea contains some exudate on the surface. Later, 3 or 4 days after onset of the disease, an erosion approximately 1 mm in diameter may develop at the center of the cornea. Corneal vascularization originating from the corneoscleral junction may be visible, and with the development of this sign most infected eyes begin to heal and recovery is uneventful. In some eyes, however, corneal opacity develops and ulceration extends into and even through the substantia propria and the membrane of Descemet forms a cone-shaped bulge from intraocular pressure. Occasionally the entire cornea perforates and the ocular contents, including the lens, may extrude through the perforation. The deeply ulcerated cornea is edematous and opaque. Because of impaired vision, photophobia, and physical discomfort, affected cattle encounter difficulty obtaining adequate feed and water, and, consequently, may lose body weight. In recovered animals a small opaque stellate scar persists on the center of the cornea.

Histopathologically, the early changes are characteristic of acute inflammation. Smears of conjunctival exudate usually show *M. bovis* and other bacteria. Epithelium may be necrosed and infiltrated with leukocytes. In ulcerated eyes the cornea is thickened from edema of the substantia propria and may also be infiltrated with leukocytes and newly-forming blood vessels. In case of corneal perforation bacteria and inflammatory exudate may be found in the eye chambers.

Among feedlot cattle the morbidity rate is commonly 60% and may reach 90%; but the mortality rate is very low. Only rarely does an animal develop fatal meningitis. One to 2 weeks following onset of the disease most individual cases recover. Animals with severe ulceration or perforation of the cornea usually recover vision after a course of 5 to 6 weeks.

Diagnosis. Bovine contagious keratoconjunctivitis is distinctive and, with the evidence of clinical signs and lesions, readily diagnosed. Conjunctivitis, photophobia, ocular discharge, corneal erosion, rapid spread and impaired vision are important diagnostic signs. Deep corneal ulceration and perforation also indicate the disease. In the laboratory the diagnosis can be confirmed by the isolation and identification of *M. bovis* on bacterial media and/or the filtrable virus in tissue cultured cells.

The differential diagnosis requires consideration of ocular trauma, viral bovine rhinotracheitis and malignant catarrh. Mechanical injuries are usually unilateral and limited to one or a few animals; discontinuity of tissue is often apparent. Viral bovine rhinotracheitis virus in some outbreaks of the disease causes granular conjunctivitis without keratitis. Respiratory signs accompany the ocular changes. In malignant catarrh several signs are present: panophthalmitis with the accumulation of exudate in the anterior chamber; severe conjunctivitis and corneal opacity; high body temperature; eroded oral membranes and inflammation of the respiratory system.

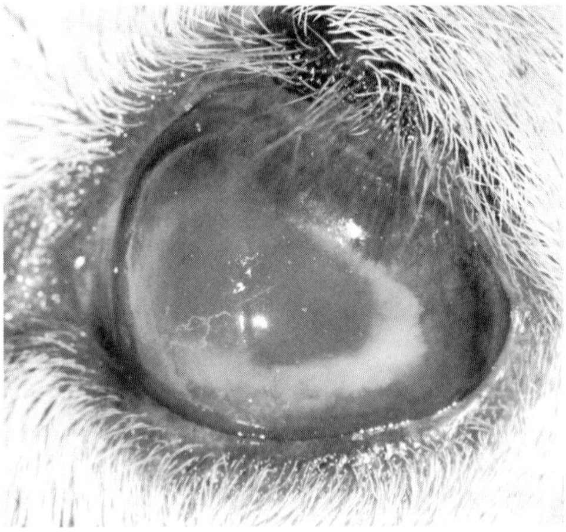

FIG. 4-23. *Beginning corneal opacity and vascularization.* × 1.2.

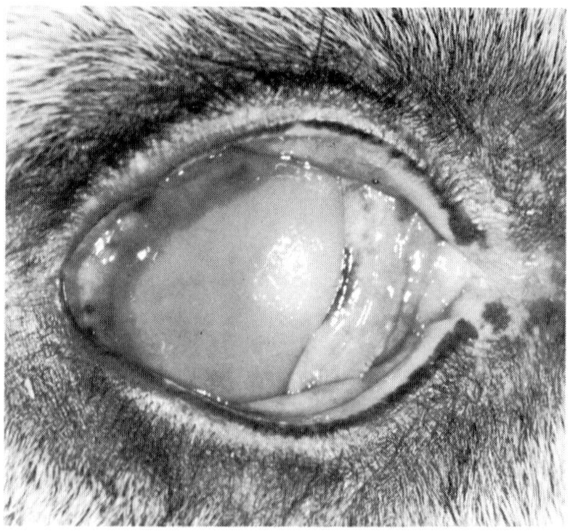

FIG. 4-24. *Keratoconjunctivitis with corneal opacity.* × 1.2.

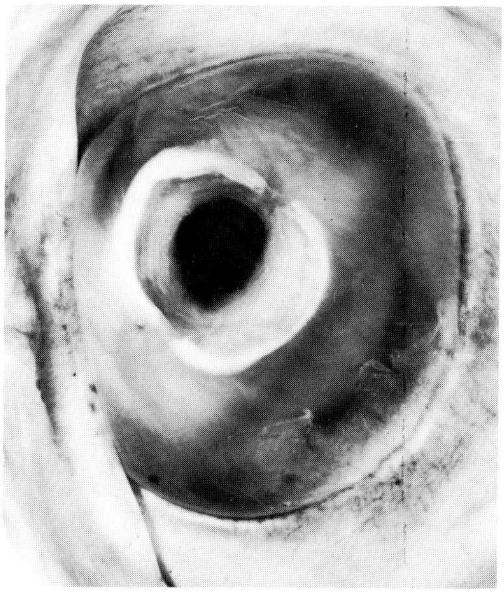

FIG. 4-25. *Perforated cornea.* × 1.3.

Prevention and Treatment. Since bovine keratoconjunctivitis is a contagious disease, animals from known infected or suspected herds should not be added to disease-free herds until they are known not to carry *M. bovis.* During early stages of an outbreak, affected animals should be removed from the feedlot and isolated. The control of house flies, face flies and stable flies, by dipping in a 0.125% aqueous Coumaphos, by spraying with 0.05 to 0.1% emulsifiable concentrate of pyrethrins or by applying with rubbers 5% oily solution of DDT or toxaphene, help to reduce the rate of spread among animals of a feedlot.

Affected animals should be kept in cool, darkened pens where fresh water and appetizing feed are readily available. Both eyes should receive topical treatments with chemotherapeutic or antibiotic agents. Powder, containing 5% sulfathiazole, ointment containing antibiotic, or pressurized sprays containing chemotherapeutic drugs and/or antibiotics, may be applied daily into the conjunctival sacs for 5 to 7 days. Eyes with severe panus and inflammation may be treated with cortical steroids injected subconjunctivally and with foreign protein, such as sterile milk, swine serum and lipoproteins, injected intramuscularly. Vitamin A administered at the rate of one million units per animal may also be beneficial. Corneal ulcers may be cauterized with tincture of iodine or dilute silver nitrate and protected against light, dust and flies. Following medication, infected eyes should be closed for 5 to 7 days. This enforced rest and protection can be achieved by mechanically applying wide adhesive tape to the closed eyelids. Position of the adhesive material can be maintained by passing the tape around the head, but loosely across the throat, and back over the closed eye.

References

Abinanti, F. R. and Plumer, G. J.: The Isolation of Infectious Bovine Rhinotracheitis Virus From Cattle Affected With Conjunctivitis—Observations on the Experimental Infection. AJVR, *22* (1961): 13–17.

Allen, J. A.: Infectious Keratitis. JAVMA, *54* (1918): 307–313.

Baldwin, E. M.: A Study of Bovine Infectious Keratitis. AJVR, *6* (1945): 180–187.

Billings, F. S.: Keratitis Contagiosa in Cattle. Bull. 10, Agr. Exp. Station, Nebr. June 1889.

Coles, J. D. W. A.: A Rickettsial-like Organism of the Conjunctival Epithelium of Cattle. J. So. Afr. Vet. Med. Assoc., *4* (1936): 221–225.

Cooper, B. S.: Treatment of Conjunctivo-keratitis of Cattle and Sheep With Ethidium Bromide. Part I. Infectious Bovine Keratitis. Vet. Rec., *72* (1960): 589–594.

Dimić, J., Trbić, B., Andrić, R. and Atanachovic, M.: The Mechanism of Infection in and Treatment of Infectious Keratoconjunctivitis. Vet. Glasn., *14* (1960): 81–86. [Vet. Bull., *30* (1960): 671.]

Dyml, B.: Isolation of a Virus of the Psittacosis-Lymphogranuloma Group From Cattle With Infectious Keratoconjunctivitis. Vet. Med. Praha, *7* (1965): 385–392.

Farley, H., Kliewer, I. O., Pearson, C. C. and Foote, L. E.: Infectious Keratitis of Cattle—A Preliminary Report. AJVR, *11* (1950): 17–21.

Gromov, V. P., Vershinin, I. I., Podshivalov, N. A., Novak, V. F. and Naumov, M. P.: Rickettsial Conjunctivitis of Cattle. Veterinariya, No. *8* (1963): 33–34.

Henson, J. B. and Grumbles, L. C.: Infectious Bovine Keratoconjunctivitis. I. Etiology. AJVR, *21* (1960): 761–766.

———: Infectious Bovine Keratoconjunctivitis. II. Susceptibility of Laboratory Animals to *Moraxella* (Hemophilus) *bovis*. Cornell Vet., *50* (1960a): 445–458.

Hughes, D. E., Pugh, G. W. and McDonald, T. J.: Ultraviolet Radiation and *Moraxella bovis* in the Etiology of Bovine Infectious Keratoconjunctivitis. AJVR, *26* (1965): 1331–1338.

———: Experimental Bovine Keratoconjunctivitis Caused by Sunlamp Irradiation and *Moraxella bovis* Infection: Determination of Optimal Irradiation. AJVR, *29* (1968): 821–827.

———: Experimental Bovine Infectious Keratoconjunctivitis Caused by Irradiation and *Moraxella bovis* Infection: Re-exposure With Homologous and Heterologous *Moraxella bovis*. AJVR, *29* (1968a): 829–833.

Hughes, D. E. and Pugh, G. W.: A Five-Year Study of Infectious Bovine Keratoconjunctivitis in a Beef Herd. JAVMA, *157* (1970): 443–451.

Hughes, J. P., Olander, H. J. and Wada, M.: Keratoconjunctivitis with Infectious Bovine Rhinotracheitis. JAVMA, *145* (1964): 32–39.

Jones, F. S. and Little, R. B.: An Infectious Ophthalmia of Cattle. J. Exp. Med., *38* (1923): 139–148.

———: The Transmission and Treatment of Infectious Ophthalmia of Cattle. J. Exp. Med., *39* (1924): 803–810.

Kliewer, I. O. and Gee, L. L.: The *In Vitro* Susceptibility of *Moraxella bovis* to Selected Antibiotics and Sulfonamides. Tech. Bull. Okla. Agri. Exp. Sta. (1960): T-84, p. 11.

Pugh, G. W.: and Hughes, D. E.: Experimental Bovine Infectious Keratoconjunctivitis Caused by Sunlamp Irradiation and *Moraxella bovis* Infection: Correlation of Hemolytic Ability and Pathogenicity. AJVR, *29* (1968): 835–839.

Sykes, J. A., Dmochowski, L., Grey, C. E. and Russell, W. O.: Isolation of a Virus from Infectious Bovine Keratoconjunctivitis. Proc. Soc. Exp. Biol. & Med., *111* (1962): 51–56.

Wilcox, G. E.: Isolation of Adenoviruses from Cattle with Conjunctivitis and Keratoconjunctivitis. Aust. Vet. J., *45* (1969): 265–270.

Anthrax

(SPLENIC FEVER; CHARBON; MILZBRAND)

Anthrax, an acute or subacute septicemia characterized by bloody discharges and splenic swelling, is caused by *Bacillus anthracis* and occurs in all homeothermic animals, including man. In many countries where the control of animal diseases is underdeveloped, bovine anthrax causes serious economic losses. In the United States where the disease is suppressed, bovine anthrax outbreaks occasionally occur in pastured cattle and less frequently in feedlot animals. The total annual loss to the cattle industry in the United States has been estimated at $100,000. Monetary losses result from mortality, vaccinations and expensive treatment. Additional losses come from the incapacitation of people affected with the disease.

Review of Literature. Early in the history of microbiology non-motile bodies, presumably bacteria, were observed in the blood of animals dead from anthrax (Rayer and Davaine, 1850). In 1877 transmission experiments demonstrated that bacteria, but not bacteria-free filtrates, from the blood and tissues of infected animals were the specific cause of anthrax (Pasteur and Joubert, 1877), and in 1876 the causative organism was isolated in artificial media from blood of infected animals and reinjected into healthy animals to reproduce the disease (Koch, 1876).

Since those early discoveries of *Bacillus anthracis*, many aspects of the organism and disease have been studied. In cattle, attempts to reproduce the disease by intracutaneous, intraconjunctival, subcutaneous, intravenous and intramuscular inoculations were generally unsuccessful, while oral inoculation through the feed caused septicemia and death (Schlingman *et al.*, 1956). Specific studies of virulent organisms disclosed that the bacilli grown in living tissues differed from those grown *in vitro* by being rapidly lysed in a solution of ammonium carbonate (Smith, Keppie and Stanley, 1953). The capsules formed either *in vivo* or *in vitro* were composed of polyglutamic acid (Ivanovics and Bruchner, 1937) and in the disease process protected the organisms against phagocytosis (Adami, 1909; Preisz, 1909) and against anthracidal substances in tissue. Extracts from dog leukocytes, swine pancreas, and calf thymus were shown to be anthracidal, and the extract from the bovine thymus was identified by electrophoresis as a basic polypeptide with a high content of lycine (Bloom, Watson and Cromartie, 1947). Substances which interfere with host resistance, especially with phagocytosis and with destruction of bacilli, were demonstrated in new lesions of anthrax and were named "aggressins" by the investigators (Bail and Weil, 1911).

Until recently the method by which anthrax caused death was speculative. Some investigators were of the opinion that fatality resulted from clogging capillaries with masses of bacteria and the resulting hypoxia in vital organs (Stableforth and Galloway, 1959). This theory, however, has been refuted by data obtained from the study of experimentally infected guinea pigs. Animals developing a bacteremia with more than 3 x 10^6 chains of organisms per ml of blood eventually died, even though the bacteria were removed from the blood by treatment with antibiotics. In terminal septicemic stages, the plasma of guinea pigs contained a toxic substance which was lethal to mice and neutralized by equine anthrax antitoxin. In experimental animals, anthrax toxin increased the premeability of capillaries to plasma proteins. The administration to an animal of a lethal dose of toxin was followed by a period of normal appearance and finally by the development of massive pulmonary edema. Injections of sublethal doses, however, resulted in a delay period and prolonged leakage of proteins and fluids from plasma into perivascular tissues of the lungs, peritoneum and subcutis (Beall and Dalldorf, 1966). Death came after clinical cessation of respiration. Circulation continued beyond respiratory failure (Walker, Lincoln and Klein, 1967). When Rhesus monkeys were given 1,000 toxin units into the cerebrospinal fluid, depression and death, mediated through the central nervous system, resulted from respiratory failure (Remmele *et al.*, 1968). These investigations strongly supported the concept that *Bacillus anthracis* forms *in vivo* a specific toxin (Smith and Keppie, 1955) that causes death of the host animal.

Normally, virulent anthrax organisms freshly isolated on solid media produce rough colonies. Investigations in South Africa, however, disclosed that virulent organisms grown on serum agar in an atmosphere of carbon dioxide produced smooth mucoid colonies which yielded some rough variants that were usually less virulent than the smooth parent (Sterne, 1937; 1937a; 1937b). Organisms in the rough variant colonies were non-capsulated and in general avirulent. Spore vaccines prepared from the rough colony variant produced satisfactory immunity in guinea pigs (Personeus, Cooper and Percival, 1956; Sterne, 1937), in two and one-half million cattle, and several thousands of horses and sheep (Sterne, 1939). In cattle the vaccine produced insignificant clinical reactions and retained immunizing power for at least 1 year. This type of vaccine has been used satisfactorily in cattle in the United States (VanNess, Plotkin, Huffaker and Evans, 1959).

In the United States, anthrax organisms were found to endure in neutral or alkaline soils containing considerable calcium. During 1953 and 1954, most of the outbreaks of the disease were in counties which contained soil favorable to the organisms or in alluvial soil downstream from an anthrax area (VanNess and Stein, 1956). Human cases of anthrax in the United States during a period 1934 through 1949 were in individuals engaged in industrial uses of animal hair and carpet wool imported from Asia, North Africa and Southern Europe. Eleven hundred twenty cases were reported (Wolff and Herman, 1951).

Occurrence. While anthrax is a disease of all breeds, sexes and ages of cattle, it occurs more commonly in adult animals than in calves. This difference may be due, in part, to eating habits which provide a greater opportunity for grazing adults to ingest spores from the soil. While anthrax is uncommon in feedlot cattle, the disease occurs occasionally as a result of contaminated feed or water. In addition to cattle, sheep and horses are highly susceptible. While people and swine possess considerable resistance, dogs, cats, birds and wild animals develop anthrax only under certain conditions. In the laboratory, mice, guinea pigs and rabbits can be infected. Geographically, anthrax occurs in all countries where cattle and/or sheep production are major industries. The disease is common in Asia, Southern Europe, Africa, South America and North America. In the United States, the incidence is high and recurring in South Dakota, Arkansas, Louisiana, Texas and California. From 1916 to 1944 the number of states reporting anthrax increased from 21 to 37. In 1945 through 1954, 3,447 outbreaks occurred in 17,604 animals from 39 states. Approximately 65% of these cases were cattle.

Probably because grazing provides opportunity for ingesting anthrax spores from contaminated soil, food, and water, anthrax seasonally occurs more commonly during summer months.

Etiology and Pathogenesis. *Bacillus anthracis*, the causative bacterium of anthrax, is a non-motile, capsulated spore-bearing, cylindrical, truncated, aerobic rod whose dimensions are 1 to 1.2 x 3 to 8 μ. The elliptical spore is located centrally within the cell. While young cultures are gram-positive, older ones tend to de-colorize easily. In the tissues of infected animals, especially the blood, the organism forms heavily capsulated chains.

In the laboratory, the organism grows on many common artificial media. Virulent organisms commonly form rough colonies. Freshly isolated virulent strains grown on serum agar in an atmosphere of carbon dioxide form smooth mucoid colonies. Continued cultivation in an atmosphere of carbon dioxide produces rough avirulent uncapsulated daughter colonies. Capsules when present are composed of polyglutamic acid and protect the cells against phagocytosis. In artificial media the organism forms acid but not gas from glucose, sucrose, fructose, maltose and dextrin. Fermentation does not occur in lactose, mannose, rhamnose, arabinose, raffinose, sorbitol and inositol.

On exposure to oxygen, anthrax bacilli form spores which are highly resistant to the adversity of chemical and physical agents. In soil, in buried infected tissues and in cultures, spores have endured for many years. Freshly prepared 5% sodium hydroxide is an effective disinfectant and kills spores after prolonged action. Ten% formaldehyde is lethal in 15 minutes. Resistance to heat varies with the method of heating and with the medium carrying the spores. In a water bath, spores from different strains endured 5 to 30 minutes at 80° C but were destroyed in 2 minutes at 100° C. In flowing steam from an Arnold sterilizer at 101° C, spores were killed in 5 to 15 minutes, and in the autoclave at 15 pounds pressure at 120° C, they were also killed in 5 to 15 minutes. Dry spores were destroyed by dry heat at 150° C in 60 minutes.

The organism contains two antigens: (1) capsular polypeptide, glutamic acid, and (2) somatic polysaccharide consisting of a complex molecule of glucosamine, galactose and acetic acid. Animals immune to anthrax have the ability to destroy or inhibit formation of the capsule. Without capsule, the bacteria are phagocytized and killed.

In clinical cases of anthrax, specific bacterial toxin, acting on the central nervous system, causes death of the host animal by suppressing respiration. The toxin consists of three factors designated by Roman numeral I, II, and III. Factor I alone is non-toxic, but a combination of factor I and factor II causes death in mice and dermal edema in rabbits. Factor II alone is non-toxic and immunogenic. Factor III, antigenically separate from the other factors, is innocuous when used alone, but lethal to mice and rats when combined with factor II.

Animals affected with acute anthrax may emit viable organisms to the external environment in fecal, urinary and nasal excretions. Incisions in the skin and other organs, especially at necropsy, release fantastically large numbers of viable organisms to the exterior. On exposure to the oxygen the viable cells form spores which can be disseminated mechanically to wide geographic areas. Contaminated soil, feed and water may be carried any distance by mobile vehicles. Contaminated stream water passing through a feedlot and used for drinking may expose feedlot cattle. Grain and hay grown on contaminated soil or feeds from animal tissues, such as steamed bone meal, may infect cattle. Carnivorous animals, such as dogs, cats and coyotes, may become contaminated while feeding on infected tissues and carry spores into feedlots. Biting flies and ticks after feeding on infected animals may transmit the disease through feeding on healthy susceptible cattle.

While information on anthrax is fragmentary and the pathogenesis is incompletely understood, available information suggests a sequence of associated events. Viable spores from soil, feed or water gain entrance to tissues through inhalation, abrasions of the skin, or more probably, through injuries along the alimentary tract. In the tissues the spores germinate and form capsules which protect them against phagocytosis. The elaboration of toxic substances causes local edema and protects bacteria against anthracidal substances in normal plasma, leukocytes and tissues. The organisms multiply rapidly in edematous fluid and are carried through afferent lymphatics into regional lymph nodes where lymphoid tissue is injured. Passing along efferent lymphatics, the organisms ultimately reach the circulating blood. Rapid multiplication of the bacteria results in a severe septicemia and the production of toxin which causes severe and fatal respiratory failure.

Clinical Signs and Postmortem Lesions. The signs of anthrax vary with the acuteness of the disease. After a variable incubation period from 1 to 14 days, animals without the observation of previous illness may be found dead. Body temperature rises to 106° to 108° F. Aggressive movements, such as shaking of the head, bellowing, stamping the feet and butting, are manifested. Some animals show generalized depression and muscular tremors. Following the loss of appetite, rumination ceases and bloating develops. Small amounts of blood may be mixed with nasal excretions, urine and feces. The oral mucous membranes and conjunctivae are congested and cyanotic.

In subacute anthrax, subcutaneous edema may be located over the neck, thorax, flanks, back or genital organs. Some animals may manifest severe dyspnea from edema of the larynx and pharynx. In some cattle the mucous membrane of the rectum and vagina contain edematous swellings. These cases persistently strain and excrete necrotic tissue and blood in the feces.

The course of anthrax also varies according to acuteness. In the acute and peracute forms the course is usually from 10 to 36 hours, but in exceptional cases, especially in early stages of an outbreak, death may occur after 1 to 2 hours. In the subacute form the course extends from 2 to 5 days and occasionally longer. In highly chronic cases the disease may endure 2 to 3 months and be manifested by progressive emaciation. The morbidity rate varies from low to high and the mortality rate is approximately 90%.

At necropsy of acute cases the feces, urine and nasal excretions are stained with blood and blood may actually exude from the skin. The systemic blood is dark and has a prolonged clotting time. The mucous membrane of the alimentary tract may be irregularly hemorrhagic and eroded, especially at Peyer's patches. Serosa of the endocardium and epicardium and the subcutaneous tissues contain multiple petechial and ecchymotic hemorrhages. Usually the spleen is enlarged by a factor of 2 to 4 and the parenchyma is soft and exudes from the cut surface. Lymph nodes, especially in the area of entering infection, are swollen and hemorrhagic. In the subacute form subcutaneous edema may be found over the neck, thorax, or sternum. The urinary bladder often contains blood.

Histopathologically, the blood shows large

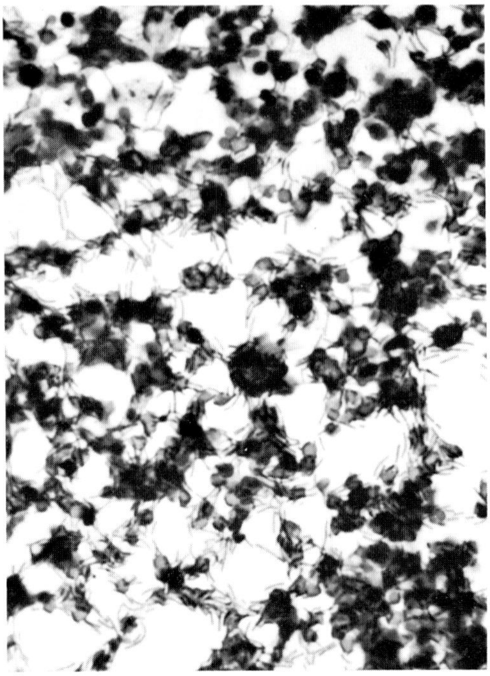

FIG. 4-26. *Abundant B. anthracis in red pulp of spleen from a steer affected with anthrax. Nocht's stain.* × 620.

numbers of bacteria, many in chains, of *B. anthracis*. The leukocyte count may be reduced. Blood capillaries and veins tend to be distended and hemorrhage is common. Germinal centers of lymph nodes and splenic corpuscles are depleted of lymphocytes. In the spleen the red pulp is filled to capacity with blood. Many erythrocytes are fragmented and hemolysed. Frequently, vast numbers of bacteria are distributed throughout the spleen. Animals with anthrax submitted for salvage slaughter should be condemned and all contaminated instruments, equipment and surfaces thoroughly disinfected.

Diagnosis. The clinical diagnosis of anthrax is made on the basis of typical signs and is usually supplemented with laboratory procedures. Important clinical signs in animals of anthrax endemic areas are the high fever, aggressiveness, bloody discharges and a short course. While necropsy should be avoided in cattle suspected of anthrax, the acute splenitis, lymphadenitis, and edema are of diagnostic importance if necropsy is performed.

In the laboratory, confirmation of the diagnosis can be obtained by the study of blood smears, by bacterial cultures and by laboratory animal inoculations. Blood smears should be obtained near time of death and stained with Giemsa or Wright's stain. In typical cases of anthrax, encapsulated single bacterial cells and chains of cells are demonstrable. With these stains the capsule is purplish-pink. Blood smears prepared after considerable autolysis are unsatisfactory for diagnosis.

Tissues submitted to the laboratory should include an amputated ear and, in case of necropsy, pieces of spleen, lymph nodes and liver. These tissues, in plastic bags to avoid leakage, should be placed along with a refrigerant in a metal container for shipment. From the ear small amounts of blood may be obtained for smears. Bacterial cultures can be made from ear blood and from other tissues submitted. In case of heavy contamination of tissues, mouse or guinea pig inoculations may be necessary. Inoculated guinea pigs usually die from anthrax in 36 to 48 hours and from the tissues *B. anthracis* can be isolated and identified.

The differential diagnosis requires consideration of acute bloat, malignant edema, blackleg, shipping fever, acute poisoning and lightning stroke. In bloat the abdomen is distended and at necropsy the spleen is normal. Blood smears do not show anthrax organisms. Malignant edema is an acute emphysematous swelling around a wound. In blackleg affected muscles are swollen and emphysematous; at necropsy, the muscles are usually dark and gaseous and the spleen is normal. The specific organisms of malignant edema and blackleg can be identified in the laboratory. Shipping fever, an acute febrile disease, is manifested by nasal discharge, depression, dyspnea and pneumonia. Acute poisonings which cause sudden death include nitrates from beet tops and oat hay, prussic acid from cyanogenic plants, insecticides, fertilizers and some metallic salts. Usually, the source of the poisoning is discernible and chemical analysis of stomach contents helps to identify the specific poison. Cattle killed by lightning stroke have singed hair and a history of death during an electric storm.

Prevention and Treatment. Cattle in or originating from an anthrax endemic area should be immunized with a viable spore vaccine, such as spore vaccine No. 3 with saponin or the Stern-strain Spore Vaccine. Considerable immunity is established within 1 week from the time of administration. A single vaccination should provide protection throughout the entire fattening period.

Outbreaks of anthrax among feedlot cattle can be controlled through the combined application of principles of sanitation and immunization. The source of exposure to virulent organisms should be determined and eliminated. Often the sources may be contaminated drinking water in a stream or contaminated flood water washed into accessibility. Hay or grain, grown on heavily contaminated soil, may contain viable spores. Rarely, feed of animal origin, such as steamed bone meal, may be contaminated with anthrax spores. Following an outbreak and to avoid disease spread, the premises should be quarantined according to state health regulations. All sick or febrile cattle should be isolated for treatment. Under no circumstances should necropsies be performed within the pens. Dead cattle and other dead animals, bones, skin, manure and bedding should be removed and disposed of by incineration or deep burial in quick lime. All pen surfaces, including soil, fences, walls, feeding equipment, watering equipment and machinery, should be disinfected by liberal application of a pressurized spray of freshly prepared 5% aqueous lye solution. Following a few weeks of vacancy and exposure to sunshine, the cleaned pen can be reoccupied. Potentially transmitting arthropods, such as ticks and biting flies, should be controlled.

Heavily exposed cattle should be passively immunized with individual doses of 50 to 100 ml of antianthrax serum given subcutaneously. The protection is for a few weeks only.

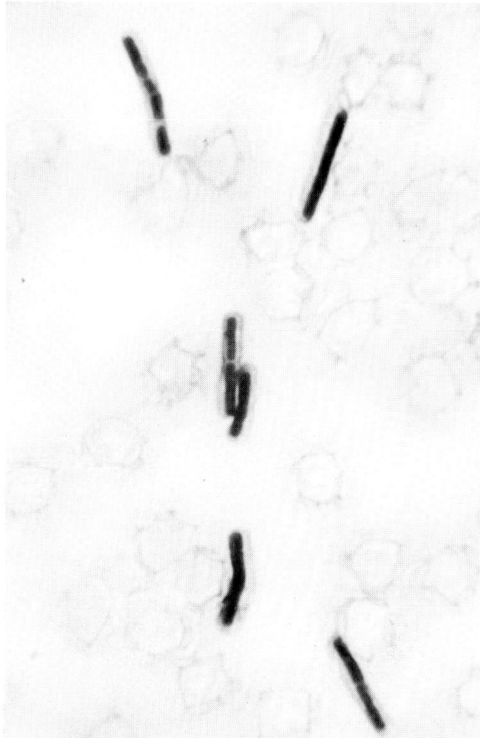

FIG. 4-27. *Capsulated cells of B. anthracis in blood smear of an inoculated mouse. Giemsa stain.* × 1550.

Often the treatment of peracute anthrax is not feasible because of death after a very short course. In many animals, however, treatment is practical and may be administered on either an individual or herd basis. The early stages of anthrax are more amenable to individual treatment. Penicillin should be administered daily at the rate of 2,000 to 4,000 units per pound of body weight. The antibiotic treatment can be supplemented with the use of 50 to 100 ml of antianthrax serum given subcutaneously and repeated at 6- to 12-hour intervals.

In case large numbers of animals are affected or heavily exposed, the entire herd or pen of cattle can be treated with oxytetracycline or chlorotetracycline in the feed or water at the rate of 1 mg per pound of body weight daily for 7 to 10 days followed by one-half this dosage for an additional 7 to 10 days.

References

Adami, G. F.: *Inflammation*. London. The Macmillan Company, 1909.

Bail, O. and Weil, E.: Beitrage Zum Stadium der Milsbrand Infection. Arch Hyg., Berl., *73* (1911): 218.

Beall, F. A. and Dalldorf, F. G.: The Pathogenesis of the Lethal effect of Anthrax Toxin in the Rat. J. Inf. Dis., *116* (1966): 377–389.

Bloom, W. L. and Prigmore, J. R.: A Method for Preparation of Antibacterial Basic Proteins of Normal Tissues. J. Bact., *64* (1952): 855–858.

Bloom, L., Watson, D. W., Cromartie, W. J. and Freed, M.: Studies on Infection with *Bacillus anthracis*. IV. Preparation and Characterization of an Anthracidal Substance from Various Animal Tissues. J. Inf. Dis., *80* (1947): 41–52.

Eurich, F. W. and Hewlett, R. T.: A System of Bacteriology. London. (Medical Research Council) *5* (1930): 439.

Hanson, R. P.: The Earliest Account of Anthrax in Man and Animals in North America. JAVMA, *135* (1959): 463–465.

Ivanovics, G. and Bruckner, V. Z.: Immun. Forsch., *90* (1937): 304.

Koch, R.: Beitr. Biol., *2* (1876): 277.

Losses in Agriculture. Agricultural Research Service. USDA. Agri. Handbook No. 291 (1965).

Pasteur, L. and Joubert, C. R.: Acad. Sci., Paris, *84* (1877): 900.

Personeus, G., Cooper, M. S. and Percival, R. C.: Studies on an Anthrax Vaccine Prepared from Noncapsulated Variants of *Bacillus anthracis*. AJVR, *17* (1956): 153–156.

Preisz, H.: Experimentelle Studien uber Virulenz Empfanglichkeit and Immunitat beim Milzbrand. Zbl. Bakt., *49* (1909): 341.

Rayer, P. F. O. and Davaine, C.: Bull. Soc. Biol. Paris. Ser. 1, 2 (1850): 141.

Remmele, N. S., Klein, F., Vick, J. A., Walker, J. S., Mahlandt, B. G. and Lincoln, R. E.: Anthrax Toxin: Preliminary Site of Action. J. Inf. Dis., *118* (1968): 104–113.

Report. Anthrax in Bonemeal. North Am. Vet., *33* (1952): 450–454.

Schlingman, A. S., Devlin, H. B., Wright, G. G., Maine R. J. and Manning, M. C.: Immunizing Activity of Alum-Precipitated Protective Antigen of *Bacillus Anthracis* in Cattle, Sheep, and Swine. AJVR, *17* (1956): 256–261.

Shrewsbury, J. F. D. and Barson, G. J.: A Bacteriological Study of the House Sparrow, *Passer domesticus*. J. Path. Bact., *64* (1956): 605.

Smith, H. and Keppie, J.: Studies on the Chemical Basis of the Pathogenicity of *Bracillus Anthracis* Using Organisms Grown *in vivo*. Mechanisms of Pathogenicity. Fifth Symposium of the Society for General Microbiology. Cambridge University Press. London. (1955): 126–155.

Smith, H., Keppie, J. and Stanley, U. L.: The Chemical Basis of the Virulence of *Bacillus anthracis*. I. Properties of Bacteria Grown *in vivo* and Preparation of Extracts. Brit. J. Exp. Path., *34* (1953): 477–485.

Stableforth, A. W. and Galloway, I. A.: *Infectious Diseases of Animals. Diseases Due to Bacteria*. Vol. 1. 1959, Academic Press. New York pp. 2–52.

Stein, C. D.: The History and Distribution of Anthrax in Livestock in the United States. Vet. Med., *40* (1945): 340–349.

Stein, C. D. and Rogers, H.: Observations on the Resistance of Anthrax Spores to Heat. Vet. Med., *40* (1945): 406–410.

Stein, C. D. and VanNess, G. B.: A Ten Year Survey of Anthrax in Livestock with Special Reference to Outbreaks in 1954. Vet. Med., *50* (1955): 579–588.

Sterne, M.: The Effects of Carbon Dioxide Concentrations on the Growth of Virulent Anthrax Strains. Pathogenicity and Immunity Tests on Guinea Pigs and Sheep with Anthrax Variants Derived from Virulent Strains. Onderstepoort. J. Vet. Sci. & An. Ind., *9* (1937): 49–67.

———: Variation in *Bacillus anthracis*. Part I. Some Effects of Carbon Dioxide on the Formation of Capsules and Spores by *B. anthracis*. Onderstepoort J. Vet. Sci. & An. Ind., *8* (1937a): 272–278.

———: Variations in *Bacillus anthracis*. Part II. Some Correlations between Colony Variation and Pathogenicity in Strains of *Bacillus anthracis*. Onderstepoort. J. Vet. Sci. & An. Ind., *8* (1937b): 279–349.

———: The Use of Anthrax Vaccines Prepared from Avirulent (Uncapsulated) Variants of *Bacillus anthracis*. Ondersteepoort. J. Vet. Sci. & An. Ind., *13* (1939): 307–312.

Stiles, G. W.: Isolation of the *Bacillus anthracis* from Spinose Ear Ticks *Ornithodorus megnini*. AJVR, *5* (1944): 318–319.

Van Ness, G. and Stein, C. D.: Soils of the United States Favorable for Anthrax. JAVMA, *128* (1956): 7–9.

Van Ness, G. B., Plotkin, S. A., Huffaker, R. H. and Evans, W. G.: The Oklahoma-Kansas Epizootic of 1957. JAVMA, *134* (1959): 125–129.

Walker, J. S., Lincoln, R. E. and Klein, F.: Proceedings of the Conference on Progress in the Understanding of Anthrax. Beaumont House, FASEB, Bethesda, Md. (1967).

Wolff, A. H. and Herman, H.: Industrial Anthrax in the United States. An Epidemic Study. Am. J. Hygiene, *53* (1951): 80–109.

Blackleg

(BLACK QUARTER; QUARTER ILL; SYMPTOMATIC ANTHRAX; CHARBON SYMPTOMATIQUE; RAUSHBRAND)

An acute infectious, but non-contagious, disease of cattle and sheep, blackleg is characterized by focal gangrenous and emphysematous myositis and is caused by *Clostridium chauvoei* and other related species of bacteria. While most young cattle from endemic areas are immunized against blackleg, some through negligence escape immunization. Consequently, losses in feedlots from this disease are due to sporadic mortality. Although total losses are low, occasional outbreaks have a high incidence.

Review of Literature. Since discovery of the cause of blackleg (Bollinger, 1875), additional causative factors in the pathogenesis of the disease and methods of immunization have been investigated sporadically (Robertson, 1929). Because *Cl. chauvoei* is evidently the main cause of blackleg, immunizing agents were prepared first from this species of organism. While the immunogenic products protected against most outbreaks of disease, an occasional heavy incidence with severe losses from blackleg occurred. In Europe bacterial cultures made from tissues of blackleg from many geographic areas revealed the presence of either or both *Cl. chauvoei* and *Cl. septicum* (Graub, 1924; Weinberg and Michailescu, 1930). In America bacteriological investigators showed that cases of blackleg commonly contain *Cl. septicum*, in addition to *Cl. chauvoei* (Breed, 1937; Breen, 1959; Scott *et al.*, 1934; Vawter, 1942); consequently, vaccines containing these two organisms were prepared commercially and used widely but still occasionally serious outbreaks of blackleg occurred in vaccinated cattle (Breen, 1959; Byrne and Armstrong, 1948). A third species of bacteria, *Cl. novyi*, was also encountered in the tissues in some outbreaks of blackleg (Scott *et al.*, 1934; Vawter, 1942). When autogenous bacterins were made containing *Cl. chauvoei*, *Cl. septicum* and *Cl. novyi* and applied to these herds, the outbreaks ceased and losses stopped but continued research produced other relevant information. In one study *Cl. sordellii* was associated with *Cl. chauvoei* in a case of blackleg (Vawter, 1942). Studies of many strains indicated variability in toxin production (Moussa, 1958); some strains of *Cl. chauvoei* produced oxygen-labile hemolysin and others produced oxygen-stabile hemolysin. *Cl. septicum* also produced oxygen-stabile hemolysin, but both species inconstantly produced necrotoxin.

After almost a century of intermittent research the means of transmission of blackleg in cattle are unknown. Experiments conducted in India disclosed that oral and intravenous inoculations of spores were innocuous. The inoculation of spores into traumatized muscle also was harmless, but the latency of spores was demonstrated by injecting spores into healthy muscle and at subsequent intervals injuring the same muscle tissue with injections of calcium chloride. By this sequence of inoculations blackleg was induced in 20 to 40 days after spore inoculation. Bacterial cultures of organs from animals recovered from blackleg disclosed spore latency for 18 days in lymphoid tissue and for 25 days in bone marrow (Minett, 1948). The predisposing influence of the nutritional plane and weather inclemency were also studied (Minett, 1948a; 1948b). Experimental animals on high and low levels of intake of carbohydrates and proteins were equally susceptible to inoculation (Minett, 1948a). Sheep subjected to local and general chilling and untreated control animals were equally susceptible to inoculations (Minett, 1948b).

Many studies have been conducted for the improvement of vaccines and for comprehension of immunization. A life-long immunity has been suggested by the fact that formalinized cultures of *Cl. chauvoei* with incorporation of *Cl. septicum* produced a high potency vaccine (Breed, 1937). Continued experience with the immunizing product has partially confirmed this finding. Using guinea pigs as experimental animals, investigators showed that two injections of vaccine were superior to one and that vaccination at young age was ineffective. Simultaneous vaccination for blackleg and hemorrhagic septicemia did not diminish the protection against blackleg (Ryff and Lee, 1941). Following the administration of a single dose of formalinized culture, protection against blackleg increased to 10 minimum lethal doses at 4 months after inoculation and then declined to 1 minimal lethal dose at 12 months. This decline of protection suggested to the investigators the advisability of repeated immunizations (Scheuber, 1944). The efficacy of high doses of penicillin in early stages as treatment was demonstrated clinically. In some animals following recovery from acute stages of the disease, the gangrenous muscle sloughed (Aitken, 1949).

Occurrence. A disease of all breeds of cattle, blackleg occurs most commonly in individual animals from 6 months to 3 years of age. The incidence, however, is low because of near universal use of vaccine. Without vaccination, a disease incidence of 2 to 3% could be expected. Despite the use of commercial vaccine, an occasional outbreak of disease has an incidence of 10 to 50%. The incidence is higher during summer and autumn than during winter. Geographically, blackleg occurs in all major cattle producing countries, but within any country, however, the distribution is not uniform. In the United States it is less common in the eastern states than in other areas of the country. Presumably the incidence of blackleg in geographic areas is related to the degree of soil contamination with spores of the causative bacteria.

Etiology and Pathogenesis. While *Cl. chauvoei* is the main cause of blackleg, occasionally *Cl. septicum* and less commonly *Cl. novyi* are also present and contribute to pathogenesis of the disease. The three species are motile, anaerobic, spore bearing and, as young cultures, gram-positive rods with a tendency to become gram-negative in older cultures. The vegetative rods measure 0.8 to 1.5 by 5 to 10 μ. The oval shaped spores are subterminal. The fermentation of some sugars are shown in table 7. In smears from the surface of liver from infected guinea pigs, *Cl. chauvoei* forms single bacilli or short chains, while *Cl. septicum* mostly forms chains; this morphologic difference is of diagnostic importance in determining species. The vegetative forms are highly susceptible to drying, high temperatures and chemical disinfectants, while the spores are resistant and withstand 120° C for 10 minutes and endure in soil and dried infected tissues for many years. Spores are killed in 15 minutes by a 3% solution of formaldehyde.

For the three main species of *Clostridium*, the antigenic structure and toxin production have been investigated. Strains of *Cl. chauvoei* appear to be of a single serologic type. Although an exotoxin is produced in liquid cultures, its concentration is low and variable. The addition of blood to broth media enhances exotoxin production. Different strains of *Cl. septicum* can be separated into four major antigenic groups. These forms produce potent exotoxins that hemolyze erythrocytes and remain stable when exposed to oxygen. *Cl. novyi* contains three serologic types of organism and possibly six types of exotoxin.

The pathogenesis of blackleg in cattle is incompletely understood. Presumably, spores from the soil are transmitted to susceptible animals by ingestion, or possibly through wound contamination. From the alimentary tract, the spores penetrate tissues through areas of discontinuity of mucous membrane, such as from trauma, or from points of tooth eruption. The spores are conveyed to muscles where some are destroyed by phagocytosis, while others remain latent for at least several weeks. Necrosis of muscle cells near the spores stimulates vegetative growth and toxin production. The growing bacteria and their toxins cause further necrosis of muscle cells and blood capillaries. In the lesions, gas

TABLE 7 *Fermentation and morphology*

	Glucose	Maltose	Lactose	Salicin	Bacteria from Guinea Pig Liver
Cl. chauvoei	AG	AG	AG	—	mostly single
Cl. septicum	AG	AG	AG	AG	mostly chains
Cl. novyi	AG	AG	—	—	
Cl. hemolyticum	AG	AG	—	—	

bodies accumulate from fermentation and hemorrhage from ruptured capillaries. Extravasated erythrocytes, and possibly red cells within the vessels, are hemolysed by toxin. Exotoxins from the bacteria and toxic substances from the lesion cause a severe systemic reaction and in most cases death. During moribund stages bacteremia is established. Following death, tissue decomposition is rapid and many of the bacteria form spores in the dehydrated tissues and soil. Recovered animals are immune.

Clinical Signs and Postmortem Lesions. Although the incubation period is difficult to determine, it is considered to vary from 2 to 5 days. Body temperature rises rapidly to 104° to 106° F. Muscular stiffness, depression, disinclination to move and anorexia are prominent. In animals affected in muscles of the limbs lameness is manifested. Affected muscles are swollen and emphysematous to palpation. Lesions are commonly located in the muscles of the shoulder, thigh, neck and back, less commonly in the crura of the diaphragm and only rarely in the tongue. The lesions in the crura of the diaphragm adversely affect breathing. In the rare infections of the tongue the swollen organ protrudes and results in dysphagia and salivation. The sporadic incidence is usually 2 to 3%, but a long sequence of cases in some outbreaks may be much higher. The mortality rate of affected and untreated animals is very high. Following successful treatment, the gangrenous muscle tissue may slough. Internal lesions may not be detectible by clinical examination.

At necropsy, most changes are limited to affected muscles. Lesions may be located in

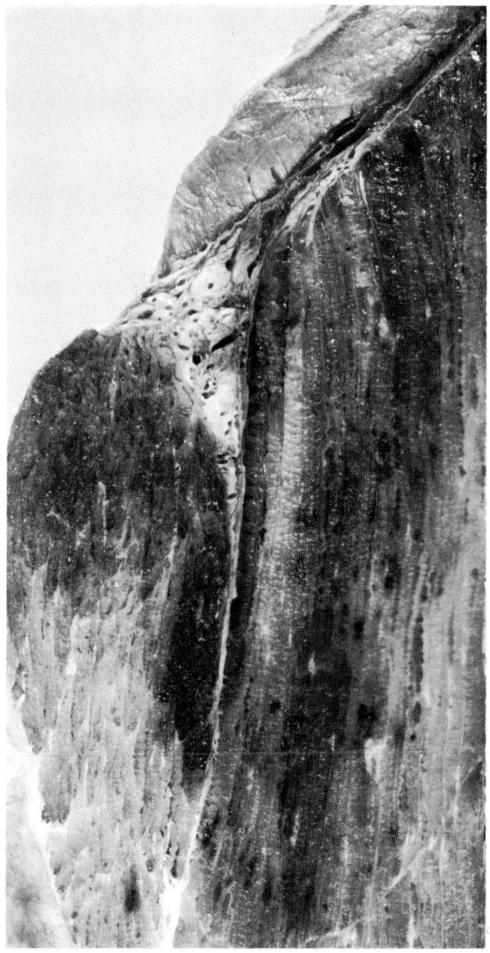

FIG. 4-28. *Muscle from a steer affected with blackleg.* × 0.7.

any muscle but are found more commonly in the thigh, shoulder, back and neck and less commonly in the tongue, crura of the diaphragm and myocardium. The affected muscle is swollen and emphysematous. Gas bodies accumulate under the skin, along

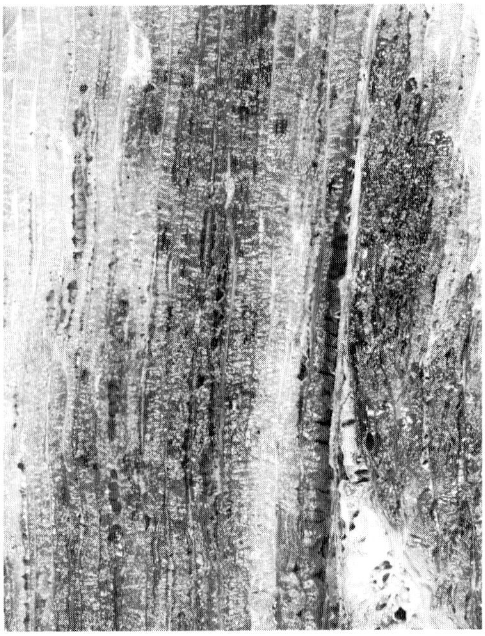

FIG. 4-29. *Blackleg in bovine muscle, showing emphysema and hemorrhage.* × 0.7.

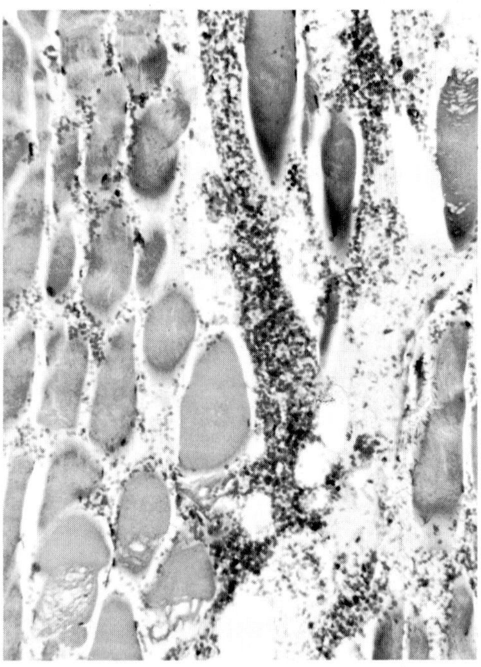

FIG. 4-30. *Acute inflammation in bovine muscle affected with blackleg. HE stain.* × 240.

fascia and between specific muscle bundles. Where hemorrhage has occurred, affected tissue is black; otherwise the muscle is pale. A butyric odor emanates from the lesion. Frequently, the muscle is dry but connective tissue at the periphery of the lesion is edematous and hemorrhagic. The serosanguineous transudate is more abundant in lesions containing *Cl. septicum.*

Histopathologically, affected tissue shows coagulative necrosis of muscle and other tissue, accumulation of serum and leukocytes and hemolysed erythrocytes. The gram-positive rods can be found throughout the lesion, but not uniformly. Some muscle bundles are separated by gas bodies.

At the time of necropsy or at inspection from salvage slaughter, the affected animal and all parts should be incinerated or disposed of with quick lime and deep burial. The contaminated surface should be disinfected with heat or chemicals.

Diagnosis. The clinical diagnosis of blackleg, although uncommon, is made from the typical signs of fever, depression, muscular stiffness, muscular swelling and crepitation. Cases in which the infection is inaccessible for palpation, such as in the crura of the diaphragm, are difficult to diagnose clinically.

At necropsy, additional evidence is the swollen, darkened, and emphysematous muscle from which the butyric odor emanates. Furthermore, the diagnosis can be confirmed in the laboratory through culture of affected tissue and by intra-muscular inoculation of guinea pigs with infected tissue. *Cl. chauvoei* and *Cl. septicum* produce a sanguineous myositis in guinea pigs. Smears from the surface of the liver show mostly single organisms, but some chains, in cases of *Cl. chauvoei* and a predominance of chains, with a few single organisms, in cases of *Cl. septicum.*

The differential diagnosis requires consideration of malignant edema, sweet clover poisoning, anthrax and shipping fever. Malignant edema is a gaseous gangrenous infection in which *Cl. septicum* enters the tissue through a wound. Usually the injury is discernible either clinically or at necropsy. In sweet clover poisoning, the affected animals have a history of having consumed spoiled sweet clover for several weeks. The enlargement in a muscular area is due to intramuscular hemorrhage. Anemia and a prolonged clotting time are discernible. Anthrax has a prolonged blood clotting time and shows typical rods of *Bacillus anthracis* in blood smears. At necropsy, the spleen is enlarged. Animals affected with shipping fever show nasal discharge, rapid respiration, and, in advanced cases, pneumonia.

Prevention and Treatment. Even though *Cl. chauvoei* and *Cl. septicum* are common in the soil in blackleg endemic areas, the degree of exposure of susceptible animals can be reduced by hygienic disposal of infected carcasses through either burning or deep burial, and by disinfection of the contaminated surface with chemicals or heat.

In most endemic areas the disease is prevented through vaccination of animals at approximately 6 months of age. One dose of vaccine is usually sufficient. In the past, immunizing agents have been aggressins prepared from infected tissues, or from artificial cultures, and vaccines prepared from dried and heated infected muscle and from formalinized whole cultures. At the present time most commercial vaccines consist of a mixture of formalinized whole cultures of *Cl. chauvoei* and *Cl. septicum.* This product usually is safe and efficacious. All cattle entering the feedlot should be vaccinated. This procedure enhances immunity in animals previously vaccinated and immunizes those that escaped earlier vaccination.

In feedlots, outbreaks of blackleg are uncommon because of earlier immunization. When the disease develops, the administration of one dose of vaccine containing *Cl. chauvoei* and *Cl. septicum* should control the disease and prevent spread. Occasionally, however, a special vaccine containing *Cl. chauvoei, Cl. septicum,* and *Cl. novyi* has been necessary to stop spread of the disease in a pen.

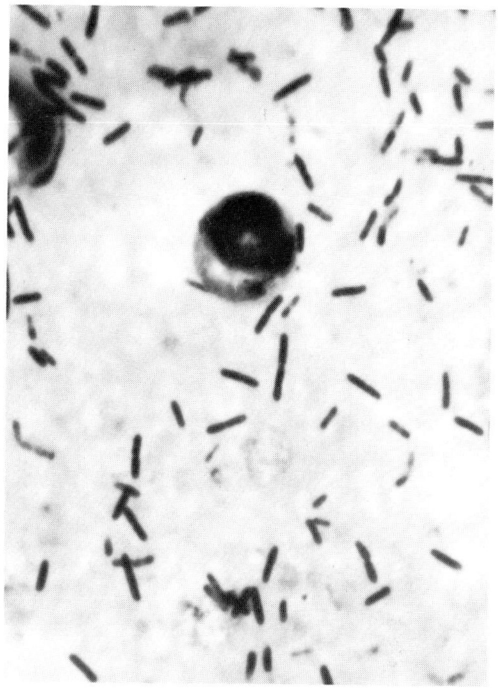

FIG. 4-31. *Clostridium chauvoei in smear from peritoneum of a guinea pig. Gram stain.* × 1550.

In early stages of the disease the use of 2,000 to 4,000 units of penicillin per pound of body weight per day administered intramuscularly has been efficacious. The gangrenous muscle tissue of surviving animals, however, may slough.

References

Aitken, W. A.: Penicillin in Blackleg. North Am. Vet., *30* (1949): 441.

Breed, F.: A Study of Blackleg and its Complications. JAVMA, *90* (1937): 521–528.

Breen, H.: Personal Communication. (1959).

Bollinger, O.: Deuts. Thiermed. vergl. Patholgie, *1* (1875): 297. (quoted by Robertson, M.: A System of Bacteriology, *3* (1929): 225–297).

Byrne, J. L. and Armstrong, J. H. O.: Blackleg with Atypical Symptoms Caused by *Cl. novyi.*: Cana. J. Comp. Med., *12* (1948): 155–160.

Graub, E.: Schweiz. Arch. Tierheilk., *66* (1924): 33.

Leclainche, E. et Vallee, H.: Sur la vaccination Centre la Charbon symptomatique. Seances Mem. Soc. Biol., *92* (1925): 1273–1276.

McEwen, A. D.: J. Comp. Path., *39* (1926): 253–283.
Minett, F. C.: Pathogenesis of Black Quarter I. Tissue Damage and Spore Latency. J. Comp. Path., *58* (1948): 201–209.
———: Pathogenesis of Black Quarter II. Influence of Nutrition and of Muscular Exercise. J. Comp. Path., *58* (1948a): 245–258.
———: Pathogenesis of Black Quarter III. Influence of Nutrition and of Muscular Exercise. J. Comp. Path., *58* (1948b): 259–266.
Moussa, R. S.: Complexity of Toxins from *Cl. septicum* and *Cl. chauvoei.* J. Bact., *76* (1958): 538–545.
Robertson, M.: Organisms Associated with Gas Gangrene. A System of Bacteriology, *3* (1929): 275–297.
Ryff, J. F. and Lee, A. M.: Blackleg Immunity. JAVMA, *111* (1941): 283–287.
Scheuber, J. R.: Some Remarks on Black Quarter Vaccines. Onderstepoort J. Vet. Science and An. Industry, *19* (1944): 17–22.
Scott, J. R., Turner, A. W. and Vawter, R. L.: Gas Edema Disease Twelfth Internal. Vet. Congress, *2* (1934): 168–182.
Stableforth, A. W. and Galloway, I. A.: Infectious Disease of Animals. Vol. 1. New York Academic Press, Inc. (1959): 160–169.
Sterne, M., Thorold, P. and Scheuber, J. R.: A Note on A New Method for Preparing a Potent Anti-Chauvoei Vaccine. J. Comp. Path., *61* (1951): 150–154.
Vawter, R. L.: Recovery of *Clostridium sordellii* from Cattle and Sheep. AJVR, *3* (1942): 382–385.
Weinberg, M. and Michailescu, M.: Ann. Pasteur, *43* (1930): 1408–1465.

Malignant Edema

(GAS GANGRENE)

An acute infectious but non-contagious disease characterized by gangrene and emphysema around a wound, malignant edema is caused by *Clostridium septicum* and related bacteria. Since the disease in feedlot cattle is uncommon and sporadic, the total economic loss to the cattle feeding industry is relatively low. The incidence following castration, dehorning or accidental wounds, however, in a single herd may be high. Economic losses result from a high mortality rate of animals in any stage of fattening.

Review of Literature. The causative organism of malignant edema, first discovered in infected animal tissues, was described under the name *Vibrion septique* (Pasteur and Joubert, 1877). Later, classified in the genus *Clostridium,* it retained the specific name *septicum. Cl. septicum* has been found as a wound contaminant in many species of domestic animals (Bouvier, 1959), including cattle, horses, sheep and swine and also in man (Robertson, 1929). Because of the opportunity for wound contamination, malignant edema in people and horses has been common during wars. In cattle and sheep, *Cl. septicum* has been found associated with *Cl. chauvoei* (Breed, 1937; Graub and Schweiz, 1924; Scott *et al.,* 1934; Weinberg *et al.,* 1930) and with *Cl. novyi* (Breen, 1959; Scott *et al.,* 1934; Vawter, 1942) in lesions of blackleg. More recent studies on the metabolism of the organism indicated that two exotoxins are produced: alpha which is lethal, necrotizing, oxygen-stabile and hemolytic; and beta which is deoxyribonuclease (Moussa, 1958; Warrack *et al.,* 1951).

Etiology and Pathogenesis. The causative bacteria of malignant edema include several species of anaerobes. While *Cl. septicum* is the main species, *Cl. novyi, Cl. perfringens, Cl. sporogenes, Cl. sordellii* and *Cl. tertium* are often associated and contribute to the cause of the disease. *Cl. septicum,* a motile spore-bearing anaerobe is found in soil, manure and alimentary tracts and on animal skin surfaces. The vegetative form measures 0.6 to 0.8 × 3 to 8 μ. The spore is oval and sub-terminal. Organisms in tissues and in young cultures are gram-positive, but in old cultures many cells become gram-negative. The tendency of the organism to form short chains is strong, but single cells are also observed. On peritoneal surfaces of infected guinea pigs, short chains predominate. The exotoxin in tissues and cultures contains two components: alpha which is necrotizing and lethal and beta which is a hemolytic deoxyribonuclease. Resistance of the organism to chemical disinfectants, heat, and light is similar to *Cl. chauvoei.*

In the pathogenesis of malignant edema,

a rapidly spreading mixed infection develops in and around a wound. Deep penetrating anaerobic wounds, such as puncture injuries, are favorable to the disease. At the time of or following the injury, spores of *Cl. septicum* and other anaerobes of soil, manure and skin surfaces are carried into the wound. Under anaerobic conditions the spores vegetate, proliferate rapidly and produce exotoxin. The necrotizing component of toxin produces necrosis of tissue, while the hemolytic component hemolyzes erythrocytes. Some gas is generated by metabolism of the bacteria. The infection spreads along loose connective tissue and fascial planes. Inflammatory edema and exudate accumulate in the affected region. Early in the disease process, the affected tissues are viable and sensitive. In advanced stages necrotic and gangrenous tissue becomes insensitive. Specific exotoxin and toxic substances from the infected tissue are absorbed and cause severe systemic depression. The high mortality results from the toxic effect on the central nervous system.

Occurrence. Malignant edema occurs in all ages, sexes and breeds of cattle. Wounds and complications from parturition predispose females to a high incidence. The soil and manure of heavily used feedlots are seeded with vast numbers of *Cl. septicum* and other clostridial bacteria; consequently, many animals injured in the environment of a feedlot become exposed to the cause of malignant edema. In addition to cattle, horses, sheep, swine, dogs, and cats of the domestic species and guinea pigs, rabbits, mice, and pigeons among the laboratory animals are susceptible. Man also is susceptible. Occurring in all seasons, the disease is universal in geographic distribution.

Clinical Signs and Postmortem Lesions. Following an incubation period from 2 to 4 days from the time of wound contamination, body temperature often rises to 106° to 108° F. In some cases body temperature remains normal. The affected animal goes off feed, breathes rapidly and is profoundly depressed. An edematous and frequently emphysematous swelling forms around the infected wound. The swelling spreads rapidly and when extending over muscles of locomotion causes lameness. In early stages the swollen tissue is painful but later becomes insensitive. A serosanguineous gaseous and malodorous fluid exudes from the wound and in addition is revealed on incision of the swollen tissue. In advanced stages of the disease the animal is prostrated and often disoriented. As the disease progresses the swelling gravitates to lower planes in the tissue. Infection of the genitalia following normal parturition or dystocia gravitates in the perineum ventrally along medial aspects of the thighs; the swollen edematous mucosa is translucent. Infection from castration wounds gravitates anteroventrally along the abdominal wall and laterally to the thighs, while infection from dehorning gravitates ventrally over the eyelid, face and neck of the infected side.

Death occurs after a course of 12 to 48 hours. While the morbidity rate is unually low, the mortality rate of affected animals is high.

At necropsy, the prominent lesion is the swelling in and around a wound. The opened affected tissue discloses an extensive serosanguineous and often gaseous transudate in the loose connective tissue and fascia around the wound. The muscles usually are intact and are invaded only slightly. Butyric and foul odors are detectible. Regional lymph nodes are swollen and hemorrhagic. During healing stages of non-fatal cases, the gangrenous skin and subcutaneous tissues may slough. Liver, kidneys and myocardium are swollen and lungs are often edematous as a result of intoxication from exotoxin and from gangrenous tissue.

Histopathologically, the tissue shows peracute inflammation. Necrosis is widespread. Hemorrhagic transudate with some leukocytes fill the interstices of the loose connective tissue between muscles and along fascial planes. In some cases muscle cells are necrotic. Gas vacuoles, gram-positive *Cl.*

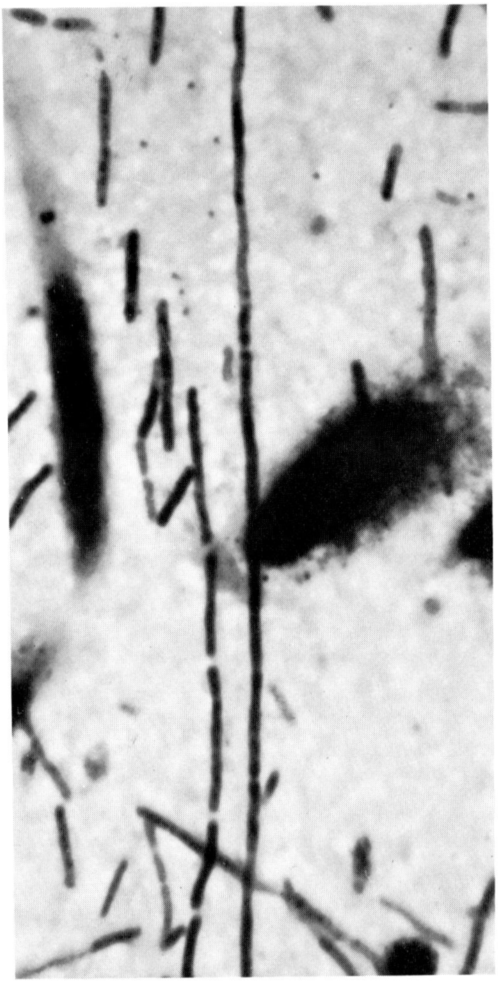

FIG. 4-32. *Clostridium septicum in smear from peritoneum of a guinea pig. Gram stain.* × 2000.

septicum and often other species of bacteria are discernible. Internally, the myocardium, liver, and kidneys show cloudy swelling. Transudate fills some alveoli and interlobular septa of the lungs.

Diagnosis. The clinical diagnosis of malignant edema is based on typical signs and lesions. Significantly important is the rapidly spreading crepitous painful swelling around a wound in a febrile animal. Additional evidence is the gaseous serosanguineous fluid in and around necrotic tissue as is revealed by incision of the swollen tissue and at necropsy.

Confirmatory evidence can be obtained in the laboratory from study of affected tissues. *Cl. septicum,* as well as *Cl. novyi, Cl. perfringens* and other bacteria, can be isolated frequently from the necrotic tissue and from the serosanguineous transudate. The intramuscular inoculation of guinea pigs with the affected tissue causes a hemorrhagic necrotizing myositis. Following death of the guinea pig, short chains of *Cl. septicum* can be demonstrated in smears from the surface of the liver.

The differential diagnosis requires consideration of blackleg. In this disease the affected animal usually has no history of injury and the necrotic muscle is dry and small bodies of gas are located between the muscle bundles, while in malignant edema the abundant serosanguineous transudate accumulates in the connective tissue between muscles in the subcutaneous tissue and in fascia. In some cases, however, the gross lesions of both malignant edema and blackleg are grossly indistinguishable and require laboratory studies for differentiation.

Prevention and Treatment. Since malignant edema is associated with contamination of wounds, the disease can be partially prevented by minimizing opportunities for injuries in a feedlot. Sharp offensive horns can be amputated or dulled to avoid puncture wounds. Protruding nails, wire and other sharp objects should be removed from fences, feeding bunks and walking areas. The vaccination of young cattle against blackleg with a vaccine containing *Cl. septicum* along with *Cl. chauvoei* gives some protection against malignant edema. To avoid wound contamination with soil bearing organisms, castration and dehorning should be performed under hygienic conditions. Antibiotics may be administered prophylactically for 4 to 5 days following surgery, injury, or parturition.

In early stages the disease is treated daily with penicillin at the rate of 2,000 to 4,000 units per pound of body weight. Supplementation with large doses of streptomycin and/or sulfonamides is beneficial. Hot flowing water may be applied daily for 30 minutes to the infected tissues for 3 to 4 days. After suppression or elimination of infection by appropriate treatment, the necrotic tissue should be incised to provide drainage and to accelerate healing.

References

Bouvier, G.: Clostridial septicemia in Calves after Dehorning. Schweiz. Arch. Tierheilk., *101* (1959): 499–501.

Breed, F.: A Study of Blackleg and its Complications. JAVMA, *90* (1937): 521–528.

Breen, H.: Personal communication. (1959).

Graub, E.: Schweiz. Arch. Tierheilk., *66* (1924): 33.

Hutyra, F., Marek, J. and Manninger, R.: *Special Pathology and Therapeutics of Diseases of Domestic Animals.* Vol. I. Alexander Eger, Inc. Chicago. 1946, pp. 49–50.

Moussa, R. S.: Complexity of Toxins from *Cl. septicum* and *Cl. chauvoei.* J. Bact. *76* (1958): 538–545.

Pasteur, and Joubert: Bull. Acad. Med. II Ser., *6* (1877): 781.

Robertson, M.: Organisms Associated with Gas Gangrene. A System of Bacteriology, *3* (1929): 225–297.

Scott, J. P., Turner, A. W. and Vawter, R. L.: Gas Edema Disease. Twelfth Internal. Vet. Congress, *2* (1934): 168–182.

Vawter, R. L.: Recovery of *Clostridium Sordellii* from Cattle and Sheep. AJVR, *3* (1942): 382–385.

Warrack, G. H., Bidwell, E. and Oakley, C. L.: The Beta-toxin (Deoxyribonuclease) of *Cl. septicum.* J. Path. & Bact., *63* (1951): 293–302.

Weinberg, M. and Mihailescu, M.: Ann. Pasteur, *43* (1930): 1408–1465.

Bovine Enterotoxemia

(OVEREATING)

Clinical enterotoxemia, an acute infectious but non-contagious disease, is characterized by sudden death, and is probably caused by the toxin of *Clostridium perfringens* type D. The toxin is formed in the small intestine and is absorbed into the blood. While this disease is often suspected and diagnosed clinically in feedlot cattle, its toxin has not been isolated from the bovine intestine nor has it been identified unequivocally. Clinical enterotoxemia, common in feedlot cattle of western and midwestern states and in many feedlots, results in serious economic losses.

Review of Literature. During and following the first World War, *Cl. perfringens* was studied intensively both *in vivo* and *in vitro.* The bacteria of this species were classified into types according to toxin production. The four common types were A, B, C, and D. Specific but common toxins formed by the different types of bacteria were designated by Greek letters, alpha, beta, and epsilon (Wilsdon, 1931).

Many important diseases have been produced by *Cl. perfringens.* During times of warfare, organisms of type A have caused gas gangrene. In Great Britain, organisms of type B, which produce beta, epsilon and alpha toxin, caused lamb dysentery, a malady of baby lambs (Dalling, 1928; 1936). In America, organisms of type C, which produce beta and alpha toxin, were identified as the cause of hemorrhagic enterotoxemia of calves up to 10 days of age. Affected calves died after a very short course (Griner and Bracken, 1953). In addition, a few outbreaks of hemorrhagic enterotoxemia of lambs from type C were diagnosed (Griner and Johnson, 1954). In Great Britain, organisms of type C produced "struck" of adult sheep (Turner and Rodwell, 1943). Bacteria of type D, producing epsilon and alpha toxin, caused enterotoxemia, a disease of primary importance in adult sheep (March, 1958). In 1932 at Australia (Bennets, 1932) and New Zealand (Gill, 1932), scientists first determined that enterotoxemia of sheep is caused by type D. Prior to the development and marketing of an effective vaccine, this disease produced an approximate mortality of 5% of young sheep fattened in feedlots of the western United States (Marsh, 1958). In a few pastured cattle, suspected cases of enterotoxemia have been diagnosed clinically, and epsilon toxin has been isolated from the small intestine (Keast and McBarron, 1954). In addition, the disease has been diagnosed in calves 7 to 8 weeks of age, and epsilon toxin has been isolated from the intestines (Griner, Eickelman and Brown, 1956).

Clostridium perfringens type D has been suspected of wide distribution in soil and manure (Bennets, 1932). From these sources, presumably, the organisms entered the digestive system through contamination of food and water. Experimentally, most washed organisms fed to adult sheep were destroyed in transit through the rumen and abomasum (Bullen and Scarisbrick, 1953). Some organisms, however, survived and entered the small intestine. In the ileum, these organisms survived temporarily and produced small amounts of toxin in sheep maintained on a ration of roughage. When host sheep suddenly ingested large amounts of high caloric concentrate, such as wheat, many starch granules passed into the small intestine. In the ileum, acting on the starch substrate, the bacteria multiplied rapidly and produced large amounts of epsilon toxin which resulted in death of the sheep (Bullen and Scarisbrick, 1957).

Clinical studies of sheep affected with enterotoxemia have demonstrated that the epsilon toxin injures the blood vessels. In the brain, the blood vessels became more permeable to plasma proteins causing the development of edema. Both neurons and myelinated tracts were injured (Griner, 1961; Griner and Carlson, 1961).

Occurrence. In feedlot cattle, enterotoxemia may occur at any stage of fattening. The incidence is highest, however, when the animals are fed rations with a very high ratio of concentrate to roughage. Both sexes and all breeds are susceptible. Animals 6 months to 2 years of age are more commonly affected. In addition to feedlot cattle, enterotoxemia occurs occasionally in pastured cattle, in calves and commonly in sheep.

Etiology and Pathogensis. Enterotoxemia is caused by the various types of *Cl. perfringens.* In feedlot cattle, *Cl. perfringens* type D has been assumed to be the cause. The specific type with its accompanying toxin has not been isolated nor identified. Table 8 presents the four principal types, the amounts, nature and actions of their toxins and the diseases produced by them.

Cl. perfringens, a gram-positive, nonmotile, anaerobic spore-bearing rod, measures approximately 4 to 8 by 0.8 to 1.5 μ. The subterminal or central spores have flattened ends. The organisms occur singly, in pairs, and in short chains and are widely distributed in soil and manure.

Although the pathogenesis of enterotoxemia in feedlot cattle has not been studied, in feedlot sheep, where the disease is common, the development of the disease has been carefully described. Probably the pathogenesis in both feedlot sheep and feedlot cattle is similar. *Cl. perfringens* type D, commonly present in soil and manure, contaminates feed and water and is ingested by feedlot cattle. In moving through the rumen and abomasum, many of the organisms are destroyed. Some, however, survive and enter the small intestine where proliferation and toxin production occur. In animals fed a ration of roughage, the environment of the small intestine is unfavorable to *Cl. perfringens* type D. Only small amounts, if any, of epsilon toxin are produced and proliferation of the organisms is limited. However, in animals maintained on a ration having a high ratio of concentrate to roughage, and especially in animals suddenly fed large quantities of high caloric concentrate of wheat, barley or corn, many undigested starch granules are transferred through the abomasum into the small intestine. In the ileum, the *Cl. perfringens* type D organisms, acting on the substrate of starch granules, proliferate rapidly and produce large amounts of nontoxic prototoxin. Trypsin from the duodenum converts the prototoxin to epsilon toxin. The latter is absorbed into the blood and is distributed to all organs.

Through its necrotizing action, epsilon toxin weakens blood capillaries which commonly rupture and produce small hemorrhages. In the brain and possibly in other organs, the walls of small vessels are rendered

TABLE 8 *Clostridium perfringens*

Type of Organism	Toxins: Types and Amounts	Nature	Action	Diseases
A	α+++	lecithinase	necrosis; hemolysis	gas gangrene
B	α+	lecithinase	necrosis; hemolysis	lamb dysentery
	β+++		necrosis	
	ϵ++	trypsin activated	necrosis	
C	α+	lecithinase	necrosis; hemolysis	1. hemorrhagic enterotoxemia, calves
	β+++		necrosis	2. "struck" of adult sheep
				3. hemorrhagic enterotoxemia, lambs
D	α+	lecithinase	necrosis; hemolysis	1. enterotoxemia of sheep
	ϵ+++	trypsin activated	necrosis	2. entertoxemia of adult cattle?
				3. enterotoxemia of feedlot cattle?
				4. enterotoxemia of calves

more permeable to protein. The toxin, diffusing from the vessels, causes serious and often fatal injury to vital neurons. Death usually occurs after a course of 1 to 2 hours. In animals which remain alive but comatose for several days, foci of necrosis develop in the brain.

Clinical Signs and Postmortem Lesions. Three clinical syndromes occur in feedlot cattle. In the first and more common form, deaths occur without evidence of previous illness. If observed clinically, affected animals suddenly become incoordinated and prostrated. Generalized convulsions, with muscular spasms of the ears and eyes, are followed by death after a course of 1 to 2 hours. In the second form, the body temperature is slightly elevated and paralysis of the posterior limbs develops. Death occurs after a course of 8 to 12 hours. In the third form, affected animals become prostrated and comatose early in the disease course. Tactile and auditory stimuli provoke convulsions with oposthotonis. Death occurs after a course of approximately 1 week. In all clinical forms hyperglycemia and glycosuria may be present. The incidence may be sporadic but in some herds within a short period the morbidity rate may reach 5 to 10%. The mortality rate of affected animals is near 100%.

At necropsy, the rumen and often the abomasum are filled with concentrate feed. The small intestine, especially the ileum, may contain considerable fluid in some segments. Petechial and ecchymotic hemorrhages are abundant in serosal membranes. The subendocardium of the left ventricle, subepicardium and thymus are common locations. Ingesta of the ileum may contain toxin and the urine glucose. The brain may exhibit demonstrable edema.

In many cases no changes are detectable histopathologically. In the brain, perivascular edema and some necrosis of neurons are often discernible. Large numbers of gram-positive *Cl. perfringens* can be found in the contents of the ileum.

Diagnosis. Enterotoxemia is diagnosed on the basis of sudden death, or a short course with typical signs, glycosuria and the demonstration of epsilon toxin and *Cl. perfringens* in contents of the small intestine. Contents of the small intestine should be transferred to a container and refrigerated within 1 hour after death. In the laboratory, toxins are identified from intestinal contents by known antitoxin neutralization and mouse inoculation. The bacteria, in large numbers, can be demonstrated in stained smears and in cultures. In case of suspected enterotoxemia, fluid contents of the small intestine, especially the ileum, should be removed from the gut, refrigerated, and transferred to a laboratory for further study.

Little positive information is currently available on enterotoxemia of feedlot cattle. Until such time, when the disease is accurately characterized and clinically collated with the presence of toxin, the diagnosis should require identification of specific toxin in the alimentary tract.

The differential diagnosis requires consideration of acute poisoning, acute bloat and thromboembolic meningoencephalitis. Poisoning may be determined from possible availability of toxic substances and from chemical analysis of ingesta of affected cattle. In acute bloat the rumen is distended with stable froth and ingesta, and the peripheral blood vessels are distended. Animals affected with thromboembolic meningoencephalitis usually remain alive, even though comatose, for many days. At necropsy foci of infection are discernible randomly distributed throughout the brain.

Prevention. In some outbreaks of enterotoxemia the development of additional cases can be prevented by reducing the amount of grain concentrate in the ration and by increasing the roughage. Relocation of the cattle to new pens and new feed may also prevent additional cases. An alternative regimen is the medication of the herd diet with chlortetracycline or oxytetracycline at the rate of 1 mg per pound of body weight for 7 to 10 days. In case of a high incidence of bloat, the use of antibiotic should be discontinued. Quaternary ammonium preparations fed in the diet at the rate of 2 grams per animal per day allegedly is beneficial. Feedlots anticipating heavy losses from enterotoxemia may vaccinate all cattle on arrival with toxoid containing *Cl. perfringens* type D. A commercial vaccine containing *Cl. chauvoei, Cl. septicum, Cl. novyi, Cl. sordelli,* and *Cl. perfringens* types C and D is available. The effectiveness of this procedure has not been verified.

The short course of enterotoxemia precludes treatment.

References

Bennets, H. W.: Infectious Entero-toxemia (the so-called Braxy-like Disease) of Sheep in Western Australia. Australia Commonwealth Council Sci. Ind. Research Bull. No. 57, 1932.

Bosworth, T. J. and Glover, R. E.: Rep. Dir. Inst. An. Path. Camb., *4* (1934): 79.

Bullen, J. J. and Scarisbrick, R.: Enterotoxemia of Sheep: The Fate of Washed Suspensions of *Cl. welchii* type D introduced into the Rumen of Normal Sheep. J. Path. & Bact., *65* (1953): 209–219.

Bullen, J. J. and Scarisbrick, R.: Enterotoxemia of Sheep: Experimental Reproduction of the Disease. J. Path. & Bact., *73* (1957): 495–509.

Dalling, T.: Lamb Dysentery. Nat. Vet. Med. Assoc. Congress. Report, New Castle-On-Tyne, Sept. 4, 1928.

———: Anaerobic Infections in Sheep. Vet. Rec., *48* (1936): 1477–1480.

Gill, D. A.: New Zealand J. Agriculture, *45* (1932): 332.

Griner, L. A. and Bracken, F. K.: *Clostridium perfringens* (type C) in Acute Hemorrhagic Enterotoxemia of Calves. JAVMA, *122* (1953): 99–102.

Griner, L. A. and Johnson, H. W.: *Clostridium perfringens* type C in Hemorrhagic Enterotoxemia of Lambs. JAVMA, *125* (1954): 125–127.

Griner, L. A. and Baldwin, E. M., Jr.: Further Work on Hemorrhagic Enterotoxemia of Infant Calves and Lambs. Proceedings Book, AVMA, 91st meeting, 1954. pp. 45–51.

Griner, L. A., Aichelman, W. W. and Brown, G. D.: *Clostridium perfringens* type D (epsilon) Enterotoxemia in Brown Swiss Dairy Calves, JAVMA, *129* (1956): 375–376.

Griner, L. A.: Enterotoxemia of Sheep. I. Effects of *Clostridium perfringens* type D Toxin on the Brains of Sheep and Mice. AJVR, *22* (1961): 429–442.

Griner, L. A. and Carlson, W. D.: Enterotoxemia of Sheep. II. Distribution of I^{131} Radioiodinated Serum Albumin in Brains of *Clostridium perfringens* type D Intoxicated Lambs. AJVR, *22* (1961): 443–446.

Keast, J. C. and McBarron, E. J.: A Case of Enterotoxemia. Aust. Vet. J., *30* (1954): 305–306.

Marsh, H.: Newsom's Sheep Diseases. 2nd ed. The Williams & Wilkins Company. Baltimore. 1958. pp. 20–26.

Montgomerie, R. F.: *Clostridium perfringens* (*Cl. welchii*) Enterotoxemia in the Ruminant. Canad. Vet. J., *2* (1951): 439–450.

Niilo, L. and Avery, R. J.: Bovine Enterotoxemia. I. *Clostridium perfringens* types Isolated from Animal Sources in Alberta and Saskatchewan. Canad. Vet. J., *4* (1963): 31–36.
Stableforth, A. W. and Galloway, I. A.: *Infectious Diseases of Animals.* Vol. I. Academic Press, Inc. New York 1959, pp. 173–195.
Turner, A. W. and Rodwell, A. W.: Aust. J. Exp. Biol. Med. Sc., *21* (1943): 17.
Wilsdon, A. J.: Observations on the Classification of *Bacillus welchii.* Univ. Cambridge. Inst. Animal Path., 2nd Rept. Director, 1931, p. 51.

Tetanus

(LOCKJAW)

An acute infectious but non-contagious neurointoxication, tetanus is characterized by muscular spasms resulting in a high mortality rate and is caused by the exotoxin of *Clostridium tetani.* Since the total incidence of the disease is low, its economic importance is minor but occasionally, however, the incidence in a herd is high. Economic losses result from high mortality rate, from loss of body weight during the course of the disease, and from expensive medical treatments.

Review of Literature. Following discovery and description of *Cl. tetani* (Nicolaier, 1884) and identification of the exotoxin (Behring and Kitasato, 1890), the organism and its toxin were studied extensively. The toxin produced by a single strain of organisms in the same medium was found to vary in complexity with the duration of incubation (Petrie, 1942–43). In addition, the toxins were potentiated by some chemicals and muscle tissue and, although requiring the same amount of antitoxin for neutralization, the potentiated toxin produced death in guinea pigs at much higher dilutions than the plain toxin. The potentiating substance in muscle was shown to be heat-stable, alcohol soluble and acetone insoluble. Potentiating chemicals included sodium acetate, citrate and glycolate (Zuger *et al.,* 1939). When mixed with fresh emulsified spinal cord and brain, the toxin was neutralized (Wasserman and Takaki, 1898). The purified toxin injected in the sub pia mater of dogs evoked convulsions for prolonged periods (Carrea and Lanari, 1962). Tetanus toxin did not traverse the placenta of rabbits when injected into the maternal blood or into the thoracic and amnionic cavities of the feti or into the uterine lumen (Fedinec, 1962).

Meticulous investigations led scientists to believe that tetanus toxin originated at a local point of infection and ascended to the central nervous system along perineural lymphatics of the axones of the motor nerve trunks. Toxins ascending the axones of sensory nerves did not enter the spinal cord because of interruption by neuron bodies of the dorsal route ganglia (Meyer and Ransom, 1903; Wright *et al.,* 1950). Within the spinal cord or medulla oblongata, receptors of the toxin were considered to be a mucolipid ganglioside within the central nervous system (van Hegningen, 1959). Toxin injected into the medulla oblongata was one thousand times more effective, as measured by survival period, than toxin injected into the blood system (Wright, 1953). While the exact mechanism by which tetanus toxin causes muscular spasm is not fully known, experimentation motivated the theory that, like strychnine, the toxin suppresses all types of synaptic inhibitions and causes muscles, both prime movers and antagonists, to contract violently, and, more or less, continuously. An opposing hypothesis suggested that tetanus toxin evokes muscular spasticity through peripheral action at the myoneural plate (Able, 1938).

The spores of *Cl. tetani* were shown to be widespread in soil. In one study they were isolated from animal feces with an occurrence rate of 15% of 53 horses, 19% of 21 cows, 26% of 23 sheep, 46% of 37 dogs, 37% of 141 rats, and 18% of 34 fowl (Kerrin, 1929; Tenbroeck and Bauer, 1922), while in another study of 21 cattle, no *Cl. tetani* were isolated from the feces (Noble, 1915).

Studies of immunization indicated that active immunity could be evoked with parenteral administration of formalinized toxin (Ramon and Descombey, 1927). Successful treatment was achieved using antitoxin and tranquilizers, such as chlorpromazine combined with heavy doses of penicillin (Gibbons, 1940; Bryer, 1958; Herlitz, 1947; Wichens *et al.*, 1960).

Occurrence. Universally distributed, the spores of *Cl. tetani* occur commonly in soil and feces of domestic animals. While most species of domestic animals are susceptible to tetanus, the descending susceptibility exists in this order: horses, swine, sheep, cattle, goats, cats, dogs and fowl. In the laboratory, mice and guinea pigs are highly susceptible. Although the incidence in cattle is low, all breeds, ages, and sexes are susceptible. During the years 1958–1963 at the Veterinary Hospital, Colorado State University, 105,670 cattle were attended, and among these animals 12 cases of tetanus occurred. While the disease occurs during all seasons, the opportunity for wound contamination is less during winter months when soil and manure are frozen.

Etiology and Pathogenesis. *Cl. tetani,* the causative agent of tetanus, is a soil-bearing, gram-positive, anaerobic, motile, spore-bearing exotoxin producing slender rod with parallel sides and rounded ends. The vegetative cell measures 0.2 to 0.6 x 2 to 5 μ. The organism, occurring usually in tissue and culture as single cells, may also form short chains which tend to separate into individual cells. The spores are terminal and spherical. The vegetative form is highly susceptible to drying, light, heat and chemical disinfectants. While the spore is highly resistant, enduring in soil and manure for many months and possibly years, aqueous phenol solution destroys most spores in 10 to 12 hours. Surface colonies on solid media are flat, feathery and elevated at the center. On blood agar they hemolyze erythrocytes. Antigenically heterogeneous, tetanus bacilli contain 10 serotypes all of which produce the same kind of exotoxin.

The toxin, a protein, contains two fractions: tetanospasmin which attacks nervous tissue and tetanolysin which hemolyses erythrocytes. Tetanus toxin is stable to freezing and thawing, is destroyed by direct sunshine in 15 hours at 40° C and in solution is destroyed in 5 minutes at 65° C. The toxin is not absorbed from the lumen of the alimentary tract.

While investigators do not agree fully on the pathogenesis of tetanus, a consensus that the toxin acts primarily through the central nervous system exists. The spores, along with pyogenic bacteria from soil and manure, enter tissues through injuries, such as foot punctures, parturition, castration, elastration, dehorning, horn punctures, nail punctures, needle perforations, dog bites and compound fractures. Professional surgery, performed under acceptable hygienic standards, does not result in tetanus. In the anaerobic wound, many tissue cells are necrotic, and the pyogenic bacteria produce exudate. Within these wound conditions the spores of *Cl. tetani* vegetate and toxin is produced. At the site of production, some of the toxin diffuses into the blood and lymph. Because of its affinity for nerve tissue, some toxin also ascends axones of the peripheral nerves and enters the spinal cord through the ventral route. Neurons of the cord and medulla are attacked. Reciprocal synaptic inhibition is abolished. Afferent stimuli are exaggerated and both prime moving and antagonistic muscles contract convulsively and, more or less, continuously. Convulsive contractions often bring physical exhaustion and respiratory failure. Death results from neuronal injury in the medulla and from respiratory failure. Non-fatal cases are immune.

Clinical Signs and Postmortem Lesions. Following a usual incubation period of 1 to 3 weeks, but occasionally longer, clinical signs, all related to muscular spasticity, are initiated in animals with a history of recent injury. In early stages of tetanus the ears are erect, the tail is stiff and elevated a few inches, the head extended, ears erect, the anxious eyes immobile and the nictitating membranes prolapsed. The rigidity and extension of the limbs makes walking difficult. The prehension of food and water is difficult and bloating is common. The temperature rises to 102° to 108° F. Sudden auditory and tactile stimuli provoke violent muscular contractions. As the disease progresses, muscular rigidity and continuous extension of the limbs make walking and other coordinated movements difficult. Frequently the reclining animal cannot rise. When assisted to the standing position, this posture can be maintained only temporarily. While walking, the limbs are abducted. Respiration accelerates and anxiety increases. The jaws are firmly set and nostrils are dilated. Death occurs after 3 to 10 days. In cattle the general mortality rate is approximately 60% of affected cases.

At necropsy, visible lesions are nonspecific and secondary to intoxication and muscular spasticity. The injury and point of infection are usually discernible. Commonly, purulent exudate from secondary infection is present. Petechial hemorrhages may be found in the voluntary muscles and on serosal surfaces, especially of the heart. Frequently, as a result of difficult breathing, the lungs show emphysema.

Histopathologically, the wound shows inflammation and necrosis. *Cl. tetani* are difficult to demonstrate.

Diagnosis. Tetanus is diagnosed from the manifestation of typical clinical signs in animals having a wound history within the previous 3 weeks. Especially important signs are the muscular spasticity and rigidity provokable with auditory and tactile stimuli. Confirmatory evidence may be obtained in the laboratory from examination of exudate from the wound. Cultures of *Cl. tetani* frequently can be isolated and occasionally tetanus exotoxin from the wound exudate can be demonstrated by inoculation of mice with tissue and exudate from the wound.

The differential diagnosis requires consideration of strychnine poisoning. While strychnine poisoning produces similar clinical signs, the course of the disease is usually a few hours. The history may reveal access to strychnine through drugs or malicious acts and the absence of recent injury. In case of poisoning by ingestion, chemical analysis of stomach contents discloses the strychnine.

Prevention and Treatment. Prevention may be partially achieved by removing from feedlots all puncture wound hazards, such as lumber with protruding nails and traumatizing pieces of glass and stone. Horns should be amputated to avoid offensive puncture wounds. All minor surgery, such as dehorning, castration and venipunctures, should be performed hygienically.

While both passive and active immunizations are possible in feedlot cattle, only passive immunization of exposed animals is practiced. At the time of acquiring and treating a deep puncture wound or other types of injury which predispose to tetanus, specific antitoxin should be administered parenterally at the rate of 1,500 units per adult animal. This passive immunization endures sufficiently long to protect against tetanus from the specific wound. The low rate of incidence of predisposing wounds and the short period of fattening does not justify active immunization.

Treatment consists of tranquilization, wound excision and cleaning and the administration of antibiotics. Affected animals should be placed in a quiet darkened room and daily receive chlorpromazine, a tranquilizing drug, at the rate of 400 mg in divided doses for several days. The puncture wound should be opened, cleaned, and irrigated with hydrogen peroxide to avoid further production of toxin. Tetanus antitoxin, although of questionable efficacy, may be administered in heavy doses to neutralize unfixed toxin in the region of the wound and elsewhere. To prevent further growth of *Cl. tetani* in the wound, penicillin in the form giving 72 to 150 hour blood level should be administered as needed. In addition, supporting therapy, such as the intravenous administration of fluids and glucose and, when possible, intragastric administration of fluids and nutrients, should be provided. Proteins, as 1 to 2 gallons of milk mixed with 6 to 12 eggs, should be given daily with a stomach tube until normal ingestion is restored. Treatment may be needed for 30 days.

References

Able, J. J., Frior, W. M. and Chalian, W.: Bull. Johns Hopkins Hosp., *63* (1938): 373.
Behring and Kitasato, S.: Dtsch. Med. Wschr., *16* (1890): 1113.
Brooks, V. B., Curtis, D. R. and Eccles, J. C.: Mode of Action of Tetanus Toxin. Nature, *175* (1955): 120–121.
Bryer, C. J., Jr.: Recovery of a Heifer with Tetanus. JAVMA, *133* (1958): 466.
Carrea, R. and Lanari, A.: Chronic Effect of Tetanus Toxin Applied Locally to the Cerebral Cortex of the Dog. Science, *137* (1962): 342-343.
Fedinec, A. A.: Transport of Tetanus Toxin Across the Rabbit Placenta and Fetal Membranes. J. Lab. & Clin. Med., *60* (1962): 606–611.
Gibbons, W. J.: Tetanus. Cornell Vet., *30* (1940): 533–537.
Haasjes, C.: Tetanus in a Cow. JAVMA, *93* (1938): 197.
Herlitz, G. H.: Successful Treatment with Penicillin of Tetanus in a Heifer. Cornell Vet., *37* (1947): 67–68.
Kerrin, J. C.: The Distribution of *B. tetani* in the Intestines of Animals. Brit. J. Path., *10* (1929): 370–373.
Magrath, L. A. and Magrath, J. M.: Tetanus in Calves from Elastration. JAVMA, *125* (1954): 451.
Meyer, H. and Ransom, F.: Arch. Path. Pharm., *49* (1903): 369.
Nicolaier, A.: Dtsch. Med. Wschr., *10* (1884): 842.
Noble, W.: Experimental Study of the Distribution and Habitat of the Tetanus Bacillus. J. Inf. Dis., *16* (1915): 132.
Petrie, G. F.: Observations on the Variable Interactions of Tetanus Toxins and Antitoxins. Bull. Health Organization, League of Nations, *10* (1942–43): 113–143.
Ramon, G. and Descombey, P.: L'Anatoxine Tetanique et la prophylaie du Tetanos Chez le Cheval et les Animaux Domestiques. Ann. Inst. Pasteur, *41* (1927): 834–849.
Tenbroeck, C. and Bauer, J. H.: The Tetanus Bacillus as an Intestinal Saprophyte in Man. J. Exp. Med., *36* (1922): 261–271.
van Hegningen, W. E.: Tentative Identification of the Tetanus Toxin Receptor in Nervous Tissue. J. Gen. Microbiol., *20* (1959): 310–320.
van Rensburg, S. J.: Tetanus in Calves as a Sequel to Elastration. J. So. African Vet. Med. Assoc., *1* (1959): 29.
Wasserman and Takaki: Berl. klin, Wchnschr., *35* (1898): 5.
Wichens, J. T. and Boswood, B.: Two Further Cases of Tetanus Treated with Chlorpromazine. Vet. Rec., *72* (1960): 162–164.
Wright, E. A., Morgan, R. S. and Wright, G. P.: Tetanus Intoxication of the Brain Stem in Rabbits. J. Path. Bact., *62* (1950): 569–583.
Wright, E. A.: The Effect of the Injection of Tetanus Toxin into the Central Nervous System of Rabbits. J. Immunology, *71* (1953): 41–44.
Zuger, B., Hollander, A. and Friedman, V.: Potentiation of Tetanus Toxin by Tissue and Chemicals. J. Inf. Dis., *65* (1939): 86–91.

Bacillary Hemoglobinuria

(RED WATER DISEASE; ICTERO-HEMOGLOBINURIA)

Bacillary hemoglobinuria, an acute febrile infectious disease of cattle, is characterized by hemoglobinuria and anemia and is caused by *Clostridium hemolyticum*. Because of limited geographic distribution of bacillary hemoglobinuria, the total economic importance of the disease is low, but in some herds within the endemic area, the incidence and mortality may be as high as 25%. Economic losses result from a high mortality rate and from the necessity for frequent vaccinations.

Review of Literature. The first account of the disease described its occurrence in cattle living in mountainous swampy pastures of California and Nevada. Clinical signs and postmortem lesions were observed (Meyer, 1916). Later the disease was seen in sheep (Records and Vawter, 1931) and swine (Records and Huber, 1931). The cause of the disease, *Cl. hemolyticum*, was identified and described as a new species and many aspects of morphology and biochemistry of the organism were determined (Vawter and Records, 1926). The exotoxin contained two components: one highly hemolytic and unstable, and the second necrotizing (Vawter and Records, 1926; Records and Vawter, 1945). While the two components have not been separated and purified, other studies indicated that the toxin contains a lecithinase similar to the lecithinase of *Cl. perfringens* type A toxin (Jasmin, 1947).

Studies of the epizootiology of the disease indicated that some animals from herds recovering from the disease contain viable organisms in the liver and kidneys. Five years following the herd outbreak of bacillary hemoglobinuria, the healthy carrier state was demonstrated in one animal (Safford and Smith, 1945; Smith and Jasmin, 1956). The transport of animals in endemic areas frequently preceded and probably provoked active cases, and when animals from endemic areas were moved to clean areas and mixed with indigenous cattle, the disease developed and spread among both introduced and indigenous cattle. Disease spread appeared to occur from direct contact with diseased animals, from healthy carrier animals, from transport of infected meat and from contaminated water (Safford and Smith, 1954).

Occurrence. Although all breeds, ages and sexes of cattle are susceptible to bacillary hemoglobinuria, animals over 6 months of age are more susceptible than calves. In addition to cattle the disease occurs, but uncommonly, in sheep and swine. In the laboratory, under experimental conditions, rabbits, guinea pigs and mice are susceptible when toxin as well as organisms, are injected parenterally. The disease occurs in feedlot cattle when animals are transported from an endemic area, where the organisms are acquired, to fattening pens. Within 10 to 20 days the disease may occur in the transported animals, as well as in other cattle with which the shipped animals cohabitate. The feedlot may be located either in endemic or clean areas.

Seasonally the disease may occur in all months, but the incidence is higher during July through December. Geographically, it has been found in Nevada, California, Florida, Idaho, Oregon, Montana, Utah, Colorado, Texas and Louisiana in the United States and in Mexico and Chile. In these particular geographic areas, the occurrence has usually been in high swampy pastures where *Fasciola hepatica* also exists.

Etiology and Pathogenesis. The causative organism, *Cl. hemolyticum*, is a motile anaerobic sporulating rod with straight parallel sides and rounded ends. Its dimensions are 1 to 1.1 x 4 to 5 μ. Spores are oval-shaped and terminal or subterminal. Capsules are not formed. In young cultures, the rods are gram-positive, while in cultures older than 12 hours many organisms become gram-negative. Presumably the spores survive in soil and water. Both vegetative cells and spores are relatively sensitive to heat. Vegetative forms are killed in 15 minutes at 65° C, while spores survive 15 minutes at 90° C but not at 95° C. The viability of sporulating cultures is maintained for as long as 3 years when stored at −75° C.

In suitable media and presumably in animal tissues, an exotoxin is produced. This substance contains two components one of which is hemolytic and unstable and begins to appear in cultures in 8 to 10 hours of incubation, reaches a maximum concentration in 16 to 20 hours, and disappears after 30 to 36 hours. Recent investigations have established that this component is similar to the lecithinase of *Cl. perfringens* type A toxin. The other component is necrotizing and stable in cultures for a week or more. In animals with bacillary hemoglobinuria, the organism is found in infarcted liver, kidneys and, in terminal stages, the blood. In endemic areas it is also found in moist soil of swampy and irrigated pastures.

While *Fasciola hepatica* coexists geographically with bacillary hemoglobinuria, and even though most cattle afflicted with bacillary hemoglobinuria are also parasitized with *F. hepatica*, no cogent evidence has been advanced to indicate that the trematode contributes essentially to the bacterial disease.

Bacillary hemoglobinuria appears to spread by direct contact with sick animals, by transport of infected tissues, by carrier animals and by contaminated feed and water. During the period of the acute disease, the organisms probably are emitted to the exterior through feces, urine and possibly nasal discharges. At the time of death, when a bacteremia is formed the organisms may escape in large numbers from the tissues into the soil, water and feed. The transport of infected tissues carries the organisms into new areas. Organisms may also be transported by moving water and vehicles. Some animals of herds where the disease has occurred carry the viable organism in liver and kidneys. Presumably, carrying animals can either develop the disease or shed organisms through feces and urine to the external environment.

Though the pathogenesis of bacillary hemoglobinuria is incompletely understood, some deductions can be made from available information. Since most cases of the disease develop during the grazing season, the organism from the soil probably is ingested with contaminated feed and water. In the small intestine, the organism produces a severe and acute duodenitis. After penetrating portal blood vessels in the duodenum, the organism is transported to the liver where it localizes and produces exotoxin. The infection and toxin result in focal necrosis and probably inflammation. When these changes are in close proximity to a large branch of the portal vein, damage to the vessel wall results in the development of an occluding thrombus. The ischemic tissue becomes infarcted and surrounded by an inflammatory reaction. In the necrotic tissue and in surrounding devitalized tissue organisms of *Cl. hemolyticum* proliferate rapidly and form large amounts of hemolytic toxin which is released into the circulatory system where rapid hemolysis of erythrocytes occurs. Hemoglobin accumulates within the plasma to the renal threshold and passes through the glomeruli into the urine. Hypoxia from anemia and toxemia from the *Cl. hemolyticum* injure endothelial cells causing increased permeability to plasma proteins; consequently, serum albumen appears in the urine and edematous fluid accumulates in body cavities. Bacteremia develops early during the course of the disease in approximately 20% of cases and terminally in the remaining cases. Death is due to hypoxia and toxemia.

Some animals from infected herds become healthy carriers of *Cl. hemolyticum*. Infection localizes in liver and kidneys and produces sufficient toxin to elicit antibodies. Presumably, carriers may shed organisms to the exterior through feces and urine.

Clinical Signs and Postmortem Lesions. Following an incubation period of indefinite length, the disease onset is sudden and animals when found may be in advanced stages of the disease or even dead. In early stages the body temperature ranges from 103° to 106° F. Ruminal movements and defecation stop. Anorexia and depression are prominent. The urine is red because of hemoglobinuria. The visible mucous membranes of eyes,

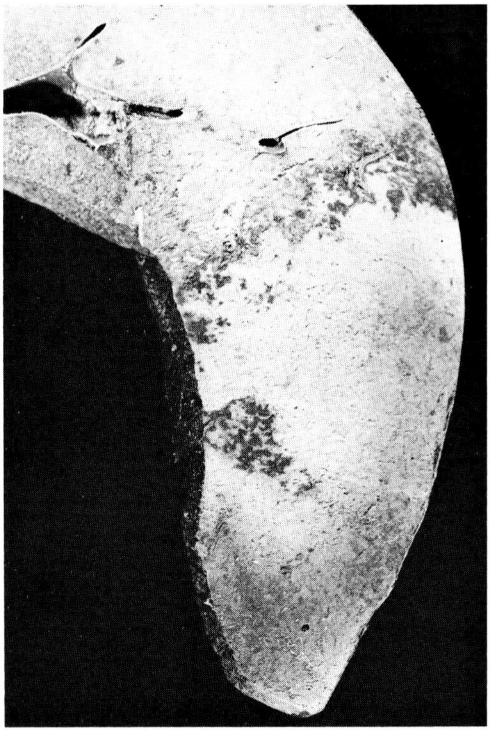

FIG. 4-33. *A liver infarct in a cow affected with bacillary hemoglobinuria.* × 0.9.

mouth and vagina become pale and icterus. The erythrocyte count declines rapidly from the normal 7 to 8 million to 2 million cells per cu ml and the hemoglobin from approximately 13 to 3.5 grams per 100 ml of blood. Respiration is rapid and mucous membranes are pale. The animal separates from the herd, has an arched posture and grunts when forced to move. In advanced stages the earlier symptoms become exaggerated. Depression is severe and constipation is replaced by a bloody diarrhea. Diuresis and diarrhea result in dehydration and loss of body weight. Terminally the body temperature declines and the animal becomes prostrated. The course varies from 1 to 4 days. The morbidity rate in unvaccinated cattle usually is from 10 to 25%, while the mortality rate of affected animals is 95%.

At necropsy, the tissues are dehydrated and body weight has diminished. Mucosal membranes, serosal surfaces and adipose tissue are icteric. The perineum may be soiled with bloody feces. Internally the blood is thin and membranes are pale. The abomasum contains petechial hemorrhages and erosions. The duodenum is swollen, hemorrhagic and edematous. Hemorrhages may have occurred into the lumen of the entire small intestine. Serous membranes often contain petechial ecchymotic hemorrhages. The body cavities, especially the peritoneal cavity, contain an abnormally large amount of blood stained fluid. In the swollen liver is an anemic infarct which measures 5 to 20 cm in diameter. This lesion is firm and pale and on cross section may reveal thrombosis of a large branch of the portal vein. Usually one or more adult flukes of *Fasciola hepatica* are in the bile ducts. The kidneys are dark colored and the urinary bladder contains red urine.

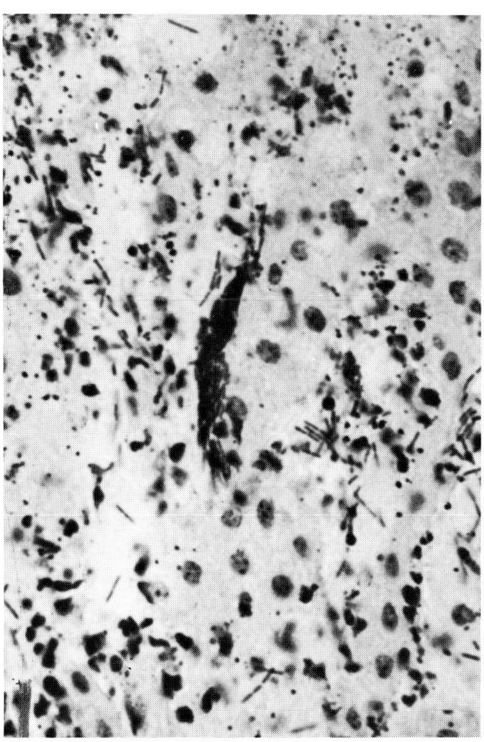

FIG. 4-34. *Cl. hemolyticum in the sinusoids of infarcted liver. Nocht's stain.* × 620.

Histopathologically, the duodenum shows acute inflammation with hemorrhage and edema. The liver infarct, a mass of necrotic tissue surrounded by a zone of inflammation, contains in the sinusoids an abundance of gram-positive rods of *Cl. hemolyticum.* Frequently the bacilli, however, are concentrated at the zone of junction of viable and necrotic tissue. The kidneys show albuminous casts and hemoglobin in collection tubules. Reabsorbed globules of hemoglobin may be found in the cytoplasm of epithelial cells of the convoluted tubules.

Diagnosis. Bacillary hemoglobinuria is diagnosed clinically on the basis of an acute febrile disease with hemoglobinuria in animals from either an endemic area or exposed to cattle from an endemic area. At necropsy, the pathognomonic liver infarction confirms a clinical diagnosis. In the laboratory *Cl. hemolyticum* can be isolated from the blood of clinical cases in approximately 20% of infected cattle. Following necropsy, the organism can be isolated from the liver infarct. Carrier animals may be identified by use of the agglutination test.

The differential diagnosis requires consideration of acute leptospirosis, anaplasmosis, piroplasmosis and postparturient hemoglobinuria. Acute leptospirosis is associated with fever, icterus and hemoglobinuria. At necropsy, however, the liver does not contain an infarct and, in some cases, leptospiras can be demonstrated in blood, urine or kidney tissues. Recovered cases may show an ascending agglutination or compliment fixation antibody titer. Anaplasmosis produces anemia and icterus, but not hemoglobinuria and not liver infarction. *Anaplasma marginale* can be demonstrated in blood smears during early stages of the disease. While piroplasmosis, or Texas fever, a febrile disease not occurring in cattle of the United States, produces hemoglobinuria and icterus, *Babesia bigemina,* the causative protozoan, can be demonstrated in erythrocytes of stained blood smears. At necropsy, the liver does not contain an infarct. Bracken fern poisoning, an acute febrile intoxication, caused by prolonged consumption of the fern *Pteris aquilina,* results in extensive hemorrhages in the visible mucous membranes but not icterus, hemoglobinuria, or liver infarction. Post-parturient hemoglobinuria, an acute disease of highly productive dairy cattle, is caused by an inadequate intake of phosphorus and occurs usually within 6 weeks following the third to sixth parturition. While the disease produces hemoglobinuria, the body temperature is near normal and no liver infarct is present.

Prevention and Treatment. In endemic areas bacillary hemoglobinuria can be prevented by vaccination. To avoid spread of disease by inoculation, a separate and clean needle should be used on each animal. In feedlot cattle one vaccination is adequate to protect duing the period of fattening. Cattle to be kept for prolonged periods should be vaccinated at 6-month intervals. Susceptible cattle should not cohabitate with cattle from an endemic area and should not be transported to endemic areas without prior vaccination. Following necropsy of an infected animal, the carcass should be burned or buried and the contaminated surface disinfected thermally or chemically.

In early stages of the disease affected cattle can be treated daily with penicillin at the rate of 2,000 to 4,000 units per pound of body weight. Blood transfusions should be administered to correct anemia. To combat dehydration, water should be administered intragastrically and fluids and glucose intravenously. Because of anemia affected animals should be handled carefully to avoid exertion and excitement. Transfusions with blood and electrolytes should be given slowly and repeated if necessary. The parenteral administration of injectable iron compounds and liver extracts accelerates recovery from anemia.

References

Jasmin, A. M.: Enzyme Activity in *Clostridium hemolyticum* Toxin AJVR, *8* (1947): 289–293.

Meyer, K. F.: Studies to Diagnose a Fatal Disease of Cattle in the Mountainous Ranges of California. JAVMA, *48* (1916): 552–560.

Quinlivan, T. D. and Wedderburn, J. F.: Bacillary hemoglobinuria in Cattle in New Zealand. New Zealand Vet. J., *7* (1959): 113–115.

Safford, J. W. and Smith, L. DS.: A Study of the Epizoology of Bacillary Hemoglobinuria. Proc. Mtg. Am. Vet. Med. Assoc., *91* (1954): 159–161.

Smith, L. DS. and Jasmin, A. M.: The Recovery of *Clostridium hemolyticum* from the Livers and Kidneys of Apparently Normal Cattle. JAVMA, *129* (1956): 68–71.

Records, E. and Huber, M.: *B. hemolyticus* Infection in a Hog. JAVMA, *78* (1931): 863–865.

Records, E. and Vawter, L. R.: Bacillary Hemoglobinuria of Cattle and Sheep (Red Water Disease). Technical Bull. 173, University of Nevada (1945): 1–48.

Vawter, L. R. and Records, E.: Recent Studies on Ictero-hemoglobinuria of Cattle. JAVMA, *68* (1926): 494–512.

Vawter, L. R.: Recovery of *Clostridium sordellii* from Cattle and Sheep., *3* (1942): 382–386.

Tuberculosis

Tuberculosis, a chronic or rarely acute contagious disease, is characterized by the formation of granulomatous lesions, occurs in man and all species of domestic and many wild animals, and is caused by *Mycobacterium tuberculosis* or some closely related species. Present and recognized in ancient and modern civilizations, this disease has caused severe suffering and extensive economic losses in people and animals.

Review of Literature. In 1882 the causative agent, *Mycobacterium tuberculosis*, was stained and visualized in affected tissue and was cultivated artificially on coagulated serum (Koch, 1882). With this impetus for research, many productive studies on the disease were initiated. Infectivity was demonstrated by inoculating guinea pigs and rabbits with tuberculous tissue from people and cattle (Villemin, 1865). Through study of the disease in laboratory animals, investigators concluded that the bovine strain is more pathogenic for rabbits than is the human strain. This information led logically to typing of the organisms and the differentiation into the human, bovine and avian strains (Smith, 1905). Following isolation of the organism, its morphology and physiology were determined (Davies, 1955; Stableforth and Galloway, 1959).

Very early in the twentieth century the disease was studied in cattle. Through the necropsy of animals that died from tuberculosis and through the study of animals that were slaughtered for food, it was determined that tubercles are located commonly in mesenteric, bronchial and mediastinal lymph nodes. In one extensive study, it was noted that in many tuberculous cattle lesions are present in hepatic lymph nodes. This observation led the investigator to postulate that the primary route of infection is by ingestion through the alimentary tract; that organisms penetrate the intestinal mucosa and enter the lymphatic system; that they are conveyed to the lymphatics, including the thoracic duct; and that by venous blood, via the right side of the heart, they enter the lungs (Behring, 1903). This postulation explains the distribution of tuberculous lesions in the mesenteric, hepatic, bronchial and mediastinal lymph nodes (Mettam, 1906). Even through the fifth decade of the century the thinking of many investigators and writers on the subject continued to support the hypothesis (Bol, 1957; Calmette, 1923; Mettam, 1906; Udall, 1954).

Other research studies, however, led the investigators to conclude that the primary route of infection in many cattle is through the respiratory system. In one study of slaughtered calves, the anatomical location of primary tuberculous lesions suggested three possible routes of primary infection: many through the lungs, some through the intestines, and a few through the umbilical veins as congenital infection (Nieberle, 1931). In another investigation abattoir reports were studied for the following tuberculous animals: 189 calves, 3,000 heifers, 3,000 tuberculous bullocks, 1,000 bulls and 3,000 cows. Again the anatomical location of primary lesions was the evidence used to indicate the routes of infection. On this basis it was concluded that calves may be infected through the umbilical veins as a congenital infection, through the intestine from the consumption of infected milk and also by inhalation of infected droplets. Data from study of the adult animals indicated that most cases contain primary lesions in the respiratory system. The dissemination of infection from the lungs was postulated to be by direct extension to adjacent alveoli, by way of lymphatics to regional lymph nodes and eventually into the blood, by erosion of bronchi to infect sputum and the alimentary system and by erosion of vessels into the blood (Stamp, 1946). In another study, 100 tuberculous cattle were investigated for primary lesions. Of these, 89 (89%) contained the primary complex in the lungs and 8 (8%) contained thoracic lesions too advanced for classification. The investigator concluded from these findings that many cattle probably become infected through inhalation of viable tubercle bacilli (Stamp, 1948).

Soon after the cultivation of tubercle bacilli in artificial media, it was discovered that growing bacteria synthesize a new protein (Koch, 1882). The injection of this protein into tuberculous animals evoked a specific allergic reaction. Technologically, this protein was concentrated and partially purified to form a diagnostic agent known as tuberculin. Because of the presence of protein derived from the original culture medium, this product, however, lacked a high degree of specificity. Through extensive experimentation tubercle bacilli were finally grown on a synthetic medium which contained no protein. The tuberculin derived from bacilli on this medium contained protein from the bacteria only and was designated PPD (Purified Protein Derivatives) tuberculin (Siebert, Aronson, Reichel, Clark and Long, 1934).

Surveys conducted in the United States during the first two decades of the twentieth century indicated that approximately 4.9% of all cattle were tuberculous and that in some heavily infected areas the incidence was much higher and varied up to 80%. In 1917, therefore, the United States Department of Agriculture initiated a program for the eradication of bovine tuberculosis. Technically, the program was based on: (1) the application of the tuberculin test to all cattle, (2) the removal and slaughter of all reactors and (3) the control of transportation of untested and reacting cattle in commerce. Each state administered its program as a federal-state project. When the incidence of bovine tuberculosis for any one state was reduced to less than 0.5% the state was designated as a modified accredited area. Finally, in 1941, after the application of 300 million bovine tuberculin tests and after the removal and slaughter of 4 million reactor cattle, the entire United States acquired the status of a modified accredited area (Simms, 1949).

Occurrence. All breeds of cattle are susceptible to tuberculosis. Animals of the dairy breeds, however, often are maintained under crowded conditions which may favor the spread of tuberculosis once the disease is established in a herd. Animals of the beef breeds are maintained on pasture and open range with little crowding; and most animals are slaughtered at a young age. The conditions of management for beef breeds are unfavorable to the spread of tuberculosis; consequently, the incidence of tuberculosis among American feedlot cattle is low. When it occurs, it is apt to be in aged dairy cattle which are placed in the feedlot for fattening prior to slaughter. Geographically, the disease is universally distributed, but because of the eradication program it has a low incidence in the United States. In an occasional herd, however, the disease may become well established before its detection. In some countries where control programs have not been instituted, the incidence of tuberculosis may be as high as 18% of all cattle. In countries where bovine tuberculosis is prevalent, the incidence increases sharply and directly with animal age.

TABLE 9

	Animal		
Type	*Guinea pig*	*Rabbit*	*Chicken*
Bovine	+	+	0
Human	+	±	0
Avian	±	+	+

Etiology. Bovine tuberculosis is caused almost entirely by the bacterium *Myobacterium tuberculosis* var. bovis. Some infections in cattle, however, have been caused by the human and avian strains. This pleomorphic organism is a slender rod which varies in length from 1.5 to 4 μ and in width from 0.2 to 0.6 μ. It is aerobic, non-motile and not spore-forming. In staining it is acid-fast and gram-positive. Many organisms, especially in old cultures, contain granules.

Mycobacterium tuberculosis, the human and bovine strains, and *Mycobacterium tuberculosis avium* are typed on the basis of pathogenicity for experimental animals as indicated in Table 9.

Outside the animal tissues this organism varies in resistance to bacteriocidal agents. When exposed to direct concentrated sunlight, it is destroyed in 2 hours. In milk heated to 70° C, it is killed in 5 minutes. In dry media such as dust, exudates and discharges, not exposed to direct sunlight, the organism may endure for several months.

Transmission. Susceptible cattle usually acquire infection from the immediate environment. Infected animals excrete the tubercle bacilli in sputum expelled by coughing and in salivary and nasal discharges. Susceptible cattle may acquire the disease by inhalation of infective aerosols or by ingestion of feed or water contaminated by infective sputum, saliva, milk or urine. In addition, cattle may become infected either by contact with tuberculous people or by exposure to human tuberculous excretions or secretions or infected human sewage.

Fetal cattle may acquire tuberculosis through the umbilical vein as a result of uterine infection. Rarely is tuberculosis of the genitalia transferred mechanically during coitus. Occasionally instruments contaminated with tubercle bacilli may inadvertently inoculate susceptible animals at the time of surgery.

Pathogenesis. Calves may acquire tuberculosis by consuming milk from a cow affected with tuberculosis of the udder. In this event the tubercle bacilli are ingested with the milk and pass into the intestine. In the ileum and the large intestine, the bacilli penetrate the mucous membrane, enter the lymphatics, and are conveyed to the mesenteric lymph nodes. While many bacilli are retained in the nodes, some pass into the efferent lymphatic channels and, via the thoracic duct, enter the venous blood which carries them into the lungs. Along this course of movement tubercles may form, especially in the lymph nodes and in the lungs. Calves in a tuberculous environment may also inhale virulent bacilli and become infected directly through the respiratory system.

In adult cattle, tuberculosis often develops in animals maintained in a tuberculous environment. Transmission of the disease is favored in dairy cattle housed in buildings which are unhygienic because of crowding, poor ventilation, and inadequate lighting. When a focus of infection develops, spread is inevitable. The route of transmission may be through the respiratory system. In some cases, however, infection may be acquired through the digestive system. A primary complex is the combination of an original organic tubercle and the near contemporaneous lesion in the regional lymph node. The anatomical location of a primary complex is evidence of the primary route of infection. Since this complex commonly occurs in the thorax, it is assumed, in the following account, that the route of infection is through the respiratory system.

Viable tubercle bacilli are expelled into the air by tuberculous animals. Susceptible cattle inhale infected droplets as an aerosol. The virulent organisms may enter the alveoli or may be arrested in the mucous membrane of the bronchial tree. In the alveoli the first tissue reaction is the accumulation of neutrophils around the bacilli. After a short period the neutrophils undergo necrosis, and epithelioid cells accumulate to form a multilayered zone around the bacteria and dead cells. Some epithelioid cells fuse to form Langhan's giant cells. Some bacilli are phagocytized and some are destroyed. A zone of lymphocytes and fibrous connective tissue forms around the zone of epithelioid cells. Vascularity is low. Towards the center of the lesion, many epithelioid cells and normal tissue cells undergo caseative necrosis. Calcium salts may be deposited in foci in the necrotic tissue. Some foci of infection coalesce and form a macroscopic tubercle. Healing of the primary lesion may occur. Some tubercle bacilli escape from the lesion and enter lymphatics which carry them to the bronchial or mediastinal lymph nodes where a new focus of infection is established.

Virulent tubercle bacilli may disseminate through the lymphatics of the subpleura and the subperitoneum and form tubercles which project onto the serous surface to cause chronic tuberculous pleuritis or "pearl disease," and chronic tuberculous peritonitis, respectively.

In some cases the initial lesion erodes into a bronchus or bronchiole. In this event, virulent bacilli enter the lumen of the bronchus. From here they may be inhaled into many alveoli to produce tuberculous pneumonia. The organisms may also be coughed up out of the infected bronchus into the atmosphere or into saliva of the mouth and nasal secretions. Infected sputum may be swallowed into the alimentary tract where secondary foci of infection are produced. In either the primary or secondary lesions, blood vessels, especially veins, may be eroded and penetrated by organisms. This creates a bacteremia and causes hematogenous dissemination of the bacilli. By this means new foci of infection may be established in any and many organs.

Metabolism of the infecting tubercle bacilli produces specific protein foreign to the host. Early in the disease and continuing through most of the course, the host tissues are sensitized to this protein. In some advanced stages, the tissues are exposed to large amounts of the protein and become desensitized. The sensitization is the basis for the tuberculin reaction used in diagnosis.

Clinical Signs and Postmortem Lesions. Since tuberculosis is often an insidious disease, clinical signs are commonly inconspicuous. Many infected animals, however, lose body weight slowly but continuously despite availability of adequate feed. Deep coughing is persistent and may become painful. In some cases tuberculous pneumonia may develop. The disease course is usually prolonged for many months and sometimes years. In case of hematogenous dissemination, the course is shortened and the termination fatal.

While the morbidity rate from tuberculosis is very low in cattle of the United States, it may be high in some countries where eradication programs have not been instituted. Eventual mortality of the diseased animals is high.

Regardless of anatomical location, tubercles possess many common characteristics. The small young tubercle, gray and translucent, usually is 1 mm or less in diameter. In miliary tuberculosis the tubercles are multiple, usually young, of near equal duration, and somewhat uniformly distributed throughout one or more organs.

The large advanced tubercles are firm nodules which vary in diameter to as much as 10 cm or more. The center of a tubercle consists of a mass of caseative necrosis which is yellowish, dry, and friable. The consistency resembles soft cheese or butter. Single or multiple foci of calcification may be present in the necrosis. The necrotic tissue is surrounded usually by a capsule of fibrous connective tissue.

Histopathologically, the caseative necrosis consists of a mass of granular acid staining cell derivatives. Some basic staining granules are present. In advanced stages, all resemblance to cells has been lost. Deposits of mineral are granular and basic staining. In actively growing tubercles, the acid fast bacilli are discernible; in static tubercles, bacilli may be scarce. Surrounding the necrosis is a zone of epithelioid cells and a few Langhan's giant cells. At the periphery of the tubercle is a zone of lymphocytes and fibrous connective tissue.

The lungs may contain single or multiple lesions which usually are caseated, encapsulated and calcified. In case of tuberculous pneumonia, multiple acini within a lobule may be filled with caseative exudate or entire lobules may be pneumonic. In many cases the pleura, both visceral and parietal, may be affected and contain single or multiple firm tubercles which project onto the surface. In some cases the pleura may contain hundreds of such tubercles and the condition is known as "pearl disease." Commonly, the regional lymph nodes of a primary lesion are also infected. The node is enlarged and firm. The advanced tubercle contains considerable caseated necrosis and often calcification. The latter, while being incised, is detectable as grittiness. The lymph node becomes infected with organisms which enter through the afferent lymphatics.

In addition to the lungs, many other organs may be infected in tuberculosis. The spleen may contain tubercles on the surface as a result of tuberculous peritonitis and in the parenchyma, as a result of bacteremia. The kidneys may contain single or multiple tubercles originating from the blood. Meat inspectors commonly examine the kidneys for evidence of tuberculous bacteremia. In some cases bones and joints are infected. Infected ribs are enlarged and weakened. The central nervous system may be infected at any point, including the meninges.

Male and female genital organs may be infected. In cows, tuberculous metritis may give rise to congenital infection of fetuses. Tuberculosis of the uterus, ovaries and testes usually is hematogenous in origin. Tuberculosis of the penis, vulva and vagina may be a venereal infection transmitted mechanically by male or female at the time of coitus.

Tuberculosis of the udder often originates from a hematogenous infection and consists of four types: acute caseating, chronic nodular, chronic diffuse, granulomatous and diffuse tuberculosis of the excretory ducts. In either type, tubercle bacilli may be shed in the milk and transmitted to consumers. At the time of postmortem inspection of tuberculous animals slaughtered for food, the inspector is required to render judgment on wholesomeness of the meat for food. A guiding principle forming a basis of decision is that no organ shall be used for food that contains tubercle bacilli or the toxic metabolites from tubercle bacilli. Since tuberculosis may be localized or generalized, affected organs only or the entire animal may be condemned. Any organ containing one or more tubercles in itself or its regional lymph node is condemned for food. If tubercles are not numerous, and if there is no evidence of hematogenous dissemination, the remaining non-infected part of the carcass is wholesome and acceptable as food. The entire animal is condemned if either one or more of the following conditions are present: (1) antemortem fever, (2) tuberculous cachexia, (3) generalized tuberculosis from hematogenous dissemination, (4) tuberculous muscles, intermuscular fascia, bone, or joints or regional lymph nodes, (5) wide distribution of tubercles in the pleural or peritoneal cavities and (6) multiple lesions, acute and progressive.

Diagnosis. Bovine tuberculosis can be diagnosed in living animals on the basis of clinical signs, tuberculin reaction, and the demonstration of tubercle bacilli in secretions and/or excretions. In dead animals, the diagnosis is based on demonstration of tubercle bacilli in typical lesions. In the United States, tuberculosis in living cattle is diagnosed almost exclusively on a positive tuberculin reaction.

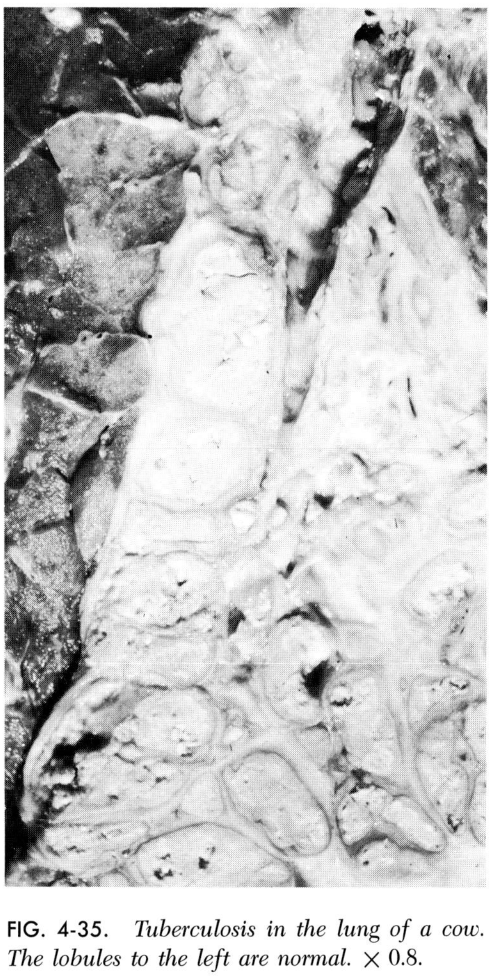

FIG. 4-35. *Tuberculosis in the lung of a cow. The lobules to the left are normal.* × 0.8.

Tuberculin is a refined biological product containing specific proteins synthesized by growing tubercle bacilli. The original tuberculins were produced by growing bacilli in media which contained protein in the substrate. Consequently, the final product contained protein from the medium and protein synthesized by the bacilli. A more refined tuberculin, PPD (Purified Protein Derivative), is produced by growing tubercle bacilli in a synthetic medium without protein. Consequently, the protein in PPD is derived entirely by synthesis from the bacilli. In the United States, PPD is used for the diagnosis of bovine tuberculosis and is supplied by the Agricultural Research Service, United States Department of Agriculture.

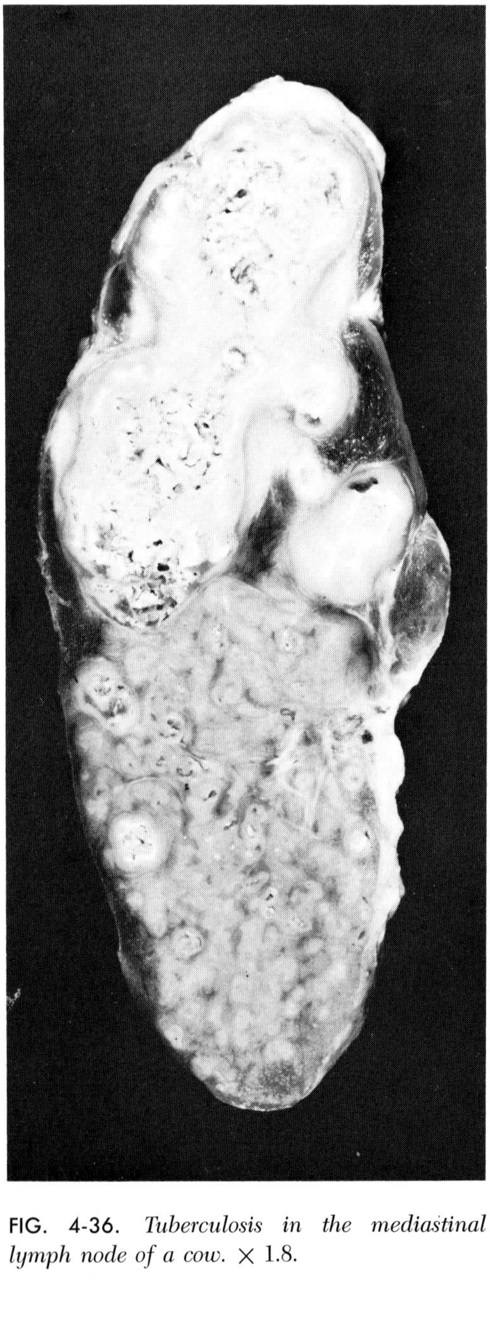

FIG. 4-36. *Tuberculosis in the mediastinal lymph node of a cow.* × 1.8.

According to the method of administration, three types of tuberculin tests are available: (1) ophthalmic, (2) subcutaneous or thermal and (3) intradermal. The ophthalmic test is the instillation of a small amount of tuberculin in the conjunctival sac. A positive reaction is the accumulation of inflammatory exudate, usually at the medial canthus, within 4 to 6 hours following application. While this test may be used in cattle, its application is uncommon. The subcutaneous or thermal test, as indicated by the name, is the subcutaneous inoculation of tuberculin and the evocation of a rise in body temperature. The body temperature is measured at hourly intervals for several readings before inoculation and at hourly intervals after inoculation. A positive reaction is a rise of 2° F or more in body temperature, between the eighth and eighteenth hour after inoculation. While this test was formerly used extensively (1900 to 1920), it has been supplanted almost entirely by the intradermal test. The intradermal test consists in the injection of 0.1 ml of tuberculin between the layers of the skin. Reading is performed 72 hours after injection. A positive reaction is indicated by firm local swelling. In the United States, the caudal fold is injected because of convenience. In England, however, injection is made at the midpoint along the lateral surface of the neck where sensitivity is maximal.

While accuracy of the intradermal test is very high, like other biological tests, errors are possible. Falsely positive reactions may result from contact of the animal with *M. tuberculosis,* human and avian types, *M.*

johnei and the acid fast bacteria associated with so-called skin tuberculosis. Falsely negative tests may result from desensitization in advanced stages of generalized tuberculosis because of tissue saturation with tuberculoproteins and in cows for a short time following parturition because of heavy excretion of antibodies in colostrum.

A positive diagnosis can also be established by demonstrating tubercle bacilli in secretions, as urine and milk, and in exudate, such as sputum. This method usually requires concentration by centrifugation and microscopic demonstration of the acid fast organisms or the inoculation of suspected materials into susceptible laboratory animals and subsequent demonstration of tubercle bacilli in lesions.

Prevention. In the United States and some other countries, as Denmark, Finland and the Netherlands, bovine tuberculosis is prevented

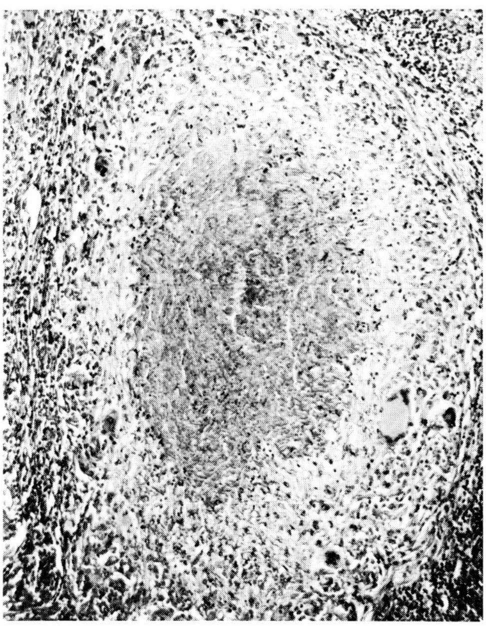

FIG. 4-37. *A tubercle in a lymph node. From the center are the following zones: caseative necrosis, epithelioid cells and Langhan's giant cells, and fibrous connective tissue and lymphocytes. HE stain.* × 116.

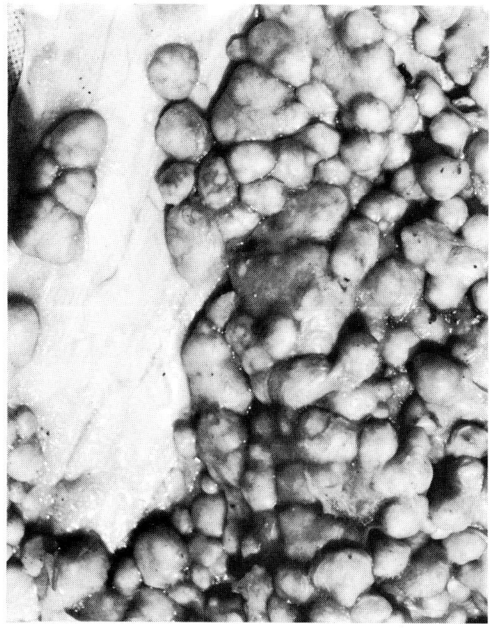

FIG. 4-38. *Chronic tuberculous pleuritis on the pleural surface of the diaphragm.* × 0.9.

currently by successful eradication of the disease from the cattle population. In the United States, this has been achieved in the individual states by the application of the intradermal tuberculin test and removal and slaughter of reactor cattle. Following removal of reactors, the premises were cleaned and disinfected. In some cases the infected property was left unoccupied for variable periods.

Providing sanitary environment also reduces spread of the disease. Housing should eliminate excessive animal crowding but provide adequately ventilated and lighted sanitary quarters.

Clean herds should be protected against the introduction of the disease. New additions to a herd should be free of tuberculosis. This status should be established by isolation and tuberculin testing prior to cohabitation with the herd. Clean cattle should not be entered in public shows or grazed on public range or pasture unless all cattle in the public assemblage are proven free of tuberculosis by proper application of the tuberculin test.

References

Behring, E. von: Dtsch. Med. Wschr., *29* (1903): 689.

Bol, B. K.: Pathoanatomical Necropsy of Domestic Animals. Government Printing Office for Agricultural Literature. Moscow. 1957. pp. 240–253.

Calmette, J.: *Tubercule Bacillus Infection and Tuberculosis in Man and Animals.* The Williams & Wilkins Co. Baltimore, 1923.

Davies, G. O.: Gaiger and Davies *Veterinary Bacteriology and Pathology.* 4th ed. Bailliere, Tindall, & Cox. London. 1955. pp. 326–375.

Koch, R.: Die Etiologie der tuberkulose. Berliner. Klin. Wchnschr., *19* (1882): 221–230.

Mettam, A. E.: Vet. Jour., *13* (1906): 551.

Nieberle, K.: Ergeb. Allg. Path. Path. Anat., *25* (1931): 631.

Siebert, F. J., Aronson, J. D., Reichel, H., Clark, E. and Long, E. T.: American Rev. Tuberculosis, *30* (1934): 707.

Simms, B. T.: Report International Vet. Congr. 1949. Vol. 2. London.

Smith, Theobald: Jour. Med. Res., *7* (1905): 253; *8* (1905): 405.

Stableforth, A. W. and Galloway, I. A.: *Infectious Diseases of Animals. Diseases Due to Bacteria.* Academic Press, Inc. New York, 1959. pp. 671–744.

Stamp, J. T.: Some Aspects of the Pathogenesis of Bovine Tuberculosis, Based on Abattoir Returns. Vet. Record, *58* (1946): 11–15.

———: Tuberculosis of the Bovine Udder. J. Comp. Path. & Therapeutics, *53* (1940–43): 220–229.

———: The Distribution of the Bronchial Tree in the Bovine Lung. J. Comp. Path. & Therapeutics, *58* (1948): 1–8.

———: Bovine Pulmonary Tuberculosis. J. Comp. Path. & Therapeutics, *58* (1948): 9–23.

Udall, D. H.: *The Practice of Veterinary Medicine.* Udall Publisher, Ithaca, New York, 1954. pp. 596–611.

Villemin, A. J.: Compte. Rend. Acad. Sc., *61* (1865): 1012.

Actinomycosis

(LUMPY JAW)

A chronic infectious but non-contagious disease, characterized by infection of the mandible and surrounding soft tissues, actinomycosis is caused by the fungus *Actinomyces bovis.* When differentiated, as it should be, from actinobacillosis, this disease has a low incidence and consequently the economic loss is relatively low. In cattle, however, the infection is progressive unless properly treated. Incapacitation of the mouth with reduced ability to utilize feed efficiently, condemnation of affected parts at slaughter and some mortality result in loss of animal values.

Review of Literature. Following the discovery of *A. bovis* in infected mandibles of cattle (Harz, 1877), actinomycosis has been observed and recognized as a cause of osteomyelitis in people (Stableforth and Galloway, 1959) and of chronic mastitis in swine (Vawter, 1946). In the United States, the U. S. Department of Agriculture accumulated statistics on the incidence of actinomycosis and/or actinobacillosis in cattle slaughtered under federal inspection. In 1967 through 1969 approximately 800 carcasses and 212,000 parts were condemned annually. These figures indicated an incidence of approximately 0.7% infection in slaughtered cattle (Federal Meat Inspection 1967–69). While most infections have been localized in osseous tissues of the head of cattle (Cohrs, 1962; Stableforth and Galloway, 1959; Vawter, 1946), actinomycosis has also been observed and studied in soft tissues, including the penis (Dieter, 1954) and testes (Kimball, Twiehaus and Frank, 1954). Attempts to reproduce the disease by parenteral inoculation of viable *A. bovis* have been often unsuccessful or have resulted in inconsequential local infection. Many investigators (Cohrs, 1962; Stableforth and Galloway, 1959) have concluded that the organism penetrates the mucosa of the mouth and the skin of the head through points of trauma. In study of the oral microflora of normal cattle, actinomycosis-like organisms were isolated (Frost, 1940). In studies of clinical treatment, considerable success was obtained from repeated applications of streptomycin (Kingman and Palen, 1951).

Occurrence. Although actinomycosis occurs occasionally in calves 6 months of age, the incidence is greater in both heifers and steers 1 to 2 years of age. Retired breeding cows and bulls being fattened are also affected. Guernsey bulls are highly susceptible and among American and Canadian cattle have a higher incidence than bulls of other dairy breeds. The disease appears in both sexes, all breeds and during all seasons. It is cosmopolitan in distribution. In addition to cattle the disease also occurs in swine, horses and people.

Etiology and Pathogenesis. The causative fungus, *A. bovis,* is pleomorphic, filamentous, branching and gram-positive in staining reaction. In infected tissues this organism grows in colonies which measure up to 2 mm in diameter and are designated "ray fungi" and sulfur granules. Within the colony the gram-positive hyphae form a tangle of branching filaments. As revealed by electron microscopy and histochemistry, the granule consists of hyphae cemented together by a polysaccharide protein complex. In this mass the tips of hyphae project from the periphery of the granule in the form of clubs. In tissue sections stained with hematoxylin and eosin, the hyphae stain blue and the cementing substance pink. The fungus can be grown on nutrient agar containing blood serum and dextrose. Growth is stimulated in an atmosphere of 10% carbon dioxide. The organsim is thought to be widely distributed in some cattle feeds and probably exists in the mouths of many healthy cattle.

A. bovis probably has little ability to penetrate healthy oral mucosa or skin. In case of injury to the oral mucosa from abrasions or penetrations, the organism enters tissues at the points of discontinuity. It may also penetrate the alveolar periosteum when teeth are expelled and when the alveolar periosteum is injured by penetration of plant fragments. Carious teeth may also be points of invasion by *A. bovis.* A high incidence of actinomycosis occasionally develops in pens of cattle within a few weeks of entry into the feedlot. This early appearance of lesions suggests that inoculation may occur on pasture or range. Once established in the deep tissues of the mandible or maxilla, the fungus slowly proliferates and evokes osteomyelitis and periostitis. Multiple colonies develop and stimulate a granulomatous reaction. At multiple points, lysis of bone creates communicating channels where fungi and exudate accumulate. New deformed bone is generated at the periosteum and endosteum. Often the teeth become loosened in the weakened bone. The affected tissue is enlarged and disfigured by granulation tissue, new bone and exudate. Eventually the exudate discharges to the surface.

In cattle, the disease usually remains localized in the head. Rarely are lymph nodes infected. In some animals, hematogenous dissemination to the lungs occurs. Unless treated, the disease is progressive, incapacitating, and eventually fatal. Impaired prehension and mastication of feed may result in loss of body weight and finally generalized cachexia.

Clinical Signs and Postmortem Lesions. Clinical signs depend on anatomical location of the infection. The slowly developing lesions cause deformity of the infected part. Infection in the head is usually unilateral. In the mandible the body may be affected, but the ramus is the more common location. In advanced stages the infected organ is enlarged and disfigured. One or more sinus tracts with intermittent discharge of exudate may communicate with a surface on skin or oral mucosa. The skin around a sinus is depillated. The lesion, firm because of new bone formation, causes increase of the transverse and vertical dimensions of the ramus. In the area of the lesion, teeth may be loosened or expelled. Although less common, similar changes may occur in the maxilla. In moderate and advanced stages of the disease, reduced mobility of the mandible and tongue, loosening of the teeth, and oral ulcers and deformations interfere seriously with prehension and mastication of feed. As a result, the infected animal is undernourished and body weight is diminished.

Infection of other organs, as the genitalia of bulls, reduces organ function but does not result in early inanition from malnutrition. The course of the disease is prolonged for many months and may endure for years. The incidence is low, but the mortality of affected cases is very high unless treatment begins early.

At necropsy, lesions in cattle are usually limited to the head. The infection may be either in the ramus or body of the mandible or in the maxilla and may result in enlargement, deformity, and hardening of the infected tissues. Exudate with grossly discernible sulfur granules may be discharging to the surface through one or more sinuses. Dimensions of the infected bone are increased. Dissection of lesions discloses extensive new bone formation from the endosteum or periosteum. Throughout the infected bone are numerous cavities and intercommunicating sinuses containing thick, translucent granulation tissue and pus. The deformed oral surface may be ulcerated. Spontaneous fracture of the infected bone may have occurred. Usually regional lymph nodes are not infected. In some cases the lungs contain metastatic foci of infection and are firm and nodular. Occasionally the disease is manifested by granulomatous lesions in soft tissues of the male genitalia.

Histopathologically, the lesions consist of multiple granulomas with replacement of some bone with granulation tissue and the formation of new bone. Each granuloma contains at the center one or more ray fungi. The colonies are surrounded successively by a zone of neutrophils, a zone of epithelioid cells, and a zone of fibrous connective tissue which increases in maturity towards the periphery. The centers of adjacent granulomas may become confluent and produce copious pus and granulation tissue.

At the time of slaughter, disposition of the carcass depends on the extent of infection. Infected organs or parts are unfit for food. Extensive infection of a mandible or maxilla renders the head unsuitable. Extensive lesions of the lungs or other viscera, accompanied by cachexia, makes the entire carcass unacceptable.

Diagnosis. Actinomycosis is diagnosed from typical gross lesions in osseous tissue and from the demonstration in exudate of sulfur granules containing gram-positive organisms. In early stages of the disease, an increased transverse diameter of the ramus of the mandible or an indurated enlargement of the maxilla without sinus formation evoke suspicion of actinomycosis. Clinically and at necropsy a diagnosis is usually established by gross demonstration of sulfur granules in exudate from infections of the mandible or maxilla. Confirmation can be obtained in the laboratory by demonstrating gram-positive fungi in stained smears of crushed sulfur granules or in sections of infected tissue. Radiographs may be used to determine the extent of bone destruction and of new bone formation.

In cattle the differential diagnosis requires consideration of actinobacillosis, nonspecific osteomyelitis and osteogenic sarcoma. Actinobacillosis affects soft tissues, especially the tongue and lymph nodes, but rarely bony tissue. Disfiguring enlargements occur in soft tissues. Pus from sinuses contains rosettes which, in stained smears of crushed rosettes, reveal gram-negative bacteria. Osteomyelitis from other and mixed bacterial infections may cause loosening and expulsion of teeth and even thickening of the transverse diameter of the mandible. Deformity and new bone formation usually, however, do not develop and sulfur granules or rosettes are not demonstrable in the exudate. The specific causative organisms can be cultivated in artificial media. The osteogenic sarcoma usually does not develop sinuses for the discharge of exudate. A histopathological diagnosis can be made from a biopsy.

Prevention and Treatment. The incidence of actinomycosis and actinobacillosis can be reduced by avoiding oral and facial injuries through which the fungi invade tissue and establish infection. Traumatic metallic bodies and excessive plant awns should be removed from feed. Protruding nails, wire and wood splinters should be removed from pen fences

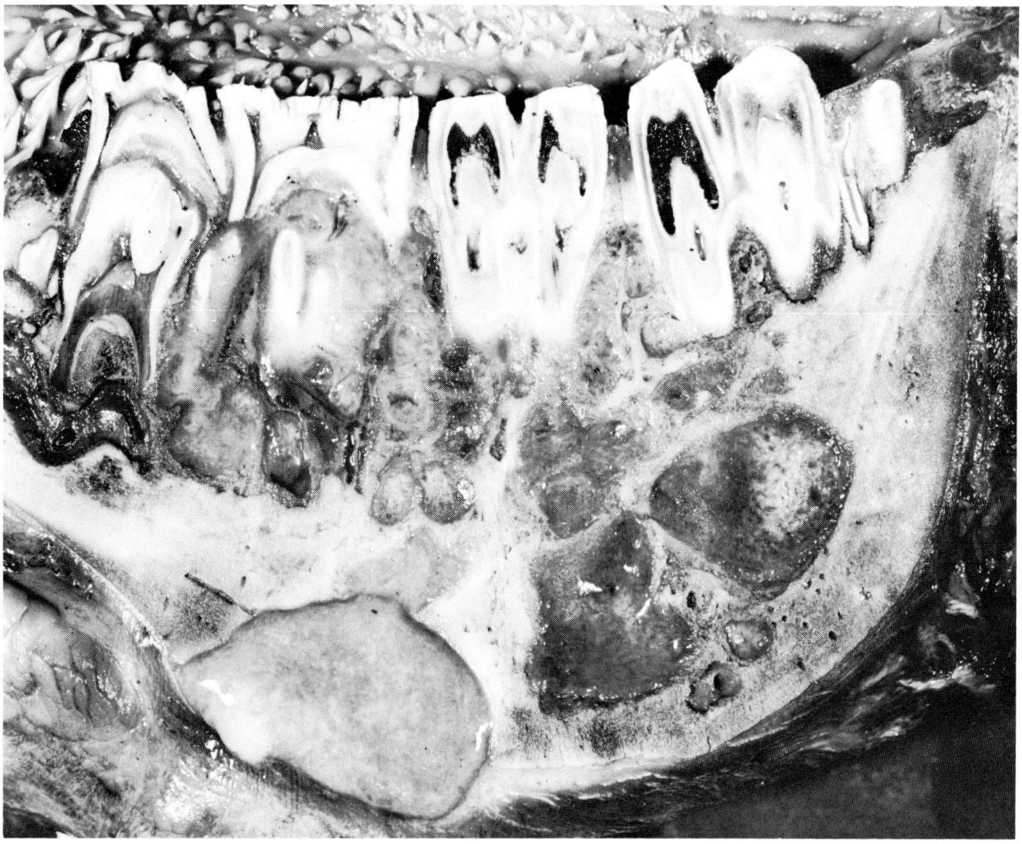

FIG. 4-39. *Saggital gross section of a bovine mandible affected with actinomycosis. Note infection around molars, bone cavities and sinuses, and the new bone.* × 1.1.

and other objects against which cattle rub. The continuous feeding as part of the diet of organic iodide compounds at the rate of 60 to 120 mg per animal per day reduces the disease incidence and may arrest developing infections.

Successful treatment can be achieved through surgical excision of infected tissue and repeated inoculation of lesions with streptomycin at the rate of 1 gram per 100 pounds of body weight per day for 7 to 10 days. Following administration of streptomycin, the affected animal should not be slaughtered for human food for at least 30 days after the last treatment. In some individual animals a series of x-radiation treatments of the lesions may be applied alone or in combination with antibiotic drug treatment.

An infected herd can be treated by medication of the diet with organic iodide compound. Calves 6 months of age should receive the drug at the rate of 1 pound per day per 300 animals for 7 days, followed by 1 pound per day per 500 animals for the remainder of the fattening period. Adult cattle should receive the drug at the rate of 1 pound per day per 100 animals for 7 days followed by 1 pound per day per 300 animals for the remainder of the fattening period.

References

Becker, R. B., Wilcox, C. J., Simpson, C. F., Gilmore, L. O. and Fechheimer, N. S.: Genetic Aspects of Actinomycosis and Actinobacillosis in Cattle. Bull. Fla. Agr. Exp. Station No. *670* (1964): 24.

Cohrs, P.: Neiberle und Cohrs, *Lehrbuch des Speziellen*

Pathologischen Anatomie der Haustiere. Vierte Auflage. Gustav Fischer, Verlag. Stuttgart. (1962).
Dieter, Von R.: Uber ein Penisgranulom beim einum Zuchtfarren. Berl. Munch. Tierarztl. Wschr., *67* (1954): 222–223.
Federal Meat Inspection. Statistical Summary. Consumer and Marketing Service. USDA. (1967–1969).
Frost, B. A.: Thesis. Cornell University Library. Ithaca, 1940.
Harz, C. O.: Ueber eine neus Pilzkrankeit beim Rinde. Zbl. Med. Wiss., *15* (1877): 481.
Kimball, A., Twiehaus, M. J. and Frank, E. R.: *Actinomyces bovis* Isolated from Six Cases of Bovine Orchitis. A Preliminary Report. AJVR, *15* (1954): 551–553.
Kingman, H. E. and Palen, J. S.: Streptomycin in the Treatment of Actinomycosis. JAVMA, *118* (1951): 28–30.
Stableforth, A. W. and Galloway, I. A.: *Infectious Diseases of Animals.* Vol. 1. Academic Press, Inc. New York. (1959): 1–15.
Vawter, L. R.: Actinomycosis in Swine. JAVMA, *109* (1946): 198–203.

Leptospirosis

(ICTEROHEMOGLOBINURIA)

A mild or severe contagious disease, leptospirosis is characterized by anorexia, loss of body weight, and in some animals, fever, hemoglobinuria, icterus and abortion. Occurring in all types of cattle, the disease has caused an estimated annual monetary loss of approximately $100 million. In 1968, 20,000 animal cases and 67 human cases were reported for the nation.

Review of Literature. Bovine leptospirosis was first discovered in the Russian Caucasus where the disease caused hemoglobinuria and icterus. The diagnosis was confirmed through isolation of a spirochaeta on artificial media (Michin and Azinov, 1935; Michin, Azinov and Solikov, 1941). Later the disease was found in Palestine where serious losses occurred in dairy cattle (Freund, 1947). In the United States, leptospirosis was first diagnosed in two herds of dairy cattle. Suspected clinically from characteristic signs, the diagnosis was confirmed by demonstrating leptospires in the kidneys and liver of affected animals (Jungherr, 1944). Later *Leptospira pomona* was isolated from infected cattle (Baker and Little, 1948). Subsequently, the disease was diagnosed in range and feedlot cattle (Marsh, 1945; Mathews, 1946; Ramirez *et al.*, 1961: Stoenner *et al.*, 1956; Stoenner, 1967; Roth, 1960). In addition to cattle, the disease has been diagnosed in swine (Bryan, 1954) and deer (Clark *et al.*, 1962; Trainer *et al.*, 1963; Reilly *et al.*, 1962) and in many other species of wild animals (Roth *et al.*, 1963; White, 1963; Martin *et al.*, 1967). The disease has been found in animals and man throughout major continents of the world (Szatalowicz *et al.*, 1969).

Studies of the pathogenic organisms of the genus *Leptospira* has resulted in the establishment of one pathogenic species, *Leptospira interrogans*, with serogroups and serotypes as subdivisions of the species (Babudieri, 1961; Classification of Leptospires, 1965; Report of the Leptospira Subcommittee, 1963). Subsequently 18 serogroups and 124 serotypes have been formed (World Health Organization, 1968). Important serotypes identified in American cattle are *L. pomona* (Stoenner *et al.*, 1956; Stoenner, 1967; Baker and Little, 1948), *L. grippotyphosa* (Hoeden, 1955; Pike, Patton, Schultze, 1961; Andrews *et al.*, 1966; Martin *et al.*, 1967), *L. hardjo* (Roth and Galton, 1960; Stoenner, 1967; Killinger *et al.*, 1969), and *L. sejroe* (Pike, Patton, Schultze, 1961); others included *L. autumnalis, L. canicola,* and *L. icterohaemorrhagiae.*

The inoculation of experimental cattle with viable *L. pomona* produced a leptospiremia followed in many animals by leptospirurea which persisted for periods varying up to 57 days (Baker and Little, 1948; Hoeden, 1955; Reinhard and Hadlow, 1954; Murphy and Jensen, 1969). Following inoculation, antibodies appeared within 8 to 9 days, reached a peak of concentration in 10 to 12 days, and then declined. In many animals a titer of 1:100 persisted for more than 18 months. Outside of bovine tissues, *L. pomona* was shown to be highly susceptible to adverse conditions. The pH values 6.0 to 8.4 were most favorable. At temperatures 20° to 26° C organisms were immobilized in 8 hours at pH 5.5, and in 2 hours at pH 8.8. Drying caused immobilization in ½ hour; slow freezing in 2 hours; drying in soil in ½ hour. Organisms remained viable in water-saturated soil for 183 days. Under simulated natural conditions organisms survived in stagnant pools for 7 days. Continuous additions of fresh water increased the survival time (Okazaki and Ringen, 1957).

Under both experimental field conditions the prophylactic and therapeutic value of hyperimmune antiserum was demonstrated in cattle and horses (Lubashenko, 1949; Stalheim, 1969). An effective vaccine consisting of a suspension of specific leptospires inactivated with oxyquinolene sulfate (Lubashenko, 1949), formol (York, 1953), or phenol (Yanagawa *et al.*, 1962) provided protection against challenge experimentally with cultures of virulent leptospires and also in the field against natural exposure. Vaccine consisting of live but attenuated *L. pomona* also protected cattle; when challenged with virulent *L. pomona,* control animals developed leptospiremia and leptospiruria while vaccinated animals were protected against these events (Stalheim, 1968).

Occurrence. Bovine leptospirosis occurs in all breeds and ages and in both sexes. Geographically, it has been observed in cattle of Europe, Japan, Australia, the United States and Canada. Predominating serotypes vary with different geographic regions.

Other species of susceptible domestic mammals include horses, sheep, dogs and swine, and wild animals, such as skunks, deer, rodents, wild carnivors and snakes, which are of epizootiologic importance to cattle. People are also susceptible. Guinea pigs, hamsters and mice are susceptible to experimental inoculation.

Etiology. Current taxonomy classifies all pathogenic leptospires in one species, *Leptospira interrogans.* These organisms differ from saprophytic leptospires by infecting mammals, provoking specific serologic reactions and being suppressed by divalent copper ions. On the basis of agglutinin-absorption reactions pathogenic leptospires are arranged to form 18 serogroups and numerous serotypes. Twelve serogroups have been identified in the United States. Important serotypes of cattle are *L. pomona, L. grippotyphosa, L. hardjo,* and *L. sejroe;* other types encountered include *L. autumnalis, L. canicola,* and *L. icterohemorrhagiae.* Table 10 lists some field hosts for serotypes.

Morphologically and culturally, serotypes of leptospires are similar. They measure approximately 7 to 40 × 0.1 μ. These long, slender organisms contain numerous coils and a hook at either or both ends. The cell consists of a central axial filament surrounded by a protoplasmic cylinder and is covered by a thin membrane. While generally stain-resistant, the organism in thin films can be differentiated with Giemsa stain and in tissue with silver impregnation methods such as Levaditi's and Warthin-Starry stains. It can be grown artificially in Korthof's and Stuart's fluid media with 5 to 10% rabbit serum. Maximal growth rate is at temperatures 28° to 30° C. The organisms are demonstrable after 7 to 15 days of incubation. In a fluid medium the highly motile leptospires rotate

TABLE 10 ***Field mammals susceptible to serotypes***

serotypes	*field hosts*
L. pomona	swine, cattle, field mice, man, deer, skunks
L. grippotyphosa	rats, cattle, mice, fox, squirrels, deer, horse, skunk
L. hardjo	cattle, deer
L. sejroe	field mice, cattle, dog, horse, swine

rapidly on their long axes. In infected cattle the pathogenic species are located in blood and liver during the leptospiremic stage, and in kidneys and urine during the leptospiruric stage. Outside the host tissues, leptospires are non-resistant to adverse environmental conditions. Highly sensitive to acidity, the optimal pH values are 6.0 to 8.4. At temperatures 20° to 26° C, they are rendered immobile at pH 5.5 in 8 hours and at pH 8.8 in 2 hours. They survive drying for ½ hour, slow freezing for 2 hours and drying in soil for ½ hour. They also survive in a soil-water mixture for 183 days, and in stagnant water for less than 7 days.

Epizootiology. Carriers of *L. pomona*, *L. grippotyphosa* and *L. hardjo*, the main causes of bovine leptospirosis, include cattle following the febrile stage and many species of domestic and wild animals. The leptospiruric stage in swine endures for several months and leptospires are heavily concentrated in the urine. The cohabitation of feedlot cattle and swine, therefore, provides opportunity for transmission of *L. pomona* from infected swine to susceptible cattle. Infected rodents for prolonged periods carry and excrete the organism through the urine. Cattle themselves, following the febrile stage of the disease, carry and excrete organisms for as long as 2 months.

Transmission of the disease to cattle may occur through direct contact and through contamination of food and water. Under feedlot conditions cattle are often crowded into small areas. Frequently several hundred cattle are confined to a pen which provides 35 to 40 square yards per animal. This crowding gives ample opportunity for direct contact of susceptible cattle with infected urine of diseased cattle. The infected urine often contacts the skin and muzzle. Infective aerosols, generated by spattering urine, enter either the lungs through inhalation, or the eyes through penetration of the conjunctiva.

Bovine leptospirosis is transmitted infrequently by other means. *Dermacentor marginatus* has been incriminated as a vector of *L. grippotyphosa*. People, especially veterinarians and meat handlers, contract leptospirosis through direct contact with infected tissues.

Pathogenesis. Following exposure to pathogenic leptospires, the organism enters the blood to produce a leptospiremia which endures for approximately 10 days and coexists with fever. In some cattle, hemolysis destroys many erythrocytes and produces hemoglobinemia and hemoglobinuria. Because of antibodies in plasma, the leptospires leave the blood and localize in liver and kidney tissue. While central lobular degeneration and necrosis develop in the liver, the infection does not endure long in that organ. In the kidneys, infection localizes in the convoluted tubules of the cortex. Following degeneration and necrosis of epithelium in infected tubules, the epithelium regenerates and proliferates. Lymphocytes, mononuclear macrophages, plasma cells and a few neutrophils infiltrate the stroma of the area. Eventually, the leptospires are transferred to the portion of the tubules at the corticomedullary junction. As a result of nephron infection, viable leptospires are shed into the urine and are voided to the exterior. The leptospiruria endures for periods up to 57 days.

From the blood of pregnant cows, leptospires traverse the placenta and enter the fetal blood. Hemolysis of erythrocytes with damaging hypoxia results in fetal death followed by abortion. Placental changes are slight.

The infection evokes antibodies which are detectable 8 to 9 days following inoculation and which reach a peak titer 10 to 12 days after inoculation. While the concentration of antibodies declines following the peak concentration, a titer of 1:100 or higher has been measured 18 months subsequent to infection. During the period of declining titer a degree of immunity gives some protection against re-infection.

Clinical Signs and Postmortem Lesions. Following an incubation period of 3 to 10 days, body temperature rises in a range, 103°

to 106° F. This febrile stage persists for approximately 10 days. While clinical signs vary considerably among cattle, some animals in an infected herd disclose hemoglobinuria, generalized icterus, and anemia. Occasionally the erythrocyte count reduces to 1,000,000 cells per cu mm of blood. Albuminuria is common. Generally throughout the herd, animals go off feed, lose body weight and develop a roughened, dry hair coat. In pregnant cattle abortions occur and the milk becomes viscid and tinged with blood and blood clots. Clinical morbidity seldom exceeds 40% with a mortality of approximately 3%. The recovery of appetite and body weight is slow.

Fatalities occur after 3 to 4 days of the febrile stage. At necropsy, icterus is generalized and anemia is evident. The cut surface of the swollen liver reveals a mottling from central lobular necrosis. Petechial and ecchymotic hemorrhages are abundant and widely distributed over serosal surfaces, especially the subepicardium and subendocardium. The swollen, congested kidneys frequently manifest perirenal edema in the adipose tissue. The renal cortex contains irregularly shaped, red foci which measure up to 0.5 mm in diameter. Petechial hemorrhages and hemoglobin-stained albuminous casts cause mottling of the renal cortices. The urinary bladder contains brown or red discolored urine. During the period ranging from 2 weeks to several months following onset of the disease, the kidney cortices contain multiple gray wedge-shaped foci several millimeters in diameter.

The histopathology varies according to the stages of disease development. During the acute stages, when most deaths occur, the liver discloses cellular degeneration and necrosis in the central zone of the lobules. Foci of necrosis may be found in other zones. Some lymphocytes, mononuclear macrophages, and even neutrophils may be discernible in the stroma around portal triads. Silver impregnation stains differentiate leptospires which, in some cases, are in colonies in the sinusoids. In the acute stages infected nephrons disclose moderate hyperemia of glomeruli, degeneration and necrosis of epithelium of convoluted tubules. A limited number of leukocytes, especially lymphocytes, infiltrate the intertubular stroma. Silver impregnation stains disclose leptospires in the lumens and in epithelial cells of infected tubules.

During the chronic stage of the disease lymphocytes, mononuclear macrophages, and plasma cells accumulate in large numbers around atrophic bile ducts. During the time 2 weeks to several months following onset of the disease, infected nephrons disclose regeneration and proliferation of tubular epithelium. Lymphocytes and mononuclear macrophages infiltrate the intertubular stroma in large numbers and the surrounded tubules show varying degrees of atrophy. Silver impregnation stains differentiate leptospires in the tubules at the corticomedullary junction.

Diagnosis. The diagnosis of leptospirosis is based on clinical signs and laboratory data, the latter including the demonstration of leptospires in blood, urine or tissue, the culturing of leptospires from urine, blood or tissues from the suspected animals, and the demonstration of specific antibodies against leptospires. Important but not pathognomonic signs are icterus, hemoglobinuria, and anemia in febrile animals. At necropsy, petechial and ecchymotic hemorrhages are widely distributed on serosal surfaces. In the chronic stage of the disease, the kidneys disclose single or multiple gray foci in the cortex.

Laboratory procedures are essential for confirmation of a clinical diagnosis of leptospirosis. Either of the following procedures may be utilized:

1. Leptospires can be demonstrated in blood, urine or tissues. During the febrile and leptospiremic stage, motile leptospires may be observed in plasma with darkfield microscopic examination. Concentration of leptospires by centrifugation increases the probability of locating organisms. After approximately 1 week from the onset of disease and continuing for as long as 2 months, lep-

tospires are in the urine and can be observed by concentration through centrifugation and microscopic examination under darkfield illumination. Greater success in demonstrating leptospires results from microscopic examination of sections of kidney and liver from fatal cases. The leptospires are differentiated by silver impregnation stains, such as Levaditi's and the Wharthin-Starry methods. In the liver the organisms are located in sinusoids and occasionally within hepatic cells. In the kidneys leptospires are located, during the acute stage of the disease, within the convoluted tubules of the cortex. In cases of long standing the organisms may be in tubules at the corticomedullary junction. The black stained organisms disclose characteristic morphology.

2. Leptospires may be cultured on fluid media, as Korthof's and Stuart's media, with 5 to 10% rabbit serum. One to 2 ml of suspected blood, urine or ground tissue are inoculated into the medium. Following aerobic incubation for 7 to 10 days at 28° to 30° C, the medium is examined at 1- to 2-day intervals for leptospires. The organisms can be demonstrated in thin Giemsa stained smears, or as viable organisms with darkfield microscopic illumination. In addition, suspected blood, urine or tissues can be inoculated intraperitoneally into young hamsters or guinea pigs. In the latter a febrile reaction develops within 3 to 7 days following inoculation. Some guinea pigs die. Petechial and ecchymotic hemorrhages are common, especially in the lungs. Leptospires can be demonstrated in blood, peritoneal exudate and tissues.

3. While the procedure is difficult to employ, the demonstration of an ascending agglutination or complement fixation antibody titer is adequate evidence for a diagnosis. The titer should be measured during the first week and again after the second and possibly fourth week from onset of the disease. During the first week of infection, before antibodies have developed, the antibody titer frequently is zero.

The differential diagnosis requires consideration of acute necrobacillosis of the liver and bacillary hemoglobinuria. Acute necrobacillosis is associated clinically with icterus and weakness. At necropsy, the swollen liver contains multiple foci of coagulative necrosis. The urine is normal. Bacillary hemoglobinuria, an acute febrile disease, is characterized by generalized icterus and hemoglobinuria. At necropsy, the liver contains a single large infarction.

Prevention and Treatment. Leptospirosis can be prevented by the administration of a bacterin which is currently available commercially. The duration of immunity is sufficient to provide protection during the period of fattening. Most vaccines contain antigens for the serotype of *L. pomona* only. While the majority of bovine leptospirosis is caused by *L. pomona*, some outbreaks are associated with other serotypes. The monovalent vaccine stimulates immunity against its own serotype and against serotypes having similar antigens. Passive immunity of short duration is established through the administration of

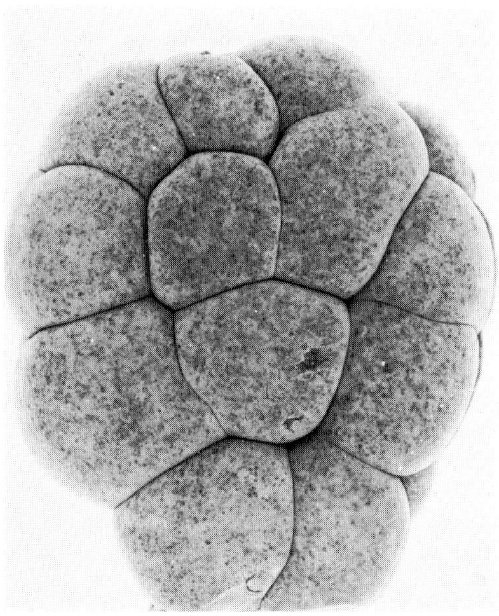

FIG. 4-40. *Kidney of a heifer affected with acute leptospirosis. The multiple small red foci in the cortex are petechial hemorrhages and convoluted tubules filled with hemoglobin.* × 0.8.

hyperimmune antiserum. Whenever feasible, cattle should be protected against exposure to leptospirosis by isolation of clinical cases and through control of feedlot rodents and other possible carrier animals.

Affected animals can be treated in the acute stage with either of the following drugs: (1) streptomycin at the rate of 1 gm per 100 pounds of body weight, and penicillin at the rate of 3,000 to 5,000 units per pound body weight, given daily, intramuscularly, in 2 divided doses for 3 to 6 days; (2) oxytetracycline, chlortetracycline or tetracycline at the rate of 5 mg per pound of body weight, given daily, intravenously, in 2 divided doses for 3 to 6 days. In addition, the administration of hyperimmune antiserum and blood transfusions for anemic animals are beneficial. Oxytetracycline or chlortetracycline can be administered in the feed at the rate of 1 mg per pound of body weight per day for 7 days. This regimen provides protection during the period of immunity development.

References

Andrews, R. D., Ferris, D. H., Hanson, L. E. and Reilley, J. R.: Leptospirosis in a Cattle-Deer Association. Zoonosis Research, *3* (1966): 79–92.

Babudieri, B.: Laboratory Diagnosis of Leptospirosis. World Health Organization Bulletin, *24* (1961): 45–58.

Baker, J. A. and Little, R. B.: Leptospirosis in Cattle. Jour. Exp. Med., *88* (1948): 295–307.

Bryan, H. S.: Studies on Leptospirosis in Domestic Animals. III. Incidence of Leptospirosis in Cattle and Swine in Illinois. JAVMA, *124* (1954): 423–427.

Clark, L. G., Kresse, J. I., Marshak, R. R. and Hollister, C. J.: *Leptospira grippotyphosa* Infections in Cattle and Wildlife in Pennsylvania. JAVMA, *141* (1962): 710–712.

Classification of Leptospires and Recent Advances in Leptospirosis. Bull. World Health Organization, *32* (1965): 881–891.

Freund, S.: Leptospirosis in Cattle in Palestine. J. Comp. Path. & Therap., *57* (1947): 62–66.

Hoeden, J. Van Der: Epizoology of Leptospirosis (Canicola) in the Bovine and Other Species in Israel. JAVMA, *126* (1955): 207–210.

Jungherr, E.: Bovine Leptospirosis. JAVMA, *105* (1944): 276–281.

Killinger, A. H., Hanson, L. E. and Mansfield, M. E.: Leptospiral Vaccination of Cattle Exposed to Infected Deer. Bull. Wildl. Dis. Assoc., *5* (1969): 182–186.

Little, R. B., Deck, J. D. and McCahon, J. V.: An Outbreak of Bovine Leptospirosis in Pennsylvania. Vet. Med., *45* (1950): 104–110.

Losses in Agriculture. USDA Agri. Research Service. Agric. Handbook No. 291. (1965).

Marsh, H.: Leptospira in Bovine Icterohemoglobinuria. JAVMA, *107* (1945): 119–121.

Martin, R. J., Hanson, L. E. and Schnurrenberger, P. R.: Leptospiral Interspecies Infection on an Illinois Farm. Publ. Health Report, Washington, *82* (1967): 75–83.

Mathews, F. P. A.: A Contagious Disease of Cattle Associated with Leptospirosis. AJVR, *7* (1946): 78–93.

Michin, N. A. and Azinov, S. A.: Spirocheatal Jaundice of Cattle in North Caucasus. Sovyet. Vet., *10* (1935): 23–27.

Michin, N. A. Azinov, S. A. and Solikov: Morphological and Cultural Characters and Virulence of *Leptospira icterohaemoglobinureae vitulorum.* Veterinariya, Moscow (1941) No. 1, 51–55.

Murphy, J. C. and Jensen, R.: Experimental Pathogenesis of Leptospiral Abortion in Cattle. AJVR, *30* (1969): 703–713.

Okazaki, W. and Ringen, L. M.: Some Effects of Various Environmental Conditions on Survival of *Leptospira pomona.* AJVR, *18* (1957): 219–223.

Pike, R. M., Paton, I. M. and Schulze, M. L.: Agglutinins for 11 Types of Leptospiras in Serum from Cattle in Northeastern Texas. AJVR, *22* (1961): 906–911.

Ramirez, M. A., Allen, R. C., Van Dresser, W. R., and Watson, D. F.: Serologic Studies Suggestive of *Leptospira hardjo* in a Beef Herd. AJVR, *22* (1961): 995–999.

Reilly, James R., Muraschi, Thelma F. and Dean, Donald J.: Experimental *Leptospira pomona* Infection in White-Tailed Deer, *Odocoileus virginianus* and in Cattle. JAVMA, *140* (1962): 53–57.

Reinhard, K. R., and Hadlow, W. J.: Experimental Bovine Leptospirosis—Pathological, Hematological and Serological Studies. Proceedings AVMA, *91* (1954): 203–216.

Report of Leptospira Subcommittee Meeting Held at Stockholm August 1958. Int. Bull. of Bact. Nomen. and Taxonomy, *13* (1963): 159–160.

Ringen, L. M., Bracken, F. K., Kenzy, S. G. and Gillespie, R. W. H.: Studies on Bovine Leptospirosis. I. Some Effects of Dihydrostreptomycin and Terramycin on the Carrier Condition in Bovine Leptospirosis. JAVMA, *126* (1955): 272–276.

Robertson, A. and Boulanger, P.: Comparison of the Complement-Fixation Test (Agglutination-Lysis) for Detection of Leptospiral Serogroup Antibodies. Canad. J. Comp. Med. & Vet. Sc., *27* (1963): 113–120.

Roth, E. E. and Galton, M. M.: Isolation and Identification of *Leptospira hardjo* from Cattle in Louisiana. AJVR, *21* (1960): 422–427.

Roth, E. E., Adams, G. E., Sanford, G. E., Greer, B., Newman, K., Moore, M., Mayeux, P. and Linder, D.: Bacteriologic and Serologic incidence of Leptospirosis Among Striped Skunks in Louisiana. Zoonoses Research, 2 (1963): 13–39.

Seibold, H. R., Keech, Herbert and Bokelman, D. L.: Histopathologic and Serologic Study of Subclinical Leptospirosis Among Cattle. JAVMA, *138* (1961): 424–430.

Stableforth, A. W. and Galloway, I. A.: *Infectious Diseases of Animals, Diseases Due to Bacteria.* Vol. 1. Academic Press, Inc. New York (1959): 346–378.

Stalheim, O. H. V.: Vaccination of Hamsters, Swine and Cattle With Viable, Avirulent *Leptospira pomona.* AJVR, *29* (1968): 1463–1468.

———: Chemotherapy of Renal Leptospirosis in Cattle. AJVR, *30* (1969): 1317–1323.

Stoenner, H. G., Crews, F. W., Crouse, A. E., Taschner, L. E., Johnson, B. S. and Wohleb, J.: The Epizoology of Bovine Leptospirosis in Washington. JAVMA, 129 (1956): 251–259.

Stoenner, H. G.: Leptospiral Abortion of Beef Cattle Caused by *Leptospira pomona* and *Leptospira hardjo.* JAVMA, 151 (1967): 1087–1090.

Sutherland, A. K. and Morrill, C. C.: An Outbreak of Leptospirosis in Cattle. JAVMA, *113* (1948): 468–471.

Szatalowicz, F. T., Griffin, T. P. and Stunkard, J. A.: The International Dimensions of Leptospirosis. JAVMA, *155* (1969): 2122–2132.

Trainer, D. O., Hanson, R. P., Pope, E. P. and Carbrey, E. A.: The Role of Deer in the Epizootiology of Leptospirosis in Wisconsin. AJVR, *24* (1963): 159–167.

Vishnevskii, P. P.: The Role of Contact in Spread of Bovine Icterohemoglobinuria. Vetinariya, Moscow (1941) No. 3, 56–61. Abst. Vet. Bull., *13* (1943): 422.

White, F. H.: Leptospiral Agglutinins in Snake Serums. AJVR, *24* (1963): 179–182.

World Health Organization: Problems in Leptospirosis. WHO Chronicle, Washington, D. C., (1968).

Yangawa, R., Hiramune, T. and Fujita, J.: The Use of Mice for Vaccination Studies of Leptospirosis. Jap. J. Vet. Sci., *24* (1962): 291–294.

York, C. J.: Aspects of Control in Bovine Leptospirosis. Proceedings of U. S. Livestock Sanitary Assoc. (1951): 295–300.

———: A Complement-Fixation Test for Leptospirosis in Cattle. AJVR, *13* (1952): 117–120.

———: Vaccination for Bovine Leptospirosis. AJVR, *14* (1953): 5–8.

5

Diseases caused by fungi

Ringworm

(BOVINE DERMATOMYCOSIS)

Characterized by scaliness and partial loss of hair, ringworm is a chronic, localized, superficial mycotic dermatitis. In cattle the fungus, *Trichophyton verrucosum*, is the usual specific cause and *T. mentagrophytes* is the unusual cause. Since the infection is superficial and localized in the skin, economic losses to the cattle industry from ringworm are low, but in feedlot cattle itching may result in restlessness and diminished rates of gain, and in areas of infection the hide may be defective for leather production. Severe generalized ringworm infection in calves may adversely affect growth rates and general thriftiness. In show cattle the infection detracts from exhibitability. Because economic losses are often trivial and slight, but annoyingly persistent, the precise total economic loss is difficult to assess and therefore unmeasured.

Review of Literature. Surveys of American (Hoerlein, 1945; Menges and Georg, 1957) and British (Ainsworth and Austwick, 1959) cattle indicated that *Trichophyton verrucosum* was the common cause of bovine ringworm and *T. mentagrophytes* the uncommon one. The former organism was readily isolated from skin lesions and grew well but slowly on Sabouraud's dextrose or maltose agar (Georg, 1954; Hoerlein, 1945a). Application of the live spores from either infected skin lesions or cultures to susceptible bovine skin produced the disease. After rubbing spores into intact or scarified skin, a lesion was discernible in 18 days, well established in 24 to 30 days, and healing in 120 days (Hoerlein, 1945; Sellers, Sinclair and LaTouche, 1956). The observation that lice were often associated with ringworm led scientists to investigate the ectoparasites as vectors of the pathogenic fungi. Lice were collected from around mycotic lesions and cultured; *T. verrucosum* was isolated from 3 of 20 specimens of *Linognathus vituli* and from 1 of 10 *Bovicola bovis* (Hajsig and Zukovic, 1961).

The incidence of bovine ringworm, although varying geographically, is high in some areas of the United States and 50% of the animals within some infected herds contained lesions. Animals 2 years or younger showed a significantly higher incidence than did other age groups (Menges and Georg, 1957). In Britain 25% of the herds were infected, and in herds consisting of 75 or more cattle the incidence was higher (McPhearson, 1957). In Denmark the herd incidence increased sharply from a few herds in 1931 to

20,000 herds in 1958 (Gierloff and Katic, 1961).

Studies of treatment efficacy, often imprecise and difficult of evaluation, demonstrated the utility of some fungicidal compounds. Captan (N-trichloromethyl-mercapto-4-cyclohexene-1,2-dicarboximide) used in a concentration of 0.45 to 0.5 pounds per 20 gallons of water was applied as a spray at 400 to 450 pounds pressure to 700 young cattle, 50% of whom contained rapidly spreading ringworm. Two applications, with an interval of 2 weeks, reduced the active lesions in all but 1 to 3% of the cattle (Baker and Davis, 1954). In a controlled experiment involving 4 infected herds griseofulvin was clinically evaluated. Orally the drug was applied daily for 7 consecutive days at the rate of 10 mg per kg of body weight. Forty days after the administration, treated cattle showed statistically significant improvement over the untreated control animals.

Occurrence. All breeds, sexes and ages of cattle are susceptible, but animals less than 2 years of age are more commonly infected than other age groups. Under crowded feedlot conditions with numerous opportunities for spread of contagious diseases, ringworm often occurs in 50 to 70% of a herd. Recently weaned young cattle entering previously infected feedlots and remaining for 5 to 6 months are exposed during periods of high age susceptibility and may become heavily infected. In addition to cattle, infection with *T. verrucosum* has been observed in dogs, horses, donkeys, sheep, goats and people, especially individuals working with infected cattle.

While general observations in the United States indicate the higher incidence of bovine ringworm during winter months, the disease occurs commonly during all seasons. In Britain a critical survey (1957) indicated no statistically significant difference in seasonal incidence. Although world-wide in distribution, the disease has attracted attention and evoked investigations in the United States, Europe, North Africa and Russia.

Etiology. Bovine ringworm is usually caused by *Trichophyton verrucosum* but rarely by *T. mentagrophytes.* These fungi grow and form hyphae in the stratum corneum of the skin and hair follicles. The hyphae divide transversely to form linearly arranged spores which measure 2 to 8 μ in diameter and are highly refractive to light. The organisms grow readily but slowly on most artificial media, but Sabouraud's dextrose or maltose agar is commonly used. While the optimum temperature is 30° to 35° C, incubation is commonly at 25° C in order to inhibit the growth of contaminating bacteria. After 2 weeks of incubation colonies are 5 to 20 mm in diameter and after 4 weeks 20 to 40 mm.

Cultural characteristics of the two species include some differentiating features. Folded colonies of *T. verrucosum* become white to yellow. Thiamin and for some strains inositol also are required for growth. The formation of macroconidia is rare. *T. mentagrophytes* forms two types of colony: downy and granular. The granular variety, usually pathogenic to cattle, horses, dogs and rodents, forms flat, powdery, white to yellow colonies that may produce some red pigment after several weeks growth. Club-shaped macroconidia with thin, smooth, walls and containing 3 or more cells are produced by most strains.

While some fungal infections fluoresce in the light of a Wood's lamp, those caused by *T. verrucosum* do not fluoresce.

The spores of *T. verrucosum* are highly resistant to dehydration and sunlight. Within the protection of animal sheds and barns spores remain viable 4½ years and in areas exposed to sunlight for many months.

Transmission. The spores of *T. verrucosum* locate in active skin lesions of cattle and on rubbing chains, posts, fences and feeding equipment. In crowded feedlots animals rub against each other and in common use rubbing, feeding and watering equipment. Once the disease is within a herd, these exercises provide opportunities for transmission of ringworm by direct contact of susceptible cattle with viable spores. Spores within a contaminated pen remain viable over periods of pen vacancy, even during summer months, and infect newly introduced cattle. Although contaminated curry combs, ropes and blankets may also transmit the disease, this equipment is not commonly used on feedlot cattle.

Pathogenesis. Following inoculation of viable spores onto the face and neck skin of susceptible cattle, localized infections may develop. Superficial scarification or rubbing of the skin, as may occur from feeding and butting, facilitates the establishment of fungal growth. The mycelia grow rapidly among the host cells of the stratum corneum. Eventually the infundibuli of hair follicles are also penetrated. The mycelial filaments segment transversely and form linearly-arranged spores which make a sheath several cells thick around the hair shaft. Penetration by some mycelia weakens the hair and causes it to break near the skin surface. A prolonged infection provokes a chronic inflammatory reaction in both the derma and epidermis. The epithelial cells proliferate, keratinize, and accumulate in excessive numbers in short papillae-like processes of the stratum corneum, and the accumulated cells become the scaly pad often grossly seen. Multiple lesions may develop from independent inoculations or spread from a primary focus. Skin lesions near the eyes may progress into non-specific keratoconjunctivitis.

The chronological changes in a developing lesion have been determined by inoculating susceptible bovine skin with viable spores. After 18 days, hair of the new lesion is disarranged and the skin is erythemic. After 24 days scaliness is obvious and spores are detected around some hair shafts. While the scaliness increases for many weeks, healing occurs approximately 4 months after inoculation.

Clinical Signs and Lesions. Following an incubation period of approximately 3 weeks, skin lesions develop. While some are mild, scaly and incompletely depillated, most lesions are discrete circular masses measuring one-half to several inches in diameter. The gray-yellow crust is dry, scaly, and firm. Projecting slightly above the surrounding skin, the crust is essentially depillated but may contain short hairs broken near the crust surface. Numerically single or multiple, the lesions may be confluent and commonly are located on the face, especially around the eyes and neck. The perineal skin often is affected. In some animals the lesions become generalized and involve large areas of the head, neck, thorax, abdomen and proximal parts of the limbs.

Active ringworm lesions annoy cattle, and the affected animals rub their lesions against fences, feeding and rubbing equipment, and other animals. When lesions are accessibly located, the animals scratch with the feet, bite the infected skin, and as a result, the lesions become deeply fissured and traumatized. While a few face and neck lesions probably have little effect on weight gains, the occasional case with a generalized infection is unthrifty and susceptible to intercurrent infections. In crowded feedlots the morbidity rate may be 50 to 70% of the herd, while the mortality rate is very low. The disease course is approximately 4 months. Recently recovered animals appear temporarily resistant to reinfection.

Histopathologically, the lesion shows chronic inflammation of the derma and epidermis. Epithelial cells of the stratum corneum increase numerically and are parakeratotic. The accumulated cells form short papillary projections above the surface of surrounding skin. Filamentous mycelia are often detectable among the cells of the stratum corneum of the skin proper and of the hair follicles. In some follicles sheaths of spores surround hair shafts which weaken and break when penetrated by mycelia. Micro-abscesses may be found in the epidermis and the derma. Lymphocytes, mononuclear macrophages and small numbers of neutrophils accumulate around infected hair follicles in the derma.

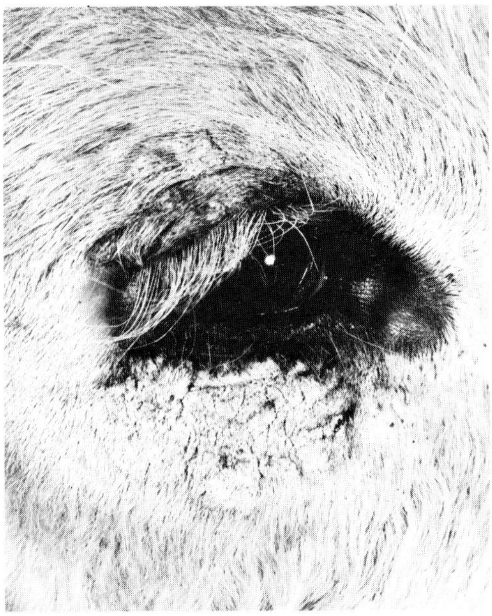

FIG. 5-1. *An active ringworm lesion on the skin near an eye of a steer.* × 0.7.

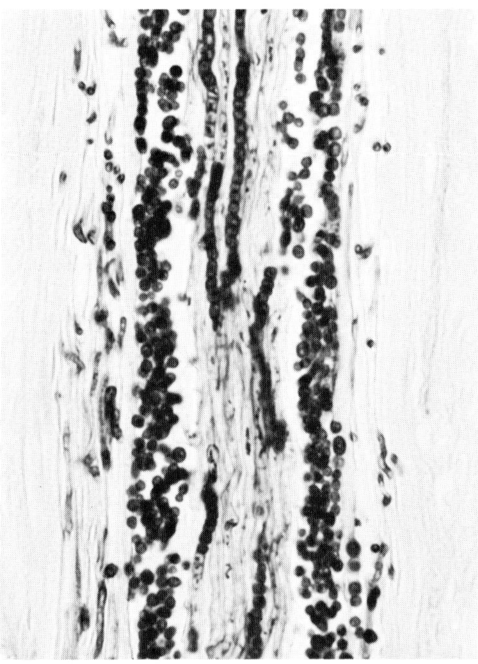

FIG. 5-2. *Spores in a bovine hair follicle and hyphae in the hair shaft. Hotchkiss-McManus stain.* × 546.

Diagnosis. The lesions of bovine ringworm are sufficiently distinctive and characteristic for accurate diagnosis. The single or multiple circular, dry, scaly, gray, depillated crust is the significant clinical sign. Laboratory confirmation can be obtained with smears, histopathologic sections, and cultures. Plucked hairs and deep scrapings may be obtained from many points at the lesion periphery. The specimens, mixed with 10 to 20% solution of sodium hydroxide, are warmed on a glass slide. After 15 to 20 minutes of clearing, the specimens are examined with a microscope. Histopathologic sections are made from the periphery of a lesion and stained with Hotchkiss-McManus or Gridley stain. The cleared unstained specimens under reduced light, microscopically show sheaths of spores surrounding some infected hair shafts. The spores are highly light refractile and measure 5 to 8 μ in diameter. In sections differentiated with Hotchkiss-McManus stain the sheaths of spores and the mycelia stain red.

Cultures of the fungus grow slowly and commonly require many weeks for final identification. Suspected scales and hairs are plucked from the lesion, ground in a mortar and pestle, and mixed with sterile water. Sabouraud's dextrose or maltose agar is inoculated and incubated at 25° to 30° C. The cultures can be identified on the evidence of morphologic characteristics.

Differential diagnosis requires consideration of focal mange lesions. In mange the crust contains considerable exudate and mites can be detected in scrapings from the lesion.

Prevention and Treatment. In heavily infected feedlots where ringworm in newly introduced cattle is anticipated, the pen contamination can be reduced by thorough cleaning, vacancy through consecutive months of spring, summer, and autumn, and by chemical disinfection of fences and feeding and rubbing equipment.

Many empirical treatments have been developed and abandoned because of limited efficacy. Most medicaments have been used as repeated topical applications. Daily applications of a mixture of equal parts of tincture of iodine and glycerin, or a tincture of iodine, or Lugol's solution have been used with considerable success. Petroleum products, such as used crank case oil, have been applied with saturated fabrics on back-rubbing equipment to treat lesions and to reduce the rate of spread. In advanced cases of ringworm, solutions of sodium iodide may be administered intravenously at the rate of 0.25 to 1.0 ounce per animal. Several specific fungicides have been developed recently but not evaluated by critical experimentation. Griseofulvin, administered orally at the rate of 10 mg per kg of body weight for 7 consecutive days has been useful. Captan as a solution of 0.45 to 0.5 pounds per 20 gallons of water can be applied as a spray with 400 to 450 pounds of pressure. The treatment should be repeated after a 2-week interval. The administration of griseofulvin or Captan is feasible under feedlot conditions.

References

Ainsworth, G. C. and Austwick, P. K. C.: Fungal Diseases of Animals. Commonwealth Agri. Bureau. Farnham Royal, England. 1959. pp. 80–91.

Baker, N. F. and Davis, D. W.: Spray Application for the Treatment of Ringworm in Cattle. Vet. Med., *49* (1954): 275–276.

Butozan, V. and Mihojlovitch, S.: Les Dermatomycoses des animaux Domestiques en Yugoslavie. Bull. Off. Epiz., *58* (1962): 733–746.

Cobb, R. W., Martin, A. R., Short, G. V. and Walley, J. K.: Griseofulvin: Controlled Field Trials in the Treatment of Naturally Occurring Ringworm in Calves. Vet. Rec., *75* (1963): 191–193.

Georg, L. K.: The Diagnosis of Ringworm in Animals. Vet. Med., *49* (1954): 157–165.

Gierloff, B. C. H. and Katic, I.: Experience with the Treatment of Ringworm in Domestic Animals by a New Fungistatic Agent Griseofulvin. Nord. Vet.-Med., *13* (1961): 571–592.

Hajsig, M. and Zukovic, M.: *Trichophyton verrucosum* Isolated from Lice. Vet. Arch., *31* (1961): 225–228.

Hoerlein, A. B.: Studies on Animal Dermatomycoses. I. Clinical Studies. Cornell Vet., *35* (1945): 287–298.

Hoerlein, A. B.: Studies on Animal Dermatomycoses. II. Cultural Studies. Cornell Vet., *35* (1945a): 299–307.

La Touche, C. J.: Some Observations on Ringworm in Calves due to *Trichophyton discoides* Sabouraud. Vet. Rec., *64* (1952): 841–843.

McPhearson, E. A.: A Survey of the Incidence of Ringworm in Cattle in Northern Britain. Vet. Rec., *69* (1957): 674–679.

Menges, R. W. and Georg, L. K.: Survey of Animal Ringworm in the United States. U. S. Public Health Service Reports, *73* (1957): 503–509.

Sellers, K. C., Sinclair, W. B. V. and LaTouche, C. J.: Preliminary Observations on Natural and Experimental Ringworm in Cattle. Vet. Rec., *68* (1956): 729–733.

Coccidioidomycosis

(COCCIDIOIDAL GRANULOMA; OIDIOMYCOSIS; VALLEY FEVER)

Chronic, asymptomatically infectious but non-contagious, coccidioidomycosis is characterized by the development of granulomatous lesions in the lungs and pulmonary lymph nodes and is caused by the fungus, *Coccidioides immitis.* The disease is distributed and limited to the western hemisphere. Cattle affected with this non-fatal disease eat and gain weight normally, and hence the disease has little economic importance to the cattle industry. Some losses result from condemnation of infected organs at slaughter, but of greater economic importance is the public health significance of the disease. The temporary and partial incapacitation of affected people requires expensive research and control programs.

Review of Literature. Since its discovery as a human disease (Posada, 1892), veterinarians inspecting carcasses at slaughter have been alert for bovine coccidioidomycosis, and they first observed it in America in animals raised and slaughtered in southern California (Giltner, 1918). Numerous subsequent studies supported the first findings and continually indicated that the disease is limited to the southwest part of the United States (Maddy, 1954; 1960; Prchal, 1948), but that in slaughtered cattle from the endemic area the disease incidence within infected herds varies from 8 to 48% (Davis and Stiles, 1937; Davis, Stiles and McGregor, 1938). During 1946–47 at Phoenix, Arizona, 38,175 cattle were slaughtered in federally inspected meat packing establishments; slaughter inspection statistics state that of these, 503 (1.3%) contained gross lesions of coccidioidomycosis, and most of the infected cattle had resided 60 to 90 days in dusty fattening feedlots of the endemic area (Prchal, 1948). To determine the percentage of cattle previously exposed to the pathogen, 11,643 home-grown cattle ranging in age from 1 to 6 years and residing at altitudes from 500 to 5500 feet, were skin-tested in Arizona. Of the tested cattle, 24.6% reacted positively, and these animals had resided at the lower altitudes (Maddy, Crecelius and Cornell, 1960).

In studies of the cause of coccidioidomycosis, lesions of lungs and of bronchial and mediastinal lymph nodes were prepared in stained smears, histopathologic sections and/or bacteriologic cultures. The fungus, *C. immitis*, was observed in 189 cattle and isolated from some specimens (Davis and Stiles, 1937). When cultured on a medium consisting mostly of an enzyme digest of lactalbumen, the organism was induced to accelerate the rate of arthrospore formation. These appeared in 12 hours (Northey and Brooks, 1962). In another study, a suspension of infected tissue inoculated intravenously into a susceptible calf caused serious illness in 1 week and death in 10 days. At necropsy, the lungs contained multiple lesions of coccidioidomycosis (Giltner, 1918). When 93 cattle were inoculated intratracheally with 500,000 to 2,000,000 viable culture particles of *C. immitis* per animal, and observed for 90 to 130 days, most animals developed skin sensitivity to coccidioidin, and some had typical lesions at necropsy (Maddy, Reed, Trautman and Snell, 1960). Viable cultures inoculated into the yolk sacs of embryonating chicken eggs resulted in marked proliferation of the fungus, and 3 to 6 days following inoculation the embryos died. Gross bovine lesions were limited to the lungs and the pulmonary and mediastinal lymph nodes (Maddy, 1954; 1962). The lymph nodal lesions, more conspicuous than the lung lesions, were caseative and active. In a study of 3,173 bovine cases, the lesions of 15.9% contained foci of calcification (Maddy, 1954). As indicated by the following, most infections in feedlot cattle were acquired in the feedlot:

In the first herd, 43 cattle were removed from the summer grazing range in Utah. Eighteen were slaughtered immediately and showed no evidence of disease. The remaining 25 were transported to a California feedlot and fattened for 64 days. At the time of slaughter 7 (28%) contained gross lesions of coccidioidomycosis.

In the second herd, 163 cattle were removed from a summer grazing range in Idaho. Thirty-two animals were slaughtered immediately, and no lesions were observed. The remaining 131 cattle were shipped to a California feedlot in an endemic area and were fattened for 57 days. At slaughter 17 (13%) contained gross lesions (Maddy, 1954).

Occurrence. All breeds, sexes and ages are susceptible, but young calves of beef breeds contain a low incidence because this age group is seldom maintained in dusty pens. Hereford steers and heifers, 6 months to 2 years of age, show a high incidence because large numbers of this breed are produced within the endemic area. During recent years, some lots of fattened cattle from Arizona have shown an incidence ranging from 5 to 20%. In addition to cattle, the disease occurs naturally in dogs, horses, burros, sheep, coyotes, llamas, monkeys, desert rodents and people. Limited in geographic distribution the disease occurs in lower Sonoran life zone of western Texas, southern New Mexico and Nevada, southwestern Utah, southern and central California where rainfall and altitudes are low and temperatures high. Other endemic areas include Mexico, Paraguay, Argentina and Venezuela. Contracted during dry dusty seasons, the lesions have a prolonged course and may be observed at slaughter during all months.

Etiology. The causative agent, *Coccidioides immitis,* is a septate fungus described as both a saprophyte and a parasite. In the saprophytic stage and under conditions of high soil humidity and moderate temperatures, the mycelia grow around decaying buried wood and feces in and near rodent burrows. Some hyphae develop specialized thickened branches which may grow to soil surfaces or soil cracks. The dry air induces formation of rectangular arthrospores and round chlamydospores in the branches. Air currents shatter the branches and disperse spores and other fungal fragments. Measuring 2 to 10 μ in diameter, the arthrospores can be grown on Sabouraud's dextrose or maltose agar enriched with cyclohexamide and chloramphenicol where the organism forms white cottony colonies, becoming tan or brown with maturity.

When inoculated into the testicles of guinea pigs, the arthrospores become enlarged, round and thick-walled spherules 10 to 200 μ in diameter.

The parasitic stage, found in lungs, bronchial lymph nodes, and mediastinal lymph nodes of infected cattle, form spherules or sporangia within the infected tissue. Containing a doubly refractile wall 2 μ thick and occasionally radiating clubs, the spherule measures 10 to 80 μ in diameter, and following maturation, it forms endospores which measure 2 to 5 μ in diameter. The endospores develop in the spherule, rupture the wall, disperse in the tissue and form new spherules. Following the inoculation of suitable artificial media, the viable parasitic organisms also grow and produce characteristic saprophytic forms.

Pathogenesis. Following the inhalation of infective dust, the viable arthrospores locate on the mucosa of bronchi or bronchioles where they enlarge and differentiate. Within 4 to 7 days mature spherules with endospores form. Eventually, the spherule ruptures, releases the endospores into surrounding tissue, and the liberated endospores develop into new generations of spherules. Through these cycles of production, the organisms increase and spread throughout the tissue, including the alveoli. Usually some spherules or endospores gain entrance to efferent lymphatics and are carried to the bronchial or mediastinal lymph nodes where secondary foci of infection develop. In cattle the organisms seldom spread beyond the regional lymph nodes.

Among individual cattle the tissue reaction to the organism varies but in most cases granulomas form, with neutrophils accumulating around the fungus. On rupture of the spherule, neutrophils enter the capsule and attempt to phagocytize endospores and other spherule contents, but in the process many neutrophilic cells are destroyed. Mononuclear macrophages also accumulate, form multinucleated giant cells, and phagocytize both spherules and endospores. Small numbers of lymphocytes and plasma cells are present. Towards the periphery of the reaction zone fibrocytes proliferate and form collagen fibers. Areas of necrosis and calcification are randomly distributed throughout the lesion. The slow growing granuloma, visible 21 days after inoculation, may grow to many centimeters in diameter. The proliferated connective tissue tends to localize the infection. In some animals the tissue reaction is excessive and in others moderate. Presumedly, the infection may be overcome, and healing may occur at any stage of lesion development.

The infection stimulates immunity, and for prolonged periods recovered animals resist reinfection. Cattle exposed to the infection develop skin sensitivity to coccidioidin as well as complement-fixing and precipitating antibodies. The lesions, minor in extent and severity, provoke no clinical signs nor alter normal rates of gain in body weight.

Postmortem Lesions. The granulomas of bovine coccidioidomycosis are encountered at postmortem inspection of organs of slaughtered cattle, or at necropsy of animals having died from other causes. Generally limited to the lungs and pulmonary lymph nodes, the lesions are commonly larger and more abundant in the bronchial and mediastinal lymph nodes than in the lung tissue proper. Numerically single or multiple, unilateral or bilateral, the young pulmonary lesion is pink and moderately firm. Measuring 0.5 to 1 inch in diameter, the mature grey or white lesions are firm. The cut surface reveals soft areas containing yellow pus. In some lesions, mineralization is detectable. The lymph nodes may contain one or many and confluent granulomatous lesions. While varying in size, the lesion may obtain a diameter of 4 inches. Young granulomas are grey, while mature ones are firm and grey-white with foci of soft yellow pus. Calcification may be detected. On the cut surface caseative necrosis and pockets of yellow pus with or without focal calcification are often apparent.

Histopathologically, the lesions are typical of infectious granulomas. Double contoured spherules, with or without endospores, are distributed widely throughout the central zone of the lesion. Some spherules contain eosinophilic clubs projecting from the surface. Ruptured spherules and fragments of capsules are often discernible. Neutrophils surround many spherules and penetrate ruptured capsules. Some lymphocytes and plasma cells are present. Peripheral to the zone of neutrophils are mononuclear macrophages and multinucleated giant cells which often phagocytize the fungus. At the lesion periphery, fibrocytes proliferate and collagen fibers are present in variable amounts. Foci of necrosis and dense accumulations of pus are common. In some areas mineralization occurs.

At postmortem inspection of slaughtered cattle, lesions from coccidioidomycosis usually are limited to the lungs and pulmonary lymph nodes, and when few in number and small in size only the infected organs are condemned. In animals having large numerous lesions throughout the lungs, the entire carcass is judged unsuitable for human food.

Diagnosis. Bovine coccidioidomycosis, not diagnosed in living cattle, is established in dead animals on the evidence of gross lesions and laboratory findings observed at postmortem examination of organs of slaughtered cattle and at necropsy of animals having died from other causes. Lesions are restricted to the lungs and pulmonary lymph nodes. Important specific features of the lesions are fibrosis, caseative necrosis, and purulent inflammation as shown on the cut surface. In the laboratory, confirmation can be obtained by finding and identifying *C. immitis* in sections, smears or microbiological cultures. Histopathologic sections stained with hematoxylin and eosin or PAS stain provide good morphologic differentiation for the diagnosis. Stained smears also enable identification of spherules. Cultures made on Sabouraud's dextrose or maltose agar require relatively long periods for complete growth and identification. Specific precipitins can be demon-

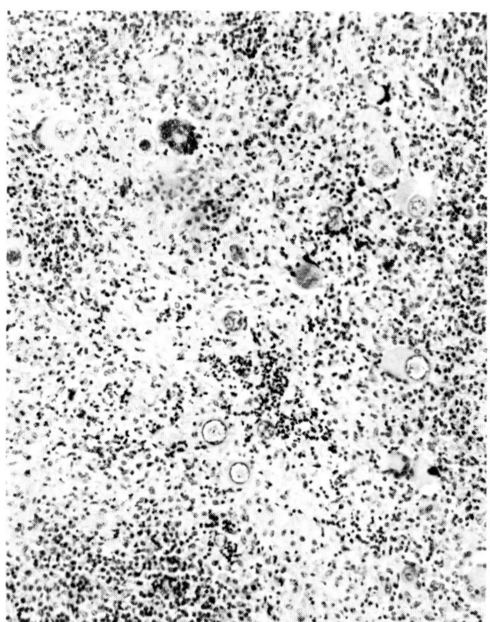

FIG. 5-3. *Spherules of C. immitis and tissue reaction in a lymph node of steer affected with coccidioidomycosis. H & E stain.* × 115.

strated in serum. In living animals a skin sensitivity test can be applied. This is achieved by intradermal inoculation in the neck region of 0.1 ml of undiluted coccidioidin. Local induration measuring 5 mm or more and appearing within 96 hours constitutes a positive reaction, and therefore indicates previous exposure of the animal to infection.

Prevention. The incidence of the disease can be lowered by any practice which diminishes feedlot dust: moistening pen surfaces and driveways, covering pen surfaces and roads with hard non-dusting material, growing grass on unused soil surfaces.

Since bovine coccidioidomycosis has never been diagnosed in live cattle, effective treatments have not been developed.

References

Crane, C. S.: Equine Coccidioidomycosis. Vet. Med., *57* (1962): 1073–1074.

Davis, C. L. and Stiles, G. W.: Pulmonary Coccodioidal Granuloma. A New Site of Infection in Cattle, JAVMA, *91* (1937): 209–215.

Davis, C. L., Stiles, G. W. and McGregor, A. N.: Coccidioidal Granuloma in Calves. JAVMA, *92* (1938): 562–563.

Giltner, L. T.: Occurrence of Coccidioidal Granuloma (Oidiomycosis) in Cattle. Jour. Ag. Res., *14* (1918): 533.

Maddy, K. T.: Coccidioidomycosis of Cattle in the Southwestern United States. JAVMA, *124* (1954): 456–464.

———: Coccidioidomycosis in a Sheep. JAVMA, *124* (1954a): 465–466.

———: Coccidioidomycosis. *Advances in Veterinary Science.* Academic Press, Publishers. New York. (1960): 251–286.

———: The Diagnosis of Coccidioidomycosis. Proc. U.S.L.S.A. (1962): 396–408.

Maddy, K. T., Crecelius, H. G., and Cornell, R. G.: Distribution of *Coccidioides immitis* Determined by Testing Cattle. U. S. Public Health Service Reports, *75* (1960): 955–962.

Maddy, K. T., Reed, R. E., Trautman, R. J. and Snell, V. N.: Experimental Bovine Coccidioidomycosis. AJVR, *21* (1960): 748–752.

Northey, W. T. and Brooks, L. D.: Studies on *Coccidioides immitis.* I. A Simple Medium for *in vitro* Spherulation. J. Bact., *84* (1962): 742–746.

Pappagianis, D., Levine, H. H., Smith, C. W., Bermen, R. V. and Kobayashi, G. S.: Immunization of Mice with Viable *Coccidioides immitis.* J. Immunology, *86* (1961): 28–34.

Posada, A.: Un nuevo caso de micosis fungoidea con psorospermias. Ann. Circ. Med. Argentina *15* (1892): 481–497.

Prchal, C. J.: Coccidioidomycosis of Cattle in Arizona. JAVMA, *112* (1948): 461–465.

Roessler, W. G., Converse, J. L. and Geating, J. A.: Virulence Assay of *Coccidioides immitis* in Embryonated Eggs. J. Bact., *81* (1961): 226–232.

Straub, M., Trautman, R. J. and Greene, J. W.: Coccidioidomycosis in Three Coyotes, AJVR, *22* (1961): 811–812.

Nasal Granuloma

(MADUROMYCOSIS; RHINOSPORIDIOSIS; SNORTING DISEASE; MYCETOMA)

A chronic mycotic but non-contagious disease, nasal granuloma is characterized by nodular thickening of the anterior nasal mucosa. The cause may be any species of a group of fungi, but *Helminthosporium* sp. appears to be the specific agent in cattle. Horses, mules and people may also be affected, but by different fungi. Because of general low herd incidence, the disease has insignificant economic importance to the cattle industry, but high morbidity rate within an affected herd may cause serious financial losses to individual owners. In people it occurs sporadically with partial incapacitation, but this adds public health significance and additional economic importance to the disease.

Review of Literature. While bovine nasal granuloma was reported earlier in India (Ainsworth and Austwick, 1959; Kirshnaumurti, 1927), the first official report in the United States was in a herd of dairy cattle maintained at an experimental station at Jeanerette, Louisiana (Creech and Miller, 1933). Other bovine cases were reported in Texas (Bridges, 1960; Robinson, 1951), Colorado (Davis and Shorten, 1936), and Oklahoma (Roberts, McDaniel, Carbray, 1963). In addition to the dairy breeds, Hereford and Santa Gertrudis have been affected (Bridges, 1960; Davis and Shorten, 1936).

Information descriptive of the causative organism, largely confined to morphology, is derived from detailed studies of the histopathology and from a limited number of isolations on artificial media. In the first studies of the infected herd at Jeanerette, Louisiana, pathogens were not isolated from the infected tissues, and injected lesion suspensions failed to produce the disease. From these facts the investigators inferred that the disease was due to an animal parasite (Creech and Miller, 1933). In further studies of the Louisiana herd, ground lesions were treated with 4% potassium hydroxide solution. In the remaining residues, numerous hyaline shells, each with a pore, were observed but no evidence suggesting animal parasitism was obtained, and investigators decided, therefore, that the causative agent was the fungus *Rhinosporidium seeberi.* More detailed investigations with specialized stains disclosed within lesions branching septate hyphae and sporangia (Bridges, 1960; Robinson, 1951). From the histopathologic demonstration of hyphae, sporangia and eosinophilia, and, from the symptoms of nasal itching, investigators postulated fungus and allergy as primary and secondary causes. They assigned the name "maduromycosis" (Bridges, 1960) to this combination of findings and symptoms. In the herd at Jeanerette, Louisiana, the treatment with iodine, administered systemically and/or topically, of infected animals was unsuccessful (Creech and Miller, 1933). From infected nasal tissue the fungus, *Helminthosporium* sp., was isolated on Sabouraud's dextrose agar in each of two investigations (Davis and Shorten 1936; Roberts, McDaniel and Carbrey, 1963).

Occurrence. Although the investigations of outbreaks of bovine nasal granuloma have been numerically few, observations suggest that all breeds and sexes are susceptible. Reports indicated that the disease incidence in feedlot cattle is very low and may occur in heifers and steers $1\frac{1}{2}$ to 2 years of age, but is more commonly found in retired breeding beef cattle being fattened for slaughter.

Although the influence of season on incidence has not been determined, clinical signs may exacerbate during summer months and abate during the winter season. Geographically, the disease has been reported among cattle of Colorado, Oklahoma and Texas, but probably occurs in other states. Outside the United States it has been reported in India and South Africa.

Etiology and Pathogenesis. While various species of fungi have been postulated as potential causes of bovine nasal granuloma, *Helminthosporium* sp. has been isolated and morphologically identified in two investigations of infected cattle. Probably other species of fungi are also capable of causing bovine rhinitis. These fungi infect the bovine nasal mucosa and evoke granulomatous lesions. Within the infected tissue they form hyphae and sporangia varying in morphologic dimensions but which stain red with periodic acid Schiff reagents. Culturing of the fungus on artificial media is difficult and the rate of growth appears to be slow. The saprophytic stage of the fungus has not been observed.

While the means of transmission has not been determined, clinical and pathological evidence suggest direct nasal contact or inhalation of pathogenic parts of the saprophytic phase of the fungus. Grass awns carrying infective spores may enter the external nares during pasture grazing or may be inhaled. In either event the nasal mucosa within 6 inches of the external nares becomes inoculated. The fungus grows slowly within the tissue and provokes a chronic granulomatous reaction. The infected mucosa thickens and forms sessile or pedunculated surface nodules; these mucosal changes diminish the caliber of the nasal meatuses and result in dyspnea accompanied with pulmonary emphysema, mouth breathing, and physical discomfort. As a chronic infection, the reaction may endure 4 years or more.

Clinical Signs and Postmortem Lesions. After a long incubation period and slow development, clinical signs relating to the nasal lesions are manifest. The affected animal sneezes frequently, and a mucopurulent discharge emanates from one or both nostrils. In early stages some necrotic tissue and blood are mixed with the discharge. In advanced stages breathing becomes difficult and stertorous. Careful study indicates that the vibrating tissues are in the anterior part of the nasal cavities, and because of itching, the nose is rubbed against fences, plants and buildings. The head is extended and breathing may be oral. From efforts to dilate the external nares, the skin over the nostril alae becomes wrinkled. With diminished appetite the rate of gain in body weight declines. Careful examination of the nasal cavities with an illuminated speculum reveals a thickened nodular mucosa covered with mucopurulent exudate.

Very few valid disease statistics are available. In the herd at Jeanerette, Louisiana, with 60 cattle, 21.6% became affected over a 4-year period. The mortality rate of affected animals is high because of complications from dyspnea and from disinclination of owners to tolerate the prolonged course. The disease may endure for 4 years or longer.

At necropsy, the primary lesions limited to the anterior 6 inches of the nasal cavities bring changes that are unilateral or bilateral and located on the nasal septum, dorsal turbinates and ventral turbinates. The affected mucosa is thickened and contains single or multiple and confluent nodules. The latter

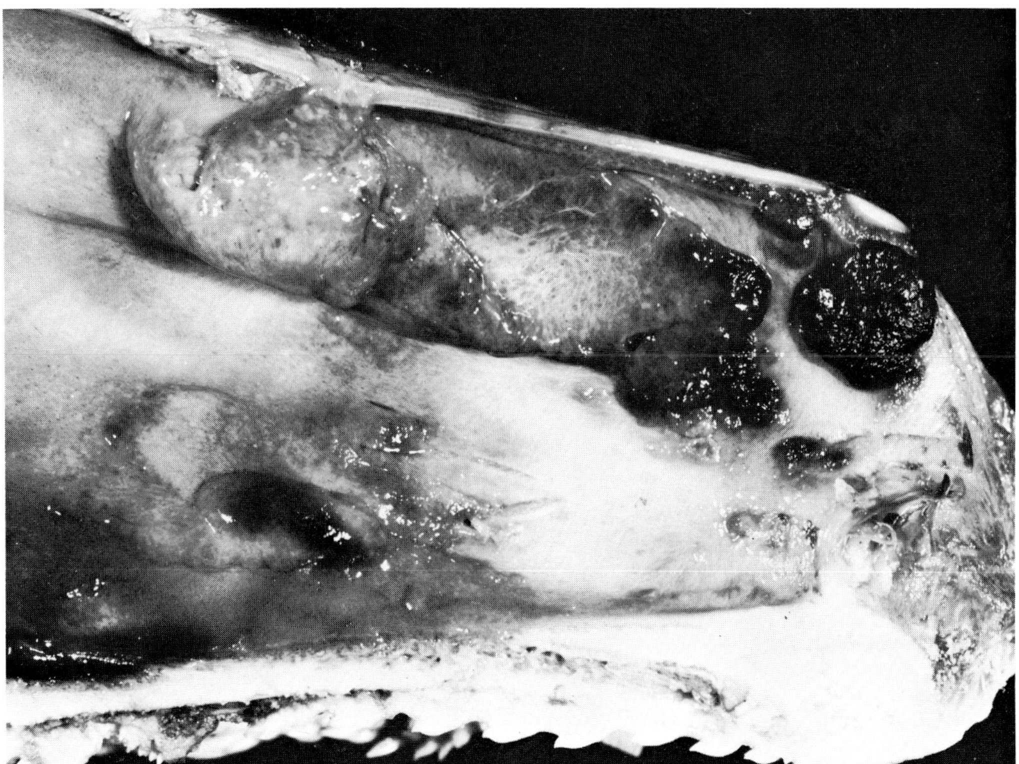

FIG. 5-4. *Thickened mucosa and sessile nodules on the dorsal and ventral turbinates of the anterior nasal cavity of a beef cow affected with nasal granuloma.* × 1.2.

are soft and often ulcerated. The points of attachment are usually sessile and less commonly pedunculated. If uncomplicated, the nodular tissue is gray with a green cast and the foci, each less than 1 mm in diameter, are yellow. In case of hemorrhage, the tissue is dark. Necrosis and sloughing may be evident. The meatuses are dimensionally diminished in amounts corresponding to the tissue enlargement. As a result of prolonged dyspnea, pulmonary emphysema may be prominent.

Histopathologically, the diseased mucosa contains widely disseminated pathogenic fungi in variable numbers. Aggregates of, or single, spores are often observed. When differentiated with PAS stain, the hyphae and sporangia are red. The hyphae are branched and contain sporangia which consist of a capsule with cytoplasm or spores. The fungi are surrounded by eosinophilic leukocytes and smaller numbers of neutrophils, lymphocytes, and plasma cells. Mononuclear macrophages forming Langhan's and foreign body giant cells are also present, and the giant cells commonly phagocytize portions of the fungi. Throughout the tissue is an increase of loose connective tissue with numerous blood capillaries. Edema is common and necrosis with surface ulceration may be present.

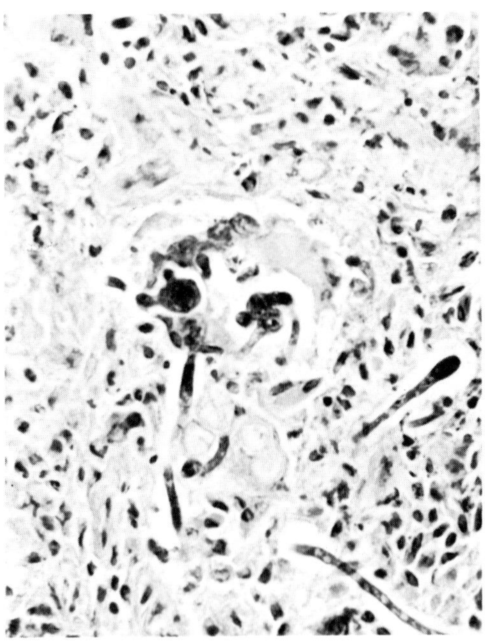

FIG. 5-5. *A granulomatous reaction around hyphae and sporangia in the nasal cavity. PAS stain.* × 431.

Diagnosis. The identification of bovine nasal granuloma is based on typical clinical signs, case history and laboratory findings. A long course of difficult breathing from partial obstruction of the anterior nasal cavities and the nasal discharge are important diagnostic signs. Additional evidence can be obtained by examining the nasal cavities with a speculum, but diagnostic confirmation may be made by finding fungi in nasal biopsies or from infected nasal tissue obtained at necropsy or slaughter.

In the laboratory the specific fungi can be located and identified in stained sections or, less reliably, in stained smears from infected tissues. Attempts to culture the fungi usually have been unsuccessful.

The differential diagnosis requires the consideration of actinobacillosis, nasal neoplasms, and the presence of foreign bodies. Actinobacillosis may cause mucosal thickening, pedunculated lesions and dyspnea, and favorably respond to treatment with streptomycin. In most cases the regional lymph nodes are also infected and enlarged, but smears from the infected mucosa or from the lymph nodes contain the clubbed rosettes of the fungus, *Actinobacillus ligniersi.* Nasal neoplasms may be primary or metastatic and are identified by histopathologic studies. The presence of foreign bodies, such as pieces of wood, metal, or glass, may be detected by careful nasal palpation and examination with a speculum.

Prevention and Treatment. Effective prevention and treatment of bovine nasal granuloma have not been developed. Since the means of transmission have not been determined with certainty, logical preventive measures have not evolved, and because of the low herd incidence, public demand for preventive programs has been slight. The topographic and/or systemic treatment with iodine and iodides was ineffective in Louisiana. Affected feedlot cattle should be slaughtered for recovery of investment as soon as the disease is diagnosed.

References

Ainsworth, G. C. and Austwick, P. K. C.: Fungal Diseases of Animals. Commonwealth Agricultural Bureaux, Farnham Royal. Bucks, England. (1959): 44–45.

Bridges, C. H.: Maduromycosis of Bovine Nasal Mucosa (Nasal Granuloma of Cattle). Cornell Vet., *50* (1960): 468–484.

Creech, G. T. and Miller, F. W.: Nasal Granuloma in Cattle. Vet. Med., *28* (1933): 279–284.

Davis, C. L. and Shorten, H. L.: Granulomatous Swellings in a Bovine. JAVMA, *89* (1936): 91–96.

Dikmans, G.: Nasal Granuloma in Cattle in Louisiana. North Am. Vet., *15* (Sept. 1934): 20–24.

Hore, D. E.: Nasal Granuloma in Victorian Dairy Cattle. Aust. Vet. J., *42* (1966): 273–278.

Krishnaumurti, A. V.: Rhinosporidiosis in Cattle. Transactions Far East. Assoc. Trop. Med., *3* (1927): 658–666.

Roberts, E. D., McDaniel, H. A. and Carbrey, E. A.: Maduromycosis of the Bovine Nasal Mucosa. JAVMA, *142* (1963): 42–47.

Robinson, V. B.: Nasal Granuloma—A Report of Two Cases in Cattle. AJVR, *12* (1951): 85–89.

6

Diseases caused by protozoa

Coccidiosis

(HEMORRHAGIC DIARRHEA)

Bovine coccidiosis, an acute contagious disease of young cattle, is characterized by mucoid and hemorrhagic diarrhea and usually is caused by *Eimeria zurnii* and *E. bovis*. Since coccidiosis causes animal losses through diminution of body weight, inefficient utilization of feed, mortality and expensive treatment, it is a disease of high economic importance. Careful estimations have suggested an annual monetary loss of somewhat over $15 million.

Review of Literature. While most adult cattle have been shown to be carriers of small numbers of coccidia (Levine, 1961), many investigations have disclosed that the disease develops in animals as old as 2 years of age (Boughton, 1945; Davis and Bowman, 1951). Even though coccidiosis, as a general disease, has been observed in many species of animals, the causative protozoa are host specific (Levine, 1961). The disease in cattle has been identified in the major cattle producing countries of the world (Christensen, 1941; Hasche and Todd, 1959; Marchenko, 1937; Supperer, 1952) with the highest incidence during autumn and winter seasons (Fitzgerald, 1962; Marquardt, 1960; Marsh, 1938).

While detailed investigations of protozoan parasites have shown that cattle contain 10 species of coccidia, only *E. bovis* and *E. zurnii* were highly pathogenic (Boughton, 1945; Davis and Bowman, 1951; 1957; Christensen, 1941; Hammond *et al.*, 1946).

In surveys *E. zurnii* and *E. bovis* were found in significant numbers in cattle (Boughton, 1942; Hasche and Todd, 1959; Marchenko, 1937; Supperer, 1952) as is indicated in Table 11. The resistance of nonsporulated oocysts to physical and chemical agents was studied using subsequent sporulation as the criterion of survival (Marquardt, Senger and Seghetti, 1960). On this basis, oocysts were highly susceptible to solutions of mercuric chloride, phenol and formaldehyde, and to direct sunlight. Following exposure to a relative humidity of 25% for 10 days, only few oocysts survived. Low temperatures significantly delayed the time of sporulation. On the other hand, oocysts were highly resistant to solutions of barium chloride, calcium chloride, cobalt chloride and cadmium chloride. They were uninhibited by a solution of copper sulfate.

Studies of the endogenous phases of the life history revealed that *E. zurnii* forms schizonts, as well as sporonts, throughout the ileum and the large intestine, while *E. bovis* develops schizonts in the ileum and the large intestine (Davis and Bowman, 1951; 1957) and *E. bovis* develops schizonts in the ileum and sporonts in the large intestine. The schizonts of *E. bovis* were visible grossly and measured approximately 0.351 x 0.299 mm (Boughton, 1942). These large schizonts were considered of diagnostic importance in *E. bovis* infection. Three to 5 weeks following heavy inoculation with *E. bovis*, experimental cattle disclosed a diminution of total plasma protein and of serum albumin, while the serum alpha globulin increased (Fitzgerald, 1962b). Cattle recovered from clinical coccidiosis have long been known to resist re-infection. When sporulated oocysts were inoculated intraperitoneally into susceptible cattle, clinical coccidiosis developed with characteristic signs and with discharge of numerous oocysts. Following recovery of these animals, they were resistant to re-infection. The intraperitoneal inoculation of 1 million unsporulated oocysts, the intramuscular inoculation of 1 million oocysts, and the intramuscular inoculation of 1 million unsporulated oocysts each failed to produce immunity (Fitzgerald, 1962a). Four lots of cattle were inoculated orally with 0, 10,000, 50,000 and 100,000 sporulated oocysts respectively. Following recovery from the disease animals of the lots receiving 50,000 and 100,000 sporulated oocysts were resistant to a challenge inoculation with 50,000 sporulated oocysts. The immunity was demonstrable for 2 to 3 months and in one group for 7 months. No immunity or resistance could be demonstrated in animals transfused with 500 ml of plasma and leukocytes from immune cattle (Senger *et al.*, 1959). Immunized and susceptible cattle were challenged by an inoculation of each animal with 800,000 to 5,000,000 sporulated oocysts. Subsequently the animals were necropsied. The numbers of schizonts were not significantly different in the two groups, while the numbers of oocysts in the immunized animals were significantly lower than in the susceptible cattle. These data suggested that the immune reaction inhibited the stages of sporogony (Hammond, Heckman *et al.*, 1958).

The efficacy of chemotherapy has been studied in both field outbreaks and in experimentally induced coccidiosis. The various sulfonamides, nicarbazine and nitrofurazone were compared for coccidiostasis and coccidiocidity as single treatments and as combinations of treatments (Gasparini *et al.*, 1958; Hammond *et al.*, 1960; 1958; 1956). Sulfamethazine, sulfamerazine, sulfaguanadine and sulfaquinoxaline were efficacious when administered at the rate of 1 gr per pound of body weight per day for 2 days and when followed by one-half the dosage for 2 additional days. Terramycin administered intramuscularly at the rate of $\frac{1}{2}$ gram daily, accompanied by sulfathiazole orally at the rate of 1 gr per pound of body weight per day gave satisfactory results (Barrows, 1957). Some experimentation, however, failed to credit popularly used compounds with any efficacy. Critical evaluation of sulfaguanadine, sulfamethazine, glycarbylamide, nitrafurazone, framycetin sulfate and zoalene was made using untreated lots for comparisons. The criterion of efficacy was the suppression of oocyst discharge in the feces. The treated animals were not significantly different from untreated cattle in oocyst production (Peardon, Bilkovich and Todd, 1963). More recently the efficacy of Amprolium was investigated. When administered to infected calves at the daily rate of 50 mg per kg of body weight for 4 consecutive days, the oocyst count rapidly decreased and the clinical condition improved. Doses of the compound several times the level used were not toxic (Horak, Raymond and Louw, 1969).

Occurrence. Coccidiosis occurs in cattle ranging in age from 1 week to 2 years but more commonly in 6-month-old animals assembled in a crowed feedlot. All breeds and both sexes are equally susceptible. In addition *E. zurnii* has been reported in deer and elk. Since most species of coccidia are highly host

TABLE 11 *Incidence of E. zurnii and E. bovis*

	Boughton (U. S.)	Hasche, Todd (Wisconsin)	Supperer (Austria)	Marchenko (USSR)
Sample size	2,492	355	130	137
E. zurnii %	42.2	25.6	11	20
E. bovis %	40.7	41.1	66	54

specific, coccidiosis is not intercommunicable between species of domestic animals. World-wide in distribution, the disease occurs more commonly in feedlot cattle during fall and winter after moistening of pens and bedding from rain, snow, or flooding followed by moderate or warm temperatures. The incidence of two pathogenic species, *E. zurnii* and *E. bovis,* is shown in Table 11.

Etiology and Pathogenesis. Cattle contain 10 species of coccidia: *E. bovis, E. zurnii, E. alabamesis, E. auburnensis, E. bukidnonensis, E. canadensis, E. cylindrica, E. ellipsoidalis, E. braziliensis* and *E. subspherica.* Two of the species, *E. bovis* and *E. zurnii,* are highly pathogenic. In clinical coccidiosis several species of coccidia are usually present, although one species may dominate. *E. bovis* and *E. zurnii* can be differentiated by morphology of the oocysts as indicated in Table 12.

In general oocysts are highly resistant to adverse factors of the external environment. The sporulation of oocysts is not inhibited by 0.1 M solution of barium chloride, calcium chloride, cobalt chloride, cadmium chloride, calcium chloride, 1 M solution of copper sulfate and 0.01 M solution of phenol. In contrast, however, sporulation does not occur in 10^{-6} M solution of mercuric chloride, in 0.05 M solution of phenol or in 0.025 M solution of formaldehyde. Exposure of oocysts to direct sunlight for 8 hours at 30° C completely inhibits sporulation. A relative humidity of 25% or less for 10 days prevents most sporulation and temperatures of 12° C and lower decelerate the rate of sporulation.

The merozoites of *E. bovis* can be grown through at least one generation in embryonic bovine tracheal epithelial cell cultures. These parasites are pathogenic for bovine intestine.

The life history consists of exogenous and endogenous phases. The exogenous phase begins with the discharge of oocysts in feces to the exterior. The oocysts sporulate and become infective in 24 to 48 hours. In the process the single cell in the oocyst discards a polar body and becomes haploid in chromosomal formula. Division of the cell forms 4 sporoblasts, each of which, through maturation, forms a sporocyst. Each of the latter contain 2 sporozoites from division of the cell within the sporoblast. At this stage of development the oocyst is infective.

The endogenous phase of the life cycle begins with ingestion of the sporulated oocyst with feed and water. In the lumen

TABLE 12 *Comparison of E. zurnii and E. bovis*

Species	Distribution	Hosts	Oocysts: Mean Dimensions Microns	Oocysts: Shape
E. zurnii	world-wide	cattle, water buffalo, deer, elk	17.8 × 15.6	spherical to ellipsoidal; no microphyle; colorless
E. bovis	world-wide	cattle, water buffalo	27.7 × 20.3	ovoid, blunted; brown-yellow

of the small intestine, excystation releases the sporozoites which penetrate the mucosa. The sporozoites of *E. zurnii* enter the epithelial cells and occupy a position between the nucleus and the distal end of the cell, while sporozoites of *E. bovis* penetrate endothelial cells of the lacteals of villi in the ileum. In the cytoplasm of these cells, the sporozoites become spherical and increase in size to form schizonts which subdivide to form numerous first generation merozoites. Schizonts of *E. zurnii* form 24 to 36 merozoites in the first of several generations, while the large schizont of *E. bovis* forms one generation of approximately 120,000 merozoites. At the end of the process of schizogony some merzoites penetrate new eipthelial cells and differentiate into female macrogametocytes which enlarge and mature. Other merzoites penetrate epithelial cells and form male microgametocytes which, on maturation, form many biflagellated microgametes. Following release from the cell the microgametes fertilize the macrogametes to form zygotes which have the diploid chromosomal formula.

The zygote contains granules of mucoprotein which form a firm wall at the periphery of the cell. The round to oval flattened cell, surrounded by the wall of mucoprotein, is the oocyst which is released into the lumen of the intestine where it mixes with feces.

Information pertinent to the endogenous phase of *E. zurnii* and *E. bovis* are given in Table 13.

Many epithelial cells of the mucosa are destroyed as a result of penetration by and growth of sporozoites and merozoites. Capillaries of denuded lamina propria hemorrhage into tissue and into the intestinal lumen. The hemorrhage causes anemia, hypoproteinemia and loss of electrolytes. Bacteria of the intestinal lumen may penetrate the injured mucosa and establish secondary infection. Occasionally the intestinal wall becomes perforated. Frequently, secondary pneumonia develops. The loss of blood constituents, intestinal injury, and secondary infection commonly cause fatality. Animals which survive are immune for at least several months. The injuries from severe coccidiosis may permanently impare the capacity of recovered cattle for efficient use of feed and for economic gains in body weight.

Clinical Signs and Postmortem Lesions. Following an incubation period of approximately 2 weeks, the clinical signs are initiated with diarrhea. In early stages the fluid feces are mixed with mucus and small amounts of blood. Later, the feces contain large amounts of blood. The fluid feces and blood either red or black often soil the tail and perianal skin and help to identify sick and oocyte shedding animals. Affected animals strain and defecate frequently. Straining often causes prolapse of the rectum. Dehydration and anemia develop to a degree which is proportionate to the severity of diarrhea and to the amount of blood in the feces. Anorexia, weakness and loss of body

TABLE 13 *Comparison of endogenous phase of E. zurnii and E. bovis*

	Anatomical Location		*Days After Inoculation to First Appearance of*			
Species	*Schizonts*	*Sporonts*	*Macrogametes*	*Microgametes*	*Oocysts*	*Days of Continuous Heavy Shed of Oocysts*
E. zurnii	ileum, large intestine	ileum, large intestine	12	15	12	8
E. bovis	ileum	large intestine	17	17	16–21	5–7

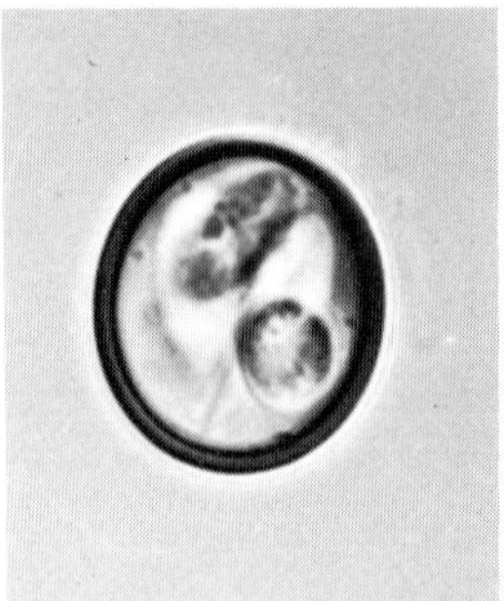

FIG. 6-1. *Eimeria zurnii oocyst.* × 1,000.

weight develop rapidly. Frequently the body temperature is elevated slightly. Anemia and pneumonia cause acceleration of respiration. Some animals develop convulsions from toxemia and anemia and some peritonitis from intestinal perforation. The clinical course varies from 4 to 14 days. Death may occur as early as the fourth day and is often due to hemorrhage, dehydration, and intercurrent pneumonia. Clinically recovered animals often fail to make normal rates of gain in body weight during the fattening period.

At necropsy the tissues are dehydrated, body weight is diminished, and the posterior skin is soiled with fluid hemorrhagic feces. The primary organic changes are in the ileum, cecum, colon and rectum. The degree of injury varies considerably. In severe and fatal cases, hemorrhage has occurred into the lumen of the alimentary tract. The bloody feces may be fluid and bright red from recent hemorrhage, or tarry and brown from dehydration and less recent hemorrhage. The affected mucous membrane is swollen, hyperemic, and occasionally edematous. The epithelial surface is eroded and pitted and may be perforated. Irregular hemorrhages give a variegated color. A diptheritic membrane of fibrin, blood clot, mucus and necrotic tissue sometimes is formed on the surface. Petechial hemorrhages may occur in the subserosa of the intestine and other organs. Lymph nodes, regional to the infection, are swollen. In animals heavily infected with *E. bovis*, white foci, 0.2 to 0.3 mm in diameter, are discernible along the infected mucosa of the ileum. Fatal cases frequently show bilateral bronchopneumonia.

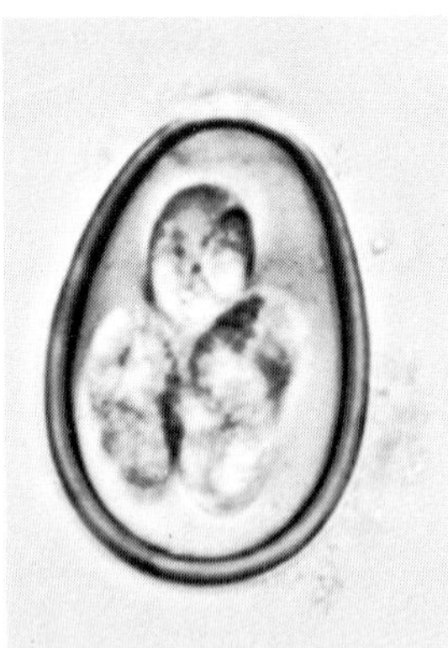

FIG. 6-2. *E. bovis oocyst.* × 1,000.

When viewed microscopically, fecal smears, except in early stages of the disease, may contain oocysts, merozoites and sporozoites. Smears of mucosal scrapings and sections of mucosa disclose schizonts, microgametes, macrogametes, oocysts, merozoites and sporozoites; depending on the stage of the disease, some or all of the parasitic forms are discernible. Many epithelial cells are destroyed and extravasated blood cells are commonly in the mucosa. Leukocytosis, due largely to bacterial invasion, may have occurred.

Diagnosis. Coccidiosis is diagnosed from the clinical signs and from laboratory findings. Important signs are the mucoid and hemorrhagic diarrhea in young cattle assembled in crowded, unsanitary conditions. In the laboratory the microscopic examination of fecal smears frequently discloses oocysts. In some cases the oocysts should be concentrated through sugar flotation or other methods. In early stages of coccidiosis, oocysts may be absent from the feces; in these cases the diagnosis may be confirmed through microscopic study of smears of scrapings and sections from the mucosa of the ileum, cecum and colon, or from subsequent fecal examinations. In scrapings and sections, schizonts, and sexual forms of the parasite can be identified.

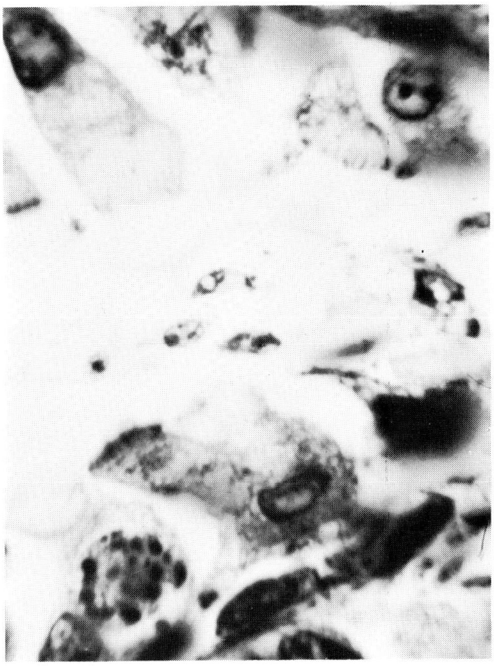

FIG. 6-3. *Sporozoites in intestinal lumen approaching epithelial cells. Haidenhain Stain.* × 1,100.

The differential diagnosis requires consideration of salmonellosis and urolithiasis. In salmonellosis the feces are more fluid, especially during early stages. Oocysts are not present in significant numbers in the feces, and schizonts, as well as gametocytes, are not present in scrapings or sections of the affected mucosa. *Salmonella typhimurium* or other species can frequently be isolated. Urolithiasis, a metabolic disease, results in occlusion of the male urethra, urine retention, and finally rupture of the urinary tract. Affected steers strain and may excrete blood in the feces. Rectal palpation reveals the distended and later ruptured bladder.

Prevention and Treatment. Bovine coccidiosis can be prevented or reduced in severity by avoiding excessive crowding and by maintaining good sanitation within the pens. Dispersal of young cattle in field, pasture, or large pens avoids exposure to heavy concentrations of sporulated oocysts. The drinking water and feed should be protected against contamination with feces. Susceptible cattle should never be fed directly on the ground where feces and urine directly contaminate the feed. Excessive moisture should be drained and moist manure and mud should be removed from the pen and replaced with ample dry bedding. Infected animals should be isolated to avoid exposure of susceptible cattle to excessive numbers of sporulated oocysts.

Treatment should begin early and not later than the thirteenth day following exposure to the infection. Individual animals may be medicated orally with sulfamethazine, or sulfaquinoxaline at the rate of 1 grain per pound of body weight per day for 3 days, followed by one-half the dosage for an additional 3 days. Animals which have suffered severe hemorrhage should receive blood transfusion to restore erythrocytes, plasma proteins, electrolytes and iron compounds.

Animals straining excessively and passing

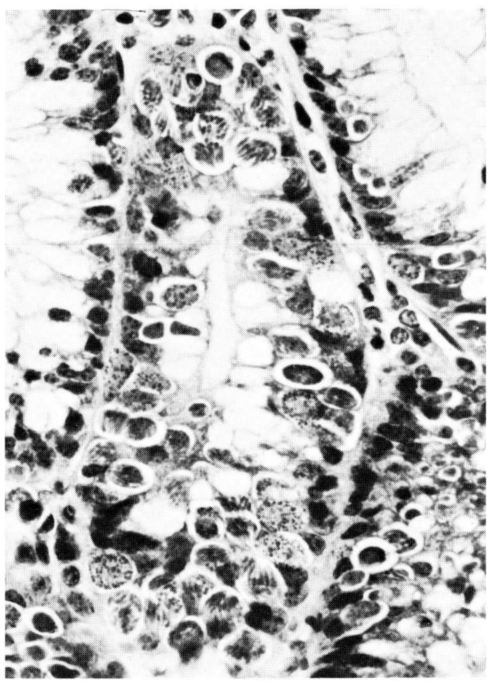

FIG. 6-4. *Merozoites of E. zurnii in intestinal epithelial cells. HE Stain.* × 359.

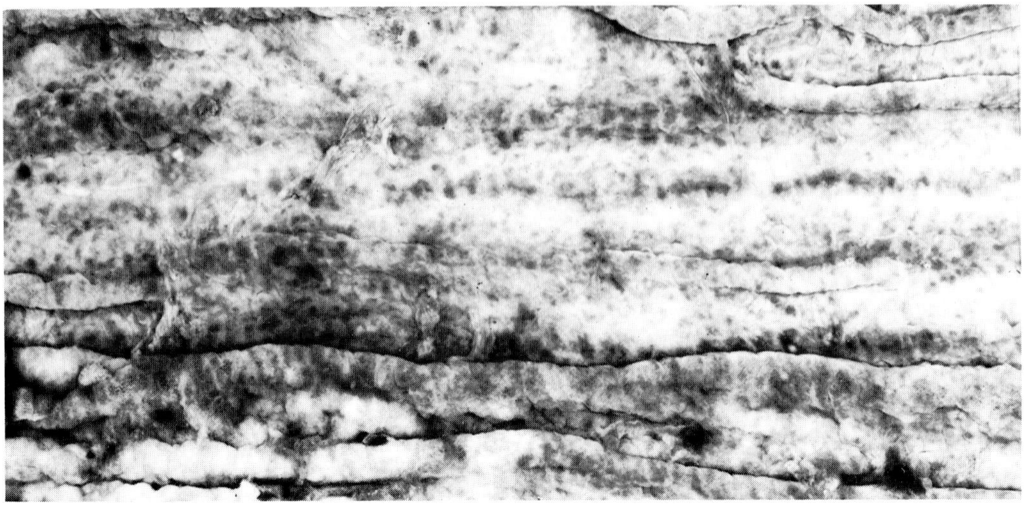

FIG. 6-5. *Colonic mucosa of a bovine infected with E. zurnii.* × 1.6.

large amounts of blood should receive a long acting epidural local anesthetic to relieve the tenesmus. Hemorrhage and irritation may be partially controlled with one of the three following enema mixtures:

No. 1—RX
- ½ gal. luke warm water
- 2 oz. sulfaquinoxaline solution
- 1 tablespoon potassium permangamate

No. 2—RX
- ½ gal. luke warm water
- 2–3 oz. tincture of iodine
- 1 oz. furacin soluble powder

No. 3—RX
- 1 quart of mineral oil
- 2–3 oz. of powdered tannic acid.

The enema solution should be administered with a Koroseal tube which is inserted gradually for a distance of 3 feet as the solution is pumped into the rectum. Care should be exercised to avoid perforation of the intestinal wall with the tube, or rupture with excessive solution pressure. At least 1 quart of the solution should remain in the rectum from 3 to 5 minutes.

When large numbers of cattle are affected the entire pen of animals should be treated through medication of the water or feed. Sulfonamides can be placed in the drinking water at the rate of 1 pound of drug per 100 gallons of water for 2 to 3 days followed by one-half the dose for 2 to 3 more days. Electrolites and arsenical compounds can be added to the drinking water for 7 to 10 days. Quaternary ammonium compounds, such as Dynafac which is prepared in pellet form, can be added to the feed at the rate of ½ to 1 once per animal daily for 5 to 7 days.

Following development of the disease, the diet should be modified to a high level of protein and low level of carbohydrates. Corn silage and 50% of the alfalfa should be removed and substituted with grass hay, straw, or stack-burnt alfalfa. The grain should consist of ⅔ oats and ½ bran for 3 to 7 days.

The entire herd can be treated by placing in the drinking water one of the sulfonamides at the rate of 1 pound per 100 gallons of water for 2 to 3 days, followed by one-half the dose for 2 to 3 more days.

References

Barrows, E. D.: Treatment of Coccidiosis in Beef Cattle. Vet. Med., *52* (1957): 164–166.

Boughton, D. C.: An Overlooked Macroscopic Intestinal Lesion of Value in Diagnosing Bovine Coccidiosis. North Am. Vet., *23* (1942): 173–175.

———: Bovine Coccidiosis: From Carrier to Clinical Case. North Am. Vet., *26* (1945): 147–153.

Christensen, J. F.: The Oocysts of Coccidia from Domestic Cattle in Alabama (U.S.A.) With Descriptions of Two New Species. J. Parasit., *27* (1941): 203–220.

Davis, L. R. and Bowman, G. W.: Coccidiosis in Cattle. Proceedings 55th annual meeting United States Lvst. Sanitary Assoc. (1951): 39–50.

———: The Endogenous Development of *Eimeria zurnii*, a Pathogenic Coccidium of Cattle. AJVR, *18* (1957): 569–574.

Fitzgerald, P. R.: Coccidia in Hereford Calves on Summer and Winter Ranges and in Feedlots in Utah. J. Parasit., *48* (1962): 347–351.

———: The Results of Intraperitoneal or Intramuscular Injections of Sporulated or Unsporulated Oocysts of *Eimeria bovis* in Calves. J. Protozoology, *9* (1962a): supplement pp. 21–22.

———: Deviations in Serum Proteins Associated with *Eimeria bovis* Infections in Calves. J. Parasit., *48* (1962b): supplement pp. 38–39.

Gasparini, G. Roncalli, R. and Ruffini, G. F.: Comparative Trials With Ammonium Sulphate, Sulfonamides, and Antibiotics in Natural Bovine Coccidiosis. Vet. Rec., *70* (1958): 787–789.

Hammond, D. M., Bowman, G. W., Davis, L. R. and Simms, B. T.: The Endogenous Phase of the Life Cycle of *Eimeria bovis*. J. Parasit., *32* (1946): 409–427.

Hammond, D. M., Fayer, R. and Miner, M. L.: Further Studies on *In Vitro* Development of *Eimeria bovis* and Attempts to Obtain Second Generation Schizonts. J. Protozoology, *16* (1969): 298–302.

Hammond, D. M., Heckman, R. A., Miner, M. L., Senger, C. M. and Fitzgerald, P. R.: The Effect of the Immune Reaction in Calves on the Number of Schizonts of *Eimeria bovis*. J. Protozoology, *5* (1958): supplement p. 8.

Hasche, M. R. and Todd, A. C.: Prevalence of Bovine Coccidia in Wisconsin. JAVMA, *134* (1959): 449–451.

Horak, I. G., Raymond, S. M. and Louw, J. P.: Use of Amprolium in the Treatment of Coccidiosis in Domestic Ruminants. J. So. Afr. Vet. Med. Assoc., *40* (1969): 293–299.

Levine, N. D.: *Protozoan Parasites of Domestic Animals and Man*. Burgess Publishing Co., Minneapolis, (1961).

Losses in Agriculture. Agricultural Research Service, USDA. Agricultural Handbook No. 291. (1965): 79.

Marchenko, G. F.: Collection of Publication. Governmental Veterinary Institute of Leningrad 1937, pp. 155–159.

Marquardt, W. C.: Oocyst Production in Subclinical Infections with Coccidia in Cattle. J. Parasit., *40* (1960): supplement p. 46.

Marquardt, W. C., Senger, C. M. and Seghetti, L.: The Effects of Physical and Chemical Agents on the Oocyst of *Eimeria zurnii*. (Protozoa, Coccidia). J. Protozoology, *7* (1960): 186–189.

Marsh, H.: Healthy Cattle as Carriers of Coccidia. JAVMA, *92* (1938): 184–194.

Peardon, D. L., Bilkovich, F. R. and Todd, A. C.: Trials of Candidate Bovine Coccidiostats. AJVR, *23* (1963): 743–748.

Senger, C. M., Hammond, D. M., Thorne, J. L., Johnson, A. E. and Wells, G. M.: Resistance of Calves to Reinfection With *Eimeria bovis*. J. Protozoology, *6* (1959): 51–58.

Supperer, R. Aster: Zool. Ztscher., Wien, *3* (1952): 591–601.

7

Diseases caused by metazoan parasites

Gastrointestinal Parasitism

(HELMINTHOSIS)

An acute or chronic and clinical or subclinical disease of cattle and other domestic animals, gastrointestinal parastism is characterized by gastroenteritis, unthriftiness and anemia. The disease is caused by several species of helminths. Often insidious in its variable degrees of infection, gastrointestinal parasitism results in either barely perceptible discomforts in some herds or severe and fatal illnesses in others. Animal losses come from anemia, anorexia, injury to the gastrointestinal tract, reduced efficiency of feed utilization, reduced growth rate, limited mortality and occasionally from diminished utility of heavily infested pastures. The total annual economic loss to the United States livestock industry has been estimated at $100 million (Losses in Agriculture, 1965), but because many widespread losses are imperceptible and unmeasured, the total probably far exceeds the estimates.

In cattle, gastrointestinal parasitism is ubiquitous, since few and probably no cattle escape parasitism. Infective larvae, along with contaminated feed, are ingested whenever forage becomes a part of the diet. In the United States (1961, 1962) surveys indicated the presence of several species of roundworms in most cattle on pasture (Becklund, 1962; Zimmerman and Hubbard, 1961). In some herds the degree of infection was low and of little clinical significance, while in others severe gastroenteritis with deaths occurred (Dickmans, 1939). Even though the disease was more severe in young animals, some adult cows on pasture suffered prolonged injury and mortality (Bailey and Herlich, 1953).

The effects of diet on parasitism have been noted under pasture husbandry and feedlot conditions. Observations of infected pasture utilization of three levels—overgrazing, moderate grazing, and undergrazing—indicated that, in general, the heavier use levels gave greater opportunity for larval parasite ingestion and produced higher incidence and more severe parasitism (Ciordia *et al.*, 1962). In a series of experiments, one lot of cattle was maintained on a feedlot diet of second cutting fescue hay and other lots on alfalfa hay. When the animals were adjusted to their respective diets, each was inoculated with the same number of infective gastrointestinal larvae. At termination of the experiment the cattle maintained on the diet of fescue hay contained 16% more worms than did the cattle maintained on alfalfa (Goldberg, 1959). In other experiments, different lots of cattle were fattened on infested pastures. The diets of some animals were supplemented with corn, and feeding continued from 2 to 4 months. At the time of slaughter, animals fed the corn supplement contained fewer gastrointestinal parasites (Vegors, Sell, Baird and Stewart, 1955). With dissimilar results, feedlot cattle divided into equal lots were fattened on diets of high and low levels of total digestible nutrients, and during the fattening period each animal was fed large numbers of infective gastrointestinal larvae. At the time of slaughter, the animals fattened on the lower feed level contained 10% more parasites than did the cattle fattened on the higher feed level. By comparison the adverse effect of the parasitism was shown when the uninfested control cattle gained 14.4 pounds more in body weight per 100 pounds of total digestible nutrients consumed than the infected cattle (Goldberg, 1962).

While the full significance of gastrointestinal nematode infection has not been determined for feedlot cattle, some evaluative research has been conducted. In one experiment the effects of subclinical parasitism from a mixture of *Ostertagia ostertagi* and *Cooperia* spp. on performance was studied. Thirty-nine genetically related and similar Angus steers were arranged into three equal lots and managed as follows: lot 1 infected and non-treated, lot 2 infected and treated, and lot 3 not infected. Animals of lots 1 and 2 were each given 3,000 infective larvae per kg body weight. Animals of lot 2 were treated with Thiabendazole 15 days after exposure. All cattle were fattened on a diet of alfalfa, corn silage, flaked corn, dried beet pulp and protein supplement. After 22 days of fattening, fecal egg counts had declined 80% in lot 1 and 99% in lot 2. During the fattening period of 189 days the uninfected cattle of lot 3 gained in body weight 0.1 kg (0.22 lb) per animal daily more than the other cattle. The adverse effect of parasitism appeared to be due to anorexia of the infected cattle (Ames, Rubin and Matsushima, 1969). In another investigation, 6 feedlot tests, involving 1899 treated cattle and 1840 control animals, were conducted. At the beginning of the tests egg counts per gram of feces varied from 50 to 100 and the principal cattle were treated with Thiabendazole. Throughout the experiment the average daily rate of gain in body weight did not significantly differ, but the treated cattle required 0.44 pound less feed per pound of gain in body weight and cost $0.80 less per 100 pounds of gain in body weight than did untreated animals (Flack, Frank, Easterbrook and Brown, 1967).

Cattle grazing parasite infested pastures continuously ingest infective larvae and universally suffer more severe parasitism than cattle fed in feedlots. Under pasture conditions, viable eggs are continuously excreted and infective larvae are repeatedly ingested; consequently, the degree of parasitism tends to augment and host injury to increase until clinical disease is established and recognizable.

In contrast, feedlot cattle usually are infected mildly. Because animals for fattening are chosen on the basis of their apparent or expected ability to make rapid and economic gains in body weight, this selection tends to exclude from the feedlot animals chronically sick or unthrifty for any cause, including heavy parasitism. Despite selection, most animals, however, contain some gastrointestinal parasites when admitted to the feedlot. At the fattening enterprise, all feed is not only harvested usually without larval contamination, but is presented to the animals in equipment which tends to exclude fecal and parasite contamination; as a consequence of precautions, feedlot cattle do not ingest infective larvae and the worm load present on entrance into the feedlot tends to diminish. The highly nutritious diet probably enables the host to more successfully combat the parasites and the degree of parasitism diminishes continuously throughout the period of fattening.

Etiology. Most species of gastrointestinal roundworms are classified in three families: *Trichostrongylidae*, *Ancylostomatidae* and *Strongylidae*, of the order *Strongyloidea*. Order characteristics include: a male copulatory bursa which consists of two lateral and one dorsal-rayed lobes, two equal spicules, and usually a gubernaculum and a well-developed buccal capsule. The life cycles are direct and contain both free-living and parasitic stages. While cattle are commonly infected with many species of parasites, one type may predominate within a single animal or a single herd. The important roundworms of the abomasum, small intestine, and large intestine are listed and compared in Table 14.

1. *Trichostrongylus axei*. Widespread geographically, this abomasal roundworm commonly affects cattle as a component of a mixed infection and, less commonly, as the predominating species. While all breeds and sexes are susceptible, young animals are more commonly and severely infected. Even

TABLE 14 ***Important species of gastrointestinal helminths***

Anatomical Location	Names: Scientific	Names: Common	Dimensions: Adults mm	Dimensions: Eggs Microns	Dimensions: Spicules mm
Abomasum	*Trichostrongylus axei*	small stomach worm	F 3–8 M 3–6	112–63	R 0.085–0.095 L 0.11–0.15
	Ostertagia ostertagi	medium stomach worm; brown stomach worm; brown hairworm	F 8.3–9.2 M 6.5–7.5	80–85 × 40–45	0.22–0.23
	Haemonchus contortus	stomach worm; wire worm; twisted stomach worm	F 18–30 M 10–20	70–85 × 41–48	0.46–0.50
Small intestine	*Cooperia punctata*	small intestinal worm; cooperids	F 5.7–7.5 M 4.7–5.9	65–72 × 30	0.12–0.15
	C. pectinata	small intestinal worm; cooperids	F 7.5–9.0 M 7.0	70–80 × 36	0.24–0.28
	C. oncophora	small intestinal worm; cooperids	F 6–8 M 5.5–9.0	84 ± 4.7 × 42 ± 2.5	0.24–0.3
	Nematodirus spathiger	thread-necked strongyle	F 15–23 M 10–15	150–230 × 80–110	0.7–1.21
	Bunostomum phlebotomum	hookworm	F 24–28 M 10–18	106 × 46	3.5–4.0
Large intestine	*Oesophagostomum radiatum*	nodular worm	F 16–22 M 14–17	70–76 × 36–40	0.7–0.8

though feedlot cattle may be lightly infected when entering the feedlots, the number of parasites diminishes both because of natural parasite mortality and because of little or no reinfection. In addition to cattle, the roundworm affects sheep, goats, horses and deer. Experimentally, rabbits are susceptible.

The life cycle is initiated with expulsion to the exterior of the ellipsoidal eggs. Under conditions of moderate humidity and warm temperatures, eggs hatch in 3 to 4 days and the larvae molt twice before developing the infective or third stage. In environmental conditions of the eastern United States the larvae endure 122 days or more. Following ingestion of infective larvae, the parasites enter the mucous membrane of the abomasum, molt the fourth time and reach maturity in approximately 3 weeks. The rate of parasite survival depends partially on the host diet. The addition of alfalfa to a diet of grass increased parasite survival in experimental cases involving rabbits. The invasion of the abomasal mucous membrane by large numbers of infective larvae results in severe gastritis, hemorrhage and reduced capacity for digestion. While in calves, a heavy infection provokes circulating complement-fixing antibodies, serology has not been used for diagnosing the disease.

Clinical signs vary according to the degree of infection. Mild parasitism results in unthriftiness, retarded growth rate and depression. Heavily infected cattle show persisting diarrhea, weakness, roughened haircoat, fluctuating body temperature, edema of the intermandibular tissues and an actual loss in body weight. Analysis of the blood reveals hypoproteinemia with an increase in gamma globulin. While the hemoglobin level and erythrocyte counts may diminish from normal, anemia is usually not prominent. Some animals may die from severe infection. At necropsy, the abomasum shows varying degrees of inflammation from focal to generalized. Careful examination of the mucosa and the abomasal contents reveals the worms. Histopathologically, the infected areas of the abomasum are eroded and heavily infiltrated with lymphocytes and mononuclear macrophages.

2. *Ostertagia ostertagi.* When present in large numbers, this parasite is highly pathogenic to cattle. All sexes and breeds are susceptible. While damaging infection may be found in cattle 1 to 2 years of age, calves are highly susceptible and more commonly infected. Widely distributed throughout the United States and many other countries, *O. ostertagi* inhabits the abomasum, and because of its small size and brown color is inconspicuous and requires careful observation for detection.

After expulsion to the external environment, the eggs, in moderate temperature and humidity, hatch in 24 hours. During the second day and after molting, the second stage larvae, measuring 300 to 450 μ in length, develop. During the third day, the second molt occurs and forms third stage larvae which measure 800 to 900 μ in length. Throughout the free-living periods the larvae are subjected to adverse environmental factors of dryness, heat and cold. Eggs are killed in 1 to 2 days at 45° C but survive in shallow water 22 days at −6° C. First and second stages of the free-living larvae survive in shallow water at 5° C for 1 to 2 months. The third stage, or infective larvae, survive 271 days in shallow water just above freezing, but are killed in approximately 2 weeks at −6° C. Low humidity is highly lethal to eggs and also to first and second stage larvae. At humidities 50 to 80%, eggs and first and second stage larvae survive approximately 5 days, while third stage or infective larvae endure 15 days. At 95% humidity, infective larvae remain viable for approximately 50 days. While larvae survive throughout the summer on irrigated pasture, they are rapidly killed on non-irrigated pasture. The parasitic stages begin with ingestion of the third stage or infective larvae which pass into the abomasum, attack and parasitize the mucous membrane. The larvae penetrate the mucous membrane, molt twice and after a pre-patent period of 22 to 23 days, form adult egg-producing females. The sequence of events following ingestion of infective larvae has been studied by serial sacrifice of experimentally infected calves. Within 6 to 12 hours following ingestion of larvae, plaques of erythema 1 to 2 mm in diameter form in the abomasum. Towards the end of the first day the plaques are gray and raised approximately 2 mm and larvae can be identified within the plaque. While larvae remain within the mucous membrane 25 days, the plaques are discernible for as long as 46 days. Even though exposure of calves to 400,000 infective larvae does result in the development of severe parasitism, the enteritis does not reduce the rate of absorption of such amino acids as lysine and leucine.

Clinical signs vary with degree of infection. Light to moderate parasitism produces obscure clinical signs of anorexia, unthriftiness and retarded growth rates, while severe parasitism results in diarrhea, thirst, anemia, roughened hair coat and reduced body weight. Even though the mortality rate is very low, death may result from intercurrent pneumonia. At necropsy the inflamed abomasum reveals gray plaques 1 to 2 mm in diameter. Larvae may be discernible within the plaques and adult worms can be removed from the abomasum and counted. Occasionally the duodenum is swollen and edematous. Beyond the alimentary tract the carcass may show emaciation and edema, especially of the intermandibular space.

3. *Haemonchus contortus.* Although a major cause of economic loss in sheep, *H. contortus* seldom causes serious disease and mortality in cattle. With a wide geographic distribution and as a minor parasite, some unmeasured economic losses result from subclinical infections and from predisposition to other diseases. Infections are acquired during grazing seasons of spring, summer and fall. While all breeds and sexes are susceptible, young cattle are more seriously affected than are mature animals. Sheep are more commonly and seriously parasitized than cattle. Although ovine strains and bovine strains each affect both cattle and sheep, slight morphologic strain differences have been described. The life cycle begins with expulsion of viable eggs to the exterior. Under conditions of favorable humidity and temperature, hatching occurs within 24 hours. After two successive molts and within 4 to 5 days from the time of expulsion from the host the infective larvae are formed. Since the infective larvae retain the skins from the previous molting, they are more resistant to adverse environmental conditions than are the preinfective larvae. In the presence of adequate moisture they ascend forage vegetation and await ingestion by a suitable host. The free-living stages are highly susceptible to drying and abnormal temperatures. On grass plots only 1% of larvae survive 14 to 28 days in summer, 27 to 41 in winter, 42 to 56 in fall, and 56 to 70 in spring. Pastures heavily infested with larvae of common species of round worms have been used to determine the endurance of viable larvae. After 61 days, few, and after 256 days, no larvae of *H. contortus* were present (Goldberg and Rubin, 1956). After four winter applications of *H. contortus* larvae infested feces to experimental grass plots, no viable larvae were demonstrable the following spring (Shorb, 1943). The parasitic stages of the life cycles are initiated with ingestion of viable infective larvae along with forage. Passing into the fourth stomach, the larvae attach to the mucous membrane of the abomasum, feed on blood and grow to sexual maturity through the prepatent period of 14 to 29 days. The adults continue to inhabit the abomasum. Maximal egg production occurs within 6 to 10 weeks and is followed by a rapid decline. Some egg production has been known to continue over a period of 14 months. The feeding in the mucosa of the abomasum of large numbers of larvae and/or adults causes significant loss of blood not only to the parasites but through hemorrhage. In one experiment, the minimum daily requirement of 30 ml of host blood was necessary to sustain 5,000 adult female worms (Martin, Ross and Clunies, 1934). During the prepatency period of heavy experimental infections, the erythrocyte count of the experimental calves de-

clined from a normal of 7,000,000 to 2,150,000 cells per cu mm and from 12 grams of hemoglobin per 100 ml of blood to as low as 2 grams per 100 ml of blood (Delaune and Mayhew, 1943). Some evidence of immunity development has been detected in calves during stages of adult parasitism and during prepatency periods of subsequent infection.

As with other forms of gastrointestinal parasitism, the clinical signs of hemonchosis vary directly with the degree of parasitism. Mild to moderate infections may result in some physical depression, diminished rates of growth and slight anemia. Heavy infections seldom if ever occur naturally. The adult *H. contortus* are conspicuous because of two characteristics: large size and variegation of color in the females. The latter characteristic is actually the white ovary spiraling around the red intestine. Commonly other species of gastrointestinal parasites accompany the *H. contortus*. At necropsy, the mucosa of the abomasum is swollen and hyperemic.

4. *Cooperia punctata, C. pectinata,* and *C. oncophora.* As a group, the three cooperids are major helminth pathogens of cattle. Inhabiting and damaging the small intestine, they cause economic loss by reducing rates of growth and, possibly, by predisposing to other diseases. While all breeds and sexes are susceptible, cattle under 2 years of age are more commonly affected than adult cattle. In the United States, cooperids are widely distributed, but *C. oncophora* is more common in all the northern states, *C. punctata* in the southeastern states, and *C. pectinata* in the southern states. The acute phase of cooperiosis, from the prepatent stage of infection, occurs during the grazing seasons of summer and autumn.

The life histories of *C. oncophora* and *C. punctata* have recently been studied in detail. Viable ova, mixed with feces, are expelled to the external environment. Following an incubation period of 16 to 20 hours, the eggs hatch. After hatching the first molt occurs 28 and 45 hours in *C. oncophora* and *C. punctata* and the second at 124 and 90 hours respectively. Infective third stage larvae reach a length of approximately 950 μ and 800 μ in *C. oncophora* and *C. punctata* respectively. The infective larvae ascend forage plants and are subjected to the adversities of temperature and humidity. In Texas, some larvae of *C. pectinata* survived a maximum of 138 days, but one-half of the total sample survived only 44 days (Bell, Galvin and Turk, 1960). In the eastern part of the United States, larvae of *C. punctata* survived in significant numbers 122 days but not 256 days, while larvae of *C. oncophora* endured 256 days (Goldberg and Rubin, 1956). The parasitic stages of cooperids are initiated with the ingestion of infective larvae. The latter pass through the stomachs and enter the small intestine where they invade the mucous membrane, feed on blood, molt and acquire sexual maturity after a prepatent period of 17 to 22 and 11 to 16 days for *C. oncophora* and *C. punctata* respectively. *C. punctata* has been cultured through all stages of its life cycle in artificial medium consisting of chick embryo extract, serum, sodium, caseinate, vitamins, hog liver extract, balanced salt solution, indicator and antibiotics (Zimmerman and Leland, 1969). Large numbers of larvae of adults result in severe enteritis and the loss of whole blood. The inoculation of 28,000 to 192,000 viable cooperid larvae and the resulting enteritis did not significantly alter the rate of absorption of isotope labeled lysine and leucine (Rubin and Cheney, 1962). Prepatent and patent periods of parasitism with *C. punctata* evoked immunity to the same parasite as was demonstrated by the inoculation. The experimental cattle, however, were fully susceptible to infective larvae of nodular worms (Mayhew, Miller and Torbet, 1969).

The clinical signs from cooperiosis vary according to degree of infection and resemble signs from other gastrointestinal infections. Slight to moderate infection may produce obscure anorexia and unthriftiness, while heavy parasitism results in fluctuating body temperature, diarrhea, anorexia, depressions, roughened hair coat, reduced body weight, reduced growth rate and edema. The disease causes a low rate of mortality unless complicated with intercurrent infections. At necropsy, acute enteritis may be detectable, especially in the anterior parts of the small intestine. The mucous membrane may show petechial hemorrhages and erosions. The cooperid worms can be washed from the intestine for identification. Other organs and tissues may be pale from anemia and edematous from hypoproteinemia.

5. *Nematodirus spathiger.* Having low pathogenicity, large numbers of the parasite are required to produce disease. While all breeds and sexes of cattle, and even sheep, support the parasite, calves apparently are more susceptible and also more apt to develop clinical signs. The parasite is widely distributed throughout the United States and other major cattle producing countries.

The life cycle is initiated with expulsion of the eggs to the external environment. Following hatching, the larvae are retained within the egg shell through two molts. The infective larvae escape from the shell, ascend grass, leaves and other forage, and are subjected to environmental hardships, especially desiccation. When dried at room temperature, 82% survived 2 months but none survived 5 months. When subjected to temperature 28° F, 99% survived 3 months and 25% survived 10 months (Goldberg and Rubin, 1956). Eaten with grass and other forage the third stage larvae begin parasitic stages. Passing through the stomachs, the larvae enter the small intestine, attach to the mucous membrane and grow to maturity. Since the parasite is of low pathogenicity, infected cattle seldom manifest clinical signs or postmortem lesions. The parasites may be found and identified at necropsy following death of the host usually from other causes. Reddish in color, the adults are attenuated and transversely striated anteriorly.

6. *Bunostomum phlebotomum.* Highly pathogenic parasites for cattle, hookworms exist throughout the United States, but especially in the southern states where the infection is known as hookworm disease and bunostomumosis. While all breeds and sexes of cattle are susceptible, young animals are more commonly and severely affected. Economic losses result from retarded growth rate, diminished body weight and mortality.

The free-living stages of the life cycle begin with expulsion of eggs to the exterior. Eggs and larvae live in the manure. Hatching occurs within 24 hours. Following two molts, the larvae reach the infective stage in 5 to 8 days and measure 400 to 650 μ in length. During the third stage they are highly sensitive to prolonged desiccation. Being positively thermotrophic, the larvae penetrate bovine skin from contact of infected manure by recumbent animals. Within 30 minutes the larvae enter the derma; within 60 minutes, the blood vessels; and in 10 days reach the lungs where molting takes place. The larvae ascend the trachea, enter the mouth or pharynx, and are swallowed. Some infective larvae, ingested with contaminated forage, may penetrate the wall of the alimentary tract, enter blood vessels and move to the lungs. In the small intestine each larva attaches to the mucous membrane with a strong buccal capsule. By means of two pairs of subventral lancets in the buccal capsule, the host tissue is lacerated. Blood is not only ingested by the parasites but bleeding is prolonged as a result of a parasite produced anticoagulant. The larvae continue to grow and after a prepatent period of 56 to 79 days reach sexual maturity. A single female worm may produce 600 eggs in 24 hours.

Clinical signs result from both moderate and heavy infections. Affected animals are unthrifty and lose body weight. Anemia with an erythrocyte count as low as 4 million cells per cu mm and a hemoglobin value of 4 gm % develops. Both edema, especially of the intermandibular tissue, and diarrhea, often with blood in the feces, develop within 4 to 5 weeks. A standard fecal examination reveals the parasite eggs. The mortality rate may be high unless the affected animals are properly treated. At necropsy, the small intestine is inflamed and hemorrhagic, and the adult hookworms are readily discernible. The connective tissue is edematous and fluid may accumulate in the body cavities. The blood is thin and membranes are pale.

7. *Oesophogostomum radiatum.* A parasite of medium pathogenicity, *O. radiatum* must be present in large numbers to produce clinical nodular worm disease in cattle. Although widely distributed in the United States, it is more common in the southern states where humidity and temperatures are high. While all breeds and sexes of cattle are susceptible, animals under 2 years of age are more commonly and severely affected.

With the discharge of eggs to the external environment, the free-living stages of the life cycle are initiated. Under moderate humidity and temperature, the eggs hatch after an incubation period of approximately 20 hours. The larvae grow, molt twice and reach the infective stage in 5 to 10 days. In the eastern United States larvae in experimental plots failed to remain infective for 61 days (Goldberg and Rubin, 1956). Parasitic stages start with the ingestion of infective larvae along with contaminated forage. The larvae pass through the stomachs and enter the small and large intestines. At any point along the alimentary tract posterior to the abomasum, but more commonly in the ileum, cecum and colon, the larvae penetrate the mucous membrane, remain for approximately 10 days before they emerge and attain sexual maturity. With a prepatent period of 37 to 41 days, the worms remain functional within the intestine for 11 to 14 months. When experimental calves were inoculated with large numbers of parasites, the larvae penetrated the wall of the intestine to variable degrees. While the submucosa was the more common point of penetration, some remained within the mucosa and some passed through the entire intestinal wall. Five days after inoculation a plaque 1 mm in diameter and dark in color from hemorrhage was formed at each point of larval penetration. In 10 days the plaques had grown to 2 mm in diameter and were white from leukocytosis. The persisting plaques are grossly detectable for 47 to 182 days.

Clinical signs of nodular disease vary with the degree of infection. Either moderate or heavy infections produce illness. The body temperature rises when the infective larvae penetrate the intestinal mucosa. Affected animals show depression and diarrhea which develop 4 to 23 days following inoculation and may persist 186 days. Anemia comes gradually, and within 5 weeks the erythrocyte numbers may descend to 50% of normal values. Infected experimental animals made one-seventh the body weight gains of uninfected control animals (Andrews and Maldonado, 1943). At the time of necropsy, inflammation is found along the ileum, cecum and colon. Gray nodules 2 to 5 mm in diameter and raised several millimeters above the surrounding surface, are found in variable numbers. During the patency periods, the adult worms attached to the mucosa can be discerned grossly and eggs microscopically in feces. The intestinal lesions are more severe in cattle receiving multiple larval inoculations. Rarely a larva penetrates the entire intestinal wall and produces peritonitis.

Diagnosis. The clinical diagnosis of gastrointestinal parasitism is inaccurate because of nonspecificity of clinical manifestations and because of unreliability of data obtained from fecal examinations. As an index to clinical parasitism egg numbers in fecal samples are highly unreliable because of variance in: (1) egg production within a parasite species, (2) egg production between strongyle species, (3) mixing and excreting eggs and feces, and (4) methodology of collecting, identifying, and enumerating the eggs. Among strongyle parasites, and only by highly skilled and specialized parasitologists, can most eggs be morphologically classified to species or even genera. The most reliable clinical diagnosis, however, is based on a combination of typical clinical signs and the demonstration of adequate numbers of parasite eggs in feces. Important clinical signs include anemia, diarrhea, unthriftiness, edema and diminished body weight.

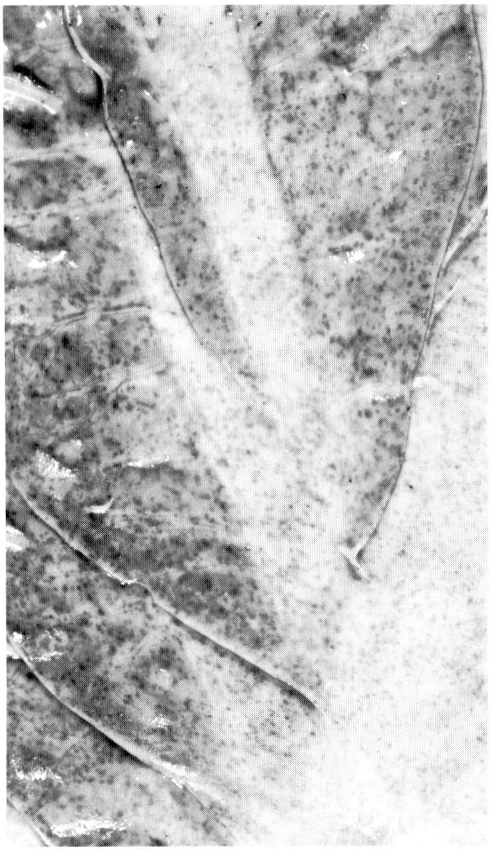

FIG. 7-1. *Multiple petechiae of the abomasum from invasion by strongyle larvae.* × 1.3.

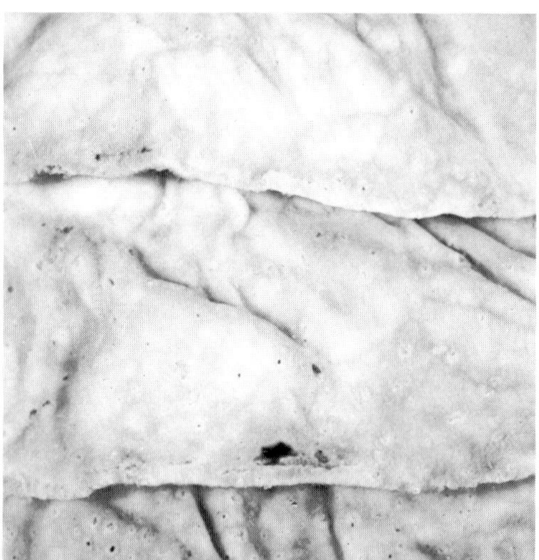

FIG. 7-2. *Advanced abomasal lesions from strongyle parasites.* × 1.0.

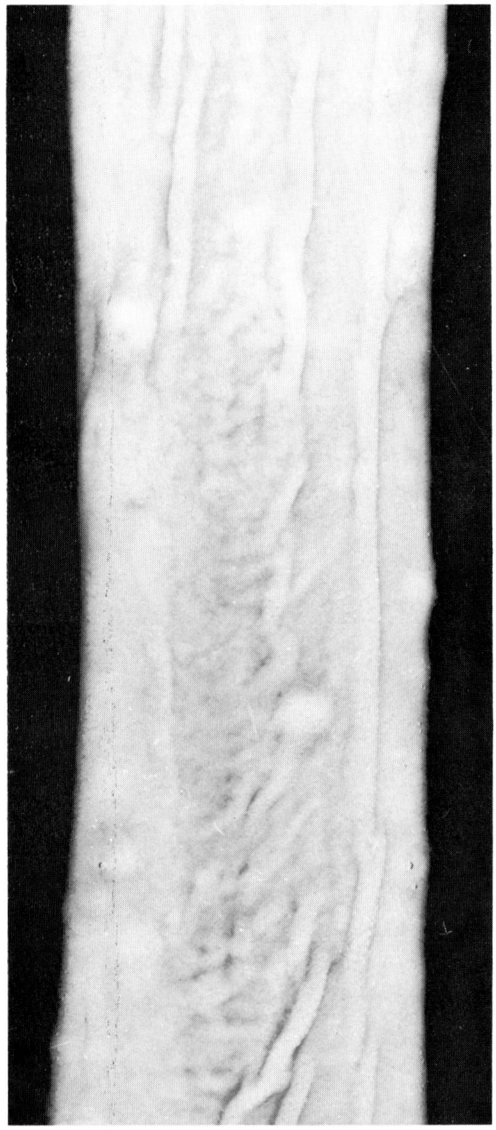

FIG. 7-3. *Nodules from Oesophagostomum radiatum in the mucosa of the small intestine.* × 1.3.

Very often clinical evidence can be supplemented with information derived from necropsy of one or more animals where the various segments of the alimentary system can be studied carefully. Adult and larval parasites frequently can be collected, identified, and enumerated. In addition, other general causes of disease can be evaluated and their interaction with parasitism assessed.

The differential diagnosis requires consideration of diseases of the alimentary system, including coccodiosis, shipping fever, Johne's disease, poisoning and founder. Coccidiosis, usually occurring in cattle under 1 year of age, results in diarrhea and hemorrhage into the feces. Several fecal examinations at different stages of disease development reveal the presence of large numbers of oocysts. At necropsy, smears from mucosal scrapings show different stages of schizogony and sporogony. Shipping fever, occurring usually within 10 days from the time of shipment into the feedlot or from the time of subjection to a stressful situation, is associated with diarrhea, fever, depression and infection of the respiratory system.

Johne's disease seldom if ever occurs in feedlots except in retired dairy cattle that have passed through the prolonged incubation period prior to admission to the feedlot. Characterized by recurring and persistent diarrhea, the disease results in loss of body weight and physical weakness. Biopsy of the rectal mucosa may reveal the causative bacterium. Chemical poisoning is extremely diverse and may be diagnosed on the basis of clinical history of exposure and chemical analysis of organs and contents of the alimentary tract. Founder, associated with consumption of excessive amounts of highly fermentable feeds, is characterized by depression and diarrhea.

Prevention and Treatment. Standard feedlot management practices provide little or no opportunity for reinfection of cattle with nematode larvae. The probability of oral inoculation is further reduced when the principles of sanitation are carefully applied. The feedlots should be drained to avoid the accumulation of stagnant water or moist mud in which parasite larvae may develop. Watering and feeding equipment should be elevated and fenced so as to avoid fecal contamination.

The prevention of gastrointestinal parasitism in pastured cattle prior to admission to the feedlot is a complex problem with many management aspects. Where parasite larval development is favored, pastures should be drained to avoid both stagnant water and mud. To reduce seeding of the pasture with parasite eggs and larvae parasitized cattle should be treated frequently. Plowing, rest from grazing periods exceeding the longevity of infective larvae and pasture crop rotation destroy most infective larvae. Heavily infected cattle should be treated for gastrointestinal parasitism prior to admission to a feedlot.

Successful treatment can be achieved with one of the following drugs: (1) thiabendazol at the rate of 4 to 5 gm per 100 pounds of body weight administered individually or in the feed for an entire lot of cattle; (2) phenothiazine at the rate of 20 gm per 100 pounds of body weight and a maximum of 60 gm per animal; or (3) Tramisol levamisole hydrochloride (Tetramisole), a broad-spectrum anthelmintic, administered individually at the daily rate of 8 mg per pound of body weight for several days. For most species of worms, thiabendazol is effective against both larvae and adults. Phenothiazine is more effective against adults than against larvae. Cooperids and *Nematodirus spathiger* possess considerable inherent resistance to either drug. The effectiveness of phenothiazine against the resistant parasites can be improved by increasing the maximal animal dose from 60 to 120 gm.

Since phenothiazine may result in photosensitization, treated cattle should be protected against intense sunshine by administration of the drug during the afternoon and by providing adequate shade. Severely parasitized cattle should be isolated from the herd, given adequate feed and water, and, if necessary, blood transfusions. The administration of medicaments as boluses should be with care to avoid pharyngeal perforation and drug deposition in the tissue.

References

Ames, E. R., Rubin, R. and Matsushima, J. K.: Effects of Gastrointestinal Nematode Parasites on Performance in Feedlot Cattle. J. An. Sc., *28* (1969): 698–704.

Andrews, J. S. and Maldonado, J. F.: Intestinal Pathology in Experimental Bovine Esophagostomiasis. AJVR, *3* (1942): 17–27.

———: Some Clinical Aspects of Experimental Esophagostomiasis in Cattle. AJVR, *4* (1943): 211–225.

Bailey, W. S. and Herlich, Harry: An Epizootic of Parasitic Gastritis in Mature Cattle. Auburn Vet., *9* (1953): 3–8.

Becklund, W. W.: Helminthiasis in Georgia Cattle—A Clinical and Economic Study. AJVR, *23* (1962): 510–515.

Bell, R. R., Galvin, T. J. and Turk, R. D.: Survival on Pasture of Infective Larvae of *Cooperia pectinata* and *Osteragia ostertagi.* AJVR, *21* (1960): 1101–1103.

Bremner, K. C.: A Study of Pathogenetic Factors in Experimental Bovine Oesophagostomosis. I. An Assessment of the Importance of Anorexia. Austral. Jour. Agri. Res., *12* (1961): 498–512.

Ciordia, H., Bizzell, M. E., Vegors, H. H., Baird, D. M., McCampbell, H. C. and Sell, O. E.: The Effect of Three Grazing Intensities of Winter Temporary Pasture on Internal Parasitism of Beef-Type Yearling Cattle. AJVR, *23* (1962): 15–20.

DeLaune, Elaine T. and Mayhew, R. L.: Studies on Bovine Gastrointestinal Parasites. VI. The Blood Picture in Stomach Worm (*Haemonchus contortus*) Infections. Trans. Amer. Micro. Soc., *62* (1943): 179–193.

Dickmans, G.: Parasitic Enteritis in Calves. Vet. Med., *34* (1939): 28–30.

Dikmans, G. and Kates, K. C.: Trichostrongylosis in Cattle. Proceed. Helminth. So. of Wash., *22* (1955): 42–46.

Dinaburg, A. G.: The Survival of the Infective Larvae of the Common Ruminant Stomach Worm, *Haemonchus contortus,* on Outdoor Grass Plots. AJVR, *5* (1944): 32–37.

Doran, David J.: The Course of Infection and Pathogenic Effect of *Trichostrongylus axei* in Calves. AJVR, *16* (1955): 401–409.

Flack, D. E., Frank, B. N., Easterbrook, H. L. and Brown, G. E.: Thiabendazole Treatment. VM/SAC, *62* (1967): 565–568.

Furman, Deane P.: Effects of Environment Upon the Free-Living Stages of *Ostertagia circumcinta* (Stadelmann) Trichostrongylidae: I. Laboratory Experiments. AJVR, *5* (1944): 79–86.

———: Effects of Environment Upon the Free-Living Stages of *Ostertagia circumcinta* (Stadelmann) Trichostrongylidae: II. Field Experiments. AJVR, *5* (1944a): 147–153.

Goldberg, A.: The Relationship of Diet to Gastrointestinal Helminth Parasitism in Cattle. AJVR, *20* (1959): 806–814.

———: Relation of Diet to Gastrointestinal Helminth Parasitism in Cattle. II. Comparison of Two Levels of Feed Intake. J. Parasitol., *48* (1962): No. 2, Sect. 2, p. 36.

Goldberg, A. and Rubin R.: Survival on Pasture of Larvae of Gastrointestinal Nematodes of Cattle. Proceed. Helminth. Soc. of Wash., *23* (1956): 65–68.

Herlich, H., Porter, D. A. and Knight, R. A.: A Study of *Haemonchus* in Cattle and Sheep. AJVR, *19* (1958): 866–872.

Isenstein, R. S.: The Life History of *Cooperia oncophora* (Railliet, 1898) Ransom 1907, a Nematode Parasite of Cattle. Jour. Parasit., *49* (1963): 235–240.

Leland, S. E., Drudge, J. H. and Wyant, Z. N.: Studies in *Trichostrongylus axei* (Cobbold, 1879). III. Blood and Plasmä Volume, Total Serum Protein, and Electrophoretic Serum Fractionation in Infected and Uninfected Calves. Exper. Parasit., *8* (1959): 383–412.

———: Studies on *Trichostrongylus axei* (Cobbold, 1879). VI. Total Serum Protein, Blood and Plasma Volume, and Electrophoretic Serum Fractionation in Infected and Uninfected Lambs. AJVR, *21* (1960): 458–463.

Losses in Agriculture. Agricultural Handbook No. 291 ARS. USDA(1965): 79.

Martin, C. J. and Ross, I. Clunies: A Minimal Computation of the Amount of Blood Removed Daily by *Haemonchus contortus.* Jour. Helminth, *12* (1934): 137–142.

Mayhew, R. L., Miller, G. C. and Torbert, B. J.: Studies on Bovine Gastrointestinal Parasites. XXI. Immunity to *Cooperia punctata* and *Oesophagostomum radiatum.* J. Parasit., *46* (1960): 859–866.

Mayhew, R. L., Torbert, B. J. and Miller, G. C.: Studies on Bovine Gastrointestinal Parasites. XX The Results of Feeding Small Amounts of Phenothiazine in Pure Infections of *Cooperia punctata.* AJVR, *20* (1959): 492–497.

Osborne, J. C., Batte, E. G. and Bell, R. R.: Pathology Following Single Infections of *Ostertagia ostertagi* in Calves. Cornell Vet., *50* (1960): 223–235.

Roberts, F. H. S.: Reactions of Calves to Infestation with the Stomach Worm, *Haemonchus placei* (Place, 1893) Ransom, 1911. Austral. Jour. Agri. Res., *8* (1957): 740–767.

Rose, J. H.: Some Observations on the Free-living Stages of *Ostertagia ostertagi,* a Stomach Worm of Cattle. Parasit., *51* (1961): 295–307.

Ross, J. G.: Experimental Infections of Calves With the Nematode Parasite *Ostertagia ostertagi.* Vet. Record, *75* (1963): 129–132.

Rubin, R. and Cheney, J. M.: Nematode Parasites of Ruminants. Annual Report, Western Regional Project W-35 (Colorado): 1962–1963.

Shorb, D. A.: Survival on Grass Plots of Eggs and Preinfective Larvae of the Common Sheep Stomach Worm, *Haemonchus contortus.* Jour. Parasit., *29* (1943): 284–289.

———: Survival on Grass Plots of Eggs and Larvae of the Stomach Worm, *Haemonchus contortus.* Jour. Agri. Res., *68* (1944): 317–324.

Sprent, J. F. A.: Some Observations on the Bionomics of *Bunostomum phlebotomum*, a Hookworm of Cattle. Parasit., *37* (1946): 202–210.

Stewart, D. F.: A Preliminary Note on a Complement Fixation Test to Detect Circulating Antibodies in Sheep Infested with *Haemonchus contortus* and *Trichostrongylus* spp. Austral. Vet. Jour., *24* (1948): 112–113.

Stewart, T. B.: The Life History of *Cooperia punctata*, a Nematode Parasitic in Cattle. Jour. Parasit., *40* (1954): 321–327.

Threlkeld, W. L.: The Life History of *Ostertagia ostertagi*. Virginia Agri. Exp. Sta. Tech. Bull. 100 (1946).

Turner, J. H.: Viability Studies on Eggs and Infective Larvae of *Nematodirus spathiger* (Railliet, 1896), A Trichostrongylid Nematode of Ruminants. Jour. Parasit. *39* (1953): 589–598.

Vegors, H. H., Sell, O. E., Baird, D. M. and Stewart, T. B.: Internal Parasitism of Beef Yearlings as Affected by Type of Pasture, Supplemental Corn Feeding, and Age of Calf. Jour. Anim. Sci., *14* (1955): 256–267.

Whitlock, J. H., Taylor, A. and Conway, D.: A Note on Exsheathing Mechanisms of Third-stage Larvae of *Haemonchus contortus*. Cornell Vet., *49* (1959): 421–422.

Zimmerman, W. J. and Hubbard, E. D.: Gastrointestinal Parasitism in Iowa Cattle. JAVMA, *139* (1961): 555–559.

Paramphistomiasis

(RUMEN FLUKE INFESTATION)

A mild parasitic disease of cattle and other ruminants, paramphistomiasis is characterized in early stages by duodenitis and, later by the presence of flukes in the rumen. The disease is caused by *Paramphistomum cervi*. In America this disease is of little importance to the cattle industry. Occasionally, however, it may cause, through illness and even mortality of affected cattle, economic loss to an individual enterprise. At slaughter rumen flukes are encountered during cleaning of the rumen for tripe.

Review of Literature. Since its early discovery, the rumen fluke has been studied morphologically, biologically, geographically and pathologically (Ershov, 1956; Boray, 1959; Olsen, 1962). The pathogenicity of the fluke for cattle was demonstrated to be dependent on numbers of flukes and anatomical location within the host. Large numbers of parasites in the duodenum caused diarrhea, loss of body weight and even mortality, but the presence of a moderate number of flukes in the rumen and/or reticulum caused little noticeable injury. Parasiticides have not been effective against the adult fluke (Boray, 1959; Ershov, 1956). In one study, however, of a small number of parasitized animals, treatment with hexachloroethane-bentonite reduced fluke egg production for at least a year (Olsen, 1949).

In South Africa the immunization of cattle with attenuated flukes was studied. Each animal received 40,000 x-irradiated metacercariae. Thirty days later each animal received 250,000 normal metacercariae and showed almost complete resistance to them (Horak, 1965).

Occurrence. In addition to cattle, the rumen fluke has been observed in sheep, goats, deer, moose, elk, and antelope. Geographically, it has wide distribution. In North America the fluke has been found in many areas, although the degree of infestation is usually not heavy.

Etiology and Pathogenesis. *Paramphistomum cervi* apparently is the more common species of rumen fluke in cattle. Other closely related species, however, have been described. The adults, light pink in color, are cone-shaped, rounded on cross section and measure 5 to 12 mm in length. With a large subterminal posterior sucker, they are slightly convex dorsally and concave ventrally.

Eggs are excreted in host feces. Under proper conditions of humidity, they hatch in approximately 1 month. The miracidia utilize, as intermediate hosts, species of snails of the genera *Fossaria, Pseudosuccinea, Bulimus, Galba, Planorbis,* and probably others. The development of cercaria within the snail requires approximately 1 month. The emerging cercariae encyst on grass or other edible vegetation. Metacercariae may endure in the encysted state for several months. When eaten by a bovine, the metacercariae pass along the alimentary system into the duodenum where excystation occurs. The young flukes penetrate the mucosa of the duodenum and migrate in the tissue anteriorally. Ultimately, they move through the lumen of the abomasum into the rumen and reticulum where, among papillae, they attach to the mucosa, the definitive position.

Pathogenicity varies directly with numbers. By severely injuring the mucous membrane in the duodenum, the larval flukes, in large numbers, interfere with digestion and provoke diarrhea. These pathologic changes may result in unthriftiness, emaciation, and even death of the host. Within the rumen, little or no injury is inflicted.

Clinical Signs and Postmortem Lesions. During the stage of heavy invasion of the duodenum, affected animals exhibit persisting diarrhea with some blood in the feces. Progressive loss of body weight and physical weakness may be followed by death. Infestation of the rumen is asymptomatic.

At necropsy of fatal cases, the inflamed and hemorrhagic duodenum may contain large numbers of flukes per square inch. In fattened cattle, the presence of flukes in the rumen is usually an incidental finding when the rumen is cleaned in the preparation of tripe. Located in the anterior dorsal sac among papillae of similar size and shape, the parasites are inconspicuous. They are conspicuous, however, if located among papillae of different color.

Diagnosis. Clinical paramphistomiasis may be suspected in endemic areas from signs of anorexia, diarrhea, and weakness. Confirmation of the diagnosis can be obtained through identification of the non-pigmented eggs in host feces. In some cases the eggs may be confused with similar eggs of fascioloid liver flukes. At necropsy, or at the time of slaughter of fat cattle, the adult flukes are found attached to the mucosa of the rumen and/or reticulum. In clinical cases larval flukes may be identified in the duodenum.

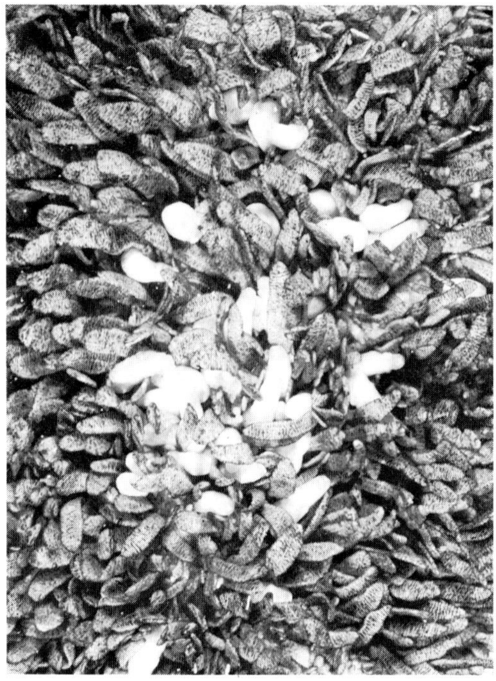

FIG. 7-4. *Adult rumen flukes among papillae of anterior dorsal sac.* × 14.

Prevention and Treatment. Prevention of paramphistomiasis can be achieved by not grazing infested pastures, by destroying snail intermediate hosts through chemical treatment, by draining pastures and by treating carrier cattle to prevent the excretion of viable fluke eggs. Infested cattle may be treated with hexachloroethane-bentonite in suspension, or with tetrachlorodifluroethane administered orally or by stomach tube at a dosage rate of 200 mg per kg of body weight.

References

Boray, J. C.: Studies on Intestinal Amphistomosis in Cattle. Austral. Vet. J., 35 (1959): 282–287.

Ershov, V. S.: *Parasitology and parasitic Diseases of Livestock.* Moscow. State Publishing House for Agricultural Literature. (1956): 54–57.

Horak, I. G.: Studies on Paramphistomiasis VII. The

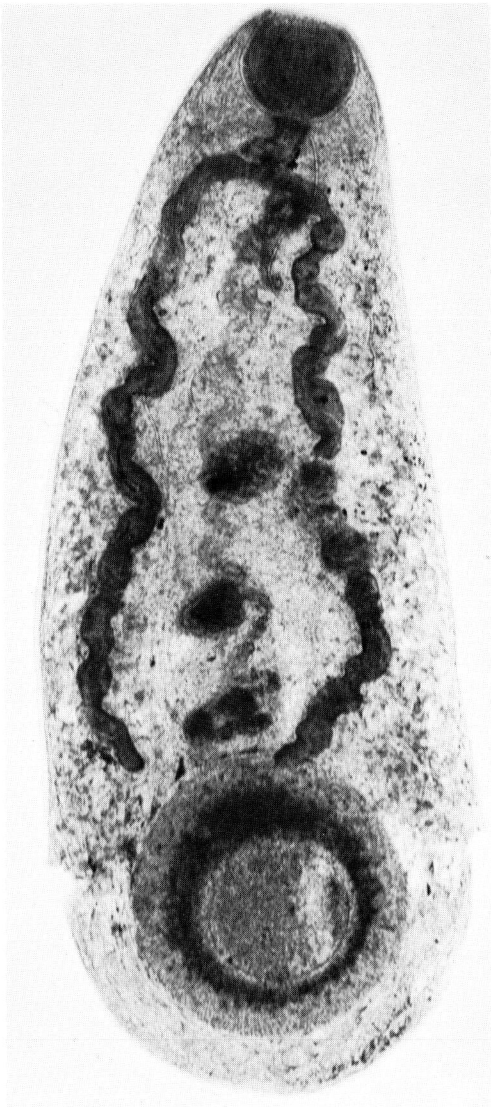

FIG. 7-5. *Adult Paramphistomum cervi.* × 14.

Immunization of Sheep, Goats, and Cattle. Preliminary Report. J. South Africa Vet. Med. Assoc., *36* (1965): 361.

La Page, G.: *Monnig's Veterinary Helminthology and Entomology.* 5th Ed. The Williams & Co. Baltimore. (1962): 83–84.

Olsen, O. W.: Action of Hexachloroethane-Bentonite Suspension on the Rumen Fluke, *Paramphistomum.* Vet. Med., *44* (1949): 108–109.

———: *Animal Parasites: Their Biology and Life Cycles.* Burgess Publishing Co., Minneapolis. (1962): 128–130.

Liver Fluke Disease

(FASCIOLIASIS; DISTOMIASIS; LIVER ROT)

Characterized by chronic cholangitis and persistent unthriftiness, liver fluke disease of cattle is caused by one or more of several species of trematodes. While this insidious disease produces extensive and unmeasured economic losses through reduced efficiency in feed utilization, assessed losses result from condemnation of infected livers at slaughter and from low mortality rates. In the United States from 1967 through 1969 approximately 3% of slaughtered cattle were infected with liver flukes. This parasitism resulted in annual condemnation at slaughter of one million livers valued at approximately $5 millions. Conservative extimates during this period indicated that condemnation of livers and diminished cattle efficiency constituted a substantial annual loss to the industry.

Review of Literature. Incredibly complex but biologically successful, the life history of the common liver fluke, *Fasciola hepatica,* slowly unraveled. The recognition of sexually mature flukes in 1737 was the first observation in an illucidating series of discoveries. By 1883 when Leukhart of Germany and Thomas of England independently described the completed life cycle, the contributions from a dozen naturalists had been made and 145 years had passed (Taylor, 1964). Subsequently, three additional species of bovine liver flukes, *F. gigantica, Fascioloides magna* and *Dicrocoelium dendriticum,* each with similar life cycles, were identified (Price, 1953).

Investigations of *F. hepatica* included many phases of the cycle. Numerous intermediate freshwater snail hosts have been identified (Taylor, 1964) and their bionomics studied (Olsen, 1944; Roberts, 1950; Boray, 1961).

Cercariae, obtained from infected snails

and fed to susceptible guinea pigs, migrated through the small intestine and, by washing, were recovered and identified from the peritoneal cavity 3 days following oral administration. Penetration of the intestinal wall produced small insignificant hemorrhages in the guinea pigs. In sheep used as experimental animals, the cercariae, after moving to the liver, penetrated Glissen's capsule, migrated through the liver parenchyma, produced grossly observable bore tracts, and were found in the bile ducts as their definitive positions (Shaw, 1932). The adult flukes, *F. hepatica*, produced a chronic mineralizing cholangitis which progressed to extensive parenchymal atrophy. Infected cattle showed a persisting eosinophilia (Morrill and Shaw, 1942).

Fascioloides magna, primarily a parasite of the livers of deer, was found also in cattle and sheep as definitive hosts. In cattle and deer slaughtered at Minnesota, approximately 30 and 21% respectively, contained this parasite (Griffiths, 1962; Olsen and Fenstermacher, 1943). After development in the molluscan intermediate host, the metacercariae were ingested along with vegetation. Cercariae penetrated the intestine, moved to and within the liver. In the definitive hosts, the adult flukes became localized by a wall of fibrous connective tissue around a parenchymal cavity containing one or more flukes, eggs, fluid, and dark pigment. In deer and sheep, the cavity communicated with bile ducts, while in cattle the cavity was completely isolated. Consequently, in deer and sheep, but not in cattle, eggs were emitted through the bile ducts to the exterior (Price, 1953).

The lancet fluke, *Dicrocoelium dendriticum*, has been studied in New York State. In that area studies indicated that the miracidia penetrate and parasitize the snail, *Cionella lubrica* (Mapes, 1951). Clusters of cercariae, surrounded by mucus and known as slime balls, were emitted from the snail. The latter were ingested by ants, *Formica fusca*, in which abdominal cysts formed. Slime balls fed to susceptible sheep failed to form adult flukes, but the ingestion of ants containing the cysts, or the ingestion of cysts dissected from ants, did produce adult lancet flukes (Krull and Mapes, 1952; Krull, Mapes, and Cortland, 1953). These findings demonstrated a three-host life cycle. In sheep, ingested metacercariae migrating through the common hepatic duct attained in 1 to 6 hours, following oral administration, the definitive position in the bile ducts (Krull, 1958).

Lesions, as observed in cattle, varied with species of fluke. *F. hepatica* produced chronic progressive cholangitis with fibroplasia, mineralization and ultimately atrophied parenchyma (Morrill and Shaw, 1942).

In diagnosing fascioliasis the technique for separating fecal plant material from fluke eggs was improved by the use of washing screens of progressively finer mesh. The eggs, concentrated by centrifugation, were stained for easy identification and rapid counting (Swanson and Hopper, 1950).

In parasitized cattle the rates of gain in weight were studied in the feedlot and on pasture. In the feedlot, with small numbers of cattle, nonparasitized animals failed to show a superior rate of gain in weight over animals infected with moderate numbers of *F. hepatica* (Morrill and Shaw, 1942; Shaw, 1944), and, on pasture, 20 cows and calves from which *F. hepatica* had been expelled by treatment failed to show superior gains over similar but parasitized cattle (Olsen, 1947). The feasibility of preventing liver fluke infection by interrupting the life cycle of the parasite has been demonstrated. The toxicity in low dilution of copper sulfate for snails was discovered (Chandler, 1920), and in infected pastures the use of this compound has been effective in preventing parasitism (Swanson, Batte and Denniss, 1952).

While the therapeutic efficacy of many drugs has been investigated, relatively few have gained practical acceptance. The toxicity of hexachlorethane for adult flukes was demonstrated in Germany (Thienel, 1926). However, the drug tended to separate rapidly from an aqueous mixture. Later, a more stable aqueous suspension was obtained by using a mixture of bentonite powder in the following formula: Hexachlorethane, 500 gm; bentonite powder 50 gm; and water, 750 ml (Olsen, 1943). When hexachlorethane was used in this mixture at the rate of 10 gm per 100 pounds of body weight in young cattle, and 20 gm per 100 pounds of body weight in adult cattle, the fecal egg counts per animal were reduced from 26 to 5 per animal (Olsen, 1947). The efficacy of carbon tetrachloride was also investigated. In cattle, an oral efficacious dose was toxic, and the effective parenteral dose produced considerable irritation and necrosis at the point of inoculation for as long as 6 months (Kendall and Parfitt, 1962; Kuttler, Matthews and Marble, 1963; Taylor, 1962). While carbon tetrachloride and hexachlorethane were effective against adult flukes, both were ineffective against immature forms (Kendall and Parfitt, 1962; Olsen, 1943; 1947).

Occurrence. Cattle of all ages, breeds and sexes are susceptible to the four species of liver flukes and immunity is not developed against subsequent exposures. While the disease is present in all seasons, new infections frequently develop during months of pasture grazing. The geographic distribution is indicated in Table 15.

Etiology and Pathogenesis. In cattle, liver fluke infection is caused by four species of trematodes: *Fasciola hepatica, Fasciola gigantica, Fascioloides magna* and *Dicrocoelium dendriticum.* Their dimensions, hosts and geographic distribution are indicated in Table 15. Because of its wide distribution and high pathogenicity for liver, *F. hepatica* causes greater total injury to cattle than any of the other species.

The complex life cycles of the different species of liver flukes have many similarities but also some differences. The life history of *F. hepatica* is typical. The hermaphroditic adult locates in the lumen of a bile duct. Discharged eggs mix with bile and eventually with the feces in which they are emitted to

TABLE 15 *Statistics on four species of liver flukes*

Species	Dimensions: Adults mm.	Dimensions: Eggs μ	Hosts: Intermediate	Hosts: Definitive	Geographic Distribution
Fasciola hepatica (common liver fluke)	20 to 30 × 8 to 15	130 to 150 × 63 to 90	*Lymnea* *Stagnicola* *Galba* *Pseudosuccinnea* *Fossaria* *Bulimus*	cattle sheep goat rabbit elk deer	cosmopolitan (U. S.: West Coast, Rocky Mtns., Gulf Coast, Great Lakes)
F. gigantica (giant liver fluke)	25 to 75 × 5 to 12	156 to 197 × 90 to 104	*Lymnea* *Physopsis* *Fossaria*	cattle deer elk	Africa India Hawaii
Fascioloides magna (large American fluke)	50 to 75 × 25 to 30	109 to 168 × 75 to 96	*Fossaria* *Galba* *Pseudosuccinea* *Stagnicola* *Lymnea*	cattle sheep deer elk	Canada U. S.: (Great Lakes, Gulf Coast, West Coast, Rocky Mtns.) Europe
Dicrocoelium dendriticum (Lancet fluke)	6 to 10 × 1.5 to 2.5	36 to 45 × 20 to 30	1. *Cionella lubrica* 2. *Formica fusca*	cattle sheep goat horse woodchuck	cosmopolitan (America: N. Y., Canada)

the exterior. In stagnant shallow water at 26° C, hatching occurs in 14 to 18 days to form the miracidium. Ciliated and free swimming, the miracidium, living only 1 to 3 hours in water, actively seeks a suitable fresh water snail which it penetrates and parasitizes as an intermediate host. Proteolytic enzymes from the miracidium probably assist in the penetration. Soon after entrance into the snail tissues, the miracidium transforms into a sac-shaped sporocyst approximately 1 mm in length. Germinal cells within the sporocyst produce 5 to 8 rediae, each of which may grow to a length of 1 to 3 mm. Under favorable conditions, daughter rediae are produced. The next larval stage is the cercaria, which is emitted from the snail approximately 50 days after snail penetration. The cercaria, consisting of body and tail, swims freely in water and within a short time, after locating on blades of grass or other objects just below the water surface, discards the tail and secretes its own protective covering. In this larval stage the metacercaria remains viable and infective for 6 months. When ingested along with vegetation by cattle and liberated in the duodenum by excystation, the cercaria penetrates through the intestinal wall and moves through the abdominal cavity to the liver. By burrowing movements and enzymatic action, the cercaria migrates through the liver parenchyma and eventually locates in a bile duct and grows to maturity. Approximately 60 days are required from ingestion for the parasite to acquire its definitive anatomical location. In cattle, the adult parasite is thought to remain productive for 3

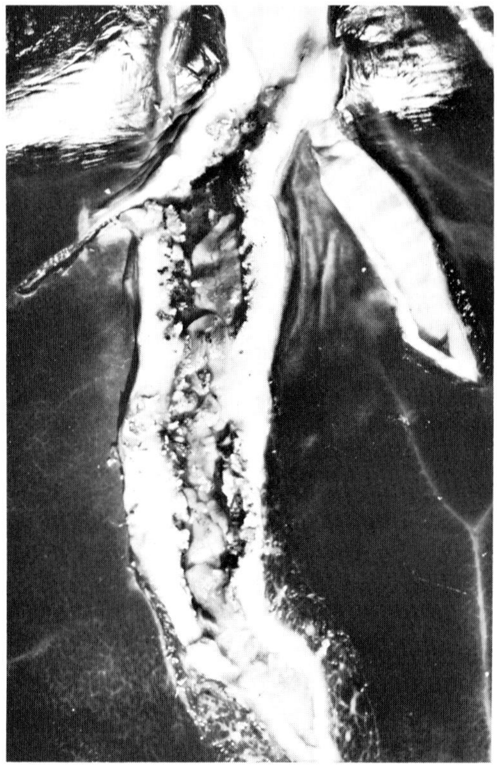

FIG. 7-6. *Fibrosis and mineralization of a bovine bile duct infected with Fasciola hepatica.* × 0.9.

TABLE 16 *Life cycle of Fasciola hepatica*

Stage	Duration
1. Adult in bile ducts	Several years
↓	
2. Eggs emitted in feces	14–18 days in water
↓	
3. Miracidium	1–3 hours in water
↓	
4. Sporocysts	35–50 days
↓	
5. Cercariae	
↓	
6. Metacercariae	6 months on vegetation
↓	60 days ingestion to bile ducts
7. Adult	

to 4 years. The cycle is summarized in Table 16.

At each stage of development the fluke encounters formidable hazards. Eggs may fail to hatch because of discharge onto dry land. Miracidia often fail to find a suitable snail which may die before sporocyst development is completed. Metacercariae may die before being consumed by a suitable host, or they may be ingested by an unsuitable host. Although many adversities decimate the fluke numbers, the large number of eggs produced compensates for subsequent losses.

While the life histories of the other liver flukes are similar to *F. hepatica,* some important differences occur. Cercariae of *Fascioloides magna* migrate through hepatic tissue of cattle, sheep and deer, and, by the formation of a confining capsule of fibrous connective tissue, the adults eventually become immobilized in a cavity. In cattle, the cavity has no luminal communication to a bile duct; consequently, cattle do not emit fluke eggs. In sheep and deer, however, the cavity containing the fluke does communicate with the bile duct and eggs are discharged to the surface. *Dicrocoelium dendriticum* is a three host trematode. Clusters of cercariae, known as slime balls, are emitted from the snail, *Cionella lubrica.* Slime balls are ingested by ants, *Formica fusca,* in which they form cysts in the abdominal cavity. Following ingestion of parasitized ants along with vegetation, the cercariae are released by excystation in the duodenum. Generally they migrate through the lumen of the hepatic duct into the numerous bile ducts, their definitive anatomical location.

Injury to the bovine host occurs at several stages of parasite development. Although petechial hemorrhages are observed, minimal injury is inflicted by passage of the immature stages of *F. hepatica* through the wall of the duodenum and the peritoneal cavity. In the liver, however, following penetration of the capsule, migration through parenchyma causes hemorrhage and necrosis. Massive simultaneous invasion of the liver by many flukes may result in hemorrhage and even rupture of the liver capsule. In the bile ducts, mature flukes feed on cells, secretions and blood. Loss of blood to the flukes, hemorrhage into the bile ducts and suppression of hemopoiesis by parasite metabolites cause

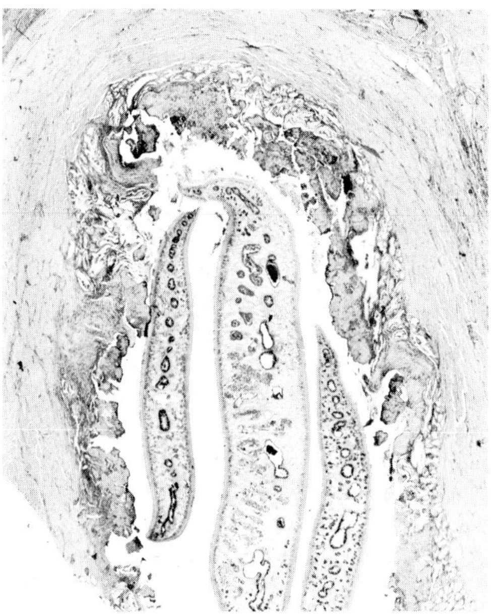

FIG. 7-7. *Bovine bile duct containing fibrosis and mineralization in the wall, and three cross sections of F. hepatica in the lumen. H&E stain.* × 6.6.

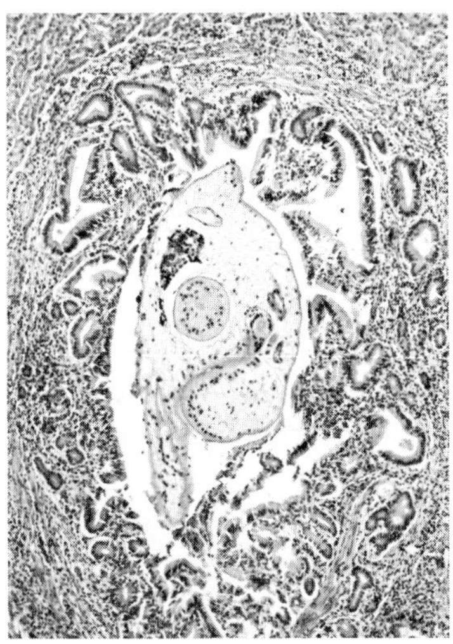

FIG. 7-8. *Bovine bile duct infected with Dicrocoelium dendriticum. H&E stain.* × 47.

anemia and hypoproteinemia in host cattle. As a result of constant irritation from the spiny fluke, the wall of the infested bile duct thickens from hyperplasia and fibrosis, and calcium phosphate precipitates in the lamina propria. The host tissue changes become progressively less favorable to the fluke, and after 3 to 4 years it dies. Following death and removal of all flukes the bile duct changes reverse and healing occurs in approximately 1 year.

Clinical Signs and Postmortem Lesions. In cattle, clinical signs vary with degree of infection and the nutritional level. A heavy infection with *F. hepatica* may be associated with roughened hair coats, constipation, unthriftiness, anemia and gradual but progressive weakness and emanciation with terminal prostration. In feedlot cattle, moderate degrees of infection frequently do not adversely affect health or rates of gain in body weight. Slight icterus may result from occlusion of a bile duct.

At necropsy, or slaughter, lesions are limited to the liver. The changes vary according to the amount of time and of infection. In acute stages of liver invasion, the organ is swollen and friable and may contain surface deposits of fibrin. Bore tracts may be discernible, and pressure on the fresh tissue may force burrowing flukes to the cut surface where they can be collected, cleaned and identified. In cases of moderate to heavy infection the liver is enlarged, rough, firm and fibrous. On the parietal surface the bile ducts are enlarged, firm and conspicuous. Incision of the ducts discloses variable amounts of mineralization and the leaf-shaped adult flukes in the lumen. The bile is often discolored and contains flakes of excrement. Dark pigment may discolor bile ducts and hepatic lymph nodes.

Histopathologically, early stages show bore tracts with or without burrowing flukes. The bore tract lumen contains blood and the walls consist of necrotic liver tissue. In chronic stages bore tracts contain fibrous connective tissue and large numbers of eosinophils, mononuclear macrophages and lymphocytes. Infected bile ducts contain adult flukes, and the bile duct walls are thickened from fibrosis, epithelial hyperplasia and leukocyte infiltration. The lamina propria is mineralized with calcium phosphate. Epithelial cells may be eroded and granules of mineral may be free in the lumen.

In cattle infected with *Fascioloides magna*, the livers have single or multiple parenchymal cysts which contain the parasites and dark fluid. Tissue surrounding the cavity often is pigmented. Histopathologically, the cavity containing flukes is surrounded by a wall of fibrous connective tissue. Large masses of fluke eggs often accumulate within the cyst and surrounding tissues.

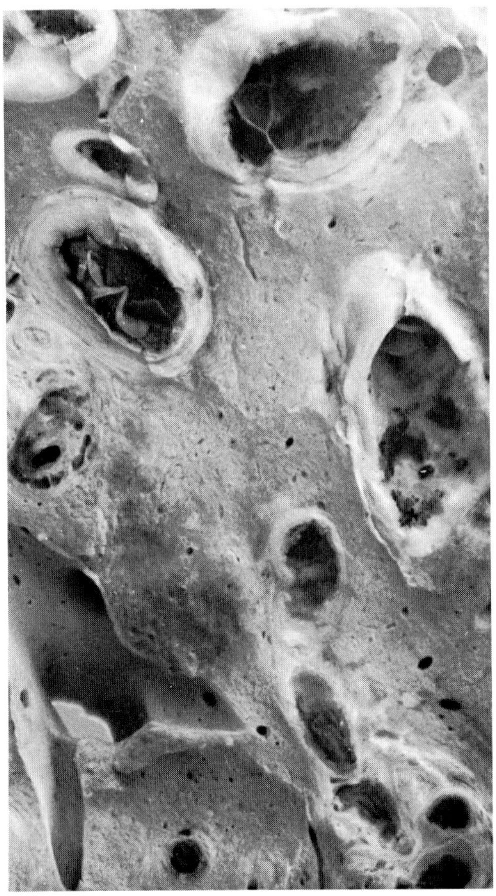

FIG. 7-9. *Fasciola hepatica. Carmine stain.* × 2.2.

In cattle infected with *Dicrocoelium dendriticum*, the bile ducts are distended. When the ducts are opened, large amounts of a mixture of mucus, exudate, cellular debris and parasites are evident. The walls of infected bile ducts are thickened and, histopathologically, they show extensive fibroplasia and hyperplasia of the epithelium forming papillary projections into the lumen and gland-like evaginations deep into the wall. In addition to flukes, the lumen contains many desquamated epithelial cells.

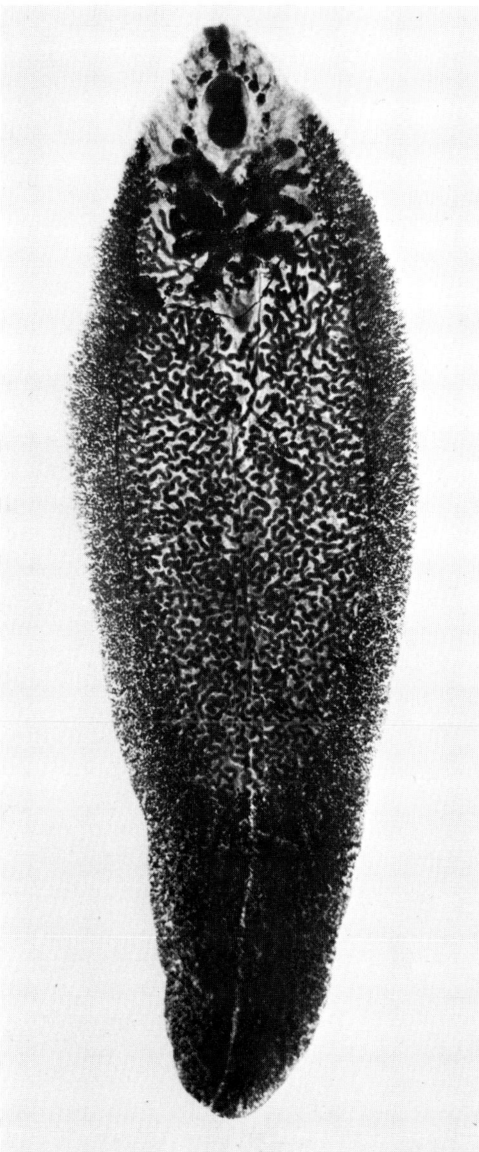

FIG. 7-10. *Fasciola gigantica in bile ducts of liver.* × 1.1.

At slaughter, cattle livers are examined carefully for fluke infection. Any amount of infection renders the organ unsuitable for human food. After cooking, livers with mild infections may be used for animal food.

Diagnosis. In endemic areas, liver fluke disease may be suspected in cattle showing typical clinical signs. The clinical diagnosis, excepting for infections with *Fascioloides magna*, can be confirmed through identifying specific fluke eggs in the feces. The thin shelled eggs of *F. hepatica* have a specific gravity only slightly greater than water and are distorted by solutions of high specific gravity. The following technique is satisfactory for concentrating fluke eggs from bovine feces:

1. Collect 300 to 500 grams of feces from the rectum.
2. Mix the sample thoroughly in a beaker.
3. Transfer 5 grams to a 250-ml flask and add 100 ml of tap water and shake thoroughly.
4. Wash the sample successively through three screens of 20, 40, and 60 appertures per linear inch into a 2000-ml beaker. Finally wash each screen into the finer screens with sufficient water to fill the beaker.
5. Allow the sample to settle for 2 hours.
6. Remove the supernatant fluid with a U-shaped siphon tube which extends to within $^3/_4$ inch from the bottom of the flask.
7. Transfer the sediment to a flask calibrated to 200 ml and agitate.
8. Transfer four 10-ml samples to each of 15-ml centrifuge tubes.
9. Centrifuge at 3000 r.p.m. for several seconds.
10. Remove the supernatant fluid with a filter pump.
11. Examine the sediment, stained or unstained, in a Petri dish with a dissection microscope. Fecal examination cannot be used for diagnosing infection in cattle from *Fascioloides magna.*

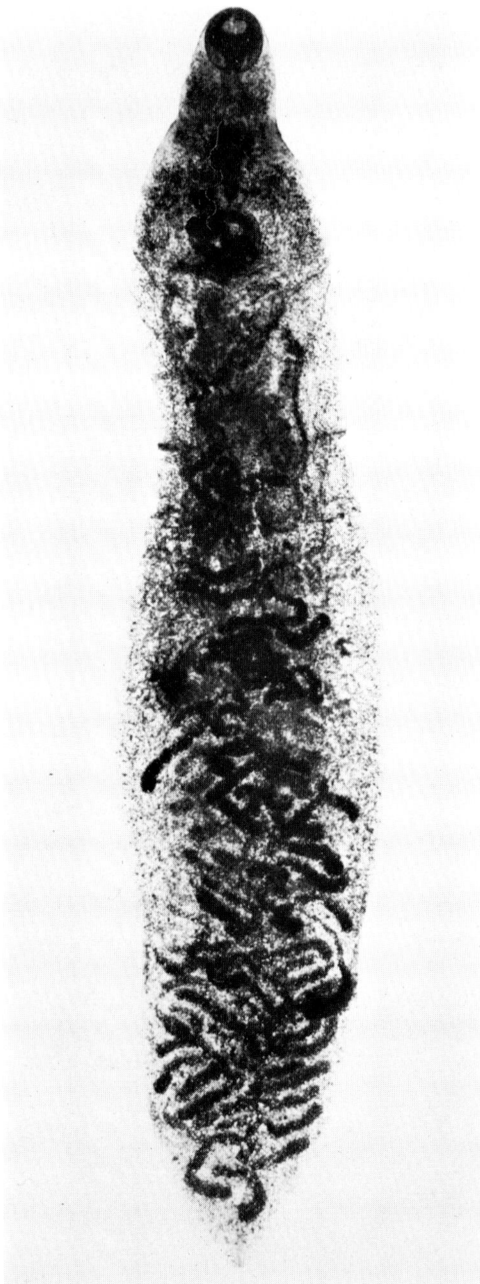

FIG. 7-11. *Dicrocoelium dendriticum. Carmine stain.* × 10.

At slaughter or necropsy, liver fluke disease is diagnosed by gross examination of the liver and by identification of adult flukes in the bile ducts or in parenchymal cysts. Light infections, especially of *D. dendriticum,* are inconspicuous and easily overlooked.

The differential diagnosis requires consideration of chronic bacterial cholangitis which causes thickening of the bile ducts without mineralization. In this disease adult flukes cannot be demonstrated at necropsy or slaughter.

Prevention and Treatment. Liver fluke disease can be prevented in a pasture area by (1) destruction of intermediate hosts and (2) treatment of infected cattle. Most programs of prevention are directed against *F. hepatica.* The intermediate molluscan host, which requires stagnant shallow fresh water for development, is eradicated wherever possible by draining ponds, ditches, puddles and other areas where stagnant water accumulates. Lumber bridges and decaying wood under which snails obtain protection against drying should be eliminated. Water sources, such as lakes, that cannot be drained should be fenced to exclude cattle from grazing at the water edges where the snails live.

An alternate method of snail eradication is the use of molluscocidal chemicals. While any of several techniques may be employed, the use of a power spray is efficient and effective when a solution of 33 pounds of copper sulfate dissolved in 400 gallons of water is applied with the power spray to all areas containing snails. Water edges of lakes and other remaining water sources should be sprayed. For effective control the spraying should be repeated in 21 days in order to insure destruction of the snail generations which were immature at the time of the first application. Following the eradication of snails from a grazing area, only nonparasitized cattle and other host animals should be admitted to the pasture. Fluke infected cattle should be treated at least twice at 21-day intervals before entering the clean pasture. This treatment avoids seeding the soil with fluke eggs. However, seeding may occur from parasitized wild animals, such as deer and rabbits.

Cattle may also be treated safely and effectively with hexachlorethane administered orally at the rate of 10 grams per 100 pounds of body weight. One treatment is sufficient for feedlot cattle. Pastured animals require the second treatment after 21 days for destruction of flukes immature at the time of the first treatment. Carbon tetrachloride, another therapeutic agent, is effective when administered intramuscularly at the dosage of 1 ml of carbon tetrachloride per 20 pounds of body weight and with a maximum of 30 ml. This route of administration, however, causes necrosis and inflammation at the point of injection. Since the muscular lesions persist for as long as 6 months, this specific therapy should be avoided in feedlot cattle.

References

Boray, J. C. and McMichael, D. F.: The Identity of the Australian Lymnaeid Snail Host of *Fasciola Hepatica* L. and its Response to Environment. Austral. Jour. Marine & Freshwater Research, *12* (1961): 150–163.

Chandler, A. C.: Control of Fluke Diseases by Destruction of the Intermediate Host. J. Agric. Research. U.S.D.A., *20* (1920): 193–208.

Federal Meat Inspection Activities. A Statistical Summary. C & MS-54 (1967, 1968, 1969).

Griffiths, Henry J.: Fascioloidiasis of Cattle, Sheep, and Deer in Northern Minnesota. JAVMA, *140* (1962): 342–347.

Holmes, P. H., Dargie, J. D., MacLean, J. M. and Mulligan, W.: The Anemia in Fascioliasis: Studies with ^{51}Cr-labelled Red Cells. J. Comp. Path., *78* (1968): 415–420.

Jensen, Paul, Mapes, Cortland R. and Whitlock, John H.: Pasture Management and Control of the Lancet Fluke (*Dicrocoelium dendriticum* Rudolphi, 1819), *45* (1955): 526–538.

Keck, G.: Investigations on the Big Fluke. II. Tissue of Infection in the Bovine Liver, Wiener Tierarztl. Monatsschr., *53* (1966): 228–231.

Kendall, S. B. and Parfitt, J. W.: The Chemotherapy of Fascioliasis. Brit. Vet. J., *118* (1962): 1–10.

Krull, Wendell H. and Mapes, Cortland R.: Studies on the Biology of *Dicrocoelium dendriticum* (Rudolphi, 1819) Looss, 1899 (Trematoda: *Dicrocoeliidae*), Including its Relation to the Intermediate Host, *Cionella lubrica* (Muller). IV. Infection Experiments Involving Definitive Hosts. Cornell Vet., *42* (1952): 276–285; 339–351; 444–489; 603–604.

———: Studies on the Biology of *Dicrocoelium dendriticum* (Rudolphi, 1819) Looss, 1899 (Trematoda: *Dicroceliidae*), Including its Relation to the Intermediate Host, *Cionella lubrica* (Muller). IX. Notes on the Cyst, Metacercaria, and Infection in the Ant, *Formica fusca.* Cornell Vet., *43* (1953): 389–410.

Krull, Wendell H.: Experiments Involving Potential Definitive Hosts of *Dicrocoelium dendriticum* (Rudolphi, 1819) Looss, 1899; *Dicrocoeliidae.* Cornell Vet., *45* (1956): 511–525.

———: The Migratory Route of the Metacercaria of *Dicrocoelium dendriticum* (Rudolphi, 1819) Looss, 1899 in the Definitive Host: *Dicrocoeliidae.* Cornell Vet., *48* (1958): 17–24.

Kuttler, K. L., Matthews, N. J. and Marble, D. W.: Comparative Therapeutic Efficacy of Carbon Tetrachloride, Hexachlorethane, and ME 3625 in *Fasciola.* AJVR, *24* (1963): 52–58.

Losses in Agriculture, ARS. USDA. Agric. Handbook 291 (1965).

Mapes, C. R.: Studies on the Biology of *Dicrocoelium dendriticum.* I. A Study of *Dicrocoelium dendriticum* and *Dicrocoelium* infection. Cornell Vet., *41* (1951): 382–432.

Morrill, Don R. and Shaw, J. N.: Studies of Pathology in Cattle Produced by Liver Fluke. Oregon State College Bul. *408* (1942): 1–30.

Ollerenshaw, C. B.: The Ecology of the Liver Fluke (*Fasciola hepatica*) Vet. Record, *71* (1959): 957–965.

Olsen, O. W. and Fenstermacher, R.: The Helminths of North American Deer. Minn. Ag. Exp. Stn. Bul. *159* (1943).

Olsen, O. W.: Preliminary Observations on Hexachlorethane for Controlling the Common Liver Fluke, *Fasciola hepatica,* in Cattle. JAVMA, *102* (1943): 433–436.

———: Bionomics of the Lymnaeid Snail, *Stagnicola Bulimoides Techelia,* the Intermediate Host of the Liver Fluke in Southern Texas. Jour. Ag. Res., *69* (1944): 389–403.

———: Hexachlorethane—Bentonite Suspension for Controlling the Common Liver Fluke, *Fasciola hepatica,* in Cattle in the Gulf Coast Region of Texas. AJVR, *8* (1947): 353–366.

Price, Emmett W.: The Fluke Situation in American Ruminants. J. Parasit., *39* (1953): 119–134.

Roberts, Enid W.: Studies on the Life-Cycle of *Fasciola hepatica* (Linnaeus) and of its Snail Host *Limnea* (Galba) *truncatula* (Muller) in the Field and Under Controlled Conditions in the Laboratory. Ann. Trop. Med. & Parasitol., *44* (1950): 187–206.

Shaw, J. N.: Studies of the Liver Fluke (*Fasciola hepatica*). JAVMA, LXXXI (1932): 76–82.

———: Hexachlorethane Treatment of Liver Fluke in Oregon Cattle. Agric. Exper. Stn. Oregon State College Bul., *7* (1944): 1–11.

Swanson, Leonard E., Batte, Edward G. and Denniss, Walter R.: Liver Fluke Disease and its Control. Agric. Exp. Stn. Florida, Bul. 502 (1952): 1–19.

Swanson, L. E. and Hopper, H. H.: Diagnosis of Liver Fluke Infection in Cattle. JAVMA, *117* (1950): 127–129.

Taylor, P. F.: The Liver Fluke Problem in Cattle and Sheep Practice, Austral. Vet. J., *38* (1962): 155–158.

Thienel, M.: Neue Arbeiten zur Medikamentosen Bekampfung der Leberegelseuche. Munich Tierarztl. Wochenshr., *77* (1926): 771–772.

Echinococcosis

(HYDATID; HYDATID CYST;

HYDATID DISEASE)

A chronic parasitic disease, echinococcosis is the invasion and the development in herbivorous and omnivorous mammals of cystic larvae of the tapeworm *Echinococcus granulosus*. As a two-host parasite, *E. granulosus* parasitizes dogs and some other members of the family *Canidae* as the definitive hosts, and ruminants, some other herbivorous mammals and man as the intermediate hosts. While the disease has caused extensive suffering and economic losses throughout most of the world, the application of sanitation has reduced the incidence to a low level in North America and some northern European countries. Occasionally in these same countries, however, an outbreak of high local incidence has formed. In the United States from 1967 through 1969, one animal per 14,600 cattle slaughtered contained hydatid cysts in the liver. These infections resulted in an average condemnation of 2,000 bovine livers annually (Federal Meat Inspection, 1967–1969). While cattle seldom die from the disease, infected organs and occasionally entire carcasses are condemned at slaughter. The reduced economic productivity in infected people is an additional loss.

Review of Literature. Since discovery of the life cycle of the parasite (1852), many aspects of the disease have been investigated. Some species of the family *Canidae* have been found to be definitive hosts (Schiller, 1960; Sweatman, 1952; Wolfgang and Poole, 1956); most domestic and wild ruminants, kangaroos and people were intermediate hosts (Animal Health Yearbook, 1968; Durie and Riek, 1952; World Health Organization, 1959). Of the bovine hydatid cysts in Africa 90% (LaPage, 1968) and in Australia 99% (Durie and Riek, 1952) were sterile. Physiologic studies of viable ova collected from infected dogs have revealed some functional peculi-

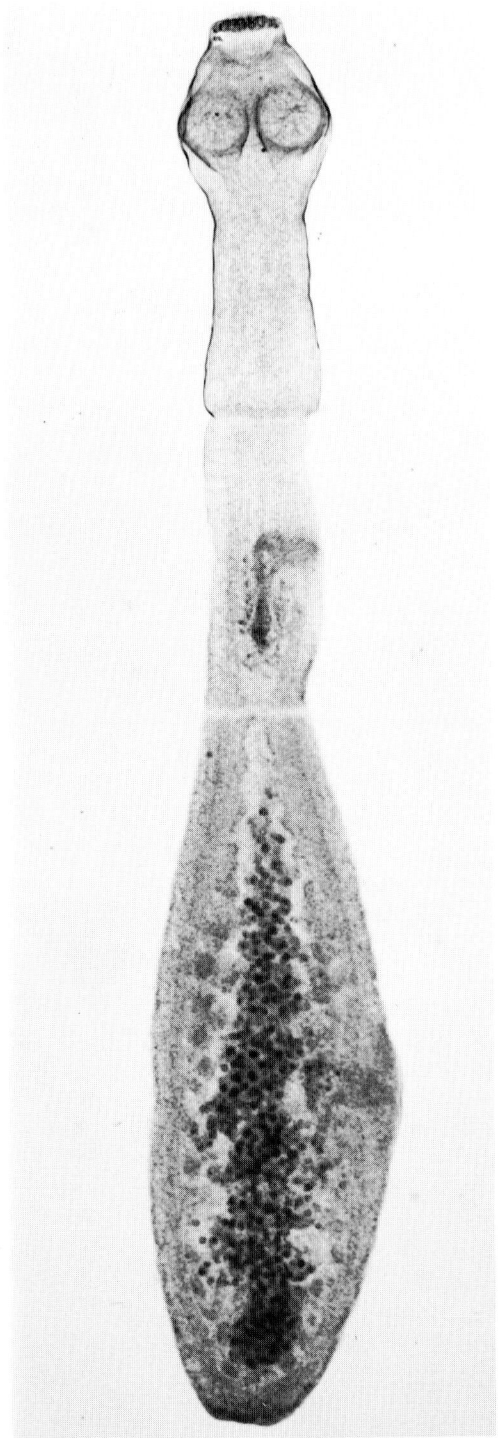

FIG. 7-12. *The adult tapeworm, Echinococcus granulosus, from the dog intestine. Carmine stain.* × 68.

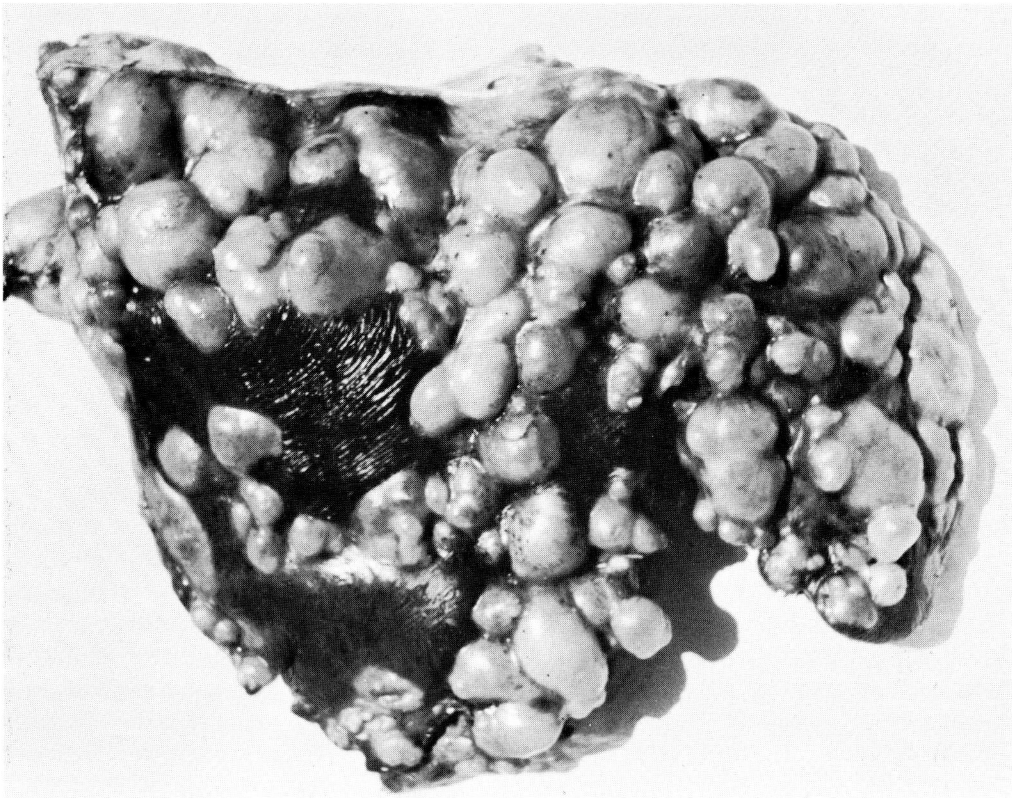

FIG. 7-13. *Multiple unopened hydatid cysts in liver.* × 0.6.

arities. Pancreatin and trypsin in *in vitro* studies caused some activation of oncospheres, but bile, bile salts and cholesterol enhanced the activating effect of pancreatin and trypsin (Meymarian, 1961). A significant number of eggs retained viability when exposed to germicides; when exposed to 70% alcohol for 60 minutes, 20 to 30% of ova were viable; when exposed to 10% aqueous Lysol for 60 minutes, 10% of the ova were viable (Meymarian and Schwabe, 1962); and exposure to 40% formaldehyde for 2 weeks failed to kill all ova (Hercus, Williams, Gemmell and Parnell, 1962).

Additional studies on culturability of the organism have yielded important information. The protoscolex, recently evaginated scolex, possessed two potentialities: to form a cyst or to develop into an adult tapeworm. In a liquid culture medium the viable protoscolex always formed a cyst. In a culture medium, however, consisting of solid substrate of heat-coagulated canine or bovine serum and supernatant nutrient liquid, the protoscolex differented into an adult tapeworm with at least three segments. While the cultured worm had many characteristics of maturity, the genitalia were not functional (Smyth, Howkins and Barton, 1966).

Occurrence. Echinococcosis, a disease caused by the larval form of the tapeworm, occurs in cattle of all breeds and sexes. Although all ages are affected, young animals apparently are more susceptible. In addition to cattle, the cysts occur in sheep, swine, camels, deer, moose, horses and people. The adult tapeworm parasitizes dogs, wolves, jackals and other related carnivores of the *Canidae* family.

Geographically, the disease is world-wide. In the United States, the incidence has been reduced to a low level, and among cattle slaughtered during 1967 through 1969, approximately 1 animal in 14,600 was affected (Federal Meat Inspection, 1967–1969). The incidence is high in southern Europe, the Mediterranean basin, Africa, the Middle East, parts of East Asia, South America and Australia. Whenever and wherever conditions favor the parasite, local areas within any country may develop a high incidence within the cattle population.

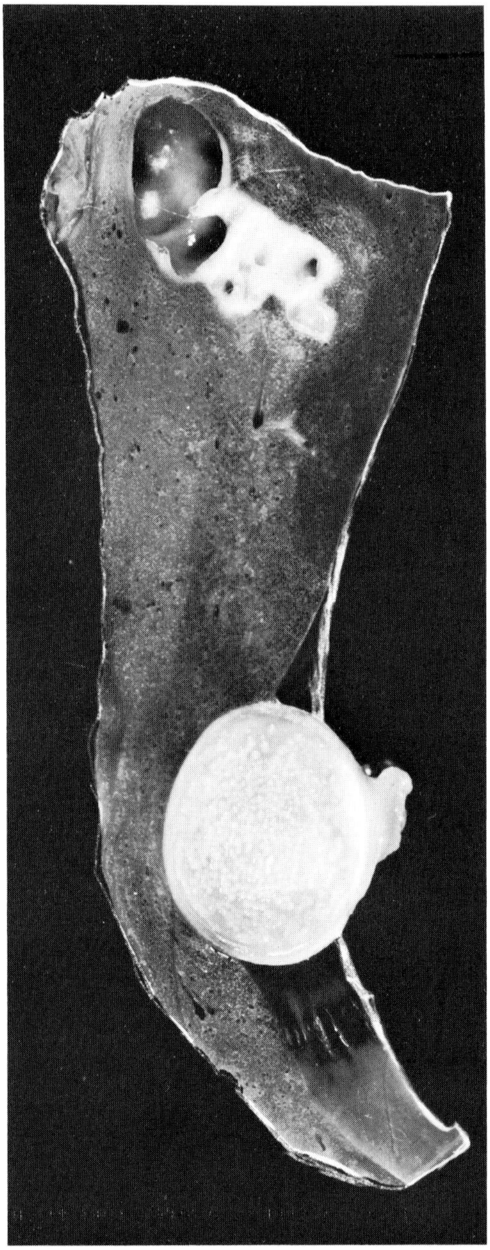

FIG. 7-14. *An opened fertile hydatid cyst in a lung. Individual endogenous brood capsules are discernible as granules.* × 2.6.

Etiology and Pathogenesis. Echinococcosis is caused by the tapeworm *E. granulosus* with the adult tapeworm infesting the small intestine of dogs and related mammalian carnivores and the cystic larvae parasitizing cattle, sheep, swine, moose, deer and man as the intermediate host. Measuring 2 to 5 mm in length, the adult worm consists of a scolex containing 4 suckers, a double row of hooklets, and few proglottids. In the intermediate host the larva forms a cyst which measures 10 to 150 mm in diameter. Usually unilocular and globular in shape, the cyst consists of a lumen and wall containing an external laminated layer and an internal germinal layer. The germinal layer produces many secondary cysts or brood capsules which project into the cyst lumen and usually contain 10 to 40 invaginated scolices. The brood capsule may maintain attachment to the germinal layer or may move freely in the fluid of the cyst as "hydatid sand."

The pathogenesis of echinococcosis varies with degree of parasitism and location of the cysts. A few small or medium sized cysts in the liver or lungs are usually innocuous. A large number in the liver, however, may cause serious or fatal hepatic insufficiency and large numbers in the lungs result in atelectasis and dyspnea. Traumatic rupture of a sterile cyst is inconsequential, but breaking of a fertile one may disseminate viable scolices through a body cavity and produce generalized echinococcosis.

The life cycle is initiated with expulsion of ova with host feces to the exterior where they may contaminate food and/or water. When ingested by a suitable intermediate bovine host, the viable eggs enter the small intestine and hatch; the larvae penetrate the intestinal wall, enter a blood vessel and are transported to the liver where many are retained, but some pass to the lungs and occasionally to other organs. Wherever a larva locates, it grows and differentiates into a cyst which consists of a germinal membrane surrounded by a laminated membrane. From the germinal membrane coenuri and brood capsules, each containing invaginated scolices, develop. When viable scolices or cysts are eaten by dogs, or other suitable mammalian host carnivores, they enter the small intestine, evaginate and attach to the mucous membrane. Here, during a prepatent period of approximately 7 to 10 weeks, the worms grow to sexual maturity and complete their life cycle. In cattle, the hydatid cyst commonly fails to form scolices. In South Africa 90% and in Australia 99% of bovine hydatid cysts were sterile. In case of sterility the life cycle is interrupted, but germicidal interruption is difficult. The ova are highly resistant to germicides and have retained viability for 2 weeks in 40% formaldehyde.

Transmission. Echinococcosis is spread by the dissemination of viable tapeworm ova from the feces of infected dogs and other definitive hosts. Infected dogs may defecate either in or near feeding or watering equipment of feedlots or in pasture grazing areas. Ingestion by cattle of the viable tapeworm ova results in the formation of hydatid cysts within the viscera.

Clinical Signs and Postmortem Lesions. Unless the parasitism is severe with cysts widely disseminated throughout the animal body, clinical signs are not produced. In feedlot cattle the cysts, usually single and located within the liver, result in little animal discomfort and no apparent alteration in the rate of gain in body weight during fattening. Since bovine hydatid cysts are usually sterile, cyst rupture does not spread viable secondary or daughter brood capsules throughout the body. Theoretically, however, a fertile bovine cyst could rupture and produce extensive and widely disseminated secondary cysts with resulting unthriftiness and even death. Cyst rupture and release of fluid from either sterile or fertile cysts may cause fatal shock. Large numbers of hydatid cysts in the lungs result in dyspnea and possible predisposition to pneumonia.

At necropsy following death of cattle from other diseases or at postmortem inspection after slaughter, the hydatid cysts are found most often in the liver, but they may be located in the lungs or other organs. While the cyst wall is strong, some areas may be thin and fragile. An opened cyst contains a single cavity filled with a transparent or translucent yellow-tinted fluid. Fertile cysts have grossly granular brood capsules attached either to the cyst wall or free in the fluid. In sterile cysts, no brood capsules are present and consequently the cyst wall is smooth.

Since fertile hydatid cysts are potentially pathogenic to people and are a source of infection to dogs, all cysts found at necropsy should be destroyed. At slaughter, organs and parts of organs infected with hydatid cyst should be condemned and destroyed.

Microscopically, the cyst wall consists of the outer layer of laminated connective

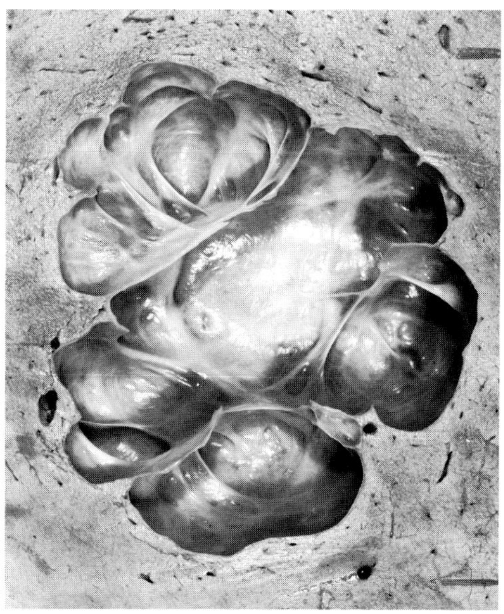

FIG. 7-15. *An opened sterile hydatid cyst in bovine liver.* × 0.4.

tissue and an inner germinal layer of cuticular cells. Fertile cysts contain brood capsules, each with many invaginated scolices, while the sterile cysts contain no brood capsules. Organ tissue surrounding the cyst is usually atrophic and may be non-functional.

Diagnosis. Since bovine echinococcosis produces no symptoms or non-specific clinical signs, the disease is not diagnosed in the living animal. The Casoni or intradermal sensitivity test for people has not been adapted to cattle. Consequently, bovine echinococcosis is recognized only at necropsy or at slaughter, and diagnosis is based on finding the grossly visible hydatid cyst. Because of their typical gross characteristics, identification of medium and large sized fertile cysts is readily achieved. Sterile cysts, however, are confused grossly with other cystic diseases. A diagnosis can be confirmed by histopathologic studies of the cyst wall. The invaginated scolices within the brood capsules identify the fertile cyst. In sterile cysts, the double layered wall is the basis for identification.

The differential diagnosis requires consideration of bovine cysticercosis, cystic bile ducts, and cystadenomas. In bovine cysticercosis the mature cyst measures approximately 9×5 mm and contains a single hookless but suckered invaginated scolex. While the cysticerci may be located in the liver, they are more commonly in the heart and voluntary musculature. Cystic bile ducts usually contain recognizable bile. Histopathologically, the wall contians cuboidal or columnar epithelial cells and cystic neoplasms usually contain solid as well as cystic portions.

Prevention and Treatment. The prevention of echinococcosis is directed at the definitive host of the parasite. Laws controlling the dog population should be enacted and enforced. Stray and unowned dogs should be impounded, and pet and work dogs confined to the owner's property. All dogs should be excluded from cattle feedlots and from meat packing establishments where infested offal might be available for consumption. For removal of the adult tapeworms, infested dogs are treated with arecoline hydrobromide administered orally at the rate of 4 mg per kg of body weight and repeated at approximately 4-month intervals. Wild dogs, wolves, jackals and foxes are also potential definitive hosts. Only by controlling the definitive host can cattle and other intermediate hosts be protected against exposure to viable ova of the parasite.

At slaughter or necropsy, carcasses should be examined carefully by competent veterinary inspectors. Cysts should be excised and sterilized to avoid ingestion by the definitive host.

The success of a preventive program is dependent upon comprehension of the parasite problem by the public. Butchers, meat establishment owners, cattle and pet owners should understand the essential features of the life cycle of the parasite. Through education, the public generally and individuals directly concerned with the parasitism should willingly cooperate in preventive programs.

Since echinococcosis is not diagnosed in living animals, cattle are not treated for the disease. At exploratory surgical operations, however, the unopened hydatid cyst should be excised.

References

Animal Health Yearbook. FAO-WHO-OIE, (1968).

Durie, P. H. and Riek, R. F.: The Role of the Dingo and Wallaby in the Infestation of Cattle with Hydatids [*Echinococcus granulosis* (Batsch, 1786) Rudolphi, 1805] in Queensland. Austral. Vet. J., *28* (1952): 249–254.

Federal Meat Inspection. A Statistical Summary C & MS-54 (1967, 1968, 1969).

Froyd, G.: The Incidence of Liver Flukes (*Fasciola gigantica*) and Hydatid Cysts (*Echinococcus granulosus*) in Kenya Cattle. Parasitology, *46* (1960): 659–662.

Hercus, C. E., Williams, R. J., Gemmell, M. A. and Parnell, I. W.: A Warning that Formalin is not a Hydatid Ovicide. Vet. Rec., *74* (1962): 1515.

Lapage, G.: *Monnig's Veterinary Helminthology and Entomology*. 5th Ed. The Williams & Wilkins Co. Baltimore. (1962). 141–145.

Meymarian, E.: Host-Parasite Relationships in Echinococcosis. VI. Hatching and Activation of *Echinococcus granulosus* ova *in vitro*. Am. J. Trop. Med. & Hygiene, *10* (1961): 719–726.

Meymarian, E. and Schwabe, C. W.:. Host-Parasite Relationships in Echinococcosis. VII. Resistance of ova of *Echinococcus granulosus* to Germicides. Am. J. Trop. Med. & Hygiene, *11* (1962): 360–364.

Ross, I. Clunies: A Note on the Development of *Echinococcus granulosus*. Jour. Council for Scientific & Indust. Res., *9* (1936): 67–68.

Simitch, T.: The Actual Situation of Echinococcic Hydatidosis in the World. Bull. Off. Internat. Epiz., *58* (1962): 756–757; 766–767.

Schiller, Everett L.: Echinococcosis in North America. Ann. Int. Med., *52* (1960): 464–476.

Smyth, J. D., Howkins, A. B. and Barton, M.: Factors Controlling the Differentiation of Hydatid Organisms, *Echinococcus granulosus*, Into Cyst or Strobilar Stages *in vitro*. Nature, *211* (1966): 1374–1377.

Sweatman, Gordon K.: Distribution and Incidence of *Echinococcus granulosus* in Man and Other Animals with Special Reference to Canada. Canad. J. Pub. Health, *43* (1952): 480–486.

Von Siebold, 1852 [quoted from Faust, E. C. and Russell, P. F.: *Craig and Faust's Clinical Parasitology*. 7th Ed. Lea & Febiger. Philadelphia. (1964): 678].

Wolfgang, R. W. and Poole, J. B.: Distribution of *Echinococcus* Disease in Northwestern Canada. Amer. Jour. Trop. Med. & Hygiene, *5* (1956): 869–871.

World Health Organization. Technical Report Series, No. 169. Joint WHO/FAO Expert Committee on Zoonoses. Geneva. (1959): 44–47.

Cysticercosis

(MEASLES; MEASLY BEEF)

A parasitic disease of cattle, cysticercosis is invasion of the musculature and viscera by larvae, *Cysticercus bovis*, of *Taenia saginata*, the beef tapeworm of man. With cattle as the intermediate host and people as the definitive host, *T. saginata* causes economic losses at two stages in its life cycle. At the time of slaughter, losses result from extensive trimming and prolonged storing of mildly infected carcasses and from condemning heavily infected carcasses. The annual loss to the United States cattle industry has been estimated. In the United States during 1967, 14,407 carcasses were condemned, while lightly infected carcasses were trimmed and stored for sterilization. The total loss, including cost for inspections, was $740,000. In many countries where the incidence is high the monetary losses are much greater. Pastures infected with tapeworm ova have lowered utility from the potential danger of infecting grazing cattle. Infections of people with the adult form of *T. saginata* cause economic losses by lowered ability to secure income from gainful work.

Review of Literature. Since determination of the life cycle of *T. saginata* (1869), the epidemiology and pathogenesis of cysticercosis have been studied extensively. Ova excreted in the feces of infected people are subjected to the environmental adversities of heat, cold, drying and sunlight. Under experimental observation, ova retained viability in liquid manure for 71 days, in city sewage for 12, in river water for 33 and on pasture for 159 (Jepson and Roth, 1949). When stored in water at 24° F, some eggs retained viability for 76 days (Lucker, 1960), and when stored in a solution of merthiolate in normal saline solution at concentration of 1:10,000 and at temperature of 4° to 5° C, viability was demonstrated as long as 168 days (Froyd, 1962). After ingestion by filth flies of the genus *Chrysomyia*, viable ova were excreted for as long as 11 days (Round, 1961). Dissected cysticerci, or cysticerci in muscle, survived heating for 3.5 to 5 minutes at 55° C but not at 56° C (Allen, 1947). In cattle, specifically, the development of cysticerci was studied by artificial inoculation with viable oncospheres and subsequent serial slaughter of infected cattle for recovery of the parasites. The disease was also produced by feeding viable ova to susceptible cattle (Froyd, 1960; McIntosh, Allen and Miller, 1960; Urquhart, 1961). Eleven days following inoculation, the tapeworm cyst was discernible while in 28 days its head or scolex began to form. By 48 days suckers formed on the scolex, and in 70 days with the neck of the scolex present, the cyst was assumed to be infective to the definitive host (McIntosh, Allen and Miller, 1960; Silverman and Hulland, 1961). While the cysticerci endured for variable periods and gradually degenerated in the intermediate host, some retained viability for as long as 639 days (Silverman and Hulland, 1961; Dewhirst, Cramer and Pistor, 1963). Cattle inoculated orally for the first time with viable ova developed significantly more cysticerci than did cattle with previous exposure to oral inoculation (Urquhart, 1961). Since previously exposed cattle developed more cysticercosis from intramuscular inoculation than from oral exposure, the resistance was considered to be located in the intestinal phase of parasitism (Froyd, 1960). Although intrauterine infection has been suspected, the experimental inoculation of 10 pregnant cattle with viable ova failed to produce any cysticercosis in the calves (Urquhart, 1961).

Occurrence. Even though all breeds and sexes of cattle are susceptible, cysticercosis occurs more commonly under 3 years of age. The lower incidence in older cattle may result from the development of resistance from earlier exposure to the disease. In the United States, although the disease incidence is low, in occasional outbreaks the herd incidence may be very high. During 1967 through 1969 more than 28 million cattle were slaughtered and inspected annually, and from these an average of only 110 carcasses were condemned and 12,585 were retained (Federal Meat Inspection, 1967–1969). In much of Europe, as in the United States, the incidence during recent decades has declined to a low level. In contrast, the incidence is very high in some countries of Africa, the Middle East, Asia and South America and probably is rising (Animal Health Yearbook, 1968).

Etiology and Pathogenesis. The cause of bovine cysticercosis is the two-host beef tapeworm, *T. saginata.* A parasite of the human small intestine, the adult worm consists of a hookless but suckered scolex and as many as 1,000 to 2,000 segments or proglottids. Usually measuring 10 to 30 feet in length, the worm detaches posterior gravid segments which are expelled to the exterior. The gravid proglottid measures 16 to 20 x 4 to 7 mm and contains approximately 100,000 eggs. Larval forms of *T. saginata*, the cysticerci, parasitize the intermuscular connective tissues of cattle. Each cysticercus consists of a cyst wall and a single scolex invaginated into the lumen. While some cysts in cattle tissue degenerate and die after a short life, some remain viable 639 days and become infective to people after residing in cattle 10 to 18 weeks. The cysts are killed in 3.5 to 5 minutes at 56° C; in 5 days at −10° C; and in 5 days in a 20 to 25% solution of salt.

The life cycle involves man as the definitive and cattle as the intermediate hosts. Gravid proglottids detach from the adult tapeworm in man and are expelled to the exterior with feces. Contaminating feed and/or water, the eggs are ingested by cattle. Within the bovine intestine the hexacanth embryo hatches, penetrates the intestinal wall, invades lacteals, traverses lymphatics and the thoracic duct, enters the systemic blood, and is transported to the musculature or other organs. The embryo leaves the blood vessel and locates in a lymphatic capillary of the connective tissue between muscles and grows to a mature larva. Within 11 days the cyst measures 0.13 to 0.15 x 0.09 to 0.13 mm and in 10 to 18 weeks, when fully grown, 7 to 9 x 5 to 6 mm. While many cysticerci degenerate and die within the bovine tissues, the ingestion of viable cysts in infected meat by man enables completion of the parasite life cycle. In the human intestine the cyst wall is digested, and the scolex evaginates, attaches to the mucous membrane, and matures in 8 to 10 weeks.

In cattle the pathogenesis of cysticercosis varies with both the number of ova ingested and the organs invaded. The presence of small or even large numbers of cysticerci in the voluntary musculature results in little or no apparent discomfort to the animal. The presence, however, of one cystercus within the sino-atrial node may result in cardiac arrhythmia and death. The invasion of the myocardium by large numbers of cysticerci may result in sufficient atrophy and destruction of myocardial cells to cause fatal heart weakness. Although cysticerci endure in bovine tissues for 2 years or longer, most cysts degenerate and die within short periods.

Transmission. Cysticercosis is transmitted to cattle by contamination of their feed and water with viable tapeworm eggs. Egg dissemination comes from deposition of infested human feces within cattle feedlots or pastures, from the conveyance of ova in human sewage, and from contamination of vehicles and other feedlot equipment.

Clinical Signs and Postmortem Lesions. Most cases of bovine cysticercosis produce few clinical signs; only rarely symptoms of heart and other organ dysfunction result from invasion of large numbers of cysticerci into vital tissues. The resulting evident clinical signs, however, are non-specific and of little diagnostic importance.

At necropsy, the cysticerci when exposed are readily discernible and are commonly located in myocardium, diaphragmatic crura, masseter muscles, tongue, and, less commonly, the skeletal muscles. Occasionally the liver is invaded, even exclusively, and may contain several hundred cysticerci. Each viable cyst is gray-yellow in color, and commonly the single scolex is visible through the translucent cyst wall. On opening the cyst, the fluid content and the scolex are distinctly evident. A degenerating cyst is usually collapsed and surrounded by inflammatory exudate and fibrous connective tissue. The number of cysticerci in any one carcass is usually small but occasionally reaches hundreds.

Histopathologically, each cyst contains a scolex invaginated into the lumen. Degener-

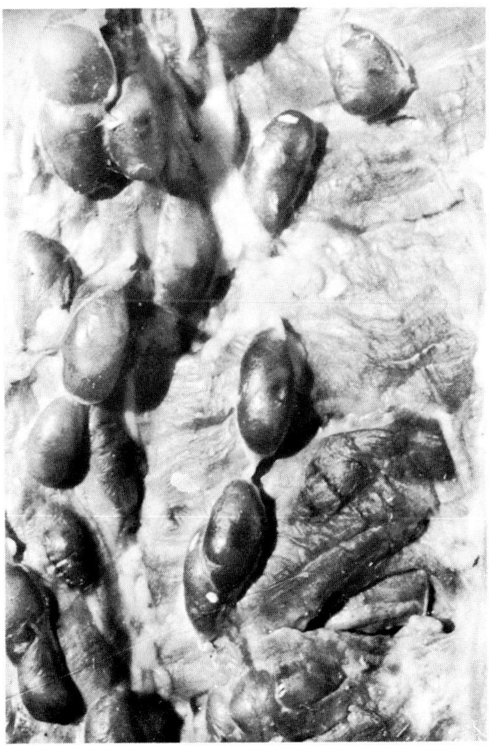

FIG. 7-16. *Numerous unopened cysticerci in muscle of the diaphragm.* × 1.1.

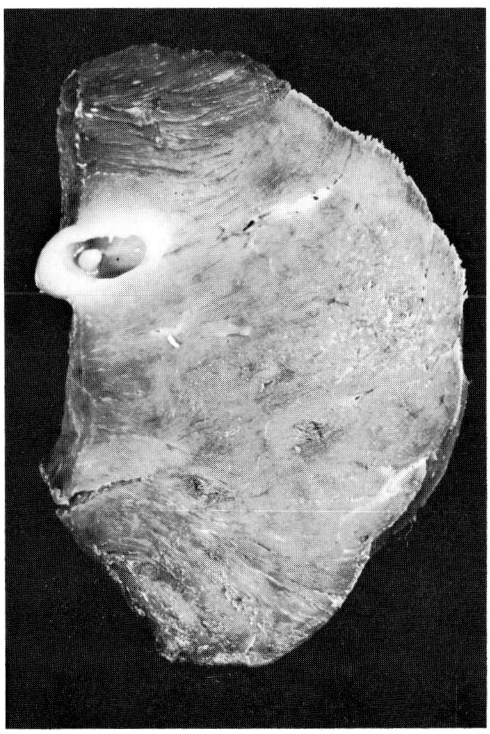

FIG. 7-17. *A single opened cysticercus in bovine heart muscle. The scolex is visible.* × 2.0.

ating cysts may be surrounded by neutrophils, eosinophils, lymphocytes, foreign body giant cells and fibrous connective tissue. Old and degenerated cysts may be mineralized with calcium salts.

At necropsy of cattle dead from intercurrent disease, cysticerci infested tissues should be destroyed by incineration or deep burial, and the contaminated surfaces disinfected. At slaughter, the decision for disposal of cysticercus infested carcasses varies with degree of infestation. In case of mild infestation, all discernible cysts should be excised and destroyed; but the remaining carcass, if in good physical condition, is satisfactory and safe for food after storage for at least 10 days at temperatures not higher than 15° F. Carcasses excessively infested are unsatisfactory as food and should be condemned.

Diagnosis. Bovine cysticercosis is not recognizable from clinical evidence alone. Diagnosis is dependent on finding and identifying cysticerci at necropsy or postmortem examination at slaughter and requires careful examination of commonly affected muscles and location of typical cysts. On the basis of diagnosing cysticercosis in a sample of slaughtered feedlot animals, the remainder of the living herd may be assumed to be affected. A sensitive and reliable serologic test has not been developed.

Prevention and Treatment. Bovine cysticercosis is preventable by the application of standard principles of sanitation for human and veterinary medicine. In endemic areas workers employed in and around feedlots, dairies, and cattle pastures should be medically examined for beef tapeworm parasitism, and infested individuals should be treated for removal of the worms. Feedlot enterprises should be provided with sanitary latrines, and the workers should avoid and be forbidden defecation within the feedlot or in pastures where cattle graze. Untreated human sewage should not be disseminated in cattle grazing or feeding areas. At the time of slaughter, carcasses should be carefully examined for cysticercosis by competent veterinary inspectors, and cysticercus infested meat should be disposed of in a manner which avoids the inclusion of viable cysticerci in human food. Meat foods should be thoroughly cooked to destroy viable cysticerci.

No effective treatment for bovine cysticercosis has been developed.

References

Allen, Rex W.: The Thermal Death Point of Cysticerci of *Taenia saginata*. Jour. Parasitol., *33* (1947): 331–338.

Animal Health Yearbook. FAO-WHO-OIE. (1968).

Dewhirst, L. W., Cramer, J. D. and Pistor, W. J.: Bovine Cysticercosis. I. Longevity of Cysticerci of *Taenia saginata*. Jour. Parasitol., *49* (1963): 297–300.

Federal Meat Inspection. A Statistical Summary. C & MS-54 (1967, 1968, 1969).

Froyd, G. and Round, M. C.: The Artificial Infection of Audlt Cattle with *Cysticercus bovis*. Res. Vet. Sci., *1* (1960): 275–282.

Froyd, G.: Longevity of *Taenia saginata* Eggs. Jour. Parasitol., *48* (1962): 279.

Ginsberg, A. and Grieve, I. M.: Two Unusual Cases of Liver Cysticercosis. Vet. Rec., *71* (1959): 618.

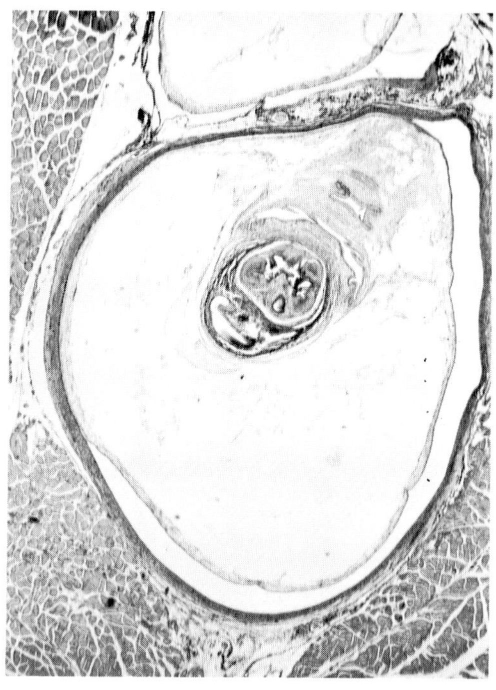

FIG. 7-18. *A cysticercus with invaginated scolex in bovine muscle. H&E stain.* × 15.

Jepson, A. and Roth, H.: Epizootiology of *Cysticercus bovis*—Resistance of the Eggs of *Taenia saginata.* Report 14th Int. Vet. Cong., London, *2* (1949): 43.
Losses in Agriculture. Agricultural Research Service U.S.D.A. Agric. Handbook 291. (1965).
Lucker, J. T.: A Test of the Resistance of *Taenia saginata* Eggs to Freezing. Jour. Parasitol., *46* (1960): 304.
McIntosh, A. and Miller, D.: Bovine Cysticercosis, with Special Reference to the Early Developmental Stages of *Taenia saginata.* AJVR, *21* (1960): 169–177.
Round, M. C.: Observations on the Possible Role of Filth Flies in the Epizootiology of Bovine Cysticercosis in Kenya. J. Hyg. Camb., *59* (1961): 505–513.
Silverman, P. H. and Hulland, T. J.: Histological Observations on Bovine Cysticercosis. Res. Vet. Sci., *2* (1961): 248–252.

Stephanofilariasis

(BOVINE FILARIAL DERMATITIS)

Stephanofilariasis, a chronic focal dermatitis of cattle, is caused by the nematode *Stephanofilaria stilesi.* While common among cattle of western and southwestern United States, the disease has little economic importance. Some losses, however, are sustained. Skin defacement may depress the market price of both slaughter and breeding animals. Because of hide damage in the anatomical area of infection, affected parts are trimmed and discarded at slaughter. In addition, affected cattle suffer continuous annoyance from the infection, and the inflamed skin attracts flies, including screw worms, during summer months. The disease may develop in young cattle and persist for several years and extend through the fattening period.

Review of Literature. While the disease probably has been endemic through much of the existence of the western cattle industry, the specific skin lesions attracted attention when high incidence and almost constant location near the umbilicus was noted. In histopathologic studies of the lesions, both adult worms and their microfilariae were observed in lymphatic vessels (Dickman, 1934; 1934a). Soon after their discovery, the parasites were isolated, described and named (Chitwood, 1934). Surveys of some western herds revealed infection in 80 to 90% of individual animals (Maddy, 1955). The disease was also identified in feedlot cattle of the midwest (Levine and Morrill, 1955) and of Hawaii (Alicata, 1947) and probably of Russia (Gnedia, 1950).

Other detailed investigations of the disease in western cattle added new information. The intermediate insect host was discovered, and larval development in the insect was described. Female and male horn flies, *Hematobium irritans,* collected from the living lesions contained filarial larvae. Laboratory-raised horn flies allowed to feed on living skin lesions subsequently contained filarial larvae, and the flies transmitted the disease by feeding on the skin of normal cattle. Within the horn fly the larvae molted twice, and after 18 to 21 days, they became infective to susceptible cattle (Hibler, 1966).

Occurrence. Filarial dermatitis occurs in all breeds and sexes. While older cattle are susceptible, animals 6 months to 3 years of age have the highest incidence. Even though transmission of the causative worm is limited to summer months, the disease, once formed, exists through all seasons. Geographically, it occurs throughout the United States but is concentrated in range cattle of the western and southwestern states where up to 90% of animals in some herds are affected. The disease has also been reported from Russia.

Etiology and Pathogenesis. Both adults and larvae of *Stephanofilaria stilesi* are parasitic in the skin lesions. The adult males, measuring 3.0 to 3.5 mm and females 5.6 to 5.8 mm in length, locate in dermal lymph cavities usually near the root of a hair follicle. The microfilariae, located in superficial lymphatics of dermal papillae, measure 45 to 60 x 2 to 4 μ and are surrounded by a delicate membrane. Within the horn fly the microfilariae grow into third stage larvae which measure 695 to 900 x 32 to 40 μ.

The life cycle of S. *stilesi* involves both cattle, the definitive host, and horn flies, the intermediate host. The horn fly frequents the skin lesion, and with its piercing mouth parts, it feeds on fresh blood and lymph, and in doing so ingests viable microfilariae. Within the fly, the microfilariae penetrate the gut wall and enter the abdominal hemocoel where they grow, undergo two molts and form mature larvae. Eventually, the larvae migrate to the salivary glands, and 18 to 21 days after entering the intermediate host, become infective. As the infected horn fly feeds on susceptible cattle, the filaroid larvae pass from the mouth of the fly into the bovine skin. The sequence of changes from inoculation of larvae until the development of adult worms in skin lymphatics is unknown. Eventually, however, microfilariae develop and locate in superficial lymphatics of dermal papillae. The presence of the irritating parasites, both adults and microfilariae, in the skin causes a chronic inflammatory reaction. Once established the disease and the parasites persist for several years.

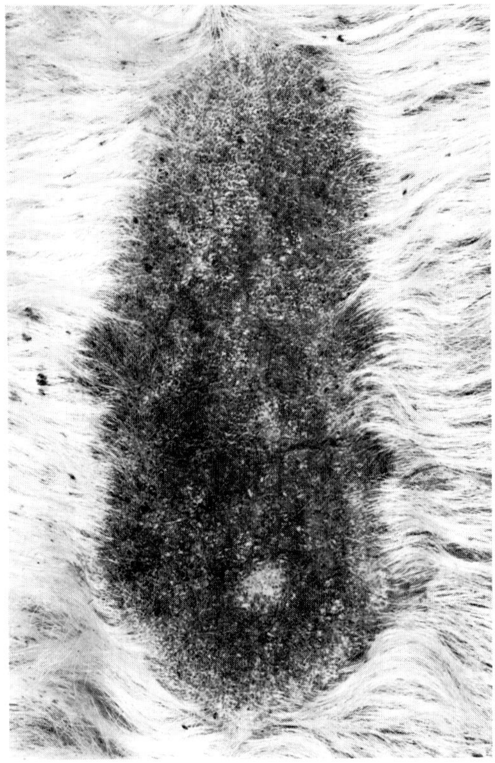

FIG. 7-19. *Stephanofilarial dermatitis near the umbilicus.* × 0.8.

Clinical Signs and Lesions. Stephanofilariasis is asymptomatic, but focal dermatitis is evident. Conspicuous dermal lesions form along the mid-ventral line. Commonly, they are at, or posterior to, the umbilicus and may be on the scrotum, prepuce and udder. On any one infected animal the lesion is usually single, often 1 to 6 inches in diameter, and its configuration may be circular, linear or oval. Inflammatory in nature, the affected skin is depillated. In early stages, serous exudate and dried blood form a deeply fissured crust. In advanced stages of the disease the crust of exudate and blood is minimal or absent, and the epithelium is thickened and scaly. During early stages of the lesions, bacteria, such as *Spherophorus necrophorus*, may penetrate the fissured skin and produce serious secondary infection.

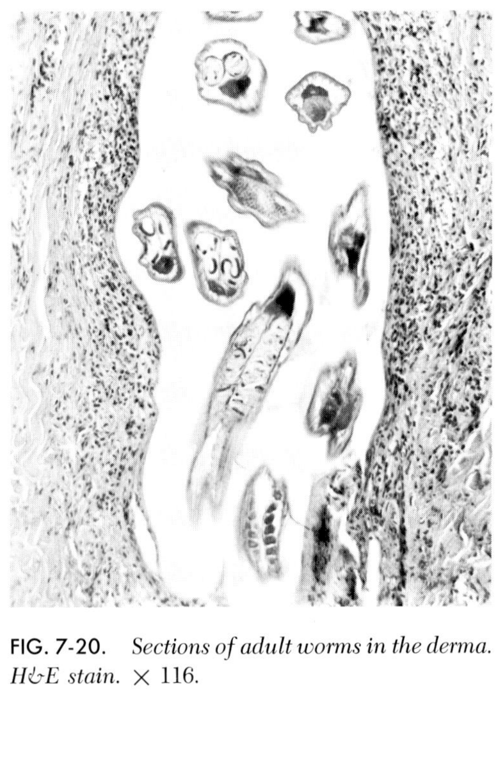

FIG. 7-20. *Sections of adult worms in the derma. H&E stain.* × 116.

Histopathologically, the causative agent and the chronic inflammatory reaction are discernible. Deep in the derma, especially around the roots of hair follicles, dilated lymphatics contain the adult worms. Lymphocytes, eosinophils, mononuclear macrophages and small numbers of neutrophils infiltrate the surrounding connective tissue. Developing eggs are usually visible in the adult female. More superficially in the lesions, the hypertrophied dermal papillae contain parasite microfilariae in dilated lymphatic vessels near the epidermis. A delicate membranous capsule surrounds the microfilariae and a few granules of proteinacious material. While microfilariae are usually single, many vessels within a single sectional plane contain parasites. Little or no inflammatory reaction forms around the larvae. Thickened in all layers, the epidermis is hypertrophied and infiltrated with some leukocytes, serum and erythrocytes. In old lesions the stratum corneum is also thickened.

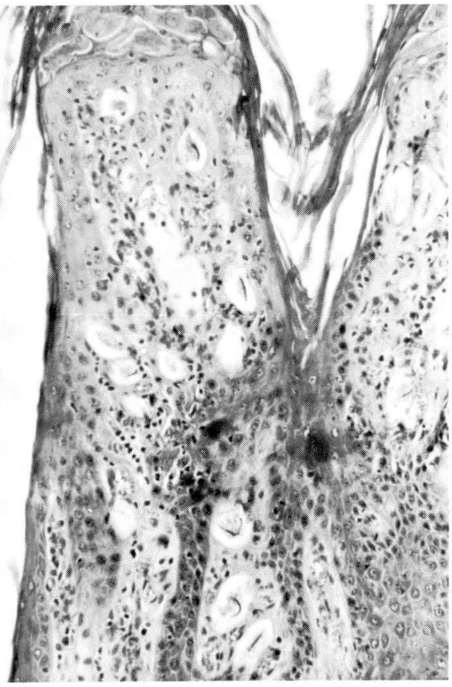

FIG. 7-21. *Microfilariae in lymphatics of a skin lesion. H&E stain.* × 145.

Prevention and Treatment. Since the intermediate host is the horn fly, the control of this and other species of flies will reduce transmission and spread of the disease. An effective treatment has not been developed and probably is not needed excepting for show animals which may be devalued by the skin lesion. Secondary bacterial infection can be successfully treated by the daily administration of streptomycin sulfate at the rate of 1 gram per 100 pounds of body weight for 3 to 4 days. Supplementary treatment is the oral or intravenous administration of sulfathiazole, sulfamethazine or sulfabromethazine at the rate of 1 to 1.5 grams per pound of body weight; after 24 to 48 hours 50% of the dose is continued for an additional 24 to 48 hours.

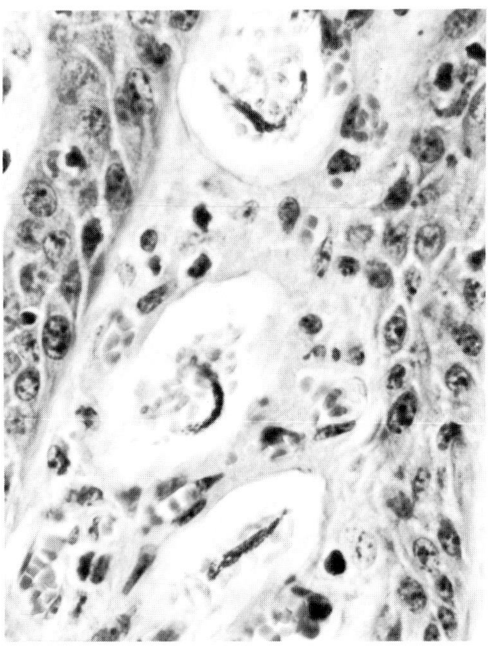

FIG. 7-22. *Microfilariae in lymphatics of a skin lesion. H&E stain.* × 593.

References

Alicata, J. E.: Parasites and Parasitic Diseases of Domestic Animals in the Hawaiian Islands. Pacific Science, *1* (1947): 69–84.

Chitwood, B. G.: A Nematode *Stephanofilaria stilesi*, New Species, from the Skin of Cattle in the United States. North Am. Vet., *15* (1934): No. 6, pp 25–27.

Dikmans, G.: Nematodes as the Cause of a Recently Discovered Skin Disease of Cattle in the United States. North Am. Vet., *15* (1934): No. 6, pp 22–25.

———: Observations on Stephanofilariasis in Cattle. Proc. Helminth. Soc. Wash., *1* (1934): 42.
Gnedina, M. P.: Discovery of *Stephanofilaria stilesi* Chitwood, 1934, in Cattle. VIGIS, *4* (1950): 82–84.
Hibler, C. P.: Life History of *Stephanofilaria stilesi* Chitwood, 1934. J. Parasitol., *50* (1964) supplement: 34.
———: Development of *Stephanofilaria stilesi* in the Horn Fly. J. Parasitol 52 (1966): 890–898.
Levine, N. D. and Morrill, C. C.: Bovine Stephanofilarial Dermatitis in Illinois. JAVMA, *127* (1955): 528–530.
Maddy, K. T.: Stephanofilarial Dermatitis of Cattle. North Am. Vet., *36* (1955): 275–278.

Ticks

As a group of arachnid arthropods, ticks are widely distributed but usually seasonal in their activities. Vectors of disease and annoyers of animals, they have public health significance and economic importance. Tick fever or bovine piroplasmosis, the first disease known to be transmitted by a living vector, was formerly widespread throughout the southern part of the United States and is still prevalent in many cattle producing countries. Because it takes position in the external ear canal, the spinose ear tick causes extreme annoyance. Tick infestations result in economic losses by transmitting diseases, such as anaplasmosis, by causing anxiety, anemia and inefficient feed utilization, and by necessitating expensive treatments. To the United States cattle industry the annual loss has been estimated at 60 million dollars. Additional, but unmeasured losses, result from incapacitation of people affected with diseases transmitted by ticks of cattle.

Review of Literature. During the ending of the nineteenth and the beginning of the twentieth century, the importance of tick parasitism to the United States cattle industry was so generally and keenly felt that the Congress enacted legislation for an eradication program against *Boophilus annulatus*, the vector of tick fever. The federal program began in 1906 and continued through 1943 when eradication was achieved (Report Cooperative Cattle Fever Activities, 1962). Since the discovery of transmission of bovine piroplasmosis, the importance of many other species of ticks has been appreciated not only to the cattle industry but to public health (Field Manual Vet. Ent., 1961). The blood feeding of large numbers of ticks on a host produced unthriftiness and anemia. In rabbits used experimentally the red cell volume descended from 43%, a normal value, to 25% on the seventh day of tick feeding. Simultaneously, the red cell count declined to 2.2 millions per cu mm. The exsanguination resulted from engorgement by female ticks (Jellison and Kohls, 1938). Points of skin puncture were attractive to gravid female screwworm flies as points for ovaposition (Report Coop. Cattle Fever Activities, 1962; Tarshis and Ommert, 1961; Tick Fever, 1960). In addition to host exsanguination, some rapidly engorging females produced in host animals tick paralysis from a neurotoxin formed in the salivary glands of the parasite. This occurred in several host species, including cattle (Jellison, Stoenner, Kramis and Beardmore, 1951), horses (Bootes, 1962), sheep, (Rosa and Gregson, 1956), dogs (Murnaghan, 1956), guinea pigs, hamsters, and groundhogs (Gregson, 1959) as well as people (Report Coop. Cattle Fever Activities, 1962). Several species of ticks were incriminated, including *Dermacentor andersoni, D. variabilis, Amblyomma americana* and *A. maculatum* in the United States, *Ixodes holocyclus* in Australia and *Ixodes rubicundus* in South Africa (Herms and James, 1961). Adult ticks feeding on the first host required 4 to 6 days to produce the paralysis, but when transferred experimentally to another host, required only 1 day (Gregson, 1959). Beginning posteriorly, the paralysis progressed forward to the medulla (Rosa and Gregson, 1956). Investigating the mode of action of the toxin, 10 male and 10 female ticks of the species *Dermacentor andersoni* were applied to 23 dogs. Of these, 9 developed paralysis. The paralyzed anterior tibial muscle contracted when stimulated directly but not when stimulated through the perineal nerve. These observations led the investigators to conclude that paralysis resulted from interference at the myoneural junction (Murnaghan, 1956).

For more than 60 years the means for controlling ticks have been actively investigated. The temporal phases of research can be divided into three periods: from 1889 to 1910 when the role of ticks as disease vectors and their control with arsenical dips were studied; from 1910 through 1940 when the feasibility and application of tick eradication programs using arsenical dips were thoroughly investigated; and from 1940 to 1959 when organic compound acaricides and tick resistance to acaricides were studied. The susceptibility of many species of ticks to newly discovered organic compounds was established (Bekker, 1959). Hexachlorocyclohexane was effective against the spinose ear tick (Kemper, Roberts and Peterson, 1947) and DDT (Stone, 1962), Dieldrin (Stone, 1962a), and Co-Ral (Stone and Webber, 1960) against *Boophilus microplus* in Australia. Tick strain resistance to acaricides was observed for the hydrocarbon compounds but not for the organophosphate compounds (Whitehead, 1959). In Australia, larvae of some strains of *Boophilus microplus* were 9 to 20 times as resistant to DDT as a susceptible reference strain, and engorged females were 700 times as resistant to Dieldrin (Stone and Webber, 1960). In this kind of study no resistance was demonstrated to the organophosphate compounds. The resistance was postulated to be due to cellular enzymes which degrade the hydrocarbon acaricide to non-toxic products (Brady and Arthur, 1962; Whitehead, 1959). Among strains of *Boophilus microplus* resistance to DDT was inherited as an incompletely recessive autosomal gene, while resistance to Dieldrin was inherited as a single dominant autosomal gene (Stone, 1962; 1962a). The effectiveness of organophosphates was demonstrated for the lone star tick and winter tick (Drummond, 1961). An organophosphate compound was ineffective against the spinose ear tick when applied to the general skin surface, but highly effective when given at a 2 to 5% concentration in a dust drench into the infected ear (Tarshis and Ommert, 1961; Drummond, Whetstone and Ernst, 1967).

Ticks of Cattle. In the United States, three species of soft ticks of the family *Argasidae* and 13 species of hard ticks of the family *Ixodidae* attack cattle. The spinose ear tick, *Otobuis megnini,* and the Rocky Mountain wood tick are of considerable importance to feedlot animals who usually acquire the ticks prior to entering the fattening pens. Table 17 presents the ticks of cattle and their distribution within the United States.

The injury to cattle from tick parasitism varies in most cases directly with numbers of parasites. The ticks feed exclusively on blood, and when several hundred parasites feed, the host becomes exsanguinated and anemic. Affected cattle are, therefore, unthrifty and may lose body weight. During warm seasons the skin injury attracts gravid screwworm flies which may cause fatal screwworm myiasis. In addition to feeding on blood and causing anemia, some engorging female ticks generate a paralyzing toxin and others, because of residence within the external ear canals, are extremely annoying.

The Spinose Ear Tick. Distributed throughout the southwestern United States, *Otobius megnini,* the spinose ear tick, is parasitic as larvae and nymphs, but free-living as adults. The bodies of nymphs are violin-shaped and spiny. The latter feature of the single host parasite and its location within the ear are the basis for the common name.

The parasitic larvae and nymphs crawl onto cattle and assemble along the inner surfaces of the ears and in the external ear canals. Several hundreds may parasitize a single host. In the process of feeding, the skin is punctured at multiple points. The resulting dermatitis generates exudate which mixes with the parasites and tends to occlude the external ear canal. The engorged and mature nymphs leave the host and, after molting,

TABLE 17 *Ticks of cattle*

Families	Name: Scientific	Name: Common	Distribution	Diseases Transmitted or Produced in Cattle
Argasidae (soft ticks)	1. *Ornithodoros coriaceus*	Pajaroello tick	Calif.; Pacific Coast of Mexico	injurious bite
	2. *Ornithodoros turicata*	relapsing-fever tick	Florida, southwest U. S., Mexico	
	3. *Otobius megnini*	spinose ear tick	Texas, New Mexico, Arizona, Calif.	Q fever and anthrax suspected
Ixodidae (hard ticks)	1. *Amblyomma americanum*	lone star tick	southeast U. S., Texas, Oklahoma, Mexico, So. America	Q fever, tularemia, tick paralysis
	2. *Amblyomma cajennense*	Cayenne tick	So. Texas; Central, So. America	Q fever
	3. *Amblyomma maculatum*	Gulf Coast tick	U. S.: Gulf Coast, Georgia, So. Carolina; Central, So. America	tick paralysis
	4. *Boophilus annulatus*	cattle fever tick	U. S.: formerly southern states; Mexico, South America, Africa	piroplasmosis anaplasmosis
	5. *Boophilus microplus*	tropical cattle tick	Florida, Mexico, Central & So. America, Australia, Africa	piroplasmosis anaplasmosis
	6. *Dermacentor albipictus*	winter tick	U. S.: northern, western states; Canada	anaplasmosis
	7. *Dermacentor andersoni*	Rocky Mountain tick	U. S.: western and northwestern states; western Canada	tularemia Q fever anaplasmosis tick paralysis
	8. *Dermacentor nigrolineatus*	brown winter tick	U. S.: wide, especially Texas, New Mexico; Mexico	anaplasmosis
	9. *Dermacentor nitens*	tropical horse tick	U. S.: So. Texas, Florida; West Indies; Mexico; So. America	
	10. *Dermacentor occidentalis*	Pacific coast tick	Calif., Oregon	anaplasmosis Q fever
	11. *Dermacentor variabilis*	American dog tick	U. S.: wide, especially east, Calif., Oregon; Canada; Mexico	tularemia anaplasmosis tick paralysis
	12. *Ixodes pacificus*	Calif. black-legged tick	U. S.: Calif., Wash., Oregon; West Canada	tularemia
	13. *Ixodes scapularis*	black-legged tick	U. S.: southeastern, southwestern states	anaplasmosis

become adults which are nonparasitic. Within a few days following mating, the female lays eggs in protected and secluded places. In addition to cattle, horses and sheep are parasitized. Cattle living in tick infested areas of the warm southern states often contain spinose ear ticks on the inner surfaces of the pinnae and in the outer part of the external ear canal. Following shipment of the infested animals to colder northern states for feedlot fattening, the ticks may move deeply into the ear canal, penetrate the tympanium, and cause middle ear infection.

Infested cattle respond to the parasites according to the degrees of their annoyance. A few ticks may evoke no clinical signs. Cattle heavily parasitized by spinose ear ticks, droop, rub and shake their ears, and turn the head to one side. Careful examination discloses the nymphal ticks in the external ear canal or on the inner inflamed surface of the pinnae.

Tick Paralysis. Ascending and progressive, tick paralysis is caused by a neurotoxin produced in and excreted from the salivary glands of some rapidly engorging female ticks. The toxin is injected into the host at the time of tick feeding. Unless the parasites are removed, the paralyzing effect progresses into the medulla and death results from respiratory failure. While the disease incidence for cattle generally is low, individual cattle herds may have as many as 50% of the animals affected. In addition to cattle, people, horses and sheep are naturally affected, and hamsters and ground hogs have been experimentally affected. Affected hamsters often manifest foaming of ocular secretions.

Tick species which cause the disease include *Dermacentor andersoni, D. variabilis, Amblyomma americanum* and *A. maculatum* in the United States, *Ixodes holocyclus* in Australia, and *I. rubicundus* in South Africa. Most cases in America have been caused by *D. andersoni.* Commonly, the parasites attach to the host skin around the head and neck. Four to 6 days of tick feeding is usually required to produce the disease. The toxin causes interruption of impulse transmissions at the myoneural junction and possibly along the spinal cord. Presumably the toxin is excreted, or detoxified rapidly, because following removal of the toxin injecting ticks, recovery is rapid.

The disease begins with weakness and incoordination of movements in the posterior

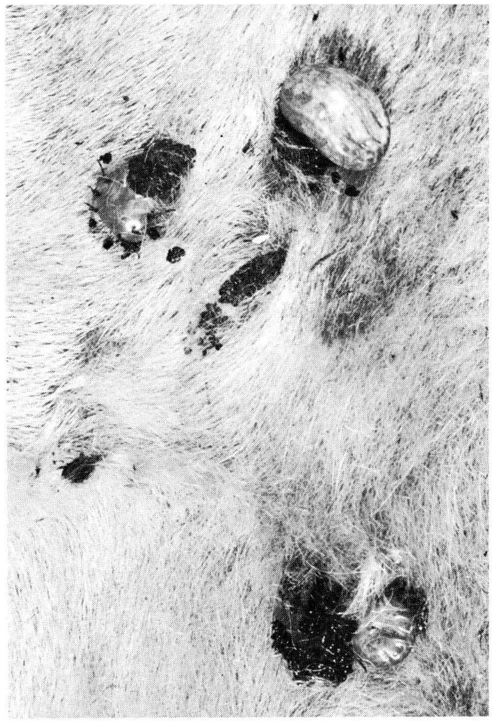

FIG. 7-23. *Dermacentor andersoni attached to the skin of a steer.* × 1.0.

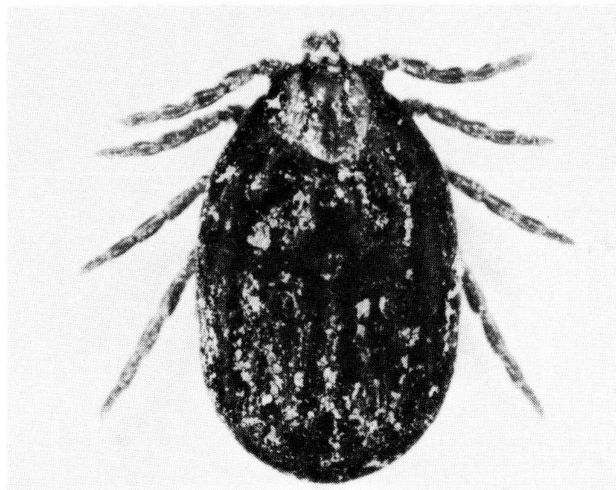

FIG. 7-24. *D. andersoni.* × 6.7.

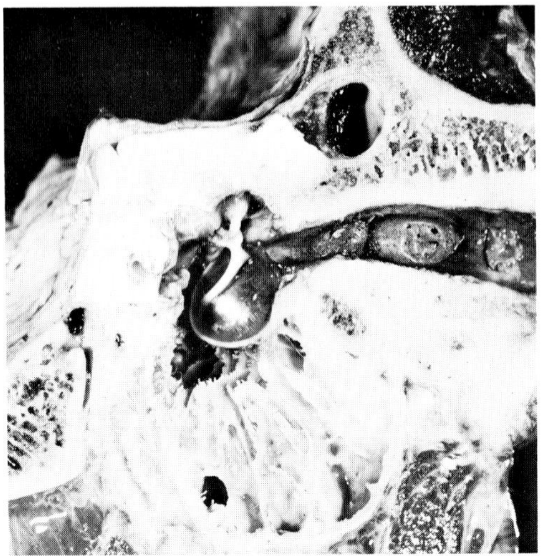

FIG. 7-25. *Spinose ear tick in the external ear canal of a steer.* × 0.7.

limbs. Within a few hours these impaired functions change into paralysis which progresses from the posterior limbs anteriorly and involves the forelimbs as well as neck and head. Some cattle may be found paralyzed without the observation of prodromal weakness. With a normal body temperature, the eyes bulge and express anxiety. The incidence is commonly low but may reach 50% in an individual herd. The course varies from 1 to 3 days and, unless the intoxicating ticks are removed early in the course of the disease, terminates fatally. At necropsy, no significant gross or microscopic changes are apparent except the presence of ticks usually attached to the skin around the neck and head. Affected cattle may harbor up to 100 or more parasites.

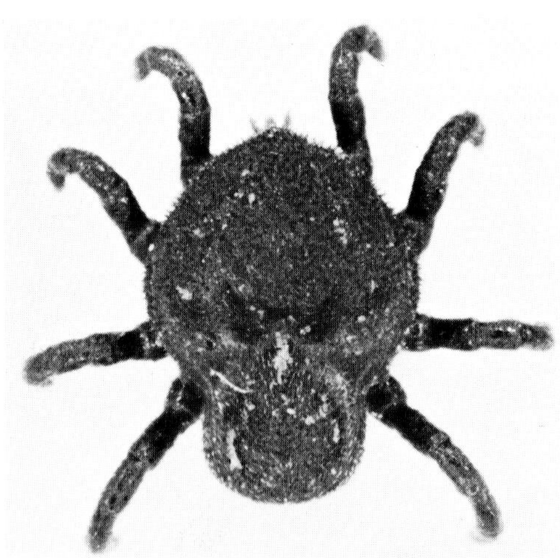

FIG. 7-26. *Nymph of spinose ear tick.* × 9.6.

Since treatment consists of removal of the engorging ticks, this may be achieved manually if only a few cattle with a small number of ticks are affected, or the use of acaricides, as sprays or dips, may destroy them. All cattle of the herd should be treated to prevent the spread of the ticks and the development of new cases of paralysis.

Prevention and Treatment. Tick parasitism can generally be prevented by avoiding grazing the cattle in infested areas during the spring season when the ticks are active. Usually this precaution is not feasible because of the necessity for utilizing available pasture and range. In tick endemic areas where paralysis is expected, cattle should be treated before the disease develops and on entrance to the feedlot, cattle should be dipped or sprayed for the destruction of ticks and other external parasites. Spinose ear tick infestation may require special medication. Many ticks can be removed manually. Dust acaricide should be injected directly into each infested ear canal with a special dose syringe. Animals with secondary middle ear infection should also receive treatment with sulfonamides and antibiotics.

Either of the medicaments presented in Table 18 is effective.

References

Bekker, P. M. P.: Dipstof En Dipping. J. So. Afric. Vet. Med. Assoc., *30* (1959): 353–380.

Bootes, B. W.: A Fatal Paralysis in Foals from *Ixodes holocyclus* Infestation. Austral. Vet. J., *38* (1962): 68–69.

Brady, V. E. and Arthur, B. W.: Absorption and Metabolism of Ruelene by Arthropods. J. Econ. Ent., *55* (1962): 833–836.

Drummond, R. O.: Tests with General Chemical 3582

TABLE 18 *Treatment for ticks*

Parasite	Tickcide	Tolerance ppm in Tissue	Min. Days Last Appl. to Slaughter	Formula and Strength	Amount of Formula/ Animal	Where and When to Apply	Safety Precautions
Ticks in general	Carboryl	—	7	WP, 0.5% spray	1 qt.	spray thoroughly repeat as needed	
	Coumaphos	1 meat fat	—	WP 0.125% dip or spray	varies with size	immerse or spray thoroughly	Do not treat sick cattle or calves under 3 months with Coumaphos
	Dioxathion	1	—	EC, 0.15% dip 0.125% spray	varies with size	if needed repeat in 2–3 weeks	
	Lindane	7	30 spray 60 dip	EC or WP 0.03% dip or spray			Do not re-apply Ronnel or Dioxathion within 2 weeks.
	Malathion	4 meat	—	EC or WP 0.5% dip or spray			
	Ronnel	0 meat	56	EC 0.75%			Do not use Lindane on weak or lactating cattle.
	Toxaphene	7	28	EC or WP 0.5% dip or spray			
Spinose ear tick	Coumaphos	1 meat fat	—	dust 5%	—	lightly inside ears with dose applicator	
	Malathion	4 meat	—	EC or WP, 0.5% spray low pressure	—	lightly inside ears	

and 4072 for the Control of Ticks Affecting Livestock. J. Econ. Ent., *54* (1961): 1050–1051.

Drummond, R. O., Whetstone, T. M. and Ernst, S. E.: Insecticidal Control of the Ear Tick in Ears of Cattle. J. Ec. Ent. *60* (1967): 1021–1025.

Federal Meat Inspection, Statistical Summary (1967, 1968, 1969).

Field Manual on Veterinary Entomology. Agricultural Research Service. U.S.D.A. June 1961.

Gregson, J. D.: Tick Paralysis in Groundhogs, Guinea Pigs, and Hamsters. Canad. J. Comp. Med. Vet. Sci., *23* (1959): 266–268.

Harvey, T. L. and Brethour, J. R.: Effectiveness of Ruelene and Ronnel for Ear Ticks Compared with Cattle Grub Control. J. Econ. Ent., *54* (1961): 814–815.

Herms, W. B. and James, M. T.: *Medical Entomology.* 5th Ed. The Macmillan Company, New York. 1961. pp. 467–469.

Guide for Use of Insecticides. Agricultural Handbook No. 331. Agri. Research Service. U.S.D.A. 1968.

Jellison, W. L. and Kohls, G. M.: Tick-Host Anemia: A Secondary Anemia Induced by *Dermacentor andersoni* Stiles. J. Parasit., *24* (1938): 143–154.

Jellison, W. L., Stoenner, H. G., Kramis, N. J. and Beardmore, H. F.: An Outbreak of Tick Paralysis in Cattle in Western Montana. Vet. Med., *46* (1951): 163–166.

Kemper, H. E., Roberts, I. H. and Peterson, H. O.: Hexachlorocyclohexane as an Acaricide for the Control of the Spinose Ear Tick on Cattle. North Am. Vet., *28* (1947): 665–668.

Losses in Agriculture, Agricultural Research Service. Agricultural Handbook No. 291. (1965): 82.

Murnaghan, M. F.: Tick Paralysis in the Dog: A Neurophysiological Study. Proceedings Tenth International Congress of Entomology, *3* (1956): 841–848.

Neitz, W. O.: Second Meeting of the FAO/OIE Expert Panel on Tickborne Diseases of Livestock, Cairo, U.A.R. December 1962.

Report of Cooperative Cattle Fever Tick Eradication Activities. Animal Disease Eradication Division. Agricultural Research Service. U.S.D.A. 1962.

Riek, R. F.: Studies on the Reactions of Animals to Infestation with Ticks. VI. Resistance of Cattle to Reinfestation with the Tick *Boophilus microplus.* Austral. J. Agr. Res., *13* (1962): 532–550.

Rosa, Ian and Gregson, J. D.: Evidence of a Neuromuscular Block in Tick Paralysis. Nature, *178* (1956): 95–96.

Stone, B. F.: The DDT-Susceptibility of Fourteen Strains of the Cattle Tick, *Boophilus microplus,* from Northern New South Wales. Austral. Vet. J., *36* (1960): 343–347.

Stone, B. F.: The Inheritance of DDT-Resistance in the Cattle Tick, *Boophilus microplus*. Austral. J. Agri. Res., *13* (1962a): 1008–1022.

———: The Inheritance of Dieldrin-Resistance in the Cattle Tick, *Boophilus microplus*. Austral. J. Agri. Res., *13* (1962): 1008–1022.

Stone, B. F. and Webber, L. G.: Cattle Ticks, *Boophilus microplus* Resistance to DDT, BHC, and Dieldrin. Austral. J. Agri. Res., *11* (1960): 105–119.

Tarshis, I. B. and Ommert, W. D.: Control of the Spinose Ear Tick, *Otobius megnini* (Duges), with an Organic Phosphate Insecticide, Combined with a Silica Aerogel. JAVMA, *138* (1961): 665–669.

Tick Fever. Farmers' Bulletin No. 1625. U.S.D.A. 1960.

Whitehead, G. B.: The Development and Mechanism of Insecticide Resistance in the Blue Tick, *Boophilus decoloratus* Koch. J. So. Afric. Vet. Med. Assoc., *30* (1959): 221–234.

Scabies

(MANGE; ITCH; BARN ITCH; SCAB; ACARIASIS)

A subacute or chronic contagious itching dermatitis, scabies is caused by four genera of ectoparasitic mites. While most species of mammals are affected with scabies, a considerable degree of host specificity prevents transfer of parasites between host species. Cattle scabies is nearly universal; in the United States, however, as well as in some other geographic areas, the incidence of some types has been reduced to a low level through eradication programs.

Although scabies is uncommon in feedlot cattle, affected enterprises suffer considerable economic loss. In one outbreak of psoroptic scabies involving 29,200 feedlot cattle, the disease daily reduced the consumption of grain from 30.2 to 23.7 pounds (21.5%) per animal and the total body weight of 150 pounds per animal (Tobin, 1962). Total annual loss to the United States cattle industry has been estimated at 3 million dollars. (Losses in Agriculture, 1965). The economic losses result from animal annoyance, reduced feed consumption, reduction in body weight, quarantine against commercial movements and costly treatments.

Types of Cattle Scabies. Bovine scabies, or mange, is classified according to the type of mite. Four genera are involved. While each scabies disease in early stages possesses differential characteristics, the positive diag-

TABLE 19 *Bovine scabies*

	Mites				*Lesions*	
Mange Type	*Name*	*Life Cycle, Days*	*Eggs/ Female*	*Length mm*	*Early Locations*	*Characteristics*
1. Psoroptic (common cattle scab)	*Psoroptes equi* var. *bovis*	10–12	15–24	F 0.8 M 0.7	withers, back, tailhead	crusty; thick; scaly; denuded
2. Sarcoptic (barn itch)	*Sarcoptes scabiei bovis*	15	10–25	F 0.5 M 0.3	escutcheon, medial surface thighs	denuded; thick; wrinkled
3. Chorioptic (symbiotic scab; tail scab)	*Chorioptes bovis* var. *bovis*	19–23	3–16	F 0.4 M 0.3	escutcheon	denuded; thickened; wrinkled; crusty
4. Demodectic (follicular mange)	*Demodex folliculorum bovis*	—	—	0.2	neck, shoulders, brisket, dewlap	nodular abscesses up to 3 cm.; content cheesy

nosis requires isolation and identification of the specific causative mite. The types of scabies, their causative agents and some specific characteristics are presented comparatively in Table 19.

1. *Psoroptic scabies* (*common cattle scab*). Until recent years, as the name suggests, psoroptic scabies has been the common form of bovine mange. Although affecting all types of cattle, beef breeds of the western ranges of the United States were often seriously parasitized and sometimes were in advanced stages of the disease before diagnosis was established. Since approximately 1935, and as a result of state-federal eradication programs, the incidence of the disease has diminished to a low level (Cattle Scab and Methods of Control, 1953). While all breeds, sexes and ages are susceptible, the disease occurs more commonly in cattle 6 months of age and older. During recent years sporadic outbreaks have occurred in both feedlot and show cattle.

The causative mite, *Psoroptes equi* var. *bovis*, is oval-shaped and white. The mouth parts are elongated, sharp and piercing, and the pedicels, or leg stalks, are relatively long and jointed.

The entire life cycle, lived on the skin of the one host, requires 10 to 12 days for completion. Survival time of the parasite away from the host varies with humidity, environmental temperature, and exposure to direct sunshine. Usually survival does not exceed 2 to 3 days, but under laboratory conditions the viability of mites separated from the host has extended beyond 2 or 3 weeks. Reproduction occurs only on the skin of the host. Following ovaposition and an incubation period of 3 to 4 days, the eggs hatch and form larvae. After two molts, the adults emerge and mate and the females complete the life cycle by ovapositing on the same host (Cattle Scab and Methods of Control, 1953).

In early stages of the disease the parasites show a predilection for the skin of the withers, back and tailhead. As the disease progresses, other anatomical areas become involved and in advanced stages the infestation may be generalized. Poorly nourished and aged cattle are more severely affected. Early lesions show acute dermatitis with crusts of dehydrated serum, blood and ex-

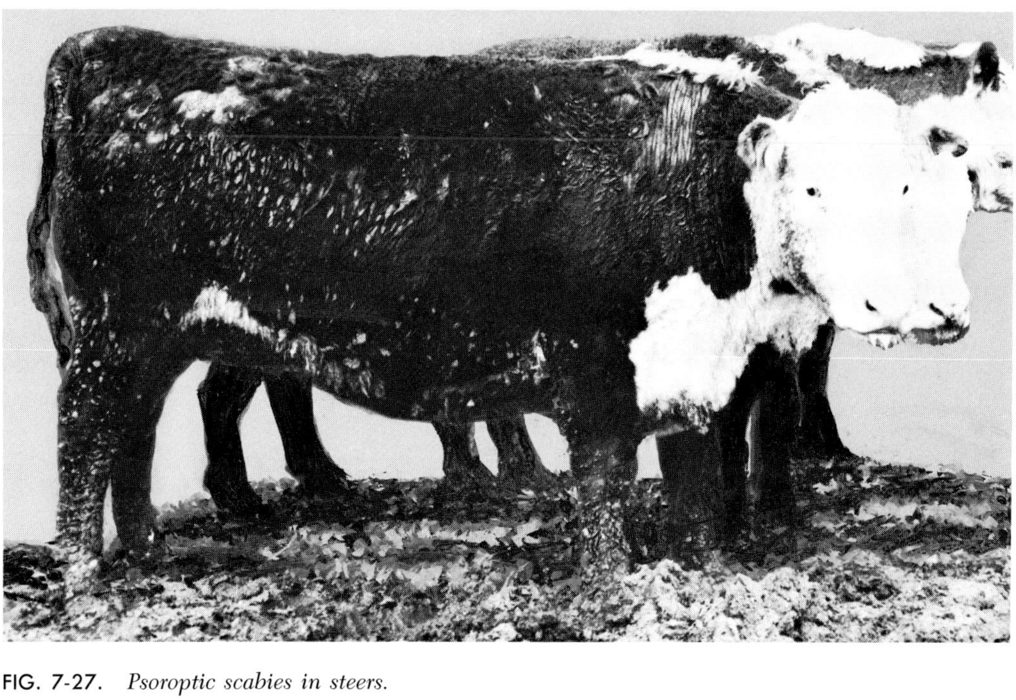

FIG. 7-27. *Psoroptic scabies in steers.*

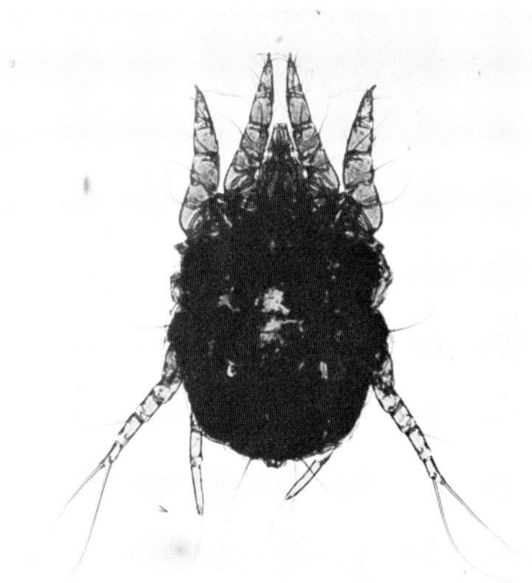

FIG. 7-28. *Psoroptes equi var. bovis.* × 83.

foliated cells among the hairs. In more advanced stages, the enlarged lesion is scaly and denuded towards the center and crusted at the periphery. The tissue changes result from feeding by the parasite. With piercing mouth parts, the parasite feeds on lymph and tissue fluids and, in the process, serum and blood escape to and accumulate on the skin surface. Irritating saliva of the parasite, injected at the time of feeding, causes a severe itching. Because the mites live on the skin surface, and feed usually at the periphery of the lesion, the infested area expands.

As a contagious disease, transmission usually occurs by direct physical contact or when the itching lesions impel affected cattle to rub against fixed objects and/or other cattle. Once the disease is introduced into feedlots, crowding facilitates the spread of scabies. While infested combs, brushes and blankets may also transmit the disease, this equipment, commonly used on show cattle, is seldom employed on feedlot animals. Frequent and common use of bedding, however, may be a means of spread. While scabies is usually host specific, it has been observed to transfer temporarily to a related foreign host. Under conditions of crowding, sheep scabies has transferred to cattle where temporary skin lesions developed (Cattle Scab and Methods of Control, 1953).

Clinical signs relate to the parasitic itching dermatitis. In early stages affected animals, even though flies are not a problem, are restless and violently switch their tails. They lick, bite, kick and scratch the infested skin. Rubbing occurs against fences, barns, trees and other cattle. As a result of rubbing and tissue changes, lesions become denuded and scaly. Affected cattle consume less feed and may lose body weight. Detectable clinical signs and skin lesions are often present 15 to 45 days following exposure. During summer, when cattle are grazing good pasture, the lesions and signs abate and during winter they augment. Unless properly treated, the disease endures indefinitely and eventually causes death.

The diagnosis is based on typical clinical signs, skin lesions and identification of the causative mite. Itching, indicated by tail switching, restlessness and violent rubbing, should direct attention to the possibility of scabies. Anatomical areas of dermatitis, especially over the withers, back and tailhead, suggest psoroptic scabies. In the search for the causative mites, deep skin scrapings, made in new lesions or at the periphery of older lesions, should be sufficiently deep to enter the derma and start hemorrhage. When the scrapings are placed on a dark smooth surface, warmed by sunshine or other means, and viewed with slight magnification through a hand lens, the light colored mites can be seen moving on the dark background. Repeated scraping may be necessary to verify or to exclude a diagnosis of scabies. Scabies dermatitis may be confused with eczema, lousiness, photosensitization and injuries from chemical irritants.

2. *Sarcoptic scabies (barn itch)*. Sarcoptic scabies or mange occurs in all breeds and sexes of cattle, but dairy animals and purebred bulls are more commonly affected. Adult cattle, especially 6 months of age and older, are susceptible. Although the total incidence is low and many states are free

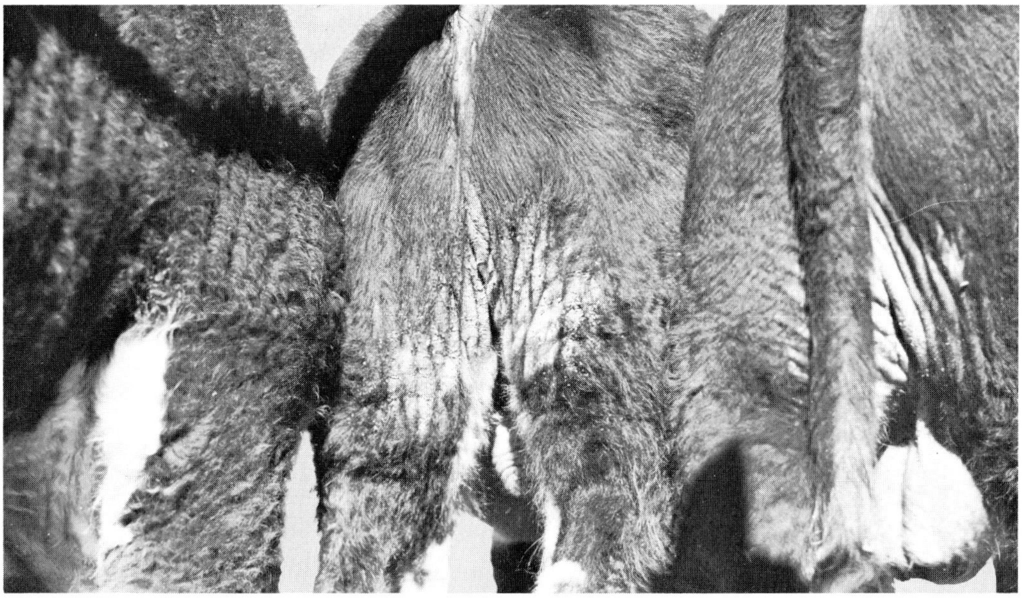

FIG. 7-29. *Sarcoptic scabies in feedlot cattle.* (*Courtesy of Dr. H. E. Kemper, ARS.*)

from the disease over prolonged periods, occasional outbreaks are encountered in most regions of the United States. In addition to cattle, other species of domestic and wild animals are attacked by sarcoptic mites which are, to a large extent, host specific. Even though the disease endures indefinitely in untreated animals, it is more severe in winter months and abates during summer when animals are provided high quality pasture.

The causative mite, *Sarcoptes scabiei bovis*, nearly round in body outline, possesses

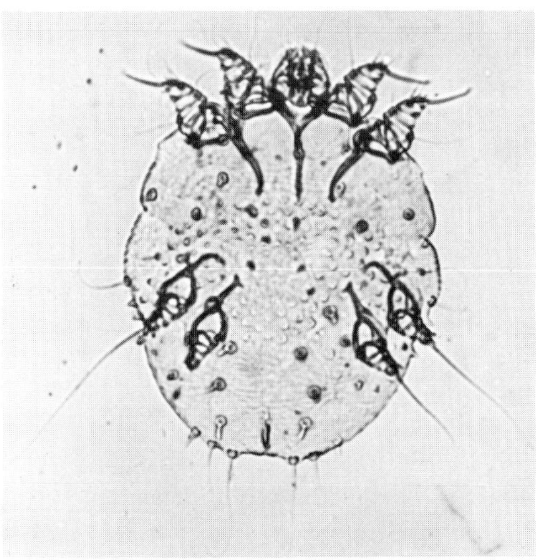

FIG. 7-30. *Sarcoptes scabiei.* × 100.

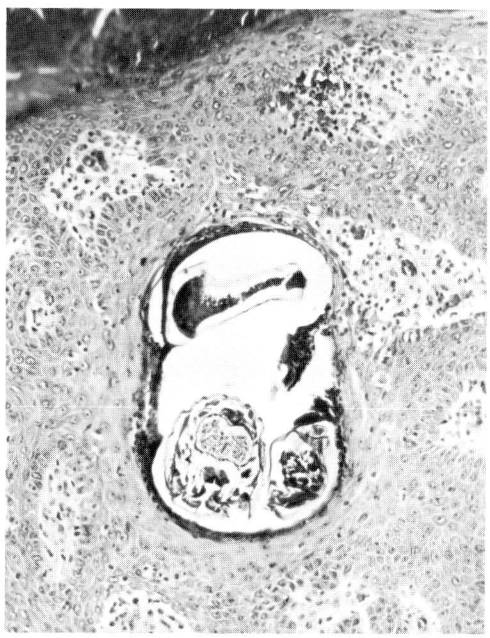

FIG. 7-31. *Skin tunnel from sarcoptic scabies. H&E stain.* × 149.

short blunt mouth parts and long unjointed pedicels or leg stalks. The four pairs of legs are short and stout.

The entire life cycle is lived in the skin of the host. After an incubation period of 3 to 10 days the eggs hatch, and approximately 11 days from hatching the parasite has matured, mated and produced new eggs. Beneath the skin surface, in tunnels created in the host epidermis, the adult mites live most of their life cycles, including mating, ovaposition and hatching. In the process of feeding they inject their irritating saliva which in turn causes severe itching, and serum and some blood exude to the surface, dehydrate, and form a crust. When separated from the natural host, the mite survives for a few days only.

Like common scabies, sarcoptic mange is transmitted largely by direct physical contact. Crowding in feedlots, frequent and common use of bedding, and rubbing against fences, barns and other cattle facilitate spread of the disease. While combs, brushes, and blankets and halters may mechanically transmit the mites from an infested to susceptible animal, these types of equipment are seldom used on feedlot animals. The disease may be transported spatially through movement of infested but undiagnosed cattle. The rate of spread is slow and some individual animals, even though in direct contact with infested cattle, may not develop the disease. The bovine mite, when transferring to a foreign host, such as sheep, horses and man, survives only temporarily, and eventually the new colony diminishes and disappears.

The clinical signs of sarcoptic mange come from the dermatitis and severe itching. Affected cattle nervously switch the tail, rub against fences, barns, posts, other cattle, and lick, bite and kick the irritated skin. Feed consumption diminishes and body weight decreases. Careful examination in early stages of the disease discloses skin lesions in the escutcheon and medial surfaces of the thighs, and the parasitized skin is swollen and contains multiple conical papillae with dried, yellowish serum. Persisting hairs stand erect. From points of predilection for early lesions, the disease spreads anteriorly along the abdomen to the brisket and neck, and posteriorly over the lateral surfaces of the limbs to the tailhead. Eventually, in advanced stages of the disease, when the mites are relatively inactive, the thickened skin is denuded, scaly, and wrinkled.

Scabies is suspected in cattle manifesting typical clinical signs and lesions of dermatitis. A positive diagnosis, however, can be made only by isolating and identifying the causative mite, *Sarcoptes scabiei bovis*. During the summer the dermatitis abates and the animals become more thrifty; in the subsequent winter, however, the disease augments and adversely affects the host.

Because of their burrowing habits, the mites are difficult to find, especially during early stages of the disease. Multiple scrapings may be necessary and should be secured from all layers of the epidermis. With the scrapings displayed on a dark warmed surface and magnified with a hand lens, the moving mites are detectable.

3. *Chorioptic Scabies* (*symbiotic scab; tail scab*). During recent years the incidence of chorioptic mange has increased, especially in the midwestern and northeastern parts of the United States (Cattle Scab and Methods of Control, 1953). This actual increase and the extensive state-federal eradication programs against common mange have made chorioptic scabies more frequently encountered than psoroptic scabies. All breeds, sexes and ages, but especially animals 6 months of age and older, are susceptible to the disease. Like other types of scabies, chorioptic mange abates during summer and increases and spreads during winter.

The mites are laterally compressed and possess short blunt mouth parts and unjointed pedicels or leg stalks. Living in colonies, the mites penetrate the skin with the piercing mouth parts and ingest lymph. The resulting spread of skin lesions is slow but inexorable.

Similar to common mange mites, *Chorioptes bovis* inhabits the host skin surface; its

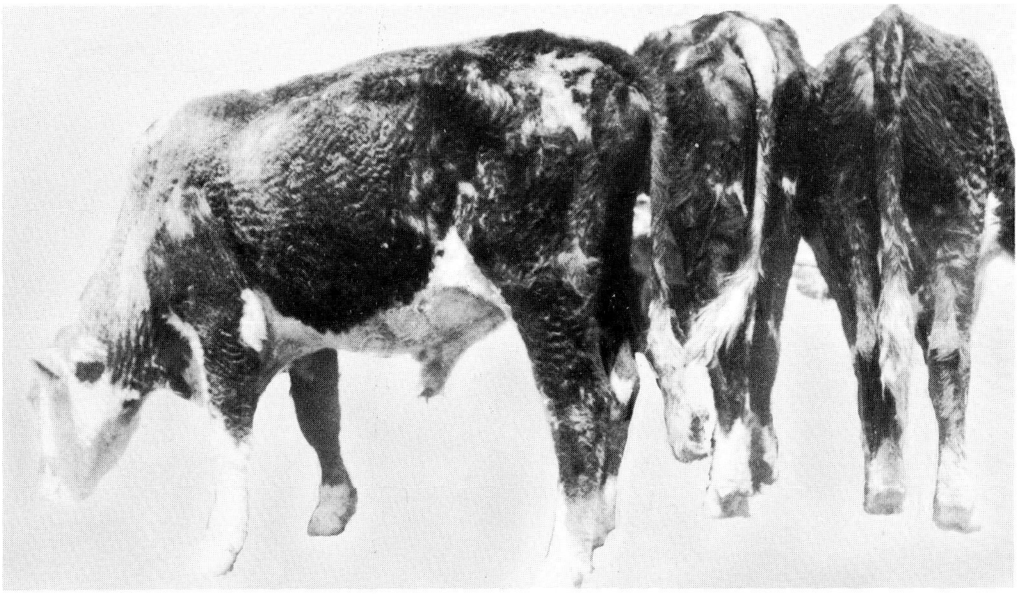

FIG. 7-32. *Chorioptic scabies in cattle.* (*Courtesy of Dr. H. E. Kemper, U.S.D.A., Albuquerque, New Mexico*)

life cycle requires 19 to 23 days for completion. When separated from the host, the mites die after a few days; but under laboratory conditions of controlled temperature and humidity, they have survived several weeks (Sweatman, 1957).

In early stages the lesions of chorioptic scabies are commonly found in the escutcheon, but have also been observed on the muzzle and around the coronary bands of feedlot cattle (Monlux, Raum, Diesch and Hunt, 1961). As the disease progresses, escutcheon lesions spread laterally onto the medial aspect of the thighs and anteriorly to the flanks and dorsally to the tail; and in advanced stages, the lesions extend over the sides of cattle. The dermatitis begins with puncture of the skin, and at each point of feeding, a papule forms and serum accumulates. As the lesion develops, the papules coalesce and the dehydrated serum forms a crust. Eventually, the parasitized skin becomes denuded, thickened and wrinkled. The crust may be fissured by flexion of the skin.

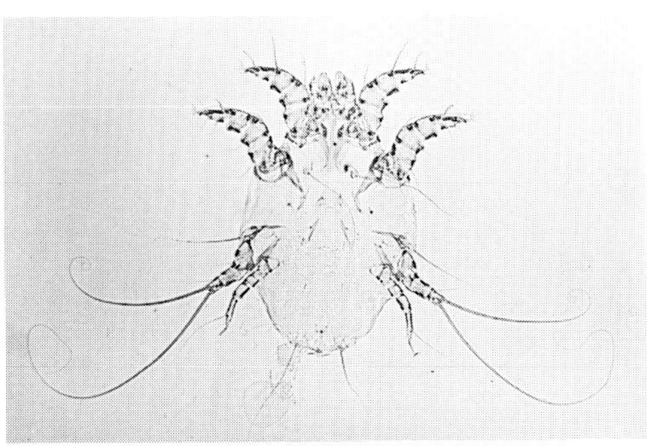

FIG. 7-33. *Chorioptes bovis.* × 66.

As with other forms of mange, chorioptic scabies evokes itching, although frequently to a less intense degree. Annoyed by the parasites and the itching, the animals shake and switch their tails, rub against fixed objects and other cattle, lick, bite and kick the irritated skin. Feed consumption declines, the rates of gain in body weight diminish and previous gains may be lost.

The diagnosis is based on the manifestation of clinical signs and typical lesions, and on the isolation and identification of the specific mite. In examining for mites, deep scrapings of the skin are made in new lesions or at the periphery of old lesions. The scrapings are placed on a smooth black surface, warmed, and examined with a hand lens for the mov-

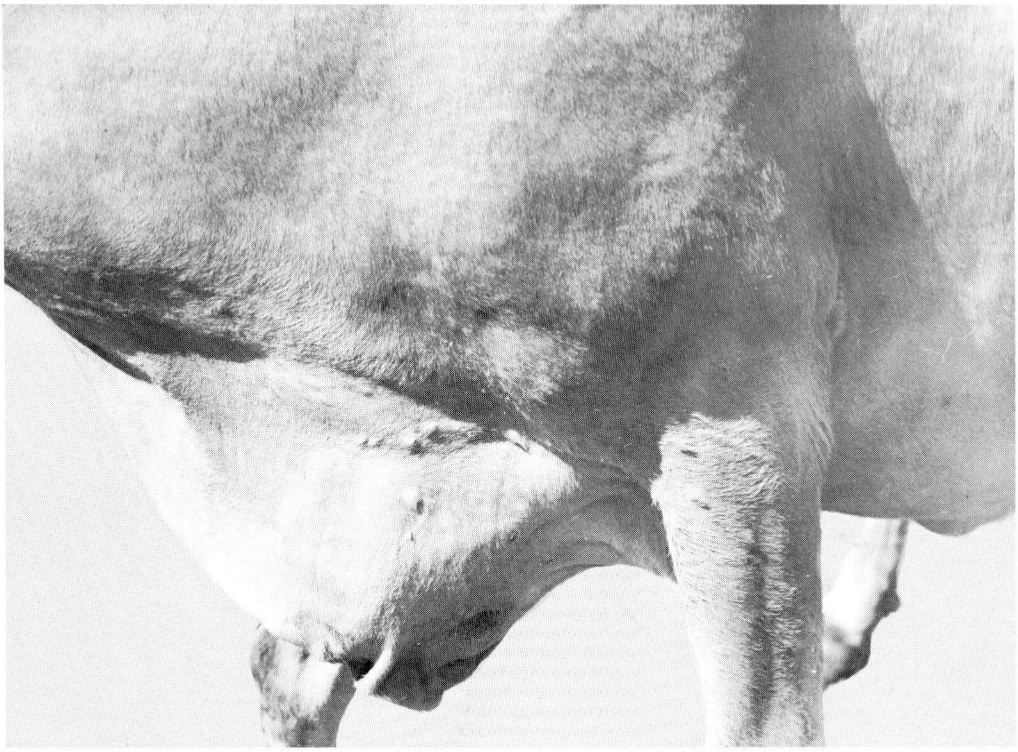

FIG. 7-34. *Demodectic scabies.* (*Courtesy, Laboratory, U.S.D.A., Agri. Res. Service, Albuquerque, New Mexico*)

ing parasites. The final identification requires microscopic examination.

4. *Demodectic scabies* (*follicular mange*). In cattle demodectic mange is inconspicuous but perhaps more common than is often suspected (Kemper and Peterson, 1952). In Canada, where the disease was seldom diagnosed, an incidence survey was conducted on 18 herds, including 828 animals. Of these, all herds but one were infested and the average herd incidence was 40.8%. Animals of all ages, excepting calves, and animals of many breeds, including Hereford, Shorthorn and Aberdeen Angus, were affected (Smith, 1961). In Germany a survey of 1620 dairy cattle identified 160 (10%) animals, all 2 years of age or older, with the disease. Incidence within herds varied from 1.5 to 48% (Schulz, Gräfner and Hiepe, 1968). And in Britain a sample of 250 slaughtered cattle were studied, and demodectic mites were found in ocular Meibomian glands of two animals (Kirkwood and Kendall, 1960). Since the disease is persistent, it occurs at all seasons, although with greater intensity during winter months.

The causative agent, *Demodex folliculorum bovis,* is approximately 0.2 mm in length and possesses four pairs of short heavy legs. Living in colonies, it parasitizes hair follicles and often with bacteria stimulates a local inflammatory reaction. The colonies of mites and bacteria, exudate and necrotic cells distend adjacent hair follicles and convert the affected tissue into a cystic mass which resembles an abscess. In dogs the mange mite occasionally invades the internal organs, but in cattle remains localized in the skin. The life cycle is unknown, but assumedly it may occur, as do the other three, entirely in the host skin. While the means of transmission are unknown, direct contact is also assumed to be one important method of spread.

In cattle, demodectic mange produces relatively few clinical signs. Most affected animals, although not all, show no evidence of itching, but when itching does occur, rubbing, scratching and biting may open the foci of infestation. Distributed in the skin of the shoulders, neck, dewlap and brisket, the lesions are multiple, nodular and easily detected by passing the hand over the surface of the parasitized skin. Large nodules are even visibly conspicuous for each nodule is covered by a thin scab and erected hair. Removal of the scab and forcible expression of the nodular contents reveal a core of firm necrotic tissue surrounded by purulent exudate.

Clinical diagnosis is based on the presence of typical skin nodules over the shoulders and neck. Confirmation can be obtained by microscopically identifying *Demodex folliculorum bovis* within the nodule contents. Movements of the living and freshly expelled mites facilitate location and identification.

Prevention and Treatment. All types of bovine scabies can be prevented by avoiding exposure of susceptible cattle to infested animals. Prior to admission to a clean feedlot all animals should be dipped or sprayed with an approved medicament. This procedure avoids the introduction of scabies into clean herds by animals in the early and inapparent stages of infestation. In addition lice and some ticks are eliminated.

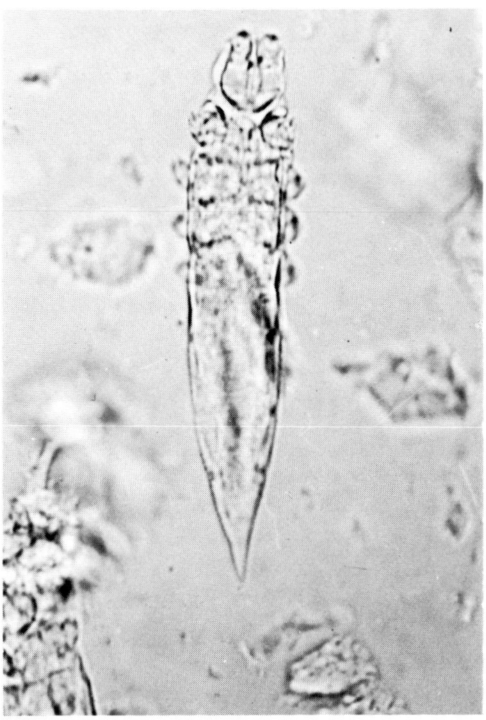

FIG. 7-35. *Demodex folliculorum bovis.* × 269.

In the United States, psoroptic, sarcoptic and chorioptic mange are contagious and reportable. In most states affected animals are quarantined until properly treated and declared free of the disease. Treatment consists of the application of a 0.5% concentration of Toxaphene spray or dip. The process is under the supervision of the state or federal government. To maintain the correct concentration the solution must be tested at frequent intervals. Usually a single application is adequate.

Historically, scabies has been officially treated with lime-sulfur dip which has been available as a commercial product used according to directions of the manufacturer or as a locally prepared mixture of:

unslaked lime	12 pounds
sulfur flour	24 pounds
soft water	100 gallons

To prepare the dip, the lime and sufficient water are mixed to form a paste. After sifting the sulfur into the paste, the mixture is thoroughly stirred and slowly added to 30 gallons of boiling water. To avoid settling of solids the mixture is stirred and boiled continuously for 1.5 to 2 hours. After dissolution of the sulfur and the formation of an amber color, the mixture is settled and the supernatant removed and added to sufficient water to make 100 gallons of concentrated solution. For use, 30 gallons of the concentrate are added to 70 gallons of water. Heated to 95° to 105° F, the dip is applied by submersion of the animals in a vat.

Demodectic mange is not reportable. A satisfactory means of treatment has not been developed. Experimentally, the use of an organophosphate compound administered systemically was ineffective (Smith, 1962).

References

Cattle Scab and Methods of Control and Eradication. Farmers' Bull. No. 1017. U. S. Dept. of Agriculture. (1953): 1–26.

Kemper, H. E. and Peterson, H. O.: Treatment of Cattle Scabies with Lindane. Vet. Med., *47* (1952): 453–455.

Kirkwood, A. and Kendall, J. B.: Demodectic Mange in Cattle. Vet. Rec., *78* (1966): 33-34.

Koutz, F. R.: *Demodex folluculorum* Studies: V. Demodectic Mange in Cattle. Vet. Med., *50* (1955): 305–306.

———: *Demodex folliculorum* Studies. VI. The Internal Phase of Canine Demodectic Mange. JAVMA, *131* (1957): 45–48.

Losses in Agriculture. Agricultural Research Service. U.S.D.A. Agricultural Handbook No. 291 (1965): 82.

Monlux, W. S., Raun, E. S., Diesch, S. J. and Hunt, J. A.: Foot Rot and a Mucosal-Type Disease. JAVMA, *138* (1961): 379–381.

Nemeséri, von L. and Széky, A.: Die Rinderdemodikose. Berl. und Munch. Tierarz. Woch., *75* (1962): 304–307.

Roberts, Irwin H. and Rogoff, Wm. M.: Organic Insecticides for the Control of Swine Mange. JAVMA, *123* (1953): 227–231.

Schulz, W., Grafner, G. and Hiepe, T.: Demodectic Mange in Cattle. Mh. Vet. Med., *23* (1968): 535–540.

Smith, H. J.: Bovine Demodicidosis. I. Incidence in Ontario, Canad. J. Comp. Med., *25* (1961): 165–169.

———: Bovine Demodicidosis. II. Clinical Manifestations in Ontario. Canad. Jour. Comp. Med., *25* (1961): 201–204.

———: Bovine Demodicidosis. III. Its Effect on Hides and Leather. Canad. Jour. Comp. Med., *25* (1961): 243–246.

———: Bovine Demodicidosis. VI. An Attempt at Treatment with a Systemic Organic Phosphate Insecticide. Canad. Jour. Comp. Med., *26* (1962): 42.

Sweatman, G. K.: Life History, Non-Specificity, and Revision of the Genus Chorioptes, a Parasitic Mite of Herbivors. Canad. J. Zool., *35* (1957): 641–689.

Tobin, W. C.: Cattle Scabies Can be Costly. JAVMA, *141* (1962): 845–847.

Flies

The arthropods herein considered are dipterous insects whose adults frequent feedlots and cause injury to cattle. Of a large number of species of dipterous flies which are agricultural pests, at least five are of economic importance to the cattle industry: horn flies, stable flies, horse flies, face flies and house flies.

As a group, these insects are active during the warm weather of spring, summer and autumn. Most of the species breed in media near feedlots and annually produce multiple generations. All species annoy cattle by frequenting the skin surface, and some cause physical injury by feeding on blood and by transmitting infectious diseases. Conservative estimates of annual losses in the United States to the cattle industry was $261 million (Losses in Agriculture, 1965). In Kansas, experiments conducted with pastured cattle demonstrated the economic importance of fly control. In seven experiments involving cows, calves and a mixture of cows and calves, lots of cattle treated to minimize fly injury were compared with cattle receiving no treatment. In each of the seven experiments the average daily gain in body weight for treated cattle exceeded the gains in untreated animals by as much as one-half pound (Laake, 1946).

While most feedlot enterprises are seasonal and concentrated during the winter, many lots are in use during the terminal autumnal fly period and during the early spring period. During recent years the number of enterprises practicing continuous feedlot fattening has increased, but in general, fly problems are most intense during July and August.

Important Species. While most species of flies frequenting feedlots either annoy or injure cattle, both effects reduce the rate of fattening and result in economic loss. Flies of great economic importance are as follows:

1. *Horn flies* (*Hematobia irritans*). During warm seasons horn flies and cattle coexist. Individual flies are approximately 4 mm in length and dark gray in color. Habitually in clusters, the flies live constantly on cattle. Frequently they rest on skin of the shoulders, neck and horns. Commonly 150 to 300 and occasionally 1,000 to 4,000 horn flies may live simultaneously on a single host. The

continuous presence and intermittent feeding by the flies disturb the cattle, and this persistent annoyance results in slower rates of gain. The flies feed on blood by penetrating the skin with piercing mouth parts. Each fly feeds 30 to 40 times daily and the total daily feeding time is 100 to 150 minutes. The intermittent feeding habit may enable mechanical transmission of some infectious diseases. In controlled experiments, dairy cattle subjected to horn fly injury decreased productivity 1.4% during the first month and 13.1% later (Freeborn, Regan and Folger, 1925). The annual loss to the cattle industry of the nation has been estimated at $115 million (Losses in Agriculture, 1965).

The fertilized females leave the host long enough to deposit eggs in fresh manure. Following hatching, the larvae live in and feed on moist manure. Pupation occurs in the same medium, and the adult fly emerges approximately 21 days following ovaposition. During summer months each bovine animal produces approximately 10 fecal boluses per day, and an average of 6 to 10 flies emerge per bolus.

2. *Stable flies* (*Stomoxys calcitrans*). Gray, with 7 spots on the abdomen, the stable fly measures approximately 6 to 7 mm in length. Although not residing continuously on the host, by penetrating the skin with the piercing mouth parts, it attacks usually twice daily to feed on blood. Commonly 8 to 10 flies simultaneously frequent a single host. Following the feeding, the fly rests on fences and building exteriors. The vicious feeding of stable flies agonize and annoy the host, and remove blood. Estimates of the annual loss in the United States to the cattle industry was $74 million (Losses in Agriculture, 1965). In Texas severe stable fly injury resulted in 40 to 60% reduction in productivity of dairy cattle and marked loss of body weight in beef animals. In northern Texas, 300 cattle and horses died from injurious effects (Bishopp, 1913). By successive feeding on a series of cattle, the stable fly has mechanically transmitted anthrax from infected to susceptible cattle.

Breeding occurs in organic material. The gravid female ovaposits in moist, decaying straw, hay, grain, other feeds and manure. After hatching, the larvae feed on the moist decaying plant tissue and grow to approximately 15 to 20 mm in length in 1 to 2½ months. After a pupation period of 1 to 3 weeks, the adult fly emerges and begins a new life cycle.

3. *Horse flies* (*Tabanus spp.*). The horse fly family, *Tabanidae*, contains many species which are important pests in cattle production. Usually gray-blue or black in color, the horse fly measures 6 to 28 mm in length. While the males feed on plants, the females with their large piercing mouth parts penetrate the skin and feed on blood from cattle, horses and other domestic animals. Horse flies breed in a moist environment. Each gravid female lays several hundred eggs which usually are deposited on vegetation overhanging swamps, ponds, streams or stagnant water. Larvae in watering tanks often cause apprehension among laymen who are unable to identify them. Following hatching, the larvae drop into the water or mud where they live and feed on plant or animal material. The length of the larval period is extremely variable. Some species overwinter as larvae. Following completion of growth, the larvae move to drier soil and pupate below the surface. Adults emerge after approximately 8 days. The total developmental period averages approximately 100 days. Horse flies are strong fliers and fierce biters. Penetration of the skin by piercing mouth parts of the female flies causes pain, anxiety and loss of blood. Following feeding the large mouth parts may contain considerable residual or contaminating blood. This characteristic enables horse flies to mechanically transmit anaplasmosis and anthrax by feeding on infected and susceptible cattle in rapid succession. Estimates of annual losses in the United States to the cattle industry were $30 million (Losses in Agriculture, 1965). Losses come from unthriftiness, injury, and annoyance.

4. *Face flies* (*Musca autumnalis*). Intro-

duced from Europe, face flies were first observed in America in Nova Scotia (Vockeroth, 1953). Since that time the flies have spread southward and westward and have been observed in most parts of the United States (Dobson and Huber, 1961; Guide for Use of Insecticides, 1968). Closely resembling other species, the face fly is gray in color and measures 6 to 7 mm in length. With their sponging mouth parts, they feed on tears, mucus, saliva and fresh manure. Even though biting does not occur, large numbers of face flies around the eyes, nostrils and mouth are extremely annoying and thereby cause economic loss estimated at $42 million annually (Losses in Agriculture, 1965). Commonly 25 to 30 and occasionally 75 to 100 face flies congregate on the face of a single host and feed on nasal and ocular secretions. Infectious keratoconjunctivitis or pink eye probably is transmitted mechanically by these insects. Its wide geographic distribution and vast numbers make this disturbing species an economically important pest of feedlot cattle.

Gravid females deposit eggs in fresh manure. Following an incubation period of approximately 24 hours, hatching occurs and the emerging larvae live in and feed on the fresh manure. Pupation also occurs in the manure. Adult flies emerge approximately 2 weeks following ovaposition (Teskey, 1960).

5. *House flies* (*Musca domestica*). Perhaps the most abundant insect pest of feedlots is the house fly. Grey in color, it measures 6 to 7 mm in length. Feeding on organic liquids and wastes, the house fly causes extreme annoyance to cattle as well as to other domestic animals. While house flies are nonbiting, they cause serious economic losses through annoyance of cattle and by disease transmission. In controlled experimentation, dairy cattle subjected to house flies reduced productivity 3.3% during the first month of experimentation (Freeborn, Regan and Folger, 1925). Since these flies frequent feedlots, barns and the interiors of human residences, they create public health problems in both sanitation and esthetics.

The gravid female deposits eggs in manure, moist decomposing hay, grain garbage and other plant material. The eggs hatch after an incubation period from 12 to 36 hours. The larvae feed on the organic medium and grow to full size in 6 to 11 days. As with all flies, pupation occurs, and adults

TABLE 20 *Morphology and habits of common species of flies*

	Hematobia irritans (horn fly)	*Stomoxys calcitrans* (stable fly)	*Tabanus spp.* (horse fly)	*Musca autumnalis* (face fly)	*Musca domestica* (house fly)
1. Life history					
eggs, days	1	3	4–7 hrs.	1	1
larvae, days	5	15	60–90	5	3–7
pupae, days	4–5	10	14–21	7	5–15
adults, days	21	20	—	—	3–10
2. Adult size mm.	4	6–7	6–28	6–7	6–7
3. Adult markings	2 stripes on thorax	gray; 7 spots on abdomen	eyes narrowly separated	median abdominal stripe	gray; 4 stripes on thorax
4. Adult mouth parts	piercing	piercing	piercing	sponging	sponging
5. Eggs/female	25	25–100	—	25	400–1000
6. Adult food	blood	blood	males, plants; females, blood	mucus, tears, saliva, manure	liquids
7. Ovaposition in:	fresh manure	fermenting straw, feed	near water	fresh manure	manure, moist decaying plants

TABLE 21 *Insecticides for fly control (Guide for Use of Insecticides, 1968)*

Insect	Insecticide	Toler. ppm	Min. Days From Last Appl. to Slaughter	Formulation Strength	Amount of Formula/ Animal	Where and When to Apply
Horse flies and stable flies	Ciodrin	—	—	EC, 0.5 to 1% spray	1 to 2 pints	Wet entire surface when cattle enter feedlot. Repeat if necessary.
Face flies	Coumaphos	1 meat and fat	—	1% in oil	—	—
	Ronnel	0 meat	14	1% in oil	1 gal/ 20 ft cable	Saturate back rubbers for face access
Horn flies	Delnav	1	—	1.5% in oil	1 gal/ 20 ft cable	Saturate back rubbers
	Toxaphene	7	28	5% in oil		
	Ronnel	0 in meat	56	EC, 0.5% spray or 0.25% dip	1–2 qt	Every three weeks
	Malathion	4 in meat	—	EC or WP, 0.5% spray	2 qt.	
	Coumaphos	1 meat and fat	—	EC, 0.06% spray WP, 0.06% spray	1–2 qt.	
				Dust bag, 1% in talc		
	Ciodrin	—	—	Dust bag, 3% in talc		

emerge after 5 to 18 days. The rate of development through the immature stages varies with temperature; from 45 days at 16° C to 10 days at 30° C. Some common features of important feedlot flies are presented in Table 20.

Control of Flies. Since most flies of the feedlot breed in wet manure and moist fermenting feed, considerable fly control can be obtained by maintaining sanitary feedlots. While manure cannot be removed from pens at frequent intervals, moisture should not be permitted to accumulate around drinking equipment or any other place in or near feedlots. During summer, excepting periods of heavy rainfall, pens can be maintained sufficiently dry to inhibit fly breeding.

During summer and autumn an insecticide, such as Coumaphos, should be administered as a spray or dip soon after the cattle arrive at the feedlot. This initial application is highly efficacious in the control of grubs and lice throughout the total fattening period and for flies through a few weeks. Subsequently, horn flies and face flies can be controlled, as indicated in Table 21, by applying insecticides by means of backrubbing devices and dust bags which provide continuous self application of the insecticides. Organophosphate insecticides should be used according to directions and precautions recommended by the manufacturer.

References

Bishopp, F. C.: The Stable Fly: How to Prevent its Annoyance and its Losses to Livestock. Farmers' Bulletin 1097. 1913.

Dobson, R. C. and Huber, D. A.: Control of Face Flies

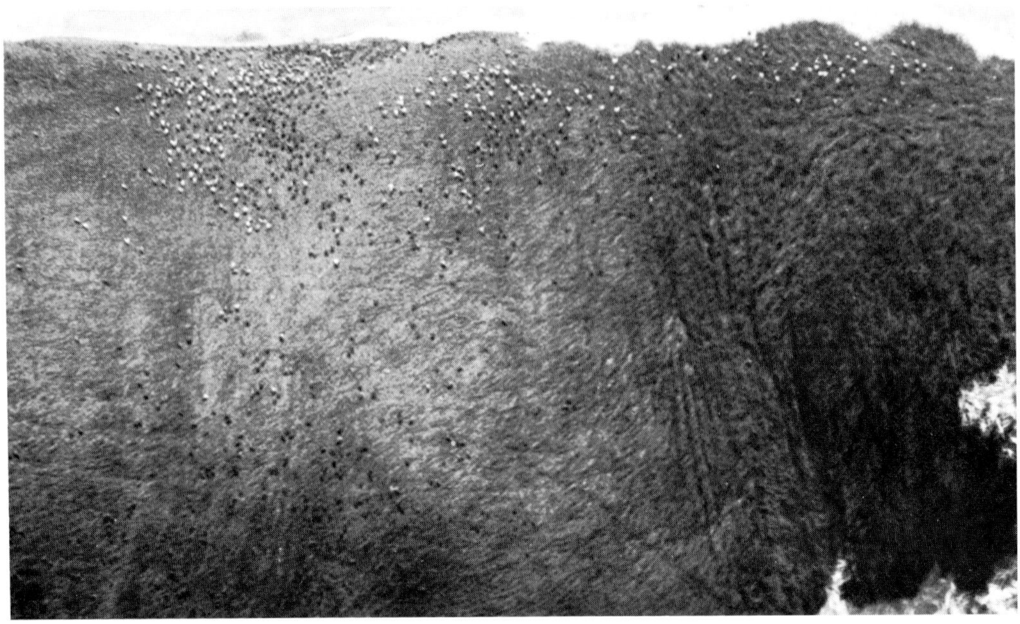

FIG. 7-36. *Horn flies on the skin.*

(*Musca autumnalis*) on Beef Cattle in Indiana. J. Econ. Ent., *54* (1961): 434–436.

Freeborn, S. B., Regan, W. M. and Folger, A. H.: The Relation of Fly Sprays to Milk Production. J. Econ. Ent., *18* (1925): 779–790.

Guide for Use of Insecticides. Agricultural Handbook No. 331. ARS and FS USDA (1968).

Horn Fly and its Control. Leaflet 205. USDA 1940.

Horn Flies on Cattle. Leaflet 388. USDA 1963.

House Fly. Leaflet 390 USDA 1963.

Howell, D. E.: Fly Control in Oklahoma. Okla. Agri. Expt. Sta. Bull. B-385. Sept. 1952.

Laake, E. W.: DDT for Control of the Horn Fly in Kansas. J. Econ. Ent., *39* (1946): 65–68.

Losses in Agriculture. Agricultural Handbook No. 291. ARS. USDA (1965): 82.

Stable Flies. How to Control Them. Leaflet 338. USDA. 1953.

Teskey, H. J.: A Review of Life-history and Habits of *Musca autumnalis* de Greer (Diptera: *Muscidae*). Canad. Ent., *92* (1960): 360–362.

Vockeroth, J. R.: *Musca autumnalis* Deg. in North America (Diptera: *Muscidae*). Canad. Ent., *85* (1953): 422–423.

Screwworm Myiasis

Screwworm myiasis is an invasion of injured but living tissues by the larvae of the dipterous fly, *Cochliomyia hominivorix.* Prior to the introduction of fly eradication programs, this parasitic disease caused to the United States cattle industry annual economic losses from attack on 1.5 million animals estimated at $100 million. Losses resulted from mortality, loss of body weight, incapacitation and disfigurement of infested animals and from expensive prevention and treatment programs.

Review of Literature. While recognized in the southwestern part of the United States and in Mexico for well over a century, in 1933 *C. hominivorax,* spreading to the southeastern United States, thrived and inflicted heavy losses until 1959 when eradicated from that geographic area (U.S.D.A., 1963; Status of Screwworms, 1962).

Basic research on the susceptibility of insects to irradiation revealed that x-irradiated cigarette beetles produced infertile eggs (Runner, 1916). With this beginning information, scientists of the United States Department of Agriculture promulgated the principle of insect eradication by wide geographic dispersal into the natural population of numerous sterile but sexually vigorous males. According to this principle, the biotic potential of a species is directly proportional to the ratio of fertile males to sterile males. The number of fertile female matings to sterile males is proportional to the ratio of sterile males to the fertile males. As an example, the natural population of flies may contain 1 million fertile females and 1 million fertile males. The introduction of 1 million sterile males would result in approximately one-half the female flies mating with sterile males and a reduction in the size of the next generation by one-half plus the progeny of the fertile matings. The continuous introduction of a million sterile males to each generation would increase the ratio of sterile males to fertile males, proportionately reduce the number of matings of fertile males to fertile females, and eventually reduce the biotic potential of the species to zero (Bushland and Hopkins, 1951; Knipling, 1955; 1959; 1963). Following the development of methods for culturing screwworms (Smith, 1960) and the discovery that exposure of screwworm pupae to 8,000 roentgens of gamma rays resulted in sterile but sexually vigorous males, the principle was tested in a pilot experiment on Curacao Island in the Netherlands Antilles. This isolated island, containing an area of approximately 170 square miles, was heavily infested with screwworms. In 1954, sterilized male flies were released weekly at the rate of 400 per square mile. After approximately 14 weeks, the last sterile eggs were found and screwworms were eradicated from the island (Baumhover *et al.*, 1955; Status of Screwworm, 1962). Because of isolation from other infected areas the island remained clean.

Because of the effectiveness of the eradication on Curacao Island, similar programs were undertaken in southeastern United States. In 1957 eradication was initiated in Florida, Alabama, Georgia and South Carolina. Sterile flies, including males and females, were released at the rate of 1,000 per square mile per week. Supplementary measures included: the establishing and operating of inspection stations at peripheral fringes for the examination for possible screwworm infestations of animals entering the area, careful examination of animals by owners, treatment for screwworm infestation, reporting of outbreaks and informing the public about the program. By 1959, screwworms were eradicated from the southeastern area (USDA, 1963; Status of Screwworms, 1962), and acting on previously gained information, a similar eradication campaign was initiated in February 1962 for the southwestern part of the United States. Sterile flies were released in the overwintering areas of southern Texas and southern New Mexico, Southern Arizona, Southern California and in northern Mexico. To avoid the importation of screwworms with infected cattle, livestock inspection stations were established along the United States-Mexican border, the coasts of Texas and Louisiana and the eastern boundaries of Louisiana and Arkansas (USDA, 1963).

Occurrence. Screwworm larvae attack all species of warm blooded animals. Screwworms occur in South America, Central America, nearby islands, and in the southwestern part of the United States. From 1933 through 1959 they were also found in the southeastern part of the United States. Overwintering occurs in climatically mild areas, especially in the southern parts of Texas, New Mexico, Arizona, California and in Mexico. From the overwintering areas, flies migrate northward during summer months and have been found in Nebraska and Colorado. The flies cannot overwinter where the average temperature is 50° F or lower for approximately 80 consecutive days. Screwworm infestation of cattle and other warm blooded animals occurs during the warm months of spring, summer and autumn when the adult female flies are active. Cattle of all breeds, ages and sexes are attacked in anatomical areas of injury.

Etiology and Pathogenesis. Screwworm infestation is caused by the larvae of *Cochliomyia hominivorax*. Blue-green in color, the adult flies measure approximately 12 to 15 mm in length. The head is orange and the dorsal thorax contains 3 longitudinal dark stripes. The mature larvae morphologically resemble a wood screw; the larval body tapers from the large posterior diameter anteriorly and possesses clusters of cuticular spines on each body segment. In the living maggot, tracheal trunks are discernible in the posterior segments.

The life history is typical of many dipterous flies. Masses of overlapping eggs are laid in or near injuries on cattle, sheep, swine, horses and other warm blooded animals. The female fly is attracted to injuries such as surgical incisions, accidental incisions, puncture wounds, tick bites, dog bites, bloody excretions from the genitalia and alimentary tracts, and the severed umbilici of newly born animals. A single female fly may lay as many as 4,000 eggs. Usually these are deposited in clusters of approximately 250 eggs cemented together. Hatching occurs in 10 to 12 hours, and the larvae bore into living tissue and at first are usually in clusters with the posterior extremities extending toward the surface. The maggots tear away and live on the live host tissue. Growing rapidly to maturity within 3 to 6 days, they drop from the host and pupate in the soil. Pupation lasts usually from 3 to 7 days but in cool temperature may extend over several weeks. The adults emerge and mate within a few days and egg laying can begin within 5 to 6 days from the time of adult emergence. With favorable temperature and climate, the average length of the life cycle is 21 days. Hibernation or overwintering occurs as pupae or adults in the mild climates of the southern parts of Texas, New Mexico, Arizona, California and in Mexico. The strong flying adults may travel 35 miles per week.

The newly hatched screwworm larvae crowd together, dig into, feed on and rapidly destroy host tissue. Infested tissue attracts additional female flies which ovaposit new batches of eggs. Toxemia and continuous destruction of tissue cause agonizing death of the host.

Clinical Signs and Postmortem Lesions. Cattle infested with screwworms manifest excruciating pain. Apprehensive and nervous, they separate from the herd and, in the seclusion of shade, bite and scratch at the infested wound. The body temperature may be elevated. Many species of flies, including female screwworm flies, are attracted to the infested wound which discharges a serosanguineous malodorous fluid. After cleaning the wound and removing the exudate, the observer sees the clusters of crowded screwworm larvae and the cavity created by the parasite. If untreated, the area of infestation continues to expand through the addition of new eggs. In terminal stages, the host is depressed, disoriented and often prostrated. Death usually occurs after a course of approximately 10 days.

At necropsy of fatally infested cattle, the prominent changes are in the area of the wound. Inflammatory exudate discharges from the infested wound and stains the surrounding skin. Following the removal of exudate, large numbers of screwworm larvae in various stages of development are observed in crowded nests. The infested cavity may be many inches in diameter. Infestations of the abdominal wall commonly extend into the peritoneal cavity. A foul odor emanates from the infested tissues and by scratching, rubbing and biting by the host, the infested wound may have been traumatized.

Beyond the area of infestation secondary changes may be discernible. Often the membranes are anemic from hemorrhage and frequently petechiated from intoxication. The liver, kidneys and myocardium may be swollen. The body cavities may have been invaded by screwworms as well as accompanying bacteria.

Diagnosis. Screwworm myiasis is diagnosed by finding and identifying larvae of *C. hominivorax* in the wound. Two signs attract attention: infested cattle isolate themselves from the herd and they scratch, rub and bite injured tissue. In endemic areas, veterinarians and livestock owners learn to detect infested animals and to identify screwworm larvae.

The differential diagnosis requires consideration of infestation with a common blowfly,

Cochliomyia macellaria. This fly deposits single eggs at random throughout the necrotic wound surface. The live larvae do not crowd together but move independently about the wound surface.

Prevention and Treatment. Screwworm infestation can be prevented to a degree by avoiding accidental injuries, such as puncture wounds from nails, wire, glass, dog bites and tick bites, and by scheduling surgery, such as castration, dehorning, ear marking, branding and calving during fly-free seasons. When injuries and surgical operations do occur during fly season, the traumatized animals should receive topical applications of preventive preparations such as Smear 62, EQ 335, or sprays of Coumaphos. The vulnerable animals should be observed at frequent intervals for the possible development of screwworm infestation. In feedlots, projecting nails, wires, bolts, wood splinters, glass and sharp stones should be removed from fences, sheds, feeding and watering equipment and the ground surface.

A more satisfactory method of prevention is regional or national eradication of screwworms. While the initial cost of the program is high, the subsequent economic savings to the livestock industry more than compensate for the initial investment. Successful eradication programs have been applied at Curacao Island off the coast of Venezuela, in the southeastern United States including Florida, Mississippi, Alabama, Georgia and South Carolina. A similar program had been initiated in southwestern states including the southern parts of Texas, New Mexico, Arizona and California. Each eradication program includes the following items:

1. The systematic and strategic release of sexually vigorous but gamma ray sterilized male flies in sufficient numbers and at frequent intervals to significantly dilute the normal fly population and to reduce the reproductive potential eventually to zero. The sterile male flies seek out and mate with normal female flies. Such matings produce infertile eggs. In the eradication program of the southeastern United States, screwworm larvae were cultivated artificially and, in the pupal stage, were sterilized by exposure to approximately 8,000 roentgens of gamma rays. Sterile male flies were released at the rate of approximately 500 per square mile per week over 80,000 square miles. Initiated in 1957, eradication was achieved by 1959.

2. All shipments of cattle into the clean area are through inspection stations where animals are carefully examined and where infestations are treated to avoid mechanical transfer of flies or larvae into the clean area. Inspection vigilance must continue as long as the danger of fly importation exists.

3. Livestock producers carefully detect and promptly report all new outbreaks of

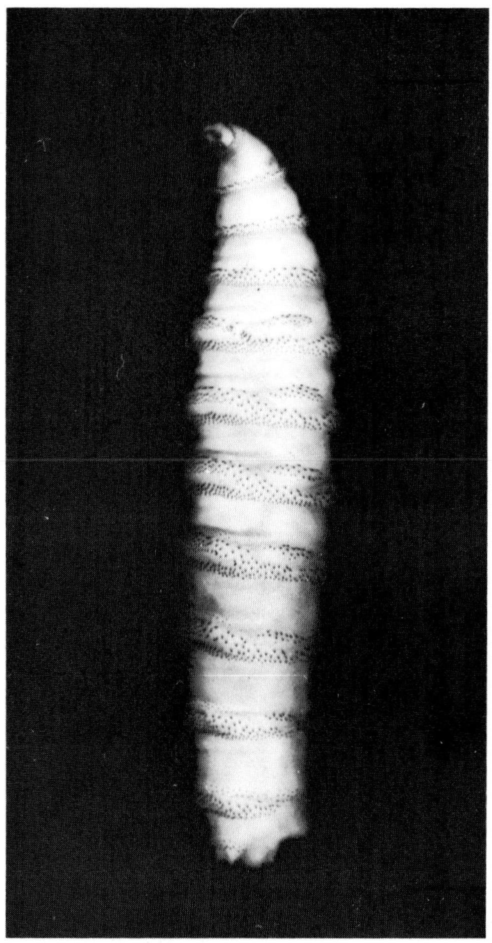

FIG. 7-37. *Mature screwworm larva.* × 11.

infestation to regulatory officials who apply eradication procedures to the new outbreaks. All livestock are protected against accidental injury and unnecessary surgery during fly seasons.

4. Livestock owners, veterinarians and others participate in disseminating relevant information to the general public. Infested wounds should be treated with Smear 62 or EQ 335 for removal of screwworms and for prevention of reinfestation.

References

Baumhover, A. H., Graham, A. J., Bitter, B. A., Hopkins, W. D., New, W. P., Dudley, F. H. and Bushland, R. C.: Screwworm Control Through Release of Sterilized Flies. J. Econ. Ent., *48* (1955): 462–468.

Bushland, R. C. and Hopkins, D. E.: Experiments with Screwworm Flies Sterilized by X-rays. J. Econ. Ent., *44* (1951): 725.

U. S. Dept. of Agriculture. Agricultural Research Service: Facts about Screwworm Eradication. ARS 91–39, Jan. 1963.

Knipling, E. F.: Possibilities of Insect Control or Eradication Through Use of Sexually Sterile Males. J. Econ. Ent., *48* (1955): 459.

———: Sterile-Male Method of Population Control. Science, *130* (1959): 902–904.

———: The Sterility Principle. Agricultural Science Review, *1* (1963): 2–12.

Losses in Agriculture. Agricultural Research Service. U.S.D.A. 1954. ARS-20-1.

Runner, G. S.: Effect of Roentgen Rays on the Tobacco, or Cigarette Beetle, and the Results of Experiments with a New Form of Roentgen Tube. J. Agr. Res., *6* (1916): 383–388.

Smith, Charles L.: Mass Production of Screwworms (*Callitroga hominivorax*) for the Eradication Program in the Southeastern States: Animal Disease Eradication. J. Econ. Ent., *53* (1960): 1110–1116.

Status of the Screwworm in the United States. ARS-22-79. Agric. Res. Serv. U.S.D.A. June 1962. pp. 1–13.

Hypodermosis

(GRUBS; OX WARBLES)

Hypodermosis, a non-febrile and parasitic disease of cattle, is caused by dipterous larvae of *Hypoderma lineatum* and *Hypoderma bovis*. Its chief characteristics are larval migrations in tissues and subcutaneous swellings in the back of the infected animal. Although widely damaging to cattle throughout the North Temperate Zone, this disease results in annual agricultural loss estimates for the United States alone at $115 million. For European agriculture, estimates are similar. Economic losses to the cattle industry result from several effects: diminished body weight, extreme harassment by female flies, unthriftiness during migration of fly larvae through tissues, trimming of expensive infected cuts of meat, devaluation of hides from multiple perforations, devaluation of trimmed carcasses and expensive prophylactic treatment.

Review of Literature. The mature larvae of *Hypoderma* spp. in the subcutis of the bovine back are macroscopic and conspicuous. Damaging and repulsive, the larval parasitism probably has existed throughout the observed historic period of the host-parasite relationship between domestic cattle and *Hypoderma* spp. Early observations (1797) of subcutaneous larvae led to the assumption that the adult female parasite, although unknown at the time, deposited eggs in the subcutis of the back where they hatched into larvae and grew to maturity (Clark, 1798). Towards the termination of the nineteenth century a sequence of important observations was made. In addition to their subcutaneous position, larvae were observed in the spinal epidural tissue and in the wall of the esophagus (Hinrichsen, 1888). Tracts considered to be caused by migrating larvae were observed in fasciae (Ruser, 1895). These additional positions of the parasite and the lesions from migrating larvae led to the conclusion that eggs or young larvae are ingested with contaminated feed and that the larvae penetrate from the lumen through the wall of the alimentary tract (Hinrichsen, 1888). Careful entomological observations recorded the deposition (Bishopp, 1926; Carpenter, Hewitt and Reddin, 1914; Riley, 1892) of numerous insect eggs on hairs, expecially of the limbs but also the bodies, of cattle, and researchers postulated that the eggs and larvae were licked from the hair and ingested by the host, and that the larvae penetrated from the lumen through the wall of the alimentary tract (Curtis, 1890). This view persisted for many years despite contrary evidence. In a research project conducted in Holland, viable larvae were removed from the spinal epidural tissues of slaughtered cattle and transplanted into the subcutaneous tissue of a goat; 12 days later dorsal subcutaneous swelling developed and eventually yielded larvae which pupated and finally metamorphosed to the adult flies. This historic event was the first observation irrefutably associating larvae and their respective adults. In the same research project, 26 viable larvae were transplanted beneath the skin of a dog. Two weeks later the larvae had migrated to other areas, including the esophagus and spinal epidural tissue of the new host (Koorevaar, 1899). In Ireland and later in the United States, ingress of the larvae was carefully investigated. Under controlled conditions, fertilized female flies were permitted to ovaposit on the hairs of experimental cattle which were restrained from licking their skins and from ingesting egg or larva contaminated food. Subsequently these cattle developed larvae in the walls of the esophagi, in the spinal epidural tissues and in the subcutis of the backs. Later the same investigators observed larvae emerge from eggs, move proximally along the hair shaft and penetrate the skin around the hair follicles. Serous exudate accumulated in the hairs around the points of penetration. Eventually larvae were observed in the wall of the esophagus, in the spinal epidural tissue and in the subcutis of the backs (Bishopp, Laake, Brundrett and Wells, 1926; Carpenter, Hewitt and Reddin, 1914).

Following elucidation of the life cycle, more attention was given to larvae in the wall of the esophagus and in the spinal epidural tissue. In Britain 3,211 larvae obtained from the walls of the esophagi from 7,440 slaughtered cattle were identified as *H. lineatum* (Beesley, 1961). In a Wisconsin project 982 larvae were removed from the spinal epidural tissues of slaughtered cattle; of these 975 were *H. bovis* and 5 were *H. lineatum*. In another sample of 982 larvae removed from the esophagi of slaughtered cattle, 981 were *H. lineatum* and 1 was *H. bovis* (Haberman, Morgan and Dickie, 1949).

Study of the invaded tissue revealed both gross and histopathologic changes. Collagenous fibers became swollen and eventually lysed. Cells underwent necrosis and exudate, consisting of leukocytes and fibrin, accumulated around parasites and bore tracts (Wolfe, 1959).

During the period of life-history studies, means of control were also being considered. Rotenone applied to the perforated back as a wash or powder was lethal to subcutaneous larvae during the period when grubs were situated in the subcutis of the back and respiring through holes in the skin. The application of rotenone at monthly intervals during the appropriate season and repeated annually reduced in 3 years in a county-wide area the incidence of grub infestation from approximately 70 to 3.7% (Spindler, Becklund and Peterson, 1955). The addition of several chlorinated hydrocarbon compounds did not increase the efficacy of the rotenone (Roberts, Lofgren and Berndt, 1953). Immediately following World War II, the efficacy of organophosphate compounds used as systemic insecticides was discovered. This group of compounds, phosphoric acid esters and derivatives, inhibit acetylcholinesterase in animal tissues. Some of these compounds were absorbed from the alimentary tract or from the skin in sufficient amounts to be toxic to migrating *Hypoderma* larvae while still being non-toxic to the cattle (Beesley, 1960; Radeleff, Woodward, Nickerson and Bushland, 1955). When the insecticides were applied orally, or dermally, the migrating larvae were destroyed, and treated cattle made superior weight gain over untreated animals (Jones, Brundrett and Radeleff, 1957; McGregor and Bushland, 1957; Raun and Herrick, 1957). In some investigations, however, even though the grubs were destroyed a superior rate of gain in body weight was not demonstrable (Baird, McCampbell, Ciordia, White and Bizzell, 1962; Marquhart and Hawkins, 1962).

Occurrence. All breeds and sexes of cattle are susceptible to hypodermosis. The phase of the disease in which mature larvae are in the subcutis of the back is found in animals 1 year of age and older. Young cattle appear to be more susceptible and may harbor 100 or more larvae. The higher incidence in young cattle may result from avoidance of ovaposition by older cattle or the development of resistance to the parasitism. The disease rarely occurs in people or horses.

Some phase of the disease occurs in all months. Ovaposition takes place during early spring and summer months and larval migration during the remaining months. The emergence of adult flies, their mating and ovaposition by the females varies with latitude, altitude and the seasons. The advent of spring weather within any geographic area varies annually. Table 22 presents the seasonal occurrence of ovaposition and the first appearance of larvae in the backs in different areas in the United States. Because of weather differences, variances from these times may be 1 month plus or minus. *H. bovis* occurs in the northern half of the United States, especially in the northeastern States, while *H. Lineatum* exists throughout the entire United States. Both species occur also in Canada, Europe and Asia.

Etiology and Pathogenesis. Hypodermosis is caused by two species of dipterous flies *H. lineatum*, the common heel fly, and *H. bovis*, the northern heel fly. Nearly 1 year is required for completion of the life cycle of both species. The robust and hairy adults contain bands of orange-yellow hairs on the thorax.

Life histories of the two species are complex and similar but with the one exception in timing. The life-history events of *H. bovis* occur a few weeks later in the season than the corresponding events in the history of *H. lineatum*. The adult flies emerge from pupae during early spring. Since functional mouth parts are absent, the adult flies do not feed. While they live from 1 to 25 days, the mean duration is 7 to 10 days. The fertilized females are active during the warm sunny days and inactive when temperatures are low. Seldom do they frequent shaded areas. The females attack cattle and ovaposit on the hairs of the distal parts of the hind limbs and also on the hocks and other parts of the body. Females of *H. lineatum* attach 5 to 7 eggs on a single hair shaft, while females of *H. bovis* attach single eggs to hair shafts. Several hundred eggs may be produced by a single female, and 100 eggs may be ovaposited on

TABLE 22 *Seasonal activities of Hypoderma spp.*

Activity	*Geographic Location*	*Time*
Ovaposition	Southwest plateau of Texas	Dec.–April 1
	North Texas, New Mexico, Arizona, So. California	Feb. 1–April 1
	Central belt of U. S.	Mar. 15–May 1
	Northern belt of U. S.	April 1–June 30
First appearance of larvae in subcutis of back	Southwest plateau of Texas	July–Aug.
	Northern Texas, Arizona, New Mex.	Oct. 10–30
	Central belt of the U. S.	Nov. 15–Dec. 15
	Northern belt of the U. S.	
	H. lineatum	Feb.–March
	H. bovis	March–April

a single bovine host. Eggs are yellow-white, smooth, glossy and ovoid. Measuring 0.76 x 0.21 mm, they form a 45° angle with the hair shaft.

Following an incubation period of 3 to 4 days the eggs hatch and the tiny larvae, 0.81 x 0.29 mm, move proximally along the hair shaft and penetrate the skin through hair follicles. Dermatitis with a serous exudate develops around points of penetration. Throughout approximately 150 days the first instar larvae migrate from the points of penetration through the subcutaneous tissue and intramuscular fasciae proximally along the limbs, and eventually into thoracic tissues. Larvae of *H. lineatum* assemble in the wall, especially the submucosa, of the esophagus, while larvae of *H. bovis* congregate in the spinal epidural fat. During periods of migration and residence in the esophagus and epidural tissues, the larvae grow to a length of 10 to 15 mm. Following approximately 3 months' residence in these locations, the larvae again migrate between muscles to a definitive position in the subcutis of the back; there they create and occupy, not cysts as is commonly stated, but cavities. Each larva cuts an aperture in the skin for respiration. Usually the posterior end of the larvae occupies the aperture, and the two posterior spiracles are visible. The larvae continue to grow, undergo two molts to form second and third instars, and acquire brown pigment in the cuticle.

Following maturation, the larvae emerge from the skin through the apertures and fall to the ground where they pupate. Some protection is usually obtained under debris or soil. After approximately 1 month the insect metamorphoses into an adult fly and a new life cycle begins. Table 23 presents the approximate number of days required for different stages of development, and Table 24 compares some characteristics of the two species.

TABLE 23 *Duration of developmental stages of Hypoderma spp.*

Event	Approximate Days
egg incubation	3–4
migration in tissues	150
residence in esophagus	90
residence in subcutis of back	40
pupation at 50° to 60° F	35
adult longevity	1–25

Occasionally, larvae, accompanied by bacteria, cause significant and damaging lesions. In the esophageal submucosa the death of larvae from systemic insecticides or other causes may stimulate an inflammatory reaction with swelling, edema and exudate. The tissue changes may be sufficient in amount to cause lumenal constriction that results in esophageal obstruction with feed. In the epidural tissues dead larvae also provoke inflammation. The swelling, edema, exudate and toxic substances may impair neural function and result in posterior paralysis. In the definitive position of the back, the subcutis containing second and their instar larvae frequently becomes secondarily infected with bacteria which enter the tissues through the skin perforations. The infection may spread along fasciae and between muscles. Purulent exudate may accumulate, surround the larvae and exude to the skin surface. In addition an occasional larva deviates from the usual course of migration and enters another organ, such as rumen, pericardium, duramater, spinal cord, brain and lymph node. The aberrant parasite finally dies and causes a granuloma with caseative necrosis resembling a tubercle.

Clinical Signs and Postmortem Lesions. While ovapositing female flies do not bite or sting, their presence and buzzing result in extreme annoyance and harassment to cattle, and attacked animals retreat in wild frenzy. The harassment results in loss of body weight, reduced milk production, and often bodily injury. Following ovaposition careful examination reveals clusters of 5 to 7 eggs, each approximately 1 mm in length, attached to a hair especially around the extremities of the posterior limbs, or single eggs

TABLE 24 *Comparison H. lineatum and H. bovis*

	H. lineatum (common heel fly)	*H. bovis* (northern heel fly)
eggs per hair	5–7	single
larvae		
1. mature body length, mm	25	27–28
2. common residence	esophagus	spinal epidura
3. posterior stigmal plates	flat	concave
adults		
1. body length, mm	12–13	15
2. body hair	black; yellow-orange thoracic bands	yellow-orange bands wider, deeper
geographic distribution, U. S.	all regions	northern half

attached to hairs. Focal dermatitis and matting of the hair with serous exudate at points of skin penetration are often discernible. Throughout the period of larval migration through tissues, the host cattle may be unthrifty and fail to grow or gain body weight at normal rates. When the larvae obtain their

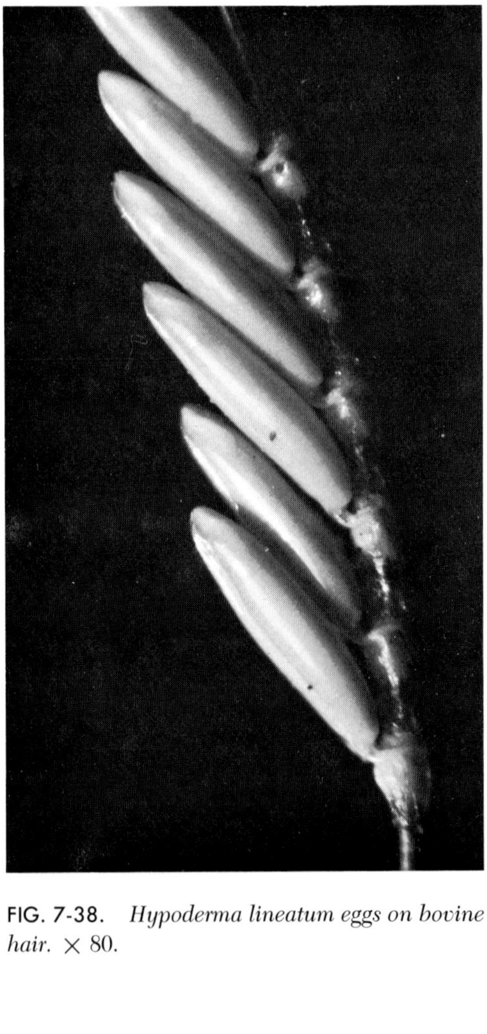

FIG. 7-38. *Hypoderma lineatum eggs on bovine hair.* × 80.

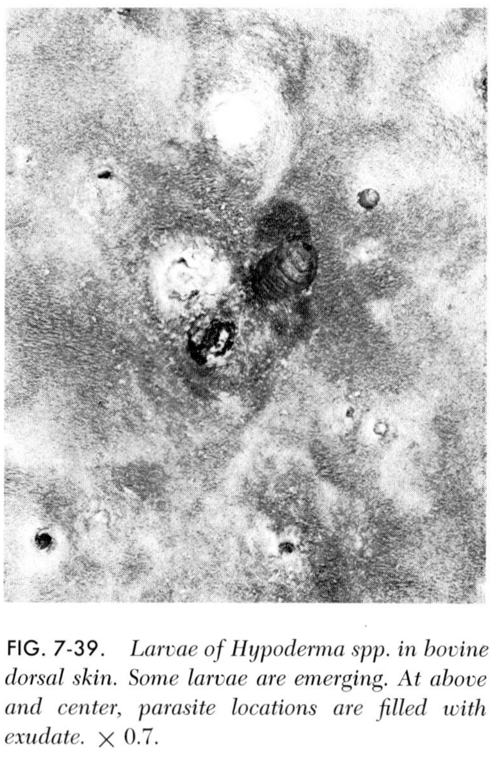

FIG. 7-39. *Larvae of Hypoderma spp. in bovine dorsal skin. Some larvae are emerging. At above and center, parasite locations are filled with exudate.* × 0.7.

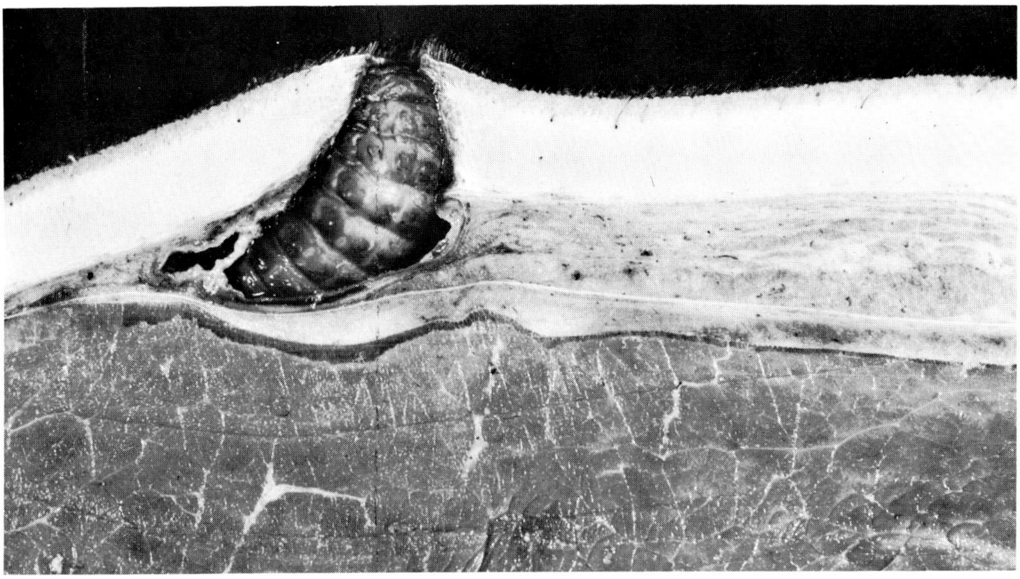

FIG. 7-40. *Hypoderma lineatum in dorsal subcutis.* × 1.6.

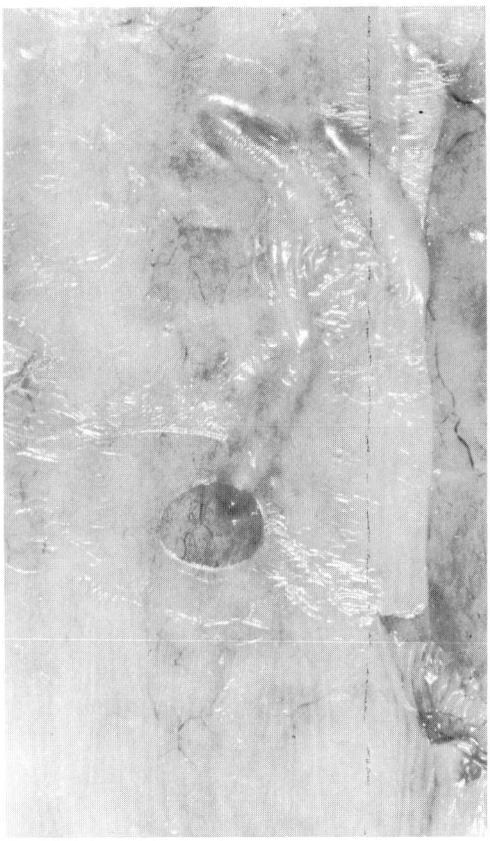

FIG. 7-41. *Mucosa of bovine esophagus containing three Hypoderma spp. larvae.* × 1.0.

definitive position in the subcutis of the back, a discrete hard swelling, usually 30 to 50 but occasionally 150 or more millimeters in diameter, is present for each larva. At each point of swelling the aperture with the posterior end of the larva is present. Serum exuding from the aperture mats the nearby hairs. Abscesses or cellulitis may form around some larvae, especially ruptured dead ones. Myelitis from larval penetration of the spinal cord or spondylitis from dead larvae may cause paralysis of the posterior limbs. Dead larvae in the esophageal wall may cause swelling and bloat.

At slaughter or necropsy, gross lesions vary with stage of larval development. Towards the midpoint of the cycle, and usually during autumn or early winter months, larvae can be found in the wall of the esophagus and in the spinal epidural tissue. As many as 100 larvae, each measuring 10 to 12 mm in length, may exist in a single host. While reaction around the parasite is usually slight, occasionally severe inflammation around dead larvae causes esophageal stricture. Green migratory tracts, often tortuous, may be discernible along intermuscular fasciae. Towards the end of the larval period, when the parasites are in the subcutis of the back the swellings, apertures and matted hair are easily palpated and observed. Digital pressure applied at the periphery of the swelling may expel the larva. When the hide is removed, the larvae are fully exposed. The parasitized subcutis contains a brown gelatinous exudate. Cavities for the larvae are surrounded by granulation tissue and open to the air through apertures, each 2 to 3 mm in diameter, in the skin. An infected parasite cavity may be 15 or more centimeters in diameter and filled with pus. From slaughtered animals, infested esophagi and spinal cords and the infested back tissues must be excised and condemned as human food.

Histopathologically acute inflammation is discernible at the points of skin penetration by the newly hatched larvae. Infested tissues of esophagi, spinal epidural tissues and the dorsal subcutis show swollen and fragmented collagen fibers, necrosis, strands of fibrin and leukocytes, especially esosinophils. The parasite cavities of the dorsal subcutis contain inflammatory exudate and are surrounded by walls of granulation tissue. Mononuclear macrophages and foreign body giant cells accumulate around discarded chiten and dead larvae. Colonies of contaminating bacteria may be present.

Diagnosis. Ovaposition can be diagnosed clinically by the frenzied excitement and wild running of attacked cattle. Careful examination of hairs of the host reveals eggs and, following penetration of newly hatched larvae, focal dermatitis. During the winter season when the larvae have acquired the definitive position in the subcutis of the back, the numerous swellings and skin perforations are readily discerned through meticulous palpation and careful inspection. Some larvae can be expelled by digital pressure around the aperture. At necropsy, the diagnosis is based on the presence of larvae in the wall of the esophagus, spinal epidural tissues or subcutis of the back.

The differential diagnosis requires the consideration of back injuries and bacterial infection. In these conditions a discrete aperture at each swelling is not present and the larvae cannot be palpated. Traumatic hematomas and sterile abscesses are soft and fluctuating. Needle centesis reveals the nature of the contents.

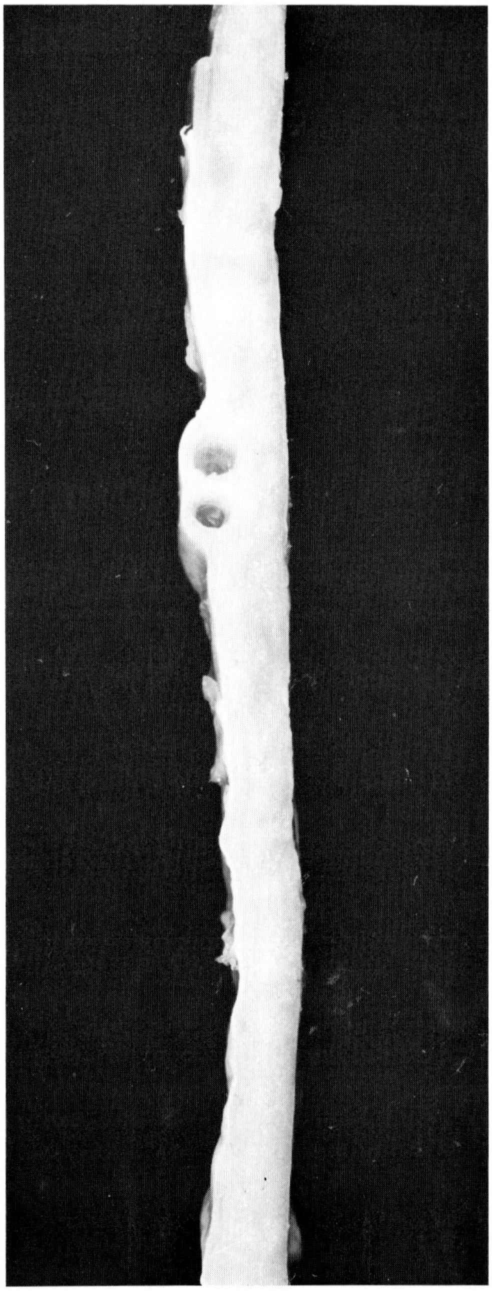

FIG. 7-42. *Gross cross section of two Hypoderma spp. in the esophageal submucosa.* × 3.

Prevention and Treatment. Hypodermosis in which mature larvae are in the subcutis of the back can be prevented by treating cattle with one of the organophosphate compounds according to directions of the manufacturer and as indicated in Table 25. Treatment must be applied during summer and fall, the interval between the end of the adult fly season and movement of the larvae to the definitive position in the subcutis of the back. In feedlot cattle the treatment is usually applied at the beginning of the fattening process but after animals have recovered from fatigue and possible illness from shipment. Ronnel should not be fed to sick or stressed animals, to lactating dairy cattle or to dry dairy animals within 60 days of parturition. Cattle should have access to both feed and water before and after treatment with Ronnel boluses. Coumaphos should not be applied to sick cattle or to calves under 3 months of age and animals 3 to 6 months of age should be sprayed lightly. The compound should not be used with synergized pyrethrum or other oral medications and should not be applied to lactating dairy cattle or to dry dairy cattle within 14 days of parturition.

Ruelene should not be administered to sick

TABLE 25 *Treatments for beef cattle against Hypoderma spp. larvae*

Insecticide	*Tolerance, ppm*	*Min. Days Last Application to Slaughter*	*Formulation and Strength*	*Amount Formula per Animal*	*Where and When to Apply*
Ronnel	0 in meat	60	0.6% in feed	0.33 lb./ 100 lb body weight	daily for 7 days at end of fly season
		28	0.26% in feed	0.3 lb./ 100 lb body weight	daily for 14 days
		21	5.5% in block or granules	0.25 lb./ 100 lb body wt./month	feed continuously for at least 75 days
Coumaphos	1 in meat and fat	—	WP 0.37–0.5% spray or 0.25% dip	varies with size	wet entire skin. Use at end of fly season
			Emuls. conc. 4%	0.5 pint/ animal	pour on back at end of fly season
Ruelene			Emuls. conc. 0.37% spray	varies with size; not more than 1 gal/animal	wet entire skin at end of fly season
		28	Emuls. conc. 8.3% in water	1 oz./100 lb. body weight; not more than 8 fl. oz./ animal.	pour evenly on back at end of fly season
Famphur		4	in feed	2.3 mg./lb. body wt. daily for 10 days	apply during grub migration

cattle, to lactating dairy animals, or to dry dairy animals within 28 days of parturition. It should not be used as a pour-on treatment in extremely hot or humid weather.

Following arrival of larvae at the definitive position in the back and perforation of the skin, rotenone can be used as a parasiticide. Treatment can be applied by either of three methods: (1) four to 5 ounces of a 1.5% rotenone dust rubbed thoroughly on the back of each animal, (2) one pint of a 5% wettable powder in water applied with a sponge or brush to the back of each animal, and (3) two to 4 quarts of 5% wettable powder in water applied to the back with a powder spray. Either method of treatment should be applied at monthly intervals for destruction of larvae arriving at the subcutis of the back at different times. Large abscesses around dead larvae in the subcutis of the back should be liberally incised for drainage and manual removal of necrotic tissue. Antibiotics help to control foci of infection.

Hypodermosis can be eradicated or reduced by systemic treatment of all cattle within a region with organophosphate insecticides. Treatment should be within a short time following termination of the adult fly season. Several successive seasons of treatment are required for eradication.

References

Baird, D. M., McCampbell, H. C., Ciordia, H., White, P. E. and Bizzell, W. E.: Two Systemic Insecticides for the Control of Cattle Grubs and Observations on their Effect on Internal Parasites. Georgia Vet., *14* (1962): 9–13.

Baxter, J. T.: A Field Trial of the Systemic Insecticide DOW ET-57 Against Warble Infestation in Cattle. Res. & Exp. Record, Ministry of Agri., Northern Ireland, *8* (1959): 73–81.

Beesley, W. N.: Field Trials with Trolene (DOW ET-57, Ronnel, Etrolene) against Warble Fly Grubs in Cattle. Vet. Record, *72* (1960): 21–23.

———: Observations on the Development of *Hypoderma lineatum* in the Bovine Host. Ann. Trop. Med. Parasitology, *55* (1961): 18–24.

Bishopp, F. C., Laake, E. W., Brundrett, H. M. and Wells, R. W.: The Cattle Grubs or Ox Warbles, Their Biologies and Suggestions for Control. U.S.D.A. Bulletin 1369. Apr. 1926.

Carpenter, G. H., Hewitt, T. R. and Reddin, T. K.: The Warbles Flies. Fourth Report on Experiments and Observations as to the Life History and Treatment. J. Dept. Agr. Tech. Instr. Ireland, *15* (1914): 105–132.

U. S. Department of Agriculture: Cattle Grubs or Heel Flies with Suggestions for Their Control. Farmers' Bulletin No. 1596. pp. 1–21.

Clark, B.: Observations on the Genus *Oestrus*. Trans. Linn. Soc. London, *3* (1797): 289–329.

Curtice, Cooper: The larvae of *Hypoderma bovis*, De Greer, U.S.D.A. Division of Entomology, Insect Life, *2* (1890): 207–208.

Guide for use of Insecticides. Ag. Handbook no. 331. ARS and FS. U.S.D.A. (1968): 166–167.

Haberman, W. O., Morgan, B. B. and Dickie, R. J.: The Occurrence of *Hypoderma* larvae in the Spinal Canal of Cattle. J. Agric. Res., *78* (1949): 637–640.

Hinrichsen: Ueber einen neuen Parasiten im Ruchenmarkskanal des Rindes. Arch Wis. und Prakt. Thierheilk, Bd., *14* (1888): 219–223.

Koorevaar, P.: De larvetoestand van *Hypoderma bovis* Tijdschr. Nederland. Dierk. Ver. (2) deel *5* (1898): 29–34. Translation in Annals and Mag. Nat. History (7) *4* (1899): 69–73.

Jones, R. H., Brundrett, H. M. and Radeleff, R. D.: Ranch Tests Against Cattle Grubs with the Insecticide DOW ET-57. Agricultural Chemicals, *12* (1957) No. 7 pp. 45, 95, 96.

Losses in Agriculture. Agricultural Handbook no. 291. ARS. USDA. (1965): 82.

Marquardt, C. and Hawkins, W. W. Jr.: Control of Cattle Grubs by the Intramuscular Injection of Bayer 29493 or CL 38023. Cornell Vet. *52* (1962): 228-236.

McGregor, W. S. and Bushland, R. C.: Tests with DOW ET-57 against Two Species of Cattle Grubs. Jour. Econ. Ent., *50* (1957): 246–249.

Mills, H. B., Marsh, H. and Willson, F. S.: Cattle Grubs in Montana. Bulletin 437. Aug. 1946. Montana State College, Agric. Exper. Station. Bozeman, Montana. pp. 1–16.

Mote, Don C.: The Ox Warble Flies, Bulletin 428, Nov. 1928. Ohio Agric. Exper. Station. Wooster, Ohio. pp. 1–45.

Radeleff, R. D.: Problems Associated with the Use of the Newer Insecticides for Livestock Pests. JAVMA, *136* (1960): 529–537.

Radeleff, R. D., Woodard, G. T., Nickerson, W. J. and Bushland, R. C.: The Acute Toxicity of Chlorinated Hydrocarbon and Organic Phosphorus Insecticides to Livestock. Tech. Bull. 1122. U. S. Dept. of Agric. Nov. 1955. pp. 1–45.

Radeleff, R. D. and Woodard, G. T.: The Toxicity of Organic Phosphorus Insecticides to Livestock. JAVMA, *130* (1957): 215–216.

Raun, E. S. and Herrick, J. B.: Feedlot Tests of the efficacy of DOW ET-57 (Trolene) for Control of Cattle Grubs. JAVMA, *131* (1957): 421–423.

Riley, C. V.: The Ox Bot in the United States. Habits and Natural History of *Hypoderma lineata.* U.S.D.A. Division Entomology, Insect Life, *4* (1892): 302–317.
Roberts, I. H., Lofgren, J. A. and Berndt, W. L.: Tests with Insecticide Formulations for the Destruction of Cattle Grubs. Jour. Econ. Ent., *45* (1953): 909–913.
Ruser, Wilhelm. Ueber das Vorkommen von Oestruslarven im Ruckenmarkskanal des Rindes. Ztschr. Fleish und Milchhyg., Jahrg. *5* (1895): 127–129.
Spindler, L. A., Becklund, W. S. and Peterson, H. O.: Cattle Grub Control in Central Washington. Proceedings U. S. Livestock Sanitary Assn. 1955. pp. 226–236.
Weidenbach, Carl P., Radeleff, R. D. and Buck, William B.: Toxicologic Studies of Ruelene. JAVMA, *140* (1962): 460–463.
Wolfe, L. S.: Observations on the Histopathological Changes Caused by the Larvae of *Hypoderma bovis* and *Hypoderma lineatum* in Tissues of Cattle. Canad. J. Animal Science, *39* (1959): 145–157.
Woodard, G. T.: The Treatment of Organic Phosphate Insecticide Poisoning With Atropine Sulfate and 2-PAM (2-Pyridine Aldoxime Methiodide). Vet. Med. *52* (1957): 571–578.

Lousiness

(PEDICULOSIS)

An insidious and seasonal parasitism, lousiness is the accumulation of pathogenic numbers of lice on the skin. While small numbers of these external parasites are innocuous, large numbers adversely affect cattle. Conservative estimates have suggested that lousiness causes to the United States cattle industry an annual loss of 47 million dollars. The losses result from anemia, unthriftiness, reduced rates of growth, inefficient feed utilization, some mortality, possible predisposition to other diseases and expensive treatment.

Review of Literature. While lice have been encountered on cattle in all seasons, they tended to increase sharply during December, January and February, and to diminish during warmer months (Gojmerac, Dicke and Allen, 1959). An exception, however, was with the tail louse, *Haematopinus quadripertusus,* which developed a high population incidence during late summer and early autumn (Creighton and Dennis, 1947). One postulated cause of seasonal fluctuation is high skin temperatures of cattle during warm seasons. Under laboratory conditions a host skin temperature of 100° F diminished the louse population, while host skin temperature of 125° F was lethal to the parasites in 1 hour. These findings relate to seasonal fluctuation of lice. When the air temperature was 78° F, bovine skin temperature varied from 100° to 125° F. The higher value developed rapidly when the skin was exposed to direct sunlight (Matthysse, 1962). Surveys have disclosed that cattle vary in external parasite load. In one study of 3,188 hides from freshly slaughtered animals, less than 2% were heavily infested (Scharff, 1962). Severely parasitized animals became anemic to variable degrees. Heavily parasitized range cattle showed approximately 50% reduction in erythrocytes and hemoglobin values, and in some animals the total leukocyte count was significantly reduced when compared to similar but nonparasitized cattle (Peterson, Roberts, Becklund and Kemper, 1953; Shemanchuk, Haufe and Thompson, 1960).

Following destruction of lice, the erythrocyte volume changed from 10 and 13% to 37 and 40% within 27 to 44 days (Peterson, Roberts, Becklund and Kemper, 1953). While the effect of lousiness on rates of gain in body weight has not been measured precisely, many investigators have logically surmised a reduction, especially from heavy parasitism (Creighton and Dennis, 1947; Cattle Lice, 1953; Kemper *et al.,* 1948; Marquardt *et al.,* 1960; Scharff, 1962; U.S.D.A. Leaflet, 1960).

The efficacy of recently discovered insecticides has been studied on many insects, including cattle lice. Benzene hexachloride as a dip was effective against sucking lice at 0.3% concentration and against chewing lice in a 0.15% concentration (Furman, 1948). Some strains of lice were susceptible to DDT, while others were highly resistant (Anthony, 1959). Organic phosphate compounds were also effective. A 0.1% concentration of General Chemical 4072 caused a 100% immediate kill of lice (Hoffman *et al.*, 1961). One hundred five recently weaned parasitized Hereford calves were treated with Bayer 21/199 by spraying. Concentrations of the compound at 0.1% destroyed most lice, while concentrations of 0.5% killed all parasites (Marquardt *et al.*, 1960). Cattle treated with 0.5% concentration of malathion remained clean of lice for 30 days (Anthony, 1959).

Occurrence. While all breeds, sexes and ages of cattle are susceptible, Hereford and Holstein breeds, bulls and cattle young and old are especially susceptible. Within a single breed, sex and age group, susceptibility varies. Within a herd of nearly uniform animals approximately 2% become heavily parasitized, while the balance of the animals are moderately or lightly infested. The cause of this variance is unknown. Crowding in pens or stalls increases vulnerability to infestation. Each species of mammal contains its host-specific species of lice.

Seasonally, lousiness occurs primarily during winter and early spring. Tail louse infestation, however, occurs more commonly during late summer and early autumn.

Geographically, lousiness appears in all countries and regions where cattle production is a major industry. Some local areas, however, may be free of some species, such as the tail louse.

Etiology and Pathogenesis. Cattle are parasitized by five species of lice as follows: *Bovicola bovis, Haematopinus eurysternus, Linognathus vituli, Solenopotes capillatus* and *Haematopinus quadripertusus.* Some morphologic and biologic characteristics of the species are presented in Table 26.

Life cycles are simple and lived entirely on the skin of the host. Single eggs are at-

TABLE 26 *Characteristics of cattle lice*

Names	Female Dimensions, mm	Color	Type of Mouth Parts	Preferred Location on Hosts	Season of High Activity	Egg Incubation, Days	Life Cycle, Days
Bovicola bovis (little red louse)	1.6–1.75 × 0.35–0.55	red-brown	chewing	shoulders, topline, tail head	winter, spring	8	20–29
Haematopinus eurysternus (short-nosed cattle louse)	3.5–4.75 × 1.53	gray-black	sucking	neck, brisket, poll, perineum	winter, spring	10–17	24–31
Linognathus vituli (long-nosed cattle louse)	1.87–2.5 × 0.6–0.8	blue-black	sucking	shoulders, neck, brisket, perineum	winter, spring	8–13	23–30
Solenopotes capillatus (little blue cattle louse)	1.75 × 0.74	blue	sucking	head, neck, brisket	winter, spring	9–13	
Haematopinus quadripertusus (tail louse)	4.4 × 2.3	brown-gray	sucking	tail brush, perineum, back	late summer, early fall		

tached to hair shafts. Following an incubation period of approximately 1 to 2 weeks, the growing nymph molts twice and produces three instars. The known life cycles vary from 20 to 30 days. The ability of the parasite to live apart from the host varies with environmental temperature and humidity. Most parasites, however, die after 2 to 7 days. One or more species may parasitize the same host, either simultaneously or sequentially. Transmission is by direct contact between cattle or rarely through infested bedding in common use by parasitized and susceptible animals.

Many aspects of the pathogenesis have not been elucidated. Presumably, some lice endure throughout warm seasons on bovine hosts. During late autumn and winter lice increase rapidly in numbers and produce light, moderate or heavy infestations. Species of sucking lice penetrate the skin and feed on whole blood of the host. Heavily infested cattle become anemic and physically weak because of continuous loss of blood to the parasites. Chewing lice consume flakes of epithelium, exudate and fragments of hairs. The presence of numerous sucking or chewing lice causes scaliness of the skin and itching. The hair may be denuded by rubbing, biting and kicking. With the advent of spring, and presumably because of elevation of temperature of the host skin, the lice diminish sharply in numbers throughout the warm season. The numerical diminution during spring and summer may be due to direct and prolonged action of sunlight on the parasites. In addition grooming by the host may help control the insects. Cattle, especially calves, maintained continuously indoors may support heavy infestations during spring and summer. During fall and winter, surface temperature of the host skin lowers and the number of lice increases. As a result of heavy parasitism during winter, growth rates of the hosts decline and cattle are predisposed to secondary diseases such as pneumonia. Death may result from severe parasitism and intercurrent diseases. Some

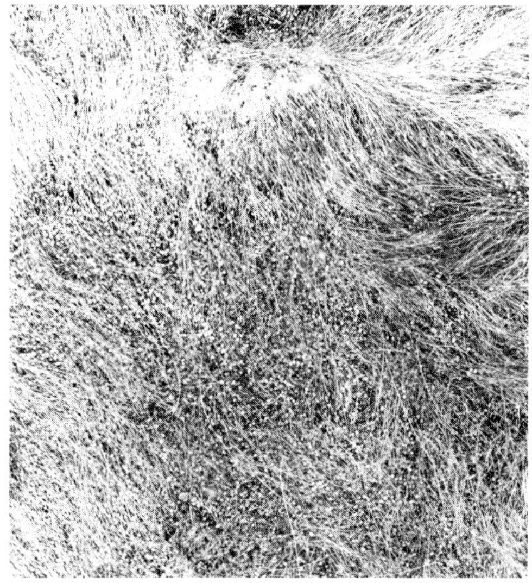

FIG. 7-43. *Skin of a steer infested with lice.* × 0.7.

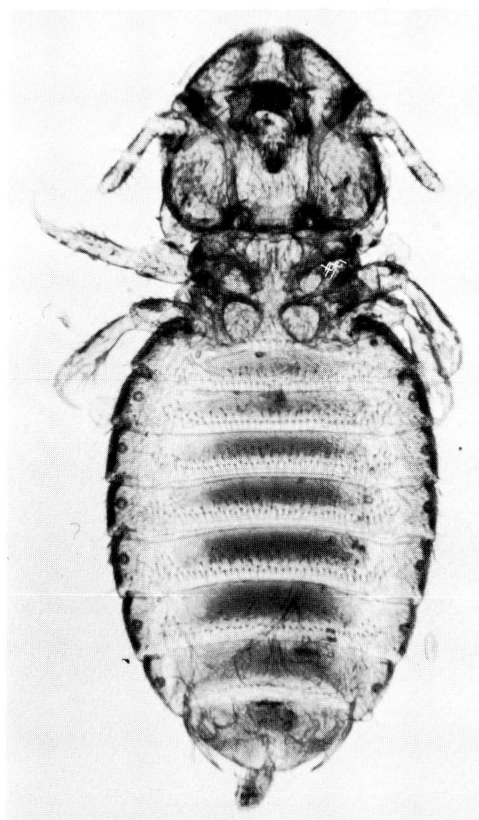

FIG. 7-44. *Bovicolis bovis.* × 55.

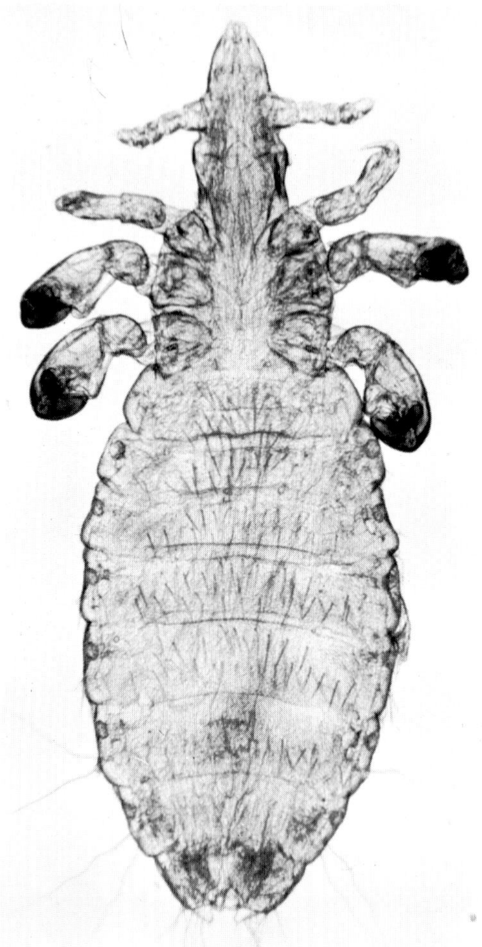

FIG. 7-45. *Haematopinus eurysternus.* × 55.

infectious diseases may be transmitted by lice.

Clinical Signs and Postmortem Lesions. Light to moderate infestations are asymptomatic and frequently escape detection. Heavily infested animals, however, lose their appetites and rub, bite and kick the irritated itching skin. With anemia the animal becomes weak and inactive. The body temperature is normal. The visible membranes of the eyes, mouth, and vulva are pale because of anemia. Hematological studies show a reduction as much as 50% of normal in the number of erythrocytes and in hemoglobin level. In anatomical areas of heavy infestation, the hair coat is discolored. Large numbers of eggs and the insects darken white hair coats, especially along the neck and brisket of Hereford cattle. Close examination of the skin reveals the dense accumulations of eggs, nymphs and adults which concentrate over the brisket, neck, face and medial aspect of the thigh. In heavy infestations the entire skin surface may be parasitized. The tail louse, *H. quadripertusus,* has a predilection for the brush of the tail. From this location infestations spread proximally along the tail to the perineum and anteriorly along the back to the neck and face.

At necropsy, the oval, nymphal and adult lice are on the skin in variable numbers. Heavily infested animals contain thin watery blood and the internal organs and membranes are pale. Dermatitis, scaliness and denudation from parasitism and rubbing may be discernible. Intercurrent diseases, such as pneumonia, may have developed and contributed to the cause of death. Histopathologically, dermatitis is apparent.

Diagnosis. Lousiness is diagnosed by finding and identifying large numbers of lice on an anemic and physically weakened animal. One or more species of lice may infest a single host. In searching for lice the skin of the neck, brisket, face, medial surface of the thighs and the tail should be examined carefully.

The differential diagnosis requires consideration of other causes of anemia and pruritus, such as infestation with ticks and mites, anaplasmosis and leptospirosis. Tick infestations are diagnosed by finding and identifying the various species of ticks which attach to the skin and engorge on blood. Mange mites are identifiable in scrapings from skin lesions. Anaplasmosis, a febrile disease, is caused by *Anaplasma marginale* which can be found in erythrocytes of blood smears prepared during early stages of the disease. Leptospirosis, also febrile, causes hemoglobinuria and an ascending agglutination titer against the leptospiral antigen. In some animals the leptospira can be isolated from the blood or organs.

Prevention and Treatment. All cattle entering the feedlot should be dipped or sprayed with one of the organophosphate compounds indicated in Table 27. This routine procedure usually prevents the establishment of lousiness during the entire period of fattening. Animals remaining in the feedlot for more than the customary 90 to 120 days may need a second treatment. Heavily parasitized cattle, as bulls, may require a second treatment in 10 to 14 days. To avoid poisoning, organophosphate insecticides should be cautiously used on full-fed cattle and during the cool part of the day. Following destruction of lice on heavily parasitized cattle, recovery from anemia is accelerated by the administration of blood transfusions, injectable iron compounds, and crude liver extracts.

References

Anthony, D. W.: Tests with DDT, Lindane, and Malathion for Control of the Long-Nosed Cattle Louse *Linognathus vituli.* J. Econ. Ent., *52* (1959): 782–784.

TABLE 27 *Treatments for lice*

Insecticide	*Tolerance, ppm*	*Min. Days Applic. to Slaughter*	*Formulation and Strength*	*Amount of Formulation per Animal*	*Where and When to Apply*	*Safety Restrictions*
Coumophos	1 meat and fat	—	EC, 0.06% spray WP, 0.06% spray or dip	varies with size of animal	Treat thoroughly Dip or spray on entrance to feedlot	Do not use on sick animals or calves under 3 mos. Do not use with synergized pyrethrins. Do not apply to lactating cows.
Dioxathion	1	—	Emuls. conc. 0.15% dip or spray	varies with size of animal		
Ronnel	0	56	EC, 0.25% dip or spray	varies with size of animal		
Ruelene	—	28	EC, 0.375% spray	varies with size of animal	Spray on entrance to feedlot	
Famphur	—	4	premix in protein supplement	1.1 mg/lb body wt daily for 30 days	mix thoroughly in feed for mort nosed louse	
Lindane	7	30 60 30	EC or WP, 0.03–0.05% spray EC or WP, 0.03% dip 1.0% Dust	varies with size of animal	immerse or spray	Repeat in 2–3 weeks if needed.
Toxaphene	7	28	EC or WP, 0.5% dip or spray	varies with size of animal	immerse or spray	
Methoxychlor	3	—	EC or WP, 0.5% spray (1–1.5% for tail louse)			

Cattle Lice and How to Eradicate Them. Farmers' Bulletin 909. U.S.D.A. 1953.

Creighton, J. T. and Dennis, N. M.: The Tail Louse in Florida. J. Econ. Ent., *40* (1947): 911–912.

Furman, D. P.: Benzene Hexachloride to Control Cattle Lice. J. Econ. Ent., *40* (1948): 672.

Gojmerac, W. L., Dicke, R. J., and Allen, N. N.: Factors Affecting the Biology of Cattle Lice. J. Econ. Ent., *52* (1959): 79–82.

Goulding, R. L. and Taylor, N. O.: Effects of Topical Applications of Dibrom Upon Cattle Lice and Cattle Grubs. J. Econ. Ent., *55* (1962): 744–746.

Guide for Use of Insecticides. Agricultural Handbook No. 331. ARS and FS. USDA (1968).

Hoffman, R. A. and Drummond, R. O.: Control of Lice on Livestock and Parasites on Poultry With General Chemical 4072. J. Econ. Ent., *54* (1961): 1052–1053.

Kemper, H. E., Cobbett, N. G., Roberts, I. H., and Peterson, H. O.: DDT Emulsions for the Destruction of Lice on Cattle, Sheep, and Goats. AJVR, *9* (1948): 373–378.

Losses in Agriculture. Agricultural Research Service. Agricultural Handbook No. 291. (1965): 82.

Marquardt, W. C., Lovelace, S. A. and Fritts, D. H.: Spray Treatment of Calves with Bayer 21/199 for Control of Cattle Grubs and Lice. JAVMA, *137* (1960): 589–594.

Matthysse, J. G.: Cattle Lice. Their Biology and Control. Cornell University Ag. Exp. Station Bulletin 832. 1946.

Peterson, H. O., Roberts, I. H., Becklund, W. W. and Kemper, H. E.: Anemia in Cattle Caused by Heavy Infestations of the Blood-sucking Louse, *Haematopinus eurysternus*, JAVMA, *122* (1953): 373–376.

Scharff, D. K.: An Investigation of the Cattle Louse Problem. J. Econ. Ent., *55* (1962): 684–688.

Shemanchuk, J. A., Haufe, W. O. and Thompson, C. O. M.: Anemia in Range Cattle Heavily Infested with Short-nosed Sucking Louse, *Haematopinus eurysternus*. Canad. J. Comp. Med. Vet. Sci., *24* (1960): 158–161.

U.S.D.A. Leaflet 456. Cattle Lice: How to Control Them. (1960).

Organophosphorus Insecticide Poisoning

(PHOSPHATE ESTER POISONING)

The phosphoric acid esters and some of their chemical derivatives are a highly insecticidal group of compounds. Because of their pharmacological properties which cause death by interference with acetylocholinesterase, they have been designated anticholinesterase compounds. Because of their action in host tissues they have been termed "systemic insecticidal compounds." Poisoning in cattle and other species of domestic animals occurs occasionally from accidental ingestion or injudicious overdosing with insecticides. While several millions of cattle have been treated with and received the benefits from these compounds, some animals have died from their lethal effects. In some herds poisoning has been associated with prolonged incapacitation and high mortality.

Review of Literature. During World War II original research was conducted in Germany on the phosphoric acid esters, popularly referred to as "nerve gases," for possible use in warfare. Following termination of the war, the data were discovered and some were made public (Metcalf and March, 1949). Earlier investigations (1943) had already indicated that triorthocresyl phosphate, a member of this group of compounds, inhibits cholinesterase, an enzyme common to most animal tissues and suggested that acetylcholinesterase inhibition is the mode of action for many phosphoric acid esters. This information also suggested the potential of this group of compounds for use as economic pesticides (Hottinger and Block, 1943). In rapid succession, many related compounds were synthesized. Those produced early in the series, such as TEPP, tetraethylpyrophosphate, were highly toxic to both insects and mammalian hosts and were restricted to use on plants. Encouraged by the initial test application of these compounds in the control of important economic insects, research chemists synthesized such compounds as parathion and malathion which proved highly lethal to insects but of low toxicity to domestic mammals (Hamblin and Golz, 1955). Later many compounds were synthesized and tested for both efficacy and safety. Products as Ruelene (Radeleff, 1960; Weidenbach, Radeleff and Buck, 1962), Ronnel and Coumaphos (Radeleff and Woodward, 1957) were developed and subsequently marketed for use against many pests of cattle. Besides being safe and efficacious these products did not appear to accumulate significantly in edible animal tissues (Guide for Use of Insecticides, 1968; Pesticide Residues, 1960). In some cases of poisoning, measurable levels of blood cholinesterase declined rapidly to 40% or less of normal (Ganong, 1963; Radeleff, 1970; Weidenback, Radeleff and Buck, 1962). Clinical signs were observed and described (Jolly, 1957; Radeleff, 1960; Raddeleff and Woodward, 1957) and rational and beneficial treatment was formulated (Hamblin and Golz, 1955; Woodward, 1957; Radeleff, 1970).

The rate of production and utilization of insecticides increased rapidly from 1940, when the chlorinated hydrocarbons were introduced, to 1962 when an estimated 350 million pounds were used in the United States. Of this amount, the organophosphate compounds were a substantial portion (Report of President's Science Adv. Committee, 1963).

Occurrence. All breeds, sexes and ages of cattle are susceptible to poisoning with phosphoric acid ester compounds; but in general, calves are more susceptible than adult cattle, and the Brahman breed appears to be more susceptible than other breeds. Since this group of insecticides is used universally, poisoning occurs in all major cattle producing countries, and while all other species of domestic animals are also susceptible, the disease occurs most commonly among cattle, sheep and horses. In feedlot cattle, poisoning occurs usually in late summer and autumn when larvae of *Hypoderma* spp. migrate and cattle, newly arrived at the feedlot, are treated for migrating grubs, lice and ticks. The disease may also occur when feedlot cattle graze harvested fields where they accidentally gain access to stores of discarded insecticide containers.

Etiology. Poisoning results from the accidental consumption of, or, an overdosing with organophosphate compounds. Some highly effective forage crop insecticides are dangerously toxic to cattle. Ingestion may result from feeding on forage having toxic insecticide residues and from ingesting insecticide stores and discarded paper or fabric containers. Some phosphoric acid esters have a narrow safety margin between therapeutic and toxic doses. Inaccurate computation of the therapeutic oral or dermal dose may cause poisoning. In addition poisoning may come from contamination during manufacture of normally safe pesticides with toxic derivatives. Table 28 presents the organophosphate compounds commonly used on cattle. Ronnel, Ruelene and Coumaphos are often used on cattle as insecticides against migrating ox warbles, lice, and ticks. Table 28 presents the maximum safe doses for those compounds.

Pharmacologic Action. The principal pharmacologic action of the organophosphate compounds is the inhibition of acetylcholinesterase. An understanding of this effect requires comprehension of the basic anatomy and physiology of the autonomic nervous system. The visceral (autonomic) system consists of the ganglia and neurons which innervate and regulate the internal organs, the blood vessels and the involuntary muscles and glands of the body in general. Organized like a reflex arc, the system conducts impulses from the viscera over afferent pathways to the central nervous system where they are integrated and transmitted by the way of efferent pathways back to the viscera. The efferent motor portions of the system consist of preganglionic and postganglionic neurons which synapse at the autonomic ganglia. Anatomically the system is subdivided into sympathetic and parasympathetic divisions. In the sympathetic division axones of the preganglionic neurons extend from the spinal cord through the first thoracic to the third or fourth lumbar spinal nerves into the paravertebral sympathetic ganglionic chain or the collateral ganglia near the viscera. The parasympathetic division consists of cranial and sacral portions. In the cranial outflow axones of preganglionic neurons leave the central nervous system through the oculomotor, facial, glossopharyngeal and vagus

TABLE 28 *Organophosphate compounds in common use for animals*

Name	Chemical Formula	Proprietary Preparations	Minimum Levels Toxic to Cattle*
Coumaphos (Bayer 21/199)	0,0-diethyl 0-(3-chloro-4-methyl-2-oxo-2H-1-benzopyran-7-yl)-phosphorothioate	Co-Ral Asuntol Muscatox	>0.5% water spray >25 mg/kg bd wt oral
Shell Compound 4294	Dimethyl 2-(alpha-methyl-benzoxyloxycarbonyl)-1-methyl vinyl phosphate	Ciodrin	0.3% spray to Brahmans >2.0% for Herefords
Cruformate	0-4-tert-butyl-2-chlorophenyl methyl methylphosphoramidate	Ruelene	50 mg/kg bd wt water spray 100 mg/kg bd wt oral
Diazinon	0,0-diethyl 0-(2-isopropyl-4-methyl-6-pyrimidenyl) phosphorothioate		>0.1% water spray
Dichlorvos (DDVP)	2,2-dichlorovinyl-dimethyl phosphate	Vapona	>2% mist spray
Dioxathion	p-dioxane-2,3,-diyl ethyl phosphorodithoate	Delnav	0.8% topical emulsion
Famophos	0-[p-(dimethyl sulfamoyl)-phenyl] 0,0-dimethyl phosphorothioate	Warbex	>50 mg/kg bd wt oral
Fenthion (Bayer 29,493)	0,0-dimethyl 0-[4-(methylthio)-m-tolyl] phosphorothioate	Baytex	>3.87% topical application @ 1 fl. oz./100 lb bd wt 25 mg/kg bd wt oral
Malathion (Compound 4049)	0,0-diamethyl-1-hydroxy-2,2,2-trichloroethyl phosphonate		2% spray 100 mg/kg bd wt oral
Ronnel (Fenchlorfos)	0,0-dimethyl-0-(2,4,5-trichlorophenyl) phosphorothioate	Ectoral Nankor	100 mg/kg bd wt oral
Trichlorfon	dimethyl(2,2,2-trichloro-1-hydroxyethyl phosphonate	Neguvon Dipterex Dylon Dyrex Freed	>2% solution topical >50 mg/kg bd wt oral

* Calves are generally more sensitive and have smaller minimum toxic doses than adult cattle.

nerves, synapse with postganglionic neurons and supply viscera of the head, thorax and abdomen. In the sacral part of the parasympathetic division axones of preganglionic neurons leave the central nervous system by way of the second to fourth sacral spinal nerves, synapse with postganglionic neurons and innervate the pelvic viscera.

The synapse is the microscopic space between the axone of one neuron and the dendrites of another neuron or between the axone and the effector end organ. Nerve impulses are conducted electrically along the axone. They cross the synaptic junctions by chemical mediators. The transmission of impulses across some synapses involves the action of acetylcholine and acetylcholinesterase. Acetylcholine, inactive from being protein bound, is concentrated at the axone terminals. The arrival of an electric impulse at the axone terminal causes release of acetylocholine which through ion movements results in membrane depolarization and transmission of the impulse across the synapse to dendrites of a postganglionic neuron or to the effector-end organ. In order that the axone membrane be repolarized the acetylcholine must be removed from the synapse. Removal is achieved by the enzyme acetylcholinesterase which hydralizes the acetylcholine into a molecule of acetate and a molecule of choline. The protein-bound and inactive acetylcholine is resynthesized. Chemical mediation of impulses by acetylcholine is achieved at (1) all synapses between preganglionic and postganglionic neurons of the autonomic system, (2) all postganglionic parasympathetic endings, (3) myoneural junctions and (4) some postganglionic sympathetic endings. In addition to many synapses, acetylcholinesterase is present in erythrocytes of cattle.

Organophosphate poisoning inhibits the action of acetylcholinesterase; consequently, following chemical mediation of an impulse, the acetylcholine not being hydralized persists and accumulates at the synapses and continues to stimulate the postganglionic neurons or the effector end organs. Continuous and hyper-stimulation of organs supplied by the parasympathetic system gives rise to clinical signs of poisoning. In fatal cases, overstimulation of the parasympathetic system causes bronchial mucous membranes to secrete fluids and bronchial muscle to contract. The two effects inhibit the movement of gas through the bronchial lumina and finally result in respiratory failure.

Clinical Signs and Postmortem Lesions. Evident clinical signs result from inhibition of acetylcholinesterase and the accumulation of acetylcholine at the junction of preganglionic and postganglionic neurons and at myoneural junctions. Following exposure of cattle to toxic amounts of organophosphate compounds onset of clinical signs is usually initiated within one-half to a few hours. Watery salivation is profuse and respirations are difficult, rapid and oral. Rales may be noticeable from excessive bronchial secretions. The pupils constrict and the tongue protrudes. Groups of muscles may contract spasmodically and, from stiffness of the limbs and eventual muscular weakness, walking is impaired. Diarrhea, sweating, bloating and convulsions may develop terminally. The measurement of acetylcholinesterase activity in the erythrocytes may show a rapid decline from normal values of 0.17 to 0.96 delta pH units per hour to values as low as 40 to 10% of normal. According to severity of the intoxication the course of the disease varies. In acute and severe poisoning death may occur within a few minutes or a few hours following onset of symptoms. In animals surviving mild poisoning, however, recovery may be complete and prompt or in poisoning from some compounds the toxic effects may persist for many days or weeks.

At necropsy, lesions are inconspicuous. The face and mouth contain excessive amounts of saliva. Secretions in the bronchi and trachea may be abundant and pulmonary edema may be apparent. The stomach and intestines are contracted and the feces may be fluid.

Diagnosis. The diagnosis of poisoning from organophosphate compounds is based on a history of possible exposure to the chemicals and the manifestation of typical clinical signs. Frequently the poisoning follows promptly after the deliberate application or accidental ingestion of organophosphate insecticides. Important signs are sudden onset with symptoms of salivation, pupillary constriction, difficult breathing and muscular spasms and stiffness. Determination of the level of acetylcholinesterase activity in the erythrocytes is of supplementary value to history and clinical signs. However, extreme variation in activity values for normal cattle renders the test of low utility excepting as supplementary information.

The differential diagnosis requires consideration of acute bloat and acute poisoning from chlorinated hydrocarbon compounds, hydrocyanic acid, heavy metals and nitrates. In case of bloat the abdomen is distended;

the pupils are not constricted and salivation is not excessive. Chlorinated hydrocarbons, also used as insecticides, cause depression, disorientation, prostration and convulsions. Hydrogen cyanide and nitrates from plants cause sudden death without premonitory signs. Histories and chemical analysis of feeds frequently are of value in diagnosing other poisons.

Prevention and Treatment. To avoid poisoning, pesticides should be used with meticulous care. Supplies of the compounds should be stored in dry places protected against access to cattle and other animals, as well as incautious and unsuspecting people. Empty containers should be destroyed to avoid chewing and consumption by livestock. Forage to which insecticide has been applied should not be fed to animals during the active life of the compounds. Before treatment cattle should be full-fed, and the drug should be used during the cool part of the day. When administering organophosphate compounds to cattle the doses for the species, size and route of administration should be accurately computed and followed. Reliable directions for use usually accompany the commercial product or can be obtained from veterinarians or the U. S. Department of Agriculture (Guide for Use of Insecticides, 1968).

For effective treatment of phosphate ester poisoning two sequences of specific drugs must be applied promptly following exposure. Adult cattle should receive 12.5 to 20 mg of atropine dissolved in 10 ml of water slowly administered intravenously. This treatment provides prompt but short effect and should be followed by 3.5 to 50 mg of atropine dissolved in 10 ml of water administered subcutaneously, along with 50 mg per kg of body weight of 2-PAM (2-formyl-1-methyl-pyridinium iodide oxime) in 100 to 125 ml of aqueous physiological salt solution administered subcutaneously in the neck region. Not more than 50 ml of the solution should be administered at any single injection site. The entire treatment should be repeated as may be necessary. If feasible, the affected animals should have residues of the compound washed from whatever surface was contacted, such as the skin or alimentary tract. In addition, cattle showing depression should receive general stimulants, and cattle exhibiting excitation should receive tranquilizers.

References

Gangong, W. F.: *Review of Medical Physiology.* Lange Medical Publication. Los Altos, Calif. (1963): 50; 148–153.

Guide for Use of Insecticides, Agricultural Handbook No. 331. ARS and FS, U.S.D.A. (1968): 162–182.

Hamblin, D. O. and Golz, H. H.: Parathion Poisoning—A Brief Review. Industrial Med. and Surg., *24* (1955): 65–72.

Hottinger, A. and Block, H.: Helv. Chim-Acta., *26* (1943): 142.

Jolly, D. W.: The Toxicity of Organic Phosphorus Insecticides. Vet. Record, *69* (1957): 796–800.

Metcalf, R. L. and March, R. B.: Studies of the Mode of Action of Parathion and Its Derivatives and Their Toxicity to Insects. J. Econ. Ent., *42* (1949): 721.

Pesticide Residues in Meat and Milk. Ag. Res. Service. U.S.D.A. ARS-33-63. Dec. 1960.

Radeleff, R. D.: Veterinary Toxicology, Lea and Febiger, Philadelphia. Second Edition. (1970): 206–233.

———: Newer Insecticides. JAVMA, *136* (1960): 529–537.

Radeleff, R. D. and Woodard, G. T.: Cholinesterase Activity of Normal Blood of Cattle and Sheep. Vet. Med., *51* (1956): 512.

———: The Toxicity of Organic Phosphate Insecticides to Livestock. JAVMA, *130* (1957): 215–216.

———: Toxicological Studies of Dow ET-57 in Cattle and Sheep. J. Econ. Ent., *50* (1957): 249–251.

Radeleff, R. D., Woodard, G. T., Nickerson, W. J. and Bushland, R. C.: The Acute Toxicity of Chlorinated Hydrocarbon and Organic Phosphorus Insecticides to Livestock. U.S.D.A. Technical Bulletin 1122. (1955).

Reik, R. F. and Keith, R. K.: Studies on Anthelmintics for Cattle. IV. The Organic Phosphorus Compound 0,0-Dimethyl2,2,2-Trichloro-1-Hydroxymethyl Phosphonate (Bayer L 13/59). Austral. Vet. J., *34* (1958): 93–103.

Report of the President's Science Advisory Committee. Use of Pesticides. The White House. Washington, D. C. May 15, 1963.

Weidenbach, C. P., Radeleff, R. D. and Buck, W. B.: Toxiologic Studies of Ruelene. JAVMA, *140* (1962): 460–463.

Woodard, G. T.: The Treatment of Organic Phosphate Insecticide Poisoning with Atropine Sulfate and 2-PAM (2-Pyridine Aldoxime Methiodide). Vet. Med., *52* (1957): 571–578.

8

Diseases having miscellaneous and unknown causes

Dental Caries

(TOOTH DECAY)

Dental caries, a focal degenerative change in tooth tissue, is characterized by progressive destruction of tooth tissue. Since the masticatory capacity of an animal is eventually reduced, the disease often leads to poor nutrition and loss of body weight. Because the disease increases with age but develops slowly, it is of relatively low economic importance in young feedlot cattle, but of considerable significance during fattening of retired cows and bulls.

Review of Literature. Tooth decay was observed and studied in both wild and domestic animals. Within the latter category, the incidence was low except for horses in which 66% in a sample of 484 animals disclosed caries to some degree (Colyer, 1963). Among cattle dental caries were found in both incisors and cheek teeth. In a sample of 7,480 young fattened cattle, the disease was observed in the permanent teeth of 4.6% of the animals but not in deciduous teeth. In the same study, 2.9% of the animals disclosed some degree of hypoplasia in permanent incisor teeth. The carious process was in enamel and dentin. In enamel the decay localized in foci of hypoplasia. In cheek teeth, enamel hypoplasis of the infundibulum created spaces where fermentable food accumulated and initiated decay which extended into the pulp cavities (Garlick, 1954). In Poland a sample of 10,000 slaughtered cattle had 1,908 animals with caries. In this group the incidence was 2% for cattle 1 to 2 years of age and 11% for animals 2 to 3 years of age. The descending order of affected teeth was incisors, premolars and molars (Kostyra, 1965).

In an investigation of environmental factors causing caries, oral bacteria and food particles were studied. Rats were used as experimental animals because of their known susceptibility to the disease. In one experiment a cariesogenic diet was fed to a lot of germ-free rats and to a lot of similar rats having conventional oral bacteria. All conventional rats and no germ-free rats developed caries of the molars (Orland, 1955). In another experiment a caries-producing diet was fed to each of two lots of conventional rats. Animals of one lot orally consumed the diet, while animals of the other lot were fed through a tube placed into the stomach. All rats fed by mouth and no rats fed by stomach tube developed molar caries (Kite *et al.*,

1955). In addition, a lot of conventional rats were fed a diet of fat and protein, while a control lot was fed a diet containing carbohydrates. Animals consuming the carbohydrate diet developed extensive caries, while animals receiving the carbohydrate-free diet developed no caries (Sognnaes, 1955). These findings established oral bacteria and carbohydrate feed as causative factors in caries.

Occurrence. While caries probably occurs equally in both sexes, the incidence varies directly with age, with both incisor and cheek teeth affected. While age incidence has not been determined accurately, 4.6% of young fattened cattle, observed in one study, contained the disease. These cases were in early stages of development and did not, in most affected animals, produce adverse effects. The disease probably occurs universally. Besides cattle, other species of domestic animals, including horses, sheep, swine and rats are affected with caries.

Etiology and Pathogenesis. Although caused by a complex interaction of many agents, some etiological factors are known. Carbohydrate foods accumulate in plaques on the enamel surface and especially in defects from focal hypoplasia and from enamel fractures. Oral bacteria, such as lactobacilli, ferment the carbohydrates to produce lactic, butyric, acetic and formic acids. At the critical pH value of approximately 5.5, demineralization of enamel occurs. The demineralized organic matrix is further decomposed by bacterial enzymes. Gradually the process of demineralization and decomposition creates a cavity which commonly extends through the enamel. In the infundibulum of cheek teeth, food accumulates in the space and ferments. As organic acids are formed, cavities develop and extend into the dentin and pulp. The resulting bacterial infection in the pulp may create an abscess at the apex of infected roots. In case of abscesses, exudate accumulates and causes swelling and sometimes ulceration of the gum. In rare cases a sinus communicates to the gum surface, the skin or into the maxillary sinus. The infected tooth and surrounding tissues are highly sensitive to thermal changes and contact pressures. The affected animal, especially in advanced disease stages, is reluctant to masticate and to drink cold water. Consequently, body weight diminishes and malnutrition develops.

Focal hypoplasia, an underdevelopment of enamel tissue, begins during embryogenesis of teeth. The probable causes include systemic infections, such as viral bovine rhinotracheitis; systemic intoxications, such as fluorosis; and systemic nutritional deficiencies, such as avitaminosis-A. These generalized adversities injure ameloblasts, the enamel-forming cells, during their formative stages and result in areas in teeth of enamel underdevelopment.

Clinical Signs and Postmortem Lesions. During early stages of development dental caries provokes few apparent clinical signs. Careful visual examination of the teeth, however, often discloses single or multiple shallow cavities in either enamel or dentin. The infected tissue is orange-brown or black. In advanced stages of caries, when the dental pulp has been invaded or when considerable dental tissue has decomposed, the animal demonstrates pain in the infected teeth. Prehension and mastication of food are not only reduced but slow and irregular. Cold drinking water is avoided. Empty chewing movements are made and a mixture of saliva and unmasticated food drips from the mouth. Masses of poorly masticated food accumulate in the buccal cavity. The affected animal becomes unthrifty and malnourished. Further examination of the teeth discloses deep cavities with black discoloration of the infected dental tissue. Often cavities are filled with fermenting feed. In cases of apical root abscesses, the gum is swollen and occasionally ulcerated. The extracted tooth reveals purulent exudate around the roots and the cavities penetrating the pulp.

Lesions vary according to stage of development of the carious process. In early

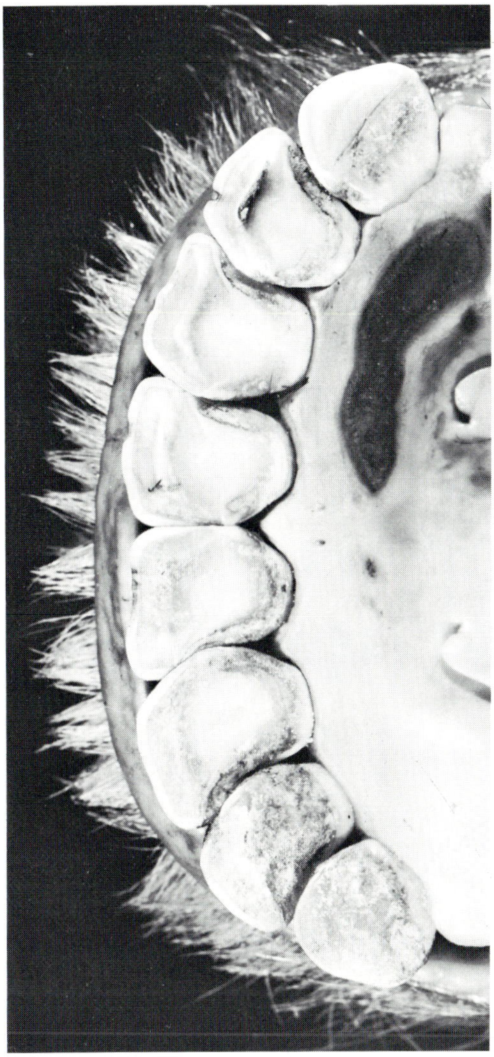

FIG. 8-1. *Dental caries in right 3rd incisor.* × 1.5.

stages, the focus of decay forms a cavity which is orange to brown. In more advanced stages an enlarging dark colored cavity forms which is usually filled with decomposing feed. If decay extends into the pulp cavity, an abscess may be present around the root. The gum, especially on the buccal side, is swollen and often ulcerated. Rarely does a sinus extend from the infected root to the mucous membrane of the mouth, the maxillary sinus or the skin. The affected tooth may be loosened.

Diagnosis. Caries is diagnosed by visual examination of the teeth and by identification of a dark cavity in the dental tissue. The cavity is located either in the enamel or dentin. In advanced stages the affected tooth in the living animal is sensitive to slight tapping and to forced movement. A large amount of the tooth may be darkened.

The differential diagnosis requires consideration of paradontal disease and actinomy-

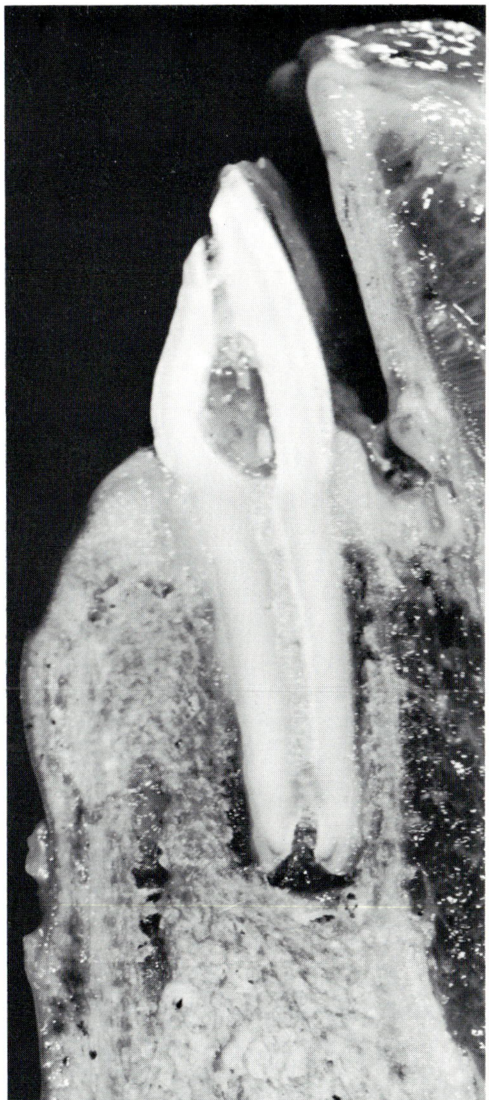

FIG. 8-2. *Same as figure 8-1, saggital section.* × 2.6.

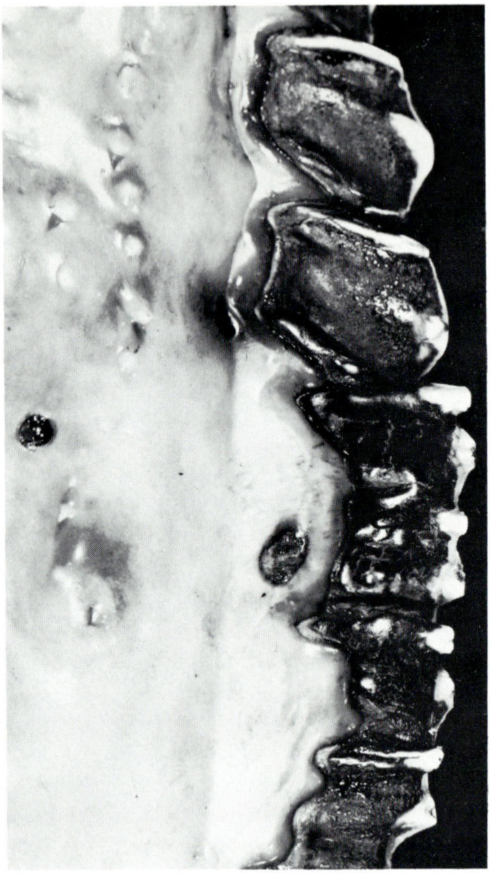

FIG. 8-3. *Ulceration of gum from caries and root abscess.* × 1.0.

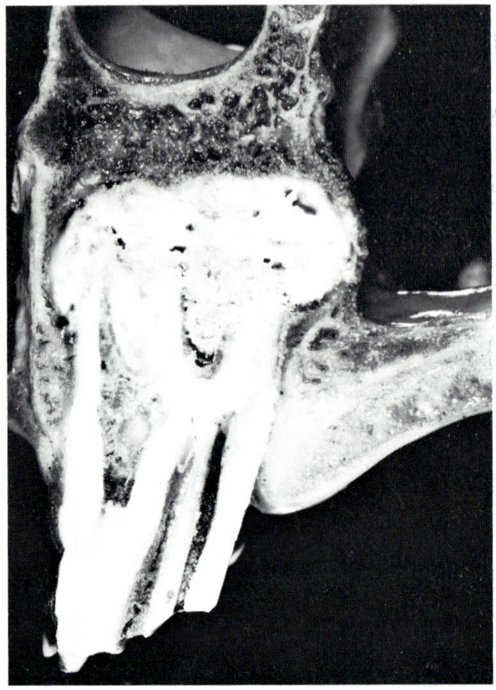

FIG. 8-4. *Caries and root abscess of right 1st maxillary molar.* × 1.1.

cosis of the mandible or maxilla. Paradontal disease is the formation of infection in the periodontal membrane. The gum recedes and the tooth becomes loosened. Actinomycosis of the mandible or maxilla causes bony deformation from bone lysis and from new bone formation. Sinuses usually discharge exudate to the surface. Typical rosettes with gram-positive filaments can be identified in the purulent exudate or tissue sections.

Prevention and Treatment. Teeth are predisposed to decay by enamel hypoplasia. The latter may be caused by systemic intoxications, systemic infections and malnutrition during the time of enamel formation. Enamel hypoplasia may be reduced and caries, in turn, prevented by providing balanced mineral nutrition and by avoiding systemic intoxications and infections during the stages of tooth formation. Since tooth decay progresses slowly and is not harmful in early stages, treatment is not necessary in most young feedlot cattle. In older cattle, however, advanced caries requires extraction of affected teeth for normal prehension, mastication, feed utilization and gain in body weight. To assist in range feed prehension, metal caps may be fitted to incisor teeth of aged breeding cows.

References

Cohrs, P.: *Lehrbuch der Speziellen pathologischen anatomie der Haustiere.* Vierte Auflage. Gustav Fischer Verlag. Stuttgart. (1962): 328–334.

Colyer, Frank: *Variations and Diseases of the Teeth of Animals.* John Bale, Sons and Danielsson, Ltd. London, (1963).

Garlick, N. L.: The Teeth of the Ox in Clinical Diagnosis. III. Developmental Anomalies and General Pathology. AJVR, *15* (1954): 500–508.

Kite, O. W., Shaw, J. H. and Sognnaes, R. F.: Prevention

of Experimental Tooth Decay by Tube Feeding. J. Nutrition, *42* (1950): 89.

Kostyra, J.: Investigations on the Occurrence, Course, and Treatment of Dental Caries in Cattle. Annals Universitatis Mariae Curie-Sklodowska, *18* (1963): 121–188.

Orland, F. J.: Chapter in book *Advances in Experimental Caries Research.* American Assoc. Advancement of Science., Washington, D.C. (1955): 169–186.

Sognnaes, R. F.: Chapter in book *Advances in Experimental Caries Research,* American Assoc. Advancement of Science., Washington, D. C. (1955): 223–225.

Paradontal Disease

(PERIODONTITIS; PARADENITIS; ALVEOLAR PERIOSTITIS)

Paradontal disease, a chronic infection of the periodontal membrane, is characterized by loosening and shedding of the teeth. In cattle, the painfulness of affected teeth reduces the capacity of the animal to prehend and masticate feed. Animals seriously affected, consequently, lose body weight, become malnourished and are marketable only as low-grade meat. While the precise disease incidence is unknown, and since most cases occur in middle-aged and old animals, the resulting economic losses are probably reduced to a low and, possibly, insignificant level.

Review of Literature. Paradontal disease has been diagnosed and studied in wild mammals, horses (Colyer, 1963) and in cattle and other ruminants (Cohrs, 1962). In sheep the disease caused serious economic losses through low productivity and mortality and reached an annual incidence of 11% in a flock of 900 ewes. The affected animals were 4 years of age and older. Both incisor and cheek teeth were affected. Studies of the assumed cause in sheep revealed the presence of numerous species of anaerobic bacteria and *Corynebacterium pyogenes* in the infected periodontal membrane. However, cultures of these organisms placed in the

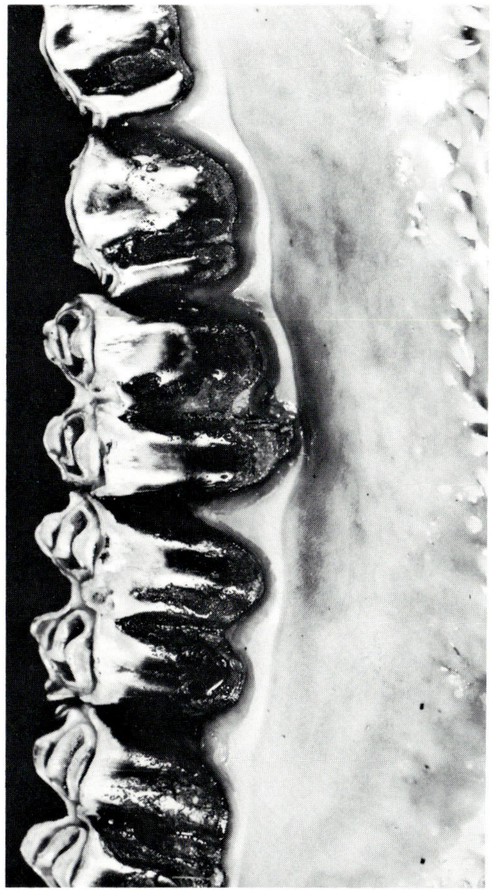

FIG. 8-5. *Recession of gum from paradontal disease.* × 1.0.

mouths of normal sheep failed to produce the disease (Heart and MacKinnon, 1958; Salisbury, Armstrong and Gray, 1953). Studies of the pathologic changes disclosed gradual but continuous destruction of the periodontal membrane with loosening of the affected teeth and extension of epithelium from the gingival membrane to form an incomplete lining in the alveolus (MacKinnon, 1959). In the study of the teeth of 7,480 young fattened cattle paradontal disease was not mentioned (Garlick, 1954).

Occurrence. While detailed and systematic studies of paradontal disease in cattle have not been made, available evidence indicates that the incidence is low, but that all breeds and both sexes are susceptible. Most cases occur in middle-aged and old animals. The geographic distribution probably is universal. Other species of affected domestic mammals include dogs, sheep and horses.

Etiology and Pathogenesis. The cause of paradontal disease presumably is a mixed bacterial infection in the periodontal membrane. Factors which predispose teeth to this disease include the deposition of dental calculus at the gingival sulcus and penetration of the gingival membrane near the teeth by foreign bodies, such as grass awns. These factors enable oral bacteria to enter the periodontal membrane.

Comprehension of the pathogenesis of paradontal disease requires some detailed knowledge of the anatomy of the teeth and the alveolus. Each tooth consists of a crown, neck and root. The crown projects beyond the gingival membrane into the oral cavity, while the root is located within and attached to the bony alveolus. The neck is that portion of the tooth at the junction of the crown and root. The crown of incisor teeth contains, from the exterior towards the center, enamel, dentin and pulp. On the root cementum replaces the enamel. In cheek teeth, both crown and root contain, from the exterior to the center, cementum, enamel, dentin and pulp. The infundibulum also contains layers of cementum and dentin. The periodontal membrane of both incisor and cheek teeth consists of many bundles of heavy collagenous fibers which firmly attach the cementum of the root to the alveolar bone. The fibers also serve as periosteum to the alveolus. The epithelial cells of the gingival membrane attach directly to the cementum at the neck of the tooth. A slight indentation of the gingival membrane near the point of attachment creates the gingival sulcus, a small crevice around the tooth.

Paradontal disease probably begins with the deposition of calculus on the cementum in the gingival sulcus or with penetration of the epithelium in the gingival sulcus by foreign bodies, such as grass awns or wood fragments. Through the points of discontinuity of epithelium in the gingival sulcus, oral bacteria penetrate into the periodontal membrane. The necrotizing infection destroys the collagenous fibers and creates a small cavity between the cementum and alveolar bone. Exudate may accumulate in the cavity. Gradually the infection extends around the tooth and towards the apex. The tooth becomes loosened and feed accumulates in the cavity. The tooth may be lost or held loosely in position by opposing teeth. The accumulation of feed in the socket may cause lateral or medial displacement of the tooth. Granulation tissue forms in the alveolus and new bone may be deposited near the alveolar bone. The infected alveolus may become epithelialized by extension of gingival epithelium. Following removal of the loosened tooth, healing usually occurs.

Clinical Signs and Postmortem Lesions. Clinical signs vary according to extent of involvement and degree of development of the disease. In early stages of the disease mastication may be near normal. Visual examination of the mouth reveals, at the point of infection, recession and atrophy of the gum. Digital pressure may express a small amount of purulent exudate from around the tooth. In advanced stages, prehension and mastication of food are quantitatively reduced because of pain and discomfort from use of the teeth. During idle chewing movements, drops of saliva and fragments of food escape from the mouth. The animal may fail to gain or may even lose body weight. Careful palpation may also disclose enlargement and firmness of tissue around the infected teeth. Oral examination reveals looseness of the infected teeth in addition to recession and atrophy of the gum. Feed may have accumulated and impacted in the alveolus to displace the loose teeth, either medially or laterally. Granulation tissue is noticeable in the alveolus and may be infected with *Spherophorus necrophorus* and/or *Actinobacillus ligniersi.* Offensive odors emanate from the necrotic tissue. Some affected teeth

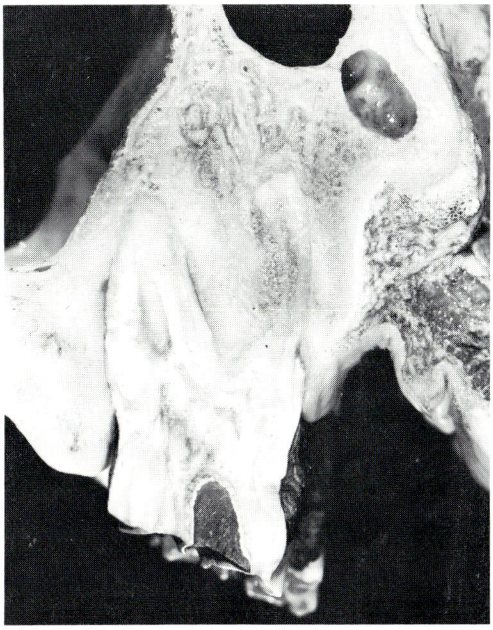

FIG. 8-6. *Cross section of maxillary 1st molar with paradontal disease.* × 1.4.

are sufficiently loose for removal without instruments.

Diagnosis. Clinically, paradontal disease is suspected in adult cattle which manifest typical signs. Slow and irregular mastication of small amounts of feed and unthriftiness are especially indicative. A positive diagnosis is obtained through oral examination which often reveals the loosened teeth, the receding gum and the periodontal infection. The differential diagnosis requires consideration of dental caries and dental fractures. In dental caries, a dark-colored cavity is in the dental tissue and an abscess may have formed near the apex of the root. Carious teeth frequently are not loosened. Dental fractures create fissures which subdivide the tooth into fragments. Caries and general infection often follow fracturing.

Treatment. During early stages the affected teeth do not adversely affect prehension, mastication and digestion and, consequently, do not require treatment. In advanced stages,

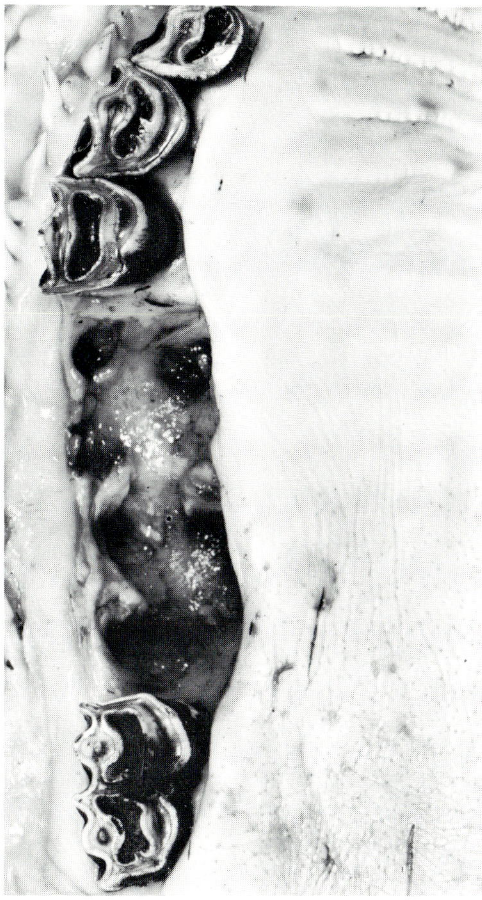

FIG. 8-7. *Teeth lost from paradontal disease.* × 0.8.

when the disease interferes with prehension and mastication, the infected teeth must be extracted by surgical procedures. Alveolar infection may be treated by the daily intramuscular administration of 1 gm of streptomycin sulfate per 100 pounds of body weight for 5 to 7 days; following treatment with this drug, slaughter must not occur for at least 30 days. If excessive granulation tissue inhibits normal mastication, emergency slaughter for recovery of investment should be performed.

References

Cohrs, P.: *Speziellen Pathologischen Anatomie der Haustiere.* Vierte Auflage. Gustav Fischer Verlag. Stuttgart. 1962. pp. 335–338.

Colyer, Frank: *Variations and Diseases of the Teeth of Animals.* John Bale Sons, and Danielsson, Ltd. London, 1963.
Garlick, N. L.: The Teeth of the Ox in Clinical Diagnosis. III. Developmental Anomalies and General Pathology. AJVR, *15* (1954): 500–508.
Hart, K. E. and MacKinnon, M. M.: Enzootic Paradontal Disease of Adult Sheep in the Bulls-Santoft Area. New Zealand Vet. J., *6* (1958): 118–123.
MacKinnon, M. M.: A Pathological Study of an Enzootic Paradontal Disease of the Mature Sheep. New Zealand Vet. J., *7* (1959): 18–26.
Salisbury, R. M., Armstrong, M. C. and Gray, K. G.: Ulcero-membranous Gingivitis in the Sheep. New Zealand Vet. J., *1* (1953): 51–52.

Esophageal Obstruction

(ESOPHAGEAL OCCLUSION; CHOKE)

Characterized by salivation and rejection of food and water, esophageal obstruction is the accidental lodgement of ingesta in the lumen. Occlusion may be partial or complete. If partial, limited amounts of fluid and gas may by-pass the static mass. If complete, gases cannot traverse the esophagus, and, consequently, accumulate within the forestomachs. Since it occurs sporadically, the disease has little economic importance to the cattle feeding industry, but under local favorable conditions the incidence and mortality may be high and economically serious to a livestock owner of a single herd.

Occurrence. Esophageal obstructions occur in all breeds and sexes. While the disease may occur in all ages, animals from 6 months to 2 years are more commonly affected. Animals under 6 months less commonly ingest choking material, and in animals older than 2 years the esophagi are fully developed and appetities more discriminating.

In late summer, autumn and early winter cattle are admitted to feedlots, but during early stages of the fattening process the animals often are allowed to graze fields for final harvesting of available animal feed. This economic salvage practice gives cattle access to particulate feed material which may obstruct the esophageal passage. Within the United States the western and midwestern states have a relatively high incidence, because geographically the disease occurs more commonly where sugar beet, potato and apple production accompany the feedlot industry.

Etiology and Pathogenesis. Esophageal obstruction follows a combination of exciting and predisposing factors. The direct, exciting agents are feeds with particulate diameters too large to pass freely through the lumen. Common offending feeds include sugar beet crowns, whole or fragments of sugar beets, table beets, ear corn, cull fruits, turnips, potatoes, corn cobs and carrots. These may be grazed from fields in the early stages of feedlot fattening, or they may be fed from crop surpluses.

Occasionally bones, wood fragments and pieces of metal or other objects may be deliberately or accidentally ingested. If the particle diameters are too large for easy passage or if their surface configurations are irregular, the foreign bodies lacerate and perforate the wall.

Predisposing factors that limit passage are congenital or acquired esophageal abnormalities, such as diverticula, strictures from scar tissue, inflammation and edema in the esophageal wall and papillomas projecting into the lumen. Scar strictures may be the residuals from trauma of previous obstructions, lacerations or perforations. Local inflammation and edema may come from death of *Hypoderma lineatum* larvae in the esophageal wall. The larvae may be killed by the administration of organophosphate insecticide. Swelling and edema may result in obstruction and cause bloat. Severe tympanites requires relief by passage of a stomach tube.

The prehended food particles such as sugar beet crowns, roots or fragments, may be too large for free passage through the esophagus or too large, tough, hard or smooth for easy mastication. When attempts at mastication are unsuccessful, the large unwieldy particle mass is forced into the pharynx, and swallowed. Because the peristolic pressures are inadequate to push the rigidly shaped food through the lumen, the food mass lodges at some part of the esophagus, and the occlusion is partial or complete. In cattle, obstructing food usually lodges immediately posterior to the anterior entrance or at some point along the cervical part of the esophagus, but in some bovine cases, the obstruction locates in the thorax near the cardia. Lodgement stimulates forceful peristaltic contractions which may eventually move the food along, but if obstruction is firm and immovable, local pressure at the points of tissue contact with the obstructing body causes necrosis of the esophageal wall. Saliva, other food, and water accumulate anterior to the obstruction and are forced either forward by overfilling, or by reversed peristalsis, into the mouth and nose. The saliva and ingesta are discharged to the exterior. Some food particles, saliva and water may enter the larynx, trachea and bronchi and precipitate foreign body pneumonia.

Normal ruminal fermentation produces gas which escapes through eructation, but as a result of esophageal obstruction the gas is retained, and bloat develops. Prolonged maceration occasionally softens or alters the feed sufficiently to enable spontaneous dislodgment.

Obstructing objects may contain surface indentations or perforations which permit the passage of some gas from the rumen through the esophagus and some fluids to enter the rumen from the esophagus. Irregularly shaped obstructing foreign bodies may lacerate the mucosa and perforate the entire wall. Unless the obstruction is relieved, death results from bloat, foreign body pneumonia or infection through injuries in the esophagus. After injury to the mucosa, correction of the obstruction may result in local scarring and constriction with predisposition to subsequent obstruction.

Clinical Signs and Postmortem Lesions. Since the onset of esophageal obstruction is sudden, the affected animal becomes quickly distressed and alarmed. Prehension of feed usually ceases immediately. The head is extended and mastication and swallowing movements are strong and repetitive. Saliva and feed particles drip from the mouth and nose. With the obstruction near the larynx, breathing may be difficult, oral and gasping. Coughing is frequent. The animal strains and often changes the position of the head and neck. Bloat develops rapidly and aggravates the animal's distress. Careful palpation along the cervical part of the esophagus may reveal the obstruction, but the thick skin and heavy musculature tend to obscure it and also make palpation inaccurate and confusing excepting for skilled, experienced veterinarians. In animals with partial occlusion, the appearance of clinical signs may be delayed several days. During the asymptomatic period the animal consumes little or no food or water, becomes dehydrated with gauntness and retraction of the eyes, constipated, and in severe cases, physically weakened and incoordinated.

In fatal cases lesions are found in the alimentary and respiratory systems. The obstructing mass is present in the esophagus, and while usually located in the cervical part, one is occasionally in the thoracic portion. In prolonged obstructions the esophageal mucosa and even musculature may be necrotic and infected, and inflammation and edema may surround the affected part of the esophagus. Anterior to the obstruction, the esophagus may be filled with saliva, feed particles and water. Lacerating and perforating points on the obstructing mass may have injured the traversed portion of the esophageal mucosa. Posterior to the obstruction the esophagus is empty. The rumen may be acutely distended with gas. The larynx and trachea may contain aspirated saliva and feed particles. Because of the entrance of the foreign material into the bronchi, bronchioles and alveoli, foreign body pneumonia may have developed.

Diagnosis. A positive clinical diagnosis requires typical signs, mechanical probing and a history of available obstructing feed particles. Important indicative signs are drooling of saliva and feed particles, repeated chewing and swallowing movements, bloating, straining and coughing. Confirmation can be obtained by dextrous palpation of cervical obstructions and by careful probing with an instrument in the cervical and thoracic parts of the esophagus. Probing should be performed carefully in order to avoid traumatic damage to the already injured esophageal wall. In fatal cases, the determination of complicating bloat or bronchopneumonia, and confirmation of the diagnosis can be obtained at necropsy.

The differential diagnosis should include the consideration of rabies, primary bloat, bronchopneumonia and polioencephalomalacia. In animals affected with rabies, the salivation and drooling comes from partial paralysis of muscles of deglutition. The animal commonly bellows in a characteristically low pitched voice, and bloat does not occur. In polioencephalomalacia, the pharyngeal muscles may be paralyzed from lesions of the central nervous system; the affected animals manifest depression and impaired vision, but no bloat. Probing of the esophagus reveals patency. A primary bloat case carries an animal history of easy access to bloat-producing feeds such as fresh legumes, and a stomach tube can be readily passed through the esophagus into the distended rumen. Animals affected with pneumonia may show dyspnea, coughing and limited bloating; salivation and repeated swallowing movements are absent; and probing of the esophagus shows complete patency.

Prevention and Treatment. By denying access to fields where obstructing food particles may be found and prehended by cattle, most cases of esophageal choke can be avoided. Potatoes, sugar beets, sugar beet crowns and other large particles of feeds should be chopped into small fragments before feeding. Following correction of occlusion, the animal is predisposed, by the local lesion, to additional choking. To avoid recurrence the original feed should be withheld for 10 to 14 days, and substituted with a diet of soft feed such as green chopped alfalfa, wet sugar beet pulp and dampened grain.

Although varying with individual cases, treatment includes both relief of acute bloat and removal of the esophageal obstructing mass. If bloat is severe and threatens fatality, the rumen should be trocarized. In animals with moderate or less bloating, attention should be directed towards removal of the obstruction. Control of the animal requires restraining, preferably in a chute, and the application of a mouth speculum. The anatomical location of the obstruction may be determined by either cervical palpation and/or careful esophageal probing. Obstructions within the cervical part of the esophagus may be manually pushed forward to the pharynx or to a position accessible to grasping instruments. In some cases the loop of a doubled wire may be passed in the esophagus beyond the obstruction, then repeatedly pulled forward to engage the obstruction and draw it forward into the pharynx and mouth. In some cases a cutting trocar may be passed through the skin and esophageal wall and used carefully to comminute the obstruction. Care must be exercised to avoid mechanical injury to the esophagus. Obstructions located in the thoracic part of the esophagus may be pushed with a stomach tube or with a firmer hose probe along the esophagus into the rumen. If probing indicates immovability of the object, lubricating mineral oil or water and detergents should be pumped against the mass, and muscle relaxants, such as Diprone, should be administered to relax the muscular esophageal wall. In some cases, rumenotomy and passing grasping instruments, such as the loop from a doubled wire, into the posterior part of the esophagus may dislodge the obstruction.

Following correction of the obstruction, bronchopneumonia if present should be treated by administering antibiotics or sulfonamides. In case of serious injury incurred

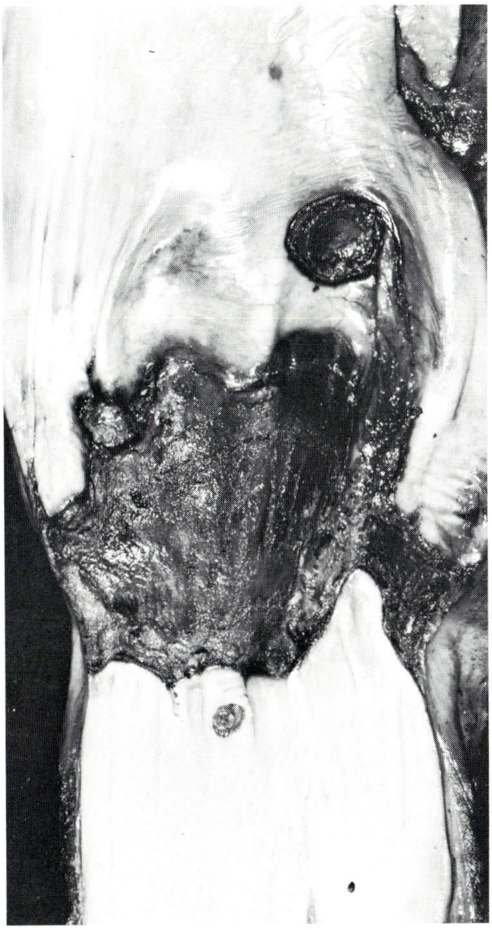

FIG. 8-8. *Necrosis of esophagus at point of obstruction. Anterior is above.* × 1.1.

during occlusion or correction, infection in and around the esophagus should be treated with equal parts of sodium bicarbonate and sulfonamides administered in gelatin capsules. If, in the process of treatment, the esophagus is ruptured, the animal should be slaughtered immediately for recovery of investment.

References

Udall, D. H.: *The Practice of Veterinary Medicine.* 6th Ed. Udall Publishing Co., Ithaca, New York. 1954. pp. 91–96.

Fincher, M. G. and Fox, F. H.: *Diseases of Cattle,* 2nd Ed. American Veterinary Publications, Inc. Wheaton, Ill. 1963. pp. 186–188.

Hutyra, F., Marek, J., and Manninger, R.: *Special Pathology and Therapeutics of the Diseases of Domestic Animals.* Vol. II. 4th Ed. Alexander Eger, Chicago. 1938. pp. 43–50.

Traumatic Reticulitis

(TRAUMATIC GASTRITIS;
TRAUMATIC PERITONITIS)

Traumatic reticulitis, an acute or chronic mechanical injury to the reticular wall, occurs in all ages of adult cattle and is caused by fragments of ingested metal. Traumatic reticulitis results in serious economic losses through mortality, reduced body weight, impaired capacity to gain weight and through condemnation of abscessed livers and stomachs at the time of slaughter.

Review of Literature. Veterinarians have long recognized that serious and numerous digestive disturbances result from the omnivorous and indiscriminating feeding habits of cattle. While traumatic reticulitis has been considered, in general, to be of paramount importance in dairy cattle (Udall, 1954), it has also been a major malady of feedlot animals. In one survey the incidence of the disease in fattened beef cattle was compared with the incidence in retired dairy cows. The stomachs and stomach contents from 2,042 prime beef cattle were examined for foreign bodies at slaughter. Of these, 670 (32.8%) contained foreign bodies capable of causing internal injuries. Of the latter number, 199 stomachs were being traumatised. The same study included 2,042 retired dairy cows. Of these, 1,698 (83.1%) contained foreign bodies within the stomachs, and 956 stomachs were injured by the metals (Fredrick, 1943). In another survey the stomachs from 1,535 adult fattened cattle were examined. Of these, 85 (5.5%) exhibited foreign body injury to the gastric wall. In many affected animals, liver abscesses were coexisting with the stomach injuries (Jensen *et al.,* 1954).

Occurrence. All adult cattle of both sexes are susceptible to gastric injury from ingested metal. At slaughter time, approximately 5 to 10% of fattened cattle manifest gastric trauma to some degree. Fragments of metal are more apt to contaminate roughage feed, especially when chopped; therefore, the disease probably begins more commonly during early periods of fattening when roughage constitutes a larger portion of the total ration.

Etiology and Pathogenesis. Injurious fragments include nails, pieces of wire and scraps of sheet metal. At the time of baling, pieces of baling-wire may accidentally enter the hay. Because occasional pieces of wire are accidentally chopped along with the hay, chopped wire-baled hay is especially dangerous. Accidentally, nails from construction may also get in the hay. Chopping machines which gather hay directly from the field may simultaneously gather and chop pieces of wire. Often small nails and tacks are present in both hay and concentrates. In the process of rolling and grinding, mills pass the feed over strong magnets to remove foreign metallic bodies. Unless the magnets are kept clean and in good condition, they are ineffective for the intended purpose.

At the time of feeding, the non-discriminating animal ingests the metallic fragments along with the feed. With little or no injury to the mouth or esophagus, the metals usually pass into the rumen or reticulum. Metals entering the rumen may, by ruminal contractions, be thrown forward into the reticulum. While many pieces of metal reside innocuously in the lumen of the reticulum, some are forced by gastric contractions and possibly by abnormal animal positions and movements, into the wall of the reticulum. Penetration of the wall may be in any direction and to variable depths. Commonly the direction is forward through the reticulum, diaphragm, pericardium and myocardium, or any fraction of that distance. Penetration of the reticular wall often immobilizes not only the reticulum but the rumen. Local peritonitis with subsequent adhesions, and occasionally generalized peritonitis, develops in the peritoneal cavity following injury. Penetration of the diaphragm and pericardium establishes pericarditis. The ingested metal may be withdrawn from one area and re-penetrate other areas. Commonly, a sinus extends from the reticulum at the point of entrance to the full depth of penetration. The resulting mechanical injury and mixed bacterial infection carried by the metal commonly evoke a persisting leukocytosis. Trauma of the reticulum may allow ruminal bacteria, especially *Spheropherus necrophorus*, to infect the subepithelial tissues, penetrate branches of the portal vein and be conveyed to the liver where abscesses may form.

Clinical Signs and Postmortem Lesions. In early stages of the disease body temperature may be elevated. Affected animals develop constipation and inappetence and lose body weight. Locomotion, performed with caution and reluctance, is painful. Pressure applied to the left anteroventral part of the abdomen provokes pain, muscular rigidity, and general discomfort. Grunting is common and bloating

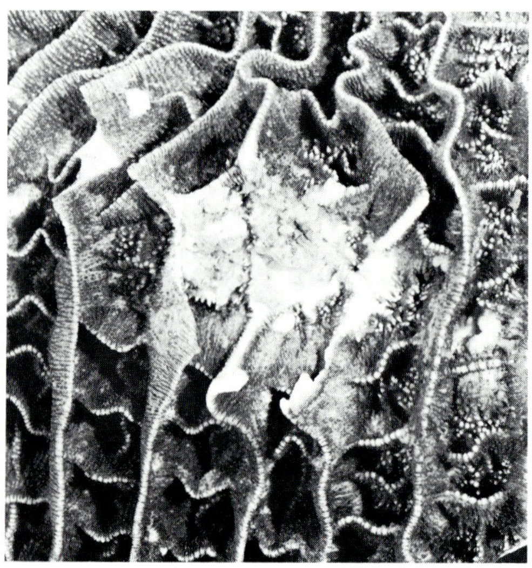

FIG. 8-9. *Reticulum traumatized by a piece of wire.* × 0.8.

may occur. The leukocyte count is persistently high. Additional signs of pericarditis or pleuritis may be associated with penetration of the foreign body into the pericardium or pleura respectively.

At necropsy, or at slaughter, metal fragments are usually found in the lumen of the reticulum. One or more pieces may penetrate the reticular wall and also may have passed into the peritoneum, diaphragm and pericardium. Adhesions between serosal surfaces are common. A sinus tract, with or without the offending metal, can usually be located. Peritonitis, pericarditis and pleuritis may be present also. As a result of pyogenic bacteria entering branches of the portal system in the area of foreign body penetration, liver abscesses may be present.

Histopathologically, granulation tissue is present around the sinus. At slaughter, traumatized stomachs are condemned for human food. In case of generalized peritonitis, pleuritis or pericarditis, the carcass also is condemned.

Diagnosis. Often accompanied with obscure clinical signs, traumatic reticulitis is difficult to diagnose. A few typical signs form the basis for diagnosis. Of special importance is the tenderness in the region of the xyphoid cartilage and the persisting leukocytosis of the blood. In case of pericarditis, auscultation reveals the presence of exudate, sometimes mixed with gas, in the pericardial sac.

The differential diagnosis requires consideration of peritonitis, abomasal ulcers, liver abscesses and pleuritis. In peritonitis the clinical signs of traumatic pericarditis are enhanced and may be caused by foreign body penetration. Abdominal tenderness and rigidity are generalized. Abomasal ulcers may be complicated with hemorrhage into the ingesta and feces, or by peritonitis from perforation of the gastric wall. Hepatic necrobacillosis and multiple liver abscesses are associated with diarrhea and yellow feces. The right anteroventral part of the abdomen is painful and rigid to palpation. Unilateral diaphragmatic pleuritis and pneumonia from foreign body penetration can be detected by auscultation.

Prevention and Treatment. In order to avoid contamination with fragments of metal, the feed is prepared with meticulous care. The baling of hay with wire should be avoided. By passage over strong magnets, which remove most of the ferrous metal, chopped feed can be decontaminated. Fields, pens, fences and feeding bunks should be cleared of loose metallic fragments.

Treatment consists in specific and supportive measures and varies with stages of the disease. In early stages a laxative, such as 1 pound of magnesium oxide, is administered to combat constipation and abomasal ulcers if present. Magnetized iron, manufactured for this specific purpose, can be placed in the reticulum via the esophagus. Adhering to the magnet, the fragments of metal are innocuous. The animal should be confined, except for brief daily exercise, for 3 to 5 days in a standing position with the fore-feet 6 to 8 inches higher than the rear-feet. This position facilitates withdrawal of metal penetrating the anterior reticular wall. Antibiotics, such as streptomycin administered at the rate of 1 gram per 100 pounds of body weight, helps to control peritonitis and pleuritis.

In severe and advanced stages, laparotomy is performed for removal of foreign bodies from the stomachs.

Animals in terminal stages of fattening and not febrile should be slaughtered for recovery of economic value.

References

Frederick, L. D.: The Economic and Nutritional Importance of Bovine Hepatic Disturbances. JAVMA, *102* (1943): 338–344.

Jensen, Rue, Deane, H. M., Cooper, J. L., Miller, V. A. and Graham, W. R.: The Rumenitis-Liver Abscess Complex in Beef Cattle. AJVR, *15* (1954): 202–216.

Udall, D. H.: *The Practice of Veterinary Medicine.* 6th ed. Udall Publishing Co. Ithaca. 1954. pp. 111–123.

Hyperkeratosis of the Rumen

(RUMINAL PARAKERATOSIS)

Ruminal hyperkeratosis, a degenerative change of the mucosa, is characterized grossly by hardening, enlargement and clumping of papillae, and microscopically by the accumulation of excessive layers of keratinized squamous epithelial cells on the papillae. The disease occurs in cattle and sheep, and is caused by fattening on finely ground feed. While of limited importance, it reduces efficiency in feed utilization and interferes at slaughter with cleaning of the rumen in the preparation of tripe.

Review of Literature. Hyperkeratosis has been observed in calves, fattened adult cattle and sheep. In calves affected with diarrhea and vitamin A deficiency, the rumen, over extensive areas including the non-papillated pillars, manifested thickening and hardening of the mucosa (Cohrs, 1962).

In fattened cattle a sample of 1,535 animals was studied. Of these, 135 (8.8%) contained varying degrees of ruminal hyperkeratosis. This lesion was manifested by thickening and hardening of some papillae, the adherence of many papillae in clumps, and by multiple foci of brown, hardened areas in the non-papillated mucosa of the rumen. The changes were more common in the mucosa over the dorsal curvature and in the anterior dorsal sac (Jensen *et al.*, 1954).

The condition was investigated in feedlot lambs under controlled experimentation, and also in commercial feedlots. In two experiments, each involving 100 lambs, the ration was finely ground and pelleted. In each experiment, at the time of slaughter, a significantly larger number of cases of ruminal hyperkeratosis were found in the lots fattened on ground feed. In a commercial feedlot, 569 lambs were fattened on coarse feed, while 1,000 lambs were fattened on ground pelleted feed. At the time of slaughter, 7.7% of the sheep fattened on coarse feed and 39.2% of the animals fattened on ground pelleted feed contained ruminal hyperkeratosis. The observations led the investigators to conclude that finely ground feeds contribute to the cause of ruminal hyperkeratosis (Jensen *et al.*, 1958).

In other investigations, the effects of ground feed on fattening cattle were confirmed. Five steers were fattened on a ration of concentrate. At slaughter, ruminal hyperkeratosis to some degree was observed in each animal. The two cattle with severe hyperkeratosis gained little body weight during the last 2 months of fattening (Tamate *et al.*, 1967). In another experiment four fistulated steers were fed alfalfa hay for 33 days followed by alfalfa pellets for 56 days. At the end of the hay-feeding period the rumens appeared normal, but after the pellet-consuming time many papillae were hyperkeratinized. Estimations of ruminal absorption of nutrients indicated that during the hay-feeding period 46% more of the volatile fatty acids were absorbed than during the pellet-feeding period (Hinders and Owens, 1965).

Occurrence. Hyperkeratosis occurs in both sexes and all ages of fattened cattle. At the time of slaughter, approximately 8.8% of fattened cattle contain ruminal hyperkeratosis to some degree. The incidence is highest among cattle fattened on rations having a high ratio of concentrate to roughage and especially in animals whose diet has been pelleted. In addition to cattle, fattened sheep commonly develop this disorder.

Etiology and Pathogenesis. The continuous and exclusive feeding for prolonged periods on finely ground ration with or without pelleting causes hyperkeratosis of the rumen. Reducing roughage in the ration to a low level may also be a contributing factor.

An important function of the rumen is the storage, mixing and digestion of fibrous roughage feeds. From such materials cellulosolytic bacteria form volatile fatty acids, a major source of available energy. Papillae provide an enormous absorptive surface area of mucous membrane where some abrasion by feed fibers occurs. If the feed is finely comminuted, abrasive action does not occur. Consequently, excessive layers of keratinized squamous epithelial cells accumulate. Colonies of bacteria, ingested hairs, plant fibers and fragments of feed accumulate in and on the layers of cells. In heavily papillated areas of the rumen, such as the anterior dorsal sac and anterior ventral sac, adjacent affected papillae adhere together to form dense clumps. Both the hyperkeratosis and the clumping of papillae reduce the absorptive efficiency of the mucosa. At the time of slaughter, the clumps of papillae prevent adequate cleaning of the rumen for the preparation of tripe. Presumably hyperkeratosis can be reversed by providing unground roughage in the ration.

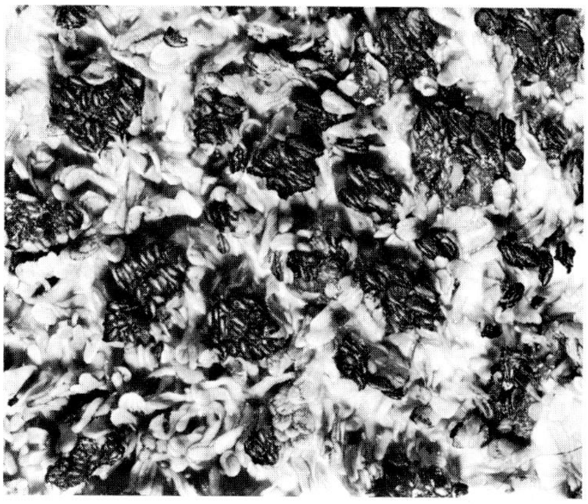

FIG. 8-10. *Clumping of ruminal papillae from hyperkeratosis.* × 1.0.

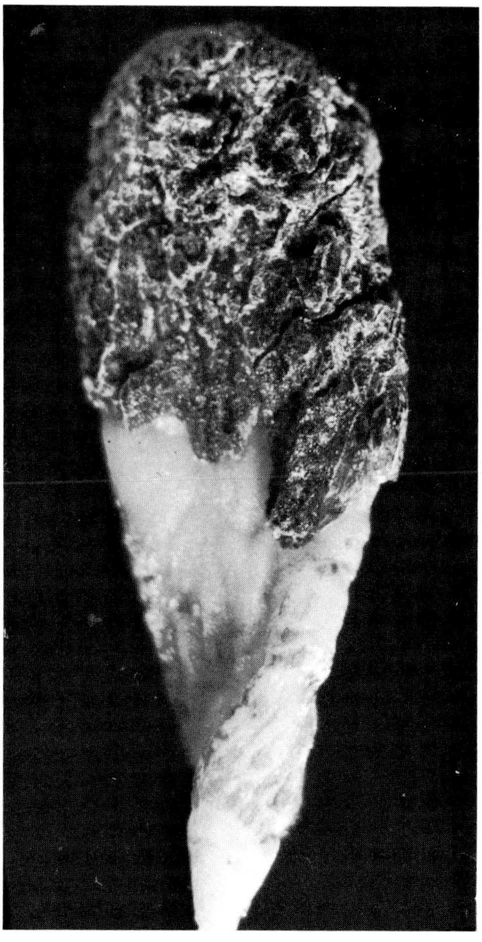

FIG. 8-11. *Hyperkeratosis of extremity of a papilla.* × 11.

Clinical Signs and Postmortem Lesions. An asymptomatic condition, hyperkeratosis of the rumen is never diagnosed clinically. At necropsy, especially at the time of slaughter, and after cleaning the rumen, foci of hyperkeratosis are apparent. Grossly, the hyperkeratosis has two manifestations: (1) Affected papillae are hardened, brown, leathery and often clumped. Individual papillae may be completely or partially hyperkeratinized. Often the distal one half or the tip is rough and hard. The detachment of hyperkeratinized papillae may significantly reduce the number of papillae within an affected part of the mucosa. (2) In the nonpapillated mucosa, especially along the dorsal curvature of the rumen, there are often multiple foci of hyperkeratosis. Each focus consists of brown firm scales which adhere to the mucosa. Removal of the scales reveals an intact mucous membrane.

Histopathologically, the surface of the mucosa contains excessive layers of keratinized squamous epithelial cells. On the surface and occasionally among the layers are fragments of feed and colonies of bacteria. Unless foreign fiber penetration has occurred, no inflammatory reaction is evoked.

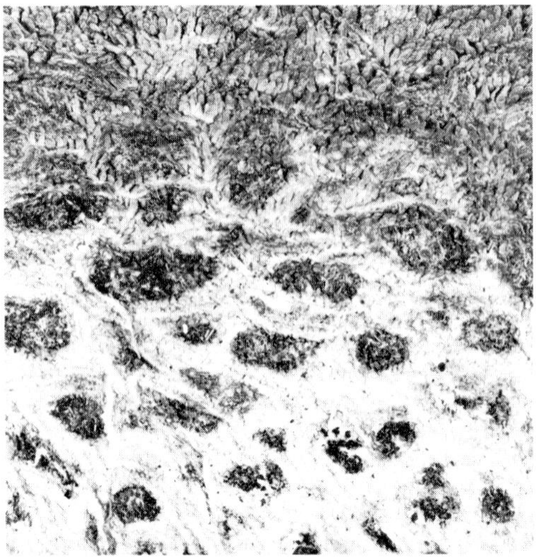

FIG. 8-12. *Focal hyperkeratosis on dorsal curvature of rumen.* × 0.6.

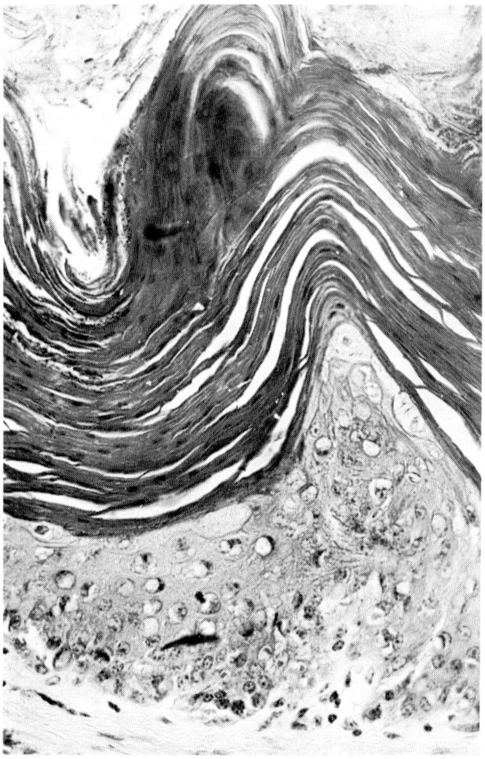

FIG. 8-13. *Hyperkeratosis. Excessive layers of keratinized cells are seen above. H&E stain.* × 200.

Diagnosis. Following washing and cleaning of the mucosa of the rumen, hyperkatosis is diagnosed at necropsy or at the time of slaughter. The firm leathery texture of tissue with clumped papillae and the foci of dark scales on the non-papillated area are the basis for diagnosis. Confirmation can be obtained by histopathologic examination of the affected rumen.

Prevention. Hyperkeratosis can be prevented to a large degree by including in the daily ration at least some unground roughage. Pelleted ration or concentrate ration should be mixed with some unground alfalfa. Feeding roughage should reduce hair-coat pulling and ingestion.

References

Cohrs, Paul: *Lehrbuch der Speziellen Pathologischen Anatomie der Haustiere.* Vierte auflage. Gustav Fisher Verlag. Stuttgart. (1962): 348.

Hinders, R. G. and Owen, F. G.: Relation of Ruminal Parakeratosis Development to Fatty Acid Absorption. J. Dairy Sc., *48* (1965): 1069–1073.

Jensen, Rue, Deane, H. M., Cooper, J. L., Miller, V. A. and Graham, W. R.: The Rumenitis-Liver Abscess Complex in Beef Cattle. JAVR., *15* (1954): 202–216.

Jensen, Rue, Flint, J. C., Udall, R. H., Deem, A. W. and Seger, C. L.: Parakeratosis of Rumens of Lambs Fattened on Pelleted Feed. AJVR, *19* (1958): 277–282.

Tamate, H., Yoneya, S., Itikawa, O., Nishimatsu, I. and Kumeno, F.: Rumen Parakeratosis in Cattle Fed a High-Concentrate Ration. Jap. J. Zootech. Sc., *38* (1967): 148–153.

Bloat

(TYMPANITES)

A metabolic disease, bloat is characterized by ruminal overdistention from pressures of feed and froth. Intra-ruminal pressures vary up to 70 mm Hg. All domestic ruminants are affected. Since bloat causes losses of more than 1.5% of the cattle production and almost equally high losses in sheep production, it is a major disease of the cattle and sheep industries. In addition, the value of many forage crops is diminished because of the danger from bloat. Except for the danger of loss from bloat, green chopped alfalfa, a feed source for inexpensive gains, would be used extensively as part of the ration for fattening cattle. The disease is classified as: (1) acute bloat in which the gas is dispersed throughout the ruminal contents as stable froth, and (2) chronic bloat in which the gas is collected in a large pocket.

Review of Literature. On the basis of duration, bloat has been classified as acute and chronic (Cole and Boda, 1960). In the chronic form, the disease recurred at frequent intervals in both feedlot and pastured cattle. Intra-ruminal pressures were moderate. Acute bloat occasionally recurred and intra-ruminal pressures varied from 45 to 70 mm Hg (Dougherty, 1953).

The cause of this disease was considered to be an interaction between diet, ruminal microflora and the ruminant animal. In pastured animals, bloat-producing diets have been shown to consist of immature, rapidly growing legumes (Cole and Boda, 1960; Dougherty, 1960; Mangan, 1959). Alfalfa and clover are especially dangerous for bloat production. In addition, bloat-producing diets for feedlot cattle have been studied. Rations consisting of barley or corn 61%, alfalfa meal 22%, soybean oil meal 16% and salt 1% have shown bloat-producing propensity. With this ration the incidence of bloat increased directly with the length of time the cattle were maintained on the ration. In the same type of ration, the substitution of 4% of the barley with soybean oil significantly increased the incidence of bloat (Elam and Davis, 1959).

Studies of the fermentation of ingesta by microflora have been made *in vivo* and *in vitro* (Cole and Boda, 1960). Results of these investigations have shown that carbon dioxide, methane and nitrogen are the major gases formed. In mixtures of ruminal liquids, legume juices and aqueous extracts of legume plants, gases evolved at different rates and in different amounts (Rosen, Fassel, Hester and Nichols, 1961). From 40 to 60% of the evolved gas was derived from citric, malonic and succinic acids. The bloat producing alfalfa had a higher content of malonic acid than non-bloat producing forage.

The formation of a stable froth, dispersed throughout the ruminal contents, depended in part on plant cytoplasmic proteins (Mangan, 1959), saponins, pectins, and low content of plant lipids (Cole and Boda, 1960; Johns, Mangan and Reid, 1957), as well as on saliva. Scrabous plant material, acting on the ruminal wall, reflexly stimulated the flow of saliva (Clark and Weiss, 1952). Microflora of the rumen have also been suspected of contributing mucopolysaccharide to the ruminal contents. The mucopolysaccharide was believed to add stability to the froth (Hungate, Fletcher, Dougherty and Barrentine, 1955).

Studies *in vitro* and *in vivo* indicated that young green legumes contain considerable pectin. The presence of Ca^{++} and HCO_3^-, pectin methylesterase converted pectin to pectic acid and carbon dioxide. The pectic acid bound with water formed stable gel which trapped bubbles of carbon dioxide as viscid froth (Gupta and Nichols, 1962). Further investigations demonstrated high bloat incidence days and low bloat incidence days. On high bloat days fresh cut legumes contained 34 to 47% more pectin methylesterase than on low bloat days (Nichols, Deese and Lang, 1968).

Physiological and anatomical animal factors have also been studied. In studies of beef cattle and of cattle twins, inherited susceptibility to bloat was suggested. The inherited mechanism was considered to be related to the reflexes for the production of saliva and eructation (Knapp, Baker and Phillips, 1943; Lindahl, Davis and Jacobson, 1957).

Causes of death from bloat have been postulated as mechanical interference to circulation and respiration from overdistention of the rumen, and also as biochemical alteration of the animal's plasma. The rumens of fistulated animals were insufflated with oxygen to respective pressures of 40, 60, 80, and 100 mm Hg for 3 continuous minutes without adverse effects. Insufflation with carbon dioxide, however, at a pressure of 60 mm Hg caused collapse of the animals in less than 3 minutes. These procedures suggested fatal biochemical changes from absorbed carbon dioxide (Dougherty, Meredith and Barrett, 1955).

Simultaneous with the study of the pathogenesis of bloat, the development of means for its prevention and treatment have been investigated. The feeding of 50 to 100 mg of procaine penicillin per animal prevented bloat for 1 to 3 days in cattle grazing on ladino clover. The effectiveness of the penicillin, however, declined after 3 to 4 weeks. The penicillin reduced the rate of gas evolution and may have altered qualitatively the ruminal microflora. Unfortunately, the use of penicillin was less effective in preventing bloat in cattle fattened on feedlot rations of concentrates (Barrentine, Shawver and Williams, 1956). In addition, the use of mineral, vegetable or animal oil administered orally at the rate of 50 to 100 grams per animal prevented bloat for 3 hours (Cole and Boda, 1960). In order to obtain a more prolonged effect, emulsified oil was sprayed on pasture at a rate that provided consumption of 2 to 4 ounces per animal per day (Reid and Johns, 1957). Also, the use of poloxalene, a non-ionic surface active substance, lowered the surface tension of ruminal fluids, and when cattle consumed at least 10 gm per animal per day, either in salt-molasses block or in grain pellet, it prevented bloat (Foote *et al.*, 1968). The effectiveness of therapeutic agents was also investigated. Froth dissipation was the principal study. Only agents having froth-dispelling capability were effective. Among these were mineral, vegetable, and animal oils (Cole and Boda, 1960; Johns, Mangan and Reid, 1957).

Occurrence. Bloat occurs as a serious problem in cattle of both sexes, and all breeds and ages. While the incidence has been especially high in cattle pastured on legume plants, it is also high among feedlot cattle fattened on rations having a high proportion of concentrates, especially barley and soybean meal. In pastured cattle bloat occurs during spring or summer when the growth rate of forage is high. Although it occurs in feedlot cattle during all months, the incidence is high during windy seasons. During recent years the practice of feeding freshly harvested legumes and grass mixtures to feedlot cattle has increased the incidence of bloat. Bloat from freshly chopped legumes has a daily variance. On high bloat days the legumes contain a larger amount of pectin methylesterase than on non-bloat days.

Etiology and Pathogenesis. Acute bloat is caused by the rapid formation, from fermentation, of stable froth in the ruminal contents and inability of the animal to eructate. Froth stability is the tendency of gas to remain as small bubbles dispersed throughout the ingesta. In an unstable froth, small gas bubbles coalesce to form a large body of free gas. Chronic recurring bloat often develops as a secondary complication to other diseases, such as diphtheria and pneumonia, which interfere with eructation. Oral administrations of antibiotics and sulfonamides may alter the ruminal microflora to a predominance of gasogenic bacteria. Bloat may also be caused by obstructive swelling of the esophageal wall following the administration of organophosphate insecticide and death of larvae of *Hypoderma lineatum.*

While the pathogenesis of bloat is incompletely understood, considerable reliable information has been obtained by careful clinical observation and by controlled experimentation. Presumably, highly fermentable feed is ingested rapidly and in large amounts. Ruminal microflora, fermenting the ingesta, form volatile fatty acids. When acidity of the ruminal contents falls to approximately pH 6, the evolution of carbon dioxide from fermentation and from salivary bicarbonate is accelerated. Bubbles of gas are disseminated throughout the contents. The produced froth is stabilized by the presence of plant proteins, pectins and saponins. Some fractions of saliva may also strengthen the viscous froth. Some free gas, accumulating in the dorsal part of the rumen, may be eructated reflexly. Froth in the cardia prevents normal eructation. With continued evolution of gas, intraruminal pressure increases to as much as 70 mm Hg. The distended rumen expands to full capacity. The pressure increases throughout the abdominal and thoracic cavities and interferes mechanically with circulation and respiration. As a result of high pressure, carbon dioxide is absorbed into the plasma where the acid base balance may be upset. The combination of mechanical and biochemical effects often are fatal after a short course.

Clinical Signs and Postmortem Lesions. Clinical signs develop rapidly during and following feeding and result from overdistention of the rumen. The intraruminal pressure causes bulging of the left paralumbar fossa. This distortion is inconspicuous and frequently overlooked in highly fattened cattle. The uneasy and uncomfortable animal stops eating. The limbs are abducted and, to facilitate breathing, the head is extended. Urination and defecation may be frequent. The eyes protrude and breathing may be accelerated and oral. Because of abdominal pain, the animal kicks the abdomen and alternates its positions of standing and recumbency. Death may occur after a course of less than 1 hour. Eructation of gas gives relief. Chronic bloat tends to recur at intervals of 6 to 24 hours.

Necropsy reveals changes which relate to overdistention of the rumen. The pauch is filled to maximal capacity. This enlargement, forcing the diaphragm forward, diminishes the size of the thoracic cavity. The rumen contents are a mixture of feed and stable froth. The upper plane of the ruminal cavity usually contains a mass of free gas. Froth and feed fill the cardia. In animals necropsied several hours after death, the wall of the rumen and even the wall of the abdomen may be ruptured because intraruminal pressure continues and increases after death.

The intra-abdominal pressure causes alteration of other organs. The blood volume in vessels and organs of the abdomen and of the thoracic cavity, including the heart, contain an abnormally small amount of blood. In contrast, the peripheral blood vasculature, especially throughout the neck and head, is distended with blood. Small veins may have ruptured to produce hemorrhage.

Diagnosis. Bloat is diagnosed clinically on the basis of typical signs. Of special importance is the distention of the abdomen. While the paralumbar fossa usually is obliterated and the wall bulges to the exterior, in highly fattened cattle this bulging is minimal and inconspicuous. In some cases experienced stockmen, deceived by the inapparent bulging, have overlooked bloating as a cause of death. The history of cattle being fattened on bloat-producing diets is also important in arriving at a diagnosis. Relief of the animal from eructation or from expulsion of gas through a stomach tube also helps to establish a diagnosis. At necropsy, especially of animals not observed in the course of the disease, the problem is to differentiate between antemortem bloat and postmortem distention of the rumen as a result of continued fermentation of ruminal content. In each case the rumen is distended with a mixture of froth and feed. The froth from antemortem bloat, however, is more stable than the froth from postmortem fermentation. In addition, the antemortem bloat causes displacement of much of the blood from the visceral vessels to the peripheral veins.

The differential diagnosis requires consideration of many poisons, including poisonous plants and acute enterotoxemia. The differentiation may require chemical analysis of stomach contents for poisons and the assaying of intestinal contents for clostridial toxins.

Prevention and Treatment. In feedlot cattle bloat may be prevented by avoiding or changing from a bloat-producing diet, especially from those rations containing barley, soybean oil, soybean meal and freshly harvested legumes. Bloating from feeding fresh plants may be reduced by diluting the succulent legume with palatable grasses. In pastured animals, bloat can be prevented for approximately 3 days by feeding 50 to 100 mg of procaine penicillin per animal. Unfortunately, however, this procedure has not been successful in feedlot cattle. The inclusion of mineral or animal oil in the ration may have a prophylactic effect. The disease may also be prevented by feeding molasses-salt block containing 30 gm of poloxalene per 454 gm of block; this practice provides approximately 10 gm of poloxalene per animal per day.

The method of treating bloat varies with the degree of distention. Frequently, emergency treatment is required to save the animal's life. If time permits, a stomach tube can be passed into the rumen to expel some gas. In more severe cases, a trocar can be passed into the rumen through the left paralumbar fossa, or a surgical opening can be established in the same anatomical area. Following relief of ruminal pressure, mineral oil and antiferments are administered for further relief and to prevent recurrence.

In chronic bloat the cause should be determined and corrected if possible; if due to excessive use of antibiotics or sulfonamides, the use of those drugs should be discontinued; if due to esophageal constriction from scar tissue, a small ruminal fistula can be established. Recurrent bloaters can be slaughtered for recovery of value.

References

Barrentine, B. F., Shawver, C. B. and Williams, L. W.: Antibiotics for the Prevention of Bloat in Cattle Grazing Ladino Clover. J. Anim. Sci., *15* (1956): 440.

Clark, R. and Weiss, K. E.: Reflex Salivation in Sheep and Goats Initiated by Mechanical Stimulation of the Cardiac Area of the Forestomachs. J. So. Afri. Vet. Med. Assoc., *23* (1952): 163–165.

Cole, H. H., Mead, S. W. and Kleiber, M.: Bloat in Cattle. Calif. Agri. Expt. Sta. Bull. 662 (1942).

Cole, H. H. and Boda, J. M.: Continued Progress Toward Controlling Bloat. A Review. Jour. Dairy Sci., *43* (1960): 1585–1614.

Dougherty, R. W.: The Continuing Quest for the Cause of Bloat in Ruminants. JAVMA, *122* (1953): 345–352.

Dougherty, R. W., Meredith, C. D. and Barrett, B. A.: Physiological Effects of Insufflation of the Stomach of Sheep. AJVR, *16* (1955): 79–90.

Elam, C. J. and Davis, R. E.: Effects of Two Levels of Soybean Oil Mixed Into a Complete Pelleted Steer Ration on the Incidence of Feedlot Bloat. J. Anim. Sci., *18* (1959): 1510.

Gupta, J. and Nichols, R. E.: A Possible Enzymatic Cause of Fiscid Ruminal Contents, Its Relationship to Legume Bloat. AJVR, *23* (1962): 128–133.

Hungate, R. E., Fletcher, D. W., Dougherty, R. W. and Barrentine, B. F.: Microbial Activity in the Bovine Rumen: Its Measurements and Relation to Bloat. Appl. Microbiol., *3* (1955): 161.

Johns, A. T., Mangan, J. L. and Reid, C. S. W.: Bloat. New Zealand Vet. J., *5* (1957): 115.

Knapp, B., Baker, A. L. and Phillips, R. W.: Variations in the Occurrence of Bloat in the Steer Progeny of Beef Bulls. J. Anim. Sci., *2* (1943): 221.

Losses in Agriculture. Agricultural Research Service, U. S. Dept. of Agriculture. Agricultural Handbook No. 291, (1965).

Mangan, J. L.: Bloat in Cattle. XI. The Foaming Properties of Proteins, Saponins, and Rumen Liquor. New Zealand J. Agr. Res., *2* (1959): 47.

Nichols, R. E., Deese, D. and Lang, J.: Relationship of Ruminal Intake of Dry Matter and Pectin Methylesterase to Bloat Producing Capacity of Irrigable Alfalfa in Heifers. AJVR, *29* (1968): 2005–2008.

Reid, C. S. W. and Johns, A. T.: Bloat in Cattle on Red Clover. III. Treatment and Prevention With Anti-foaming Agents. New Zealand J. Sci. Technol., Sec. A, *38* (1957): 908.

Rosen, W. G., Fassel, Hester and Nichols, R. E.: The Etiology of Legume Bloat-Nonvolatile Acids. AJVR, *22* (1961): 117–122.

Weiss, K. E.: The Significance of Reflex Salivation in Relation to Froth Formation and Acute Bloat in Ruminants. Onderstepoort J. Vet. Res., *26* (1953): 241–249.

———: Physiological Studies on Eructation in Ruminants. Onderstepoort J. Vet. Res., *26* (1953a): 251–283.

Gastric Erosion and Ulcer

Gastric erosion and ulcer are respectively the superficial and deep focal discontinuities of tissue in the abomasum. Erosions are never, and ulcers seldom, diagnosed clinically. Depending on specific location, ulcers may cause colic discomfort and anorexia which diminish the rate of gain in body weight. While the mortality rate is low, some cattle die from ulcers perforating the stomach wall and from eroding large blood vessels.

Review of Literature. Surveys have been conducted of slaughtered cattle to determine the incidence of gastric ulcers in cattle of varying ages. In a study of 1,500 calves the following age incidence was observed: under 4 weeks, 0%; 4 to 5 weeks, 78%; 8 weeks, 95%; 10 to 12 weeks, 95%; 12 to 14 weeks, 98%; and young cattle, 68% (Tanz, 1938). In another investigation 1,535 adult fat cattle were observed at the time of slaughter. Of these 814 (53%) contained normal abomasums, while 721 (47%) manifested injury to the mucous membrane. Of the 721 injured stomachs, 677 (44% of total sample) contained single or multiple erosions only and 28 (1.8 % of total sample) contained ulcers only, while 16 (1% of total sample) contained both erosions and ulcers. Erosions were distributed randomly throughout the fundus and pylorus, while ulcers were in the pylorus and the distal part of the fundus. Although the cause was not determined, the investigators hypothesized that erosions are caused by the stress from shipment and starvation during the period between leaving the feedlot and slaughter (Jensen, Deane, Cooper, Miller and Graham, 1954). Other sporadic cases have been studied in which death was caused by severe hemorrhage (Bartlett and Fincher, 1956) from an abomasal ulcer and in which death was caused by perforation of the abomasal wall and the establishment of peritonitis (Carey and Carey, 1958).

Occurrence. Among adult fattened cattle, approximately 45% contain abomasal erosions and 2.9% contain abomasal ulcers or ulcer scars at the time of slaughter. In calves 8 to 14 weeks of age the incidence of abomasal ulcers may be as high as 95%. All sexes and ages are susceptible and cases of ulcers may occur at any season and at any stage of fattening.

Etiology and Pathogenesis. The cause of abomasal erosions and ulcers has not been investigated in cattle. The high incidence and appearance of recent origin of erosions at the time of slaughter has led to the postulation that they are caused by stress from sudden withdrawal of a high caloric ration and transportation from feedlots to markets by either train or truck. Both erosions and ulcers in some cases may be caused by focal hemorrhage in the mucosa of the abomasum as a result of acute diseases such as viral diarrhea, viral bovine rhinotraceitis, shipping fever and diphtheria. Erosions formed at the time of shipment of cattle from the range to the feedlot may predispose the abomasum to and initiate ulceration. Occasionally, caustic substances, such as arsenic, may necrose areas of mucosa and result in ulcer.

Since the causes of erosions and ulcers are poorly understood, the pathogenesis can be only postulated. During the final stages of fattening, cattle have constant access to unlimited amounts of high caloric feed and are maintained in a peaceful environment. Suddenly, at the time of marketing, all feed is withdrawn and the animals are shipped by train or truck to markets. Crowding is severe and fright intense. This stressful situation exists for 48 to 72 hours immediately preceding slaughter and may result in gastric hyperacidity with focal hemorrhage and erosions.

Ulcers may be caused by erosions which originate at the time of shipment to the feedlots and by focal hemorrhages in the abomasal mucosa from infectious diseases. The mucosa covering the hemorrhage is devitalized by poor circulation. Gastric enzymes destroy the degenerated cells of the mucosa and the extravasated blood. This process creates discontinuity of tissue and further degeneration of tissue at the bottom of the beginning ulcer. Progressive degeneration and digestion of tissue may continue through the entire thickness of the mucosa and enter the submucosa. In a few cases the process may continue until the entire wall is perforated. Fatality may result from severe

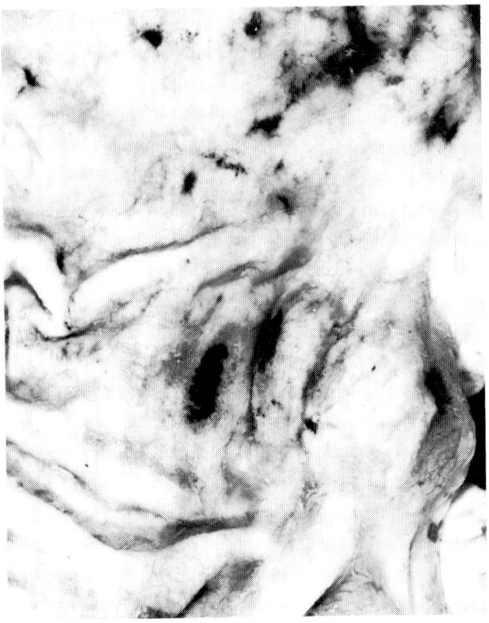

FIG. 8-14. *Erosions with hemorrhage into affected tissue.* × 0.7.

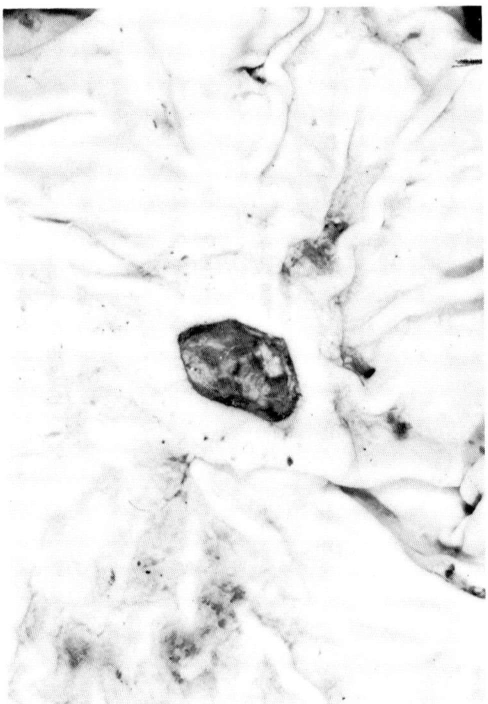

FIG. 8-15. *Ulcer which caused fatal hemorrhage.* × 1.3.

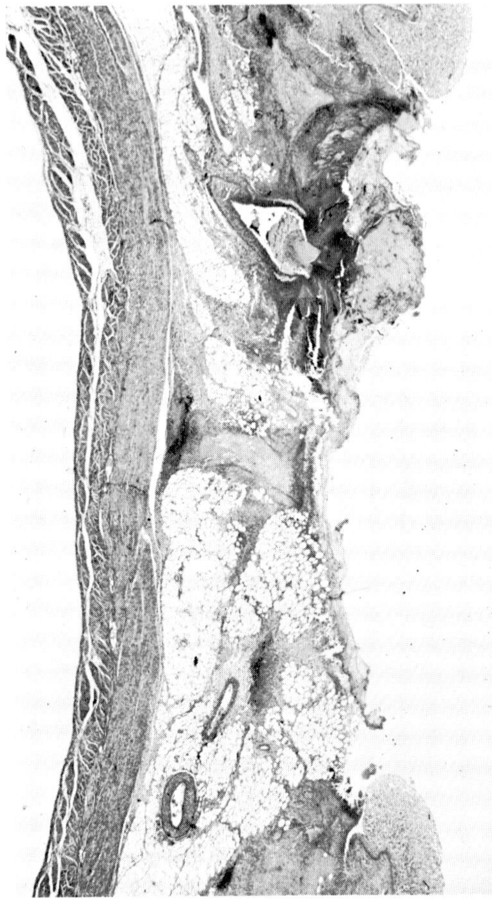

FIG. 8-16. *Same as Fig. 8-15. Note the eroded artery. H&E stain.* × 8.

hemorrhage from an eroded artery, or from peritonitis resulting from perforation of the gastric wall and the discharge of gastric contents into the peritoneal cavity. Except for the few fatalities, ulcers heal by the formation of scar tissue. Contraction of the scar causes stellate disfiguration of the mucosa.

Clinical Signs and Postmortem Lesions. Abomasal erosions produce no recognizable clinical signs. Usually ulcers also are asymptomatic. In some cases, however, ulcers cause anorexia, depression, vague pain in the region of the abomasum and abdominal tenseness. The pain does not increase with pressure and body temperature is normal.

Occasionally slow hemorrhage causes discernible black tarry blood in the feces and paleness of membranes. With ulcerous perforation of the gastric wall comes generalized peritonitis with fever, abdominal rigidity, diarrhea, depression and reluctance to move.

At the time of slaughter, erosions, single or multiple, are found in the opened and cleaned abomasum. Each erosion is a shallow cavity usually surrounded by hemorrhagic tissue. Erosions vary in size, number, location and shape. In the fundus many are on the edges of the plicae. In case of multiple erosions some hemoglobin may escape into the gastric lumen.

The ulcer is usually single and circular and is located in the distal part of the fundus or in the pylorus. The edges are sharply delimited. The ulcer measures usually 10 to 30 mm in diameter. The defect extends at least into the submucosa. The floor of the ulcer contains necrotic cells, fibrin, and ingesta. In case of fatal hemorrhage, the abomasum is distended with blood which may pass by retrograde flow into the omasum and posteriorly into the intestines. Blood clot is usually seen extending from the ulcer. In case of fatal perforation, the ulcer extends through the entire gastric wall and ingesta is present in the inflamed peritoneal cavity. Surrounding organs may be adherent to the abomasum near the point of perforation. Ulcer scars, through contraction of the connective tissue, form stellate disfigurations in the mucosa.

Histopathologically, erosions manifest focal degeneration, some digestion of cells, and hemorrhage into the lamina propria. An ulcer may be surrounded by an inflammatory reaction; the floor contains fibrin, leukocytes and granulation tissue. In case of fatal hemorrhage the eroded artery is usually discernible.

Diagnosis. Erosions are never diagnosed clinically. They are observed, however, at necropsy and slaughter after cleaning the opened abomasum. Ulcers may be diagnosed clinically on the basis of typical signs, especially abdominal rigidity, abomasal pain that does not increase from manual pressure and black tarry feces.

The differential diagnosis requires consideration of traumatic reticulitis and other causes of alimentary tract hemorrhages such as coccidiosis and salmonellosis. In traumatic reticulitis, metal is usually detectible in the region of the reticulum and manual pressure over the region of the xyphoid cartilage increases pain. In coccidiosis, oöcytes, identifiable in microscopic examination of feces, are usually present in significant numbers. In salmonellosis, the feces are extremely fluid and species of *Salmonella* can be isolated from the manure.

Treatment. Successful treatment of ulcers requires alteration in management and medication. The high caloric diet should be changed to grass hay, bran and oats. One gallon of mineral oil mixed thoroughly with 1 pound of magnesium oxide should be administered through a stomach tube. Sulfamethazine or sulfabrommethazine, administered daily at the rate of 1.5 grains per pound of body weight for 1 to 2 days followed by one-half the daily dose for several more days, may be given to control possible bacterial infection within the ulcer.

Reasonably fattened animals with severe hemorrhage may be prematurely slaughtered for recovery of monetary value.

References

Bartlett, M. P. and Fincher, M. G.: Ulcer in the Abomasum with Fatal Hemorrhage. North Am. Vet., *37* (1956): 942.

Carey, J. C. and Carey, J. W.: A Steer with a Perforated Abomasum. JAVMA, *133* (1958): 368.

Jensen, Rue, Deane, H. M., Cooper, L. J., Miller, V. A. and Graham, W. R.: The Rumentitis-Liver Abscess Complex in Beef Cattle, AJVR, *25* (1954): 202–216.

Tanz (quoted from Hutyra, F., Marek, J. and Manninger, R. *Special Pathology and Therapeutics of Diseases of Domestic Animals.* Vol. II; 4th ed. Alexander Eger, Chicago, 1938).

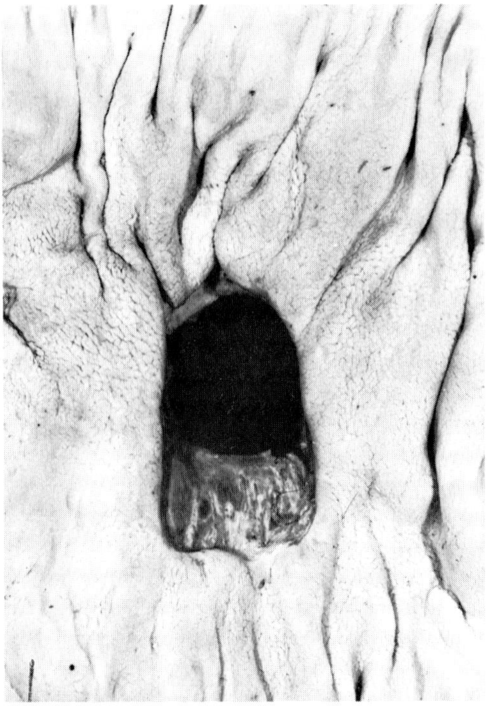

FIG. 8-17. *Perforating ulcer.* × 1.0.

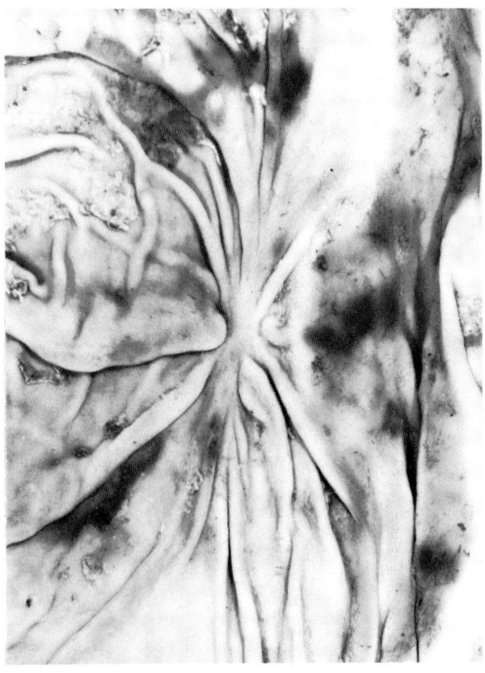

FIG. 8-18. *Scar from healed ulcer.* × 1.0.

Acute Indigestion

(FOUNDER; ACUTE IMPACTION; ACUTE ACIDOSIS)

Acute indigestion, a metabolic disease of cattle and sheep, is characterized by acidosis, prostration and coma, and is caused by sudden overeating of grain and other highly fermentable feeds. In feedlot cattle, indigestion develops commonly from rapid change of ration from roughage to concentrate and from accidental access to excessive amounts of grain. The resulting effects cause economic loss. Through acute deaths, through partial incapacitation from prolonged lameness, and from recurring digestive disturbances, the annual loss has been estimated at 1% of the total production.

Review of Literature. Veterinarians and livestock owners have long recognized the danger to cattle from sudden overeating. Engorgement on grain, silage, green corn and green fruit, especially apples, has resulted in violent illness with high mortality in cattle unaccustomed to such feed. Animals less severely affected have often developed lameness (Atkinson *et al.*, 1942; Nilsson, 1963). In affected cattle, the clinical manifestation of severe depression with a rapid and often fatal course led to the postulation that toxins formed in the rumen were the cause of death. More recent studies of rumen contents revealed that large quantities of lactic acid were formed and this led to the theory that death is caused by acidosis (Benjamin, 1961; Bond, 1959; Hungate, Dougherty, Bryant and Cello, 1952; Jensen, Deane and Cooper 1954; Meyer, 1960). Acute indigestion was produced experimentally by placing in the rumens through fistulae large amounts of grain, and/or sugar, and also by pumping into the rumen through a stomach tube ground grain with water (Jensen, Deane, Cooper and Miller, 1954). In contrast to the normal rumen acids (Elsden, Hitchcock, Marshall and Phillipson, 1946) lactic acid was formed to a concentration of 327 mM/1 and a pH of 3.8 (Bond, 1959; Hungate *et al.*, 1952; Jensen *et al.*, 1954). In addition, the ration of 8 steers was suddenly changed from roughage to grain. Within 2 to 3 days the rumen lactic acid changed from 0.1 to 100 mM/1 and the blood pH from 7.37 to 7.29. After 2 to 6 days of anorexia, feeding was resumed (Uhart and Carroll, 1967). Simultaneous studies of ruminal microflora of the same animals indicated that *Streptococcus bovis* increased rapidly to become the predominant bacterium (Hungate, *et al.*, 1952). The acidity of the rumen contents was accompanied in many cases by an increased blood level of lactic acid, inorganic phosphorus and glucose, and by a decrease of bicarbonate (Juhasz and Szegedi, 1968; Dirksen, 1965; 1967), and by the development of acid urine (Bond, 1959).

Intravenous inoculation of mice with ruminal contents from fatal cases of experimental indigestion failed to demonstrate the presence of a toxin (Hungate *et al.*, 1952; Jensen *et al.*, 1954). These observations helped to support the theory that acidosis is an important factor in the cause of death.

Occurrence. Acidosis usually develops early during the fattening process when the ration is changed too rapidly from roughage to concentrate, and the disease has a low to high morbidity rate. All ages and both sexes of cattle are susceptible to acute indigestion. Seasonally, the disease is more common during summer and autumn when grains and green feeds are more available, but it may occur from access to stored grains in any season. In addition to cattle, acute indigestion also occurs commonly in sheep.

Etiology and Pathogenesis. Acute indigestion is caused by sudden consumption of large amounts of grain, green corn, green apples or other easily fermentable feeds to which the cattle are unaccustomed. Consumption of such feed may result from a rapid rate of ration change to grain, from animals accidentally entering a field of grain, from their access to stored grain or from injudicious feeding of excessive amounts of grain.

When cattle, under normal conditions, are sustained on a ration of roughage, cellulotic bacteria predominate in ruminal microflora. Volatile fatty acids are formed in the following proportions: acetic, 67%, propionic, 19% and butyric, 14%. These acids constitute an important nutrient from cellulose digestion.

When grain, or other easily fermentable feed, is suddenly ingested in large amounts, the ruminal microflora undergo qualitative changes. *Streptococcus bovis* predominates. The microflora ferment the new feed and produce 100 or more mM/1 of lactic acid. The rumen becomes immobilized. Absorption of the acid into the blood lowers the blood pH and diminishes the content of bicarbonate and glucose. The urine becomes acidic and the heart and respiration rates accelerate. Compensation occurs by excretion of carbonic acid through rapid respiration and by excretion of hydrogen ions through the urine. Compensation may be sufficient for survival of some affected animals. In many cases, however, severe acidosis is fatal. Toxins, if present in the rumen, may be absorbed and contribute to death from respiratory failure.

High acidity of the ruminal contents is injurious to the mucosa. Some areas become swollen, vesicated and necrotic. Necrotic papillae slough from the mucous membrane. Necrosis of the epithelium enables bacteria, especially *Spherophorus necrophorus*, to enter veins and be conveyed to the liver where abscesses may form in surviving animals.

Some animals develop acute laminitis. The pathogeneses of this condition is poorly understood. Similarity of bovine laminitis and equine laminitis has not been established. Presumably, blood vessels inside the hooves dilate and engorge with blood. As a result of local increase in blood pressure, transudate accumulates in the connective tissue. Pressure on nerves inside the hooves, from engorgement and edema, causes pain.

Clinical Signs and Postmortem Lesions. Onset is sudden and body temperature is usually normal. Inappetence, depression and rumen immobility develop within 2 to 3 days following the overeating. The hair coat becomes roughened. In some animals colic causes kicking at the abdomen, stretching of muscles and frequent rolling. Borborygmus of the intestine is audible. Respiration and pulse rates are accelerated. The muzzle is dry and, in severe cases, grunting and dehydration are manifested. Ruminal and some abdominal distention may be present. As the disease progresses a mucoid diarrhea, with gray fluid feces, develops. In terminal stages physical weakness, prostration, coma, subnormal body temperature and low blood pressure with cyanosis develop rapidly. The urine is acidic. Non-fatal cases resume feeding after 2 to 6 days of anorexia but often become acutely lame from laminitis. Death may occur after a course of 1 to 3 days.

At necropsy, the most discernible gross changes are limited to the stomachs. The rumen is distended and the contents are acidic with a pH as low as 3.8. The offending feed, such as poorly masticated grain, may be present and recognizable in excessive amounts in all stomachs. The mucous membrane of the rumen exhibits localized or generalized superficial necrosis and swelling. Swollen papillae are round, friable and dark brown. Many papillae have detached from the mucosa. Congestion and inflammation may be present in the abomasum and small intestines. Serosal surfaces commonly contain petechial and ecchymotic hemorrhages. Vessels of the feet, especially in the sensitive laminae, are engorged.

Histopathologically, necrosis is extensive but ununiform through the ruminal epithelium. In some areas, especially at tips of papillae, necrosis may extend into the lamina propria. The stratified squamous epithelium is vesicated. Vesicular cavities often contain blood.

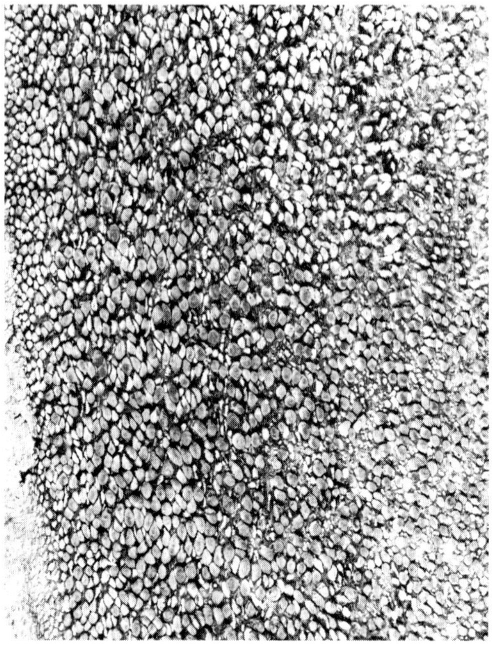

FIG. 8-19. *Acute rumenitis from a bovine with acute indigestion. Papillae are swollen and hemorrhagic; some have detached.* × 0.6.

Diagnosis. Clinically the diagnosis of indigestion is based on the presence of depression, anorexia, weakness, and a history of possible access to excessive amounts of grain or other highly fermentable concentrate. Laboratory findings usually include lowered pH of the urine, lowered pH of the plasma, reduced amount of plasma bicarbonate, and reduced amount of plasma chloride. At necropsy, confirmation of the diagnosis can be obtained by finding high acidity of the rumen contents, by the presence of grain in large amounts in any or all stomachs, and by necrosis and inflammation of the mucosa of the rumen and reticulum.

The differential diagnosis requires the consideration of traumatic reticulitis, urinary calculosis and, in dairy cattle, milk fever. Traumatic reticulitis is accompanied by leukocytosis and evidence of pain from the application of pressure in the region of the anterior abdomen. If the foreign body has penetrated into the pericardial sac, the presence of exudate may be detected by auscultation. While urinary calculosis may result in colic and associated signs, it can be diag-

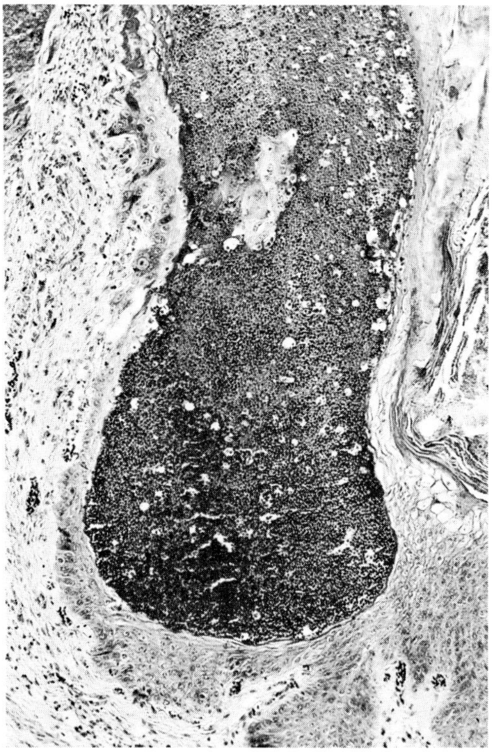

FIG. 8-20. *Hemorrhagic vesicle in ruminal mucosa of a bovine with acute indigestion. H&E Stain.* × 100.

nosed by rectal palpation and detection of distention of the urinary bladder. Milk fever is associated with constipation and responds to intravenous administration of solutions of calcium salts.

Prevention and Treatment. Acute indigestion is prevented by avoiding accidental access of cattle unaccustomed to excessive amounts of concentrate. In feedlot the ration should be changed gradually and stepwise from low to high proportion of concentrate. A minimum of 2, and preferably 4, weeks should be utilized for the transfer.

In early stages of the disease ingesta should be evacuated from the rumen by means of lavage and pumping or by rumenotomy. Following evacuation of the rumen, mineral oil, antiferments and Lentin may be administered to reduce absorption of acids and possible toxins, and to accelerate evacuation from the intestines. A solution of sodium bicarbonate may be administered orally or intravenously to restore the acid base balance. Daily intramuscular administration of antihistamines and cortical steroids for each of several days helps to prevent intoxication and laminitis.

References

Atkinson, V. T. *et al.*: Special Report on Diseases of Cattle. Government Printing Office, Washington. (1942): 218.

Benjamin, M. M.: *Outline of Veterinary Clinical Pathology.* 2nd ed. The Iowa State University Press, Ames, Iowa. (1961): 162–175.

Bond, H. E.: A Study on the Pathogenesis of Acute Acid Indigestion in Sheep. Abst. in Dissertation Abstracts, *20* (1959): 2354–2355.

Dirksen, G.: Rumen Acidosis in Cattle. Vet. Med. Rev. Leverkusen, No. 2 (1965): 98–125.

———: Biochemistry of Ruminal Acidosis in Cattle. Schweizer Arch. Tierheilk., *109* (1967): 28–34.

Elsden, S. R., Hitchcock, M. W. S., Marshall, R. A. and Phillipson, A. T.: Volatile Acids in the Digestion of Ruminants and Other Animals. J. Exp. Biol., *22* (1946): 191–199.

Hungate, R. E., Dougherty, R. W., Bryant, M. P. and Cello, R. M.: Microbiological and Physiological Changes Associated With Indigestion in Sheep. Cornell Vet., *42* (1952): 433–449.

Jensen, Rue, Deane, H. M., Cooper, J. L., Miller, V. A. and Graham, W. R.: The Rumentitis-Liver Abscess Complex in Beef Cattle. AJVR, *15* (1954): 202–216.

Juhasz, B. and Szegedi, B.: Pathogenesis of Ruminal Digestive Disorders Caused by Easily Digestible Carbohydrates. Magy. Allatorv. Lap., *23,* (1968): 60–68.

Losses in Agriculture. Agricultural Research Service, U.S.D.A. Agricultural Handbook No. 291. 1965.

Meyer, H.: Carbohydrate Metabolism in Ruminants. Dtsch. Tierarztl. Woschr, *67* (1960): 47–51.

Nilsson, S. A.: Clinical, Morphological, and Experimental Studies of Laminitis in Cattle. Acta Veterinaria Scandinavica, *4* (1963) Supplement 1.

Udall, D. H.: *The Practice of Veterinary Medicine.* Udall Publisher. Ithaca. N. Y. (1954): 102–111.

Urhart, B. A., and Carroll, F. D.: Acidosis in Beef Cattle. J. An. Sc., *26* (1967): 1195–1198.

Telangiectasis and "Sawdust" of the Liver

Telangiectasis, a degenerative change in the liver, is characterized by single or multiple dark red foci, each 1 to 5 mm in diameter, and is caused by focal dilatation and congestion of sinusoids. "Sawdust" is similar to telangiectasis except that the foci are gray. These two asymptomatic conditions are never diagnosed clinically but are encountered commonly at the time of slaughter and at necropsy. During the 3-year period, 1967 through 1969, an average of 678,000 livers were condemned annually for telangiectasis and sawdust. At a value of $5 per liver, these condemnations constituted an annual loss of over 3.4 million dollars for the nation.

Review of Literature. Annual national surveys of slaughtered cattle have indicated that approximately 1.7% of cattle livers are condemned because of extensive and generalized telangiectasis and approximately 0.7% because of extensive sawdust (Federal Meat Inspection 1967–1969).

In one experiment to determine the time during fattening when telangiectasis, sawdust and abscesses develop, random samples of cattle, with 25 animals per sample, were slaughtered at 0, 43, 80, 116, and 157 days of fattening. Telangiectasis first appeared in 36% of livers at the end of 43 days, increased to 52% at the end of 80 days, and then diminished to 8% at the end of 157 days. In the same experiment, sawdust first appeared in 4% of livers at the end of 43 days, increased to 29% at the end of 116 days, and diminished to 24% at the end of 157 days (Jensen, Frey, Cross and Connell, 1947). Bacterial cultures of telangiectasis did not reveal the presence of significant bacteria (Anderson, 1955a). In a study of pathogenesis of telangiectasis in early stages of fattening it was demonstrated that an early change is the deposition of extracellular glycogen between hepatic cells and fibers and endothelial cells lining the sinusoids. This deposit caused constriction of the sinusoids and some interference to blood flow. At these points, the sinusoidal lining was interrupted, hepatic cells were eroded, and new communicating channels were established between sinusoids. An increase in pressure dilated the sinusoid, distorted laminae and sinusoids, and interfered with circulation locally. Congestion developed in a dilated sinusoid (Anderson, 1955b; 1955c; 1955d). In case of sawdust, leukocytes infiltrated the foci of telangiectasis (Getty, 1945). This degenerated anaerobic mass, the experimenters postulated, predisposes to abscesses in case *Spherophorus necrophorus* gain access through the portal blood system (Jensen, Frey, Cross and Connell, 1947).

Occurrence. Telangiectasis and sawdust occur in both sexes of cattle at all ages, but

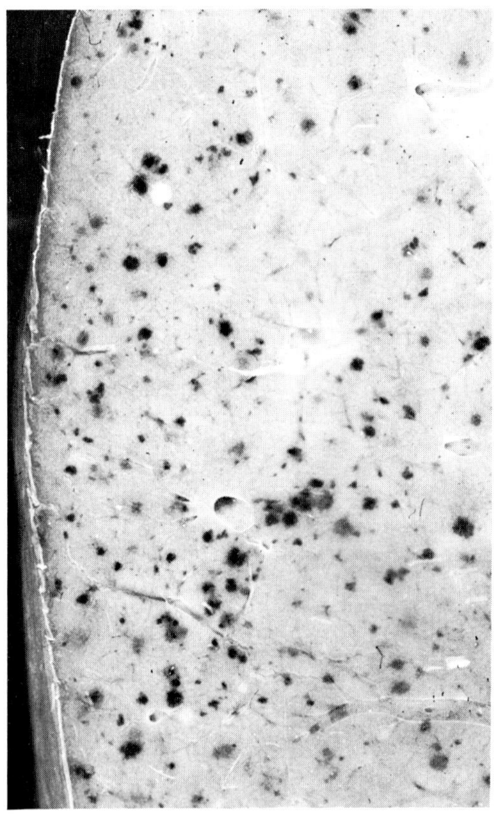

FIG. 8-21. *Multiple foci of telangiectasis on cut surface of the liver of a fattened steer.* × 1.0.

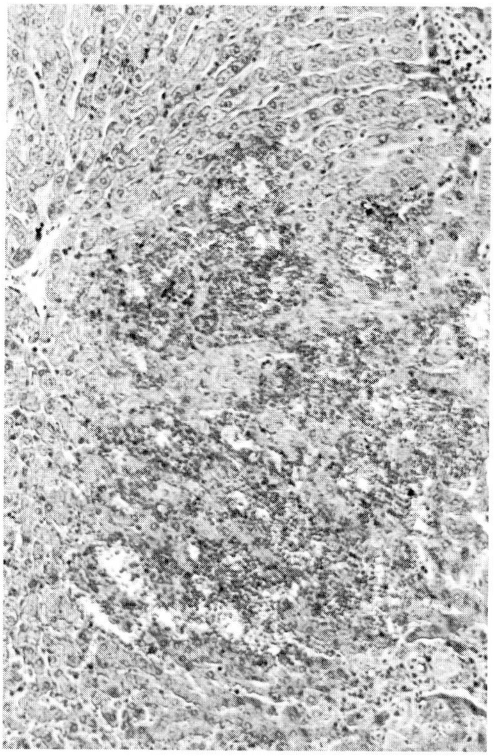

FIG. 8-22. *Telangiectasis in the liver of a steer. H&E stain.* × 156.

especially in animals 6 to 24 months of age, fattened to a high degree. Nationally, approximately 1.7% of slaughtered adult cattle have sufficient telangiectasis for liver condemnation and 0.7% contain sufficient sawdust for condemnation. An additional percentage contains lesser amounts of telangiectasis and sawdust. The two types of lesions may be concurrent.

Etiology and Pathogenesis. Telangiectasis probably is caused by a rapid rate of fattening. Extracellular glycogen, deposited focally between hepatic cells and the membrane lining the sinusoid, causes diminution of the lumen of the sinusoid. The lining membrane, composed of fibers and some endothelial cells, is broken. Blood current through the broken membrane erodes and displaces hepatic cells. This process creates new communicating channels between adjacent sinusoids. The increase in volume and pressure of blood in the confluent sinusoid distorts adjacent hepatic laminae; the distortion obstructs sinusoidal drainage, dilates the sinusoid and stagnates blood. Some blood may hemolyze. The congested mass of blood is seen grossly as a dark focus, usually 1 to 5 mm in diameter. Healing occurs by hemolysis of blood, the regeneration of hepatic laminae and the establishment of new sinusoids for circulation.

In some livers, some foci of telangiectasis probably are converted to sawdust. The congested blood hemolyzes, and hepatic cells undergo atrophy and necrosis. Leukocytes, especially neutrophils, lymphocytes and mononuclear macrophages, infiltrate the area. Grossly, such foci appear gray and measure 1 to 5 mm in diameter. Like tel-

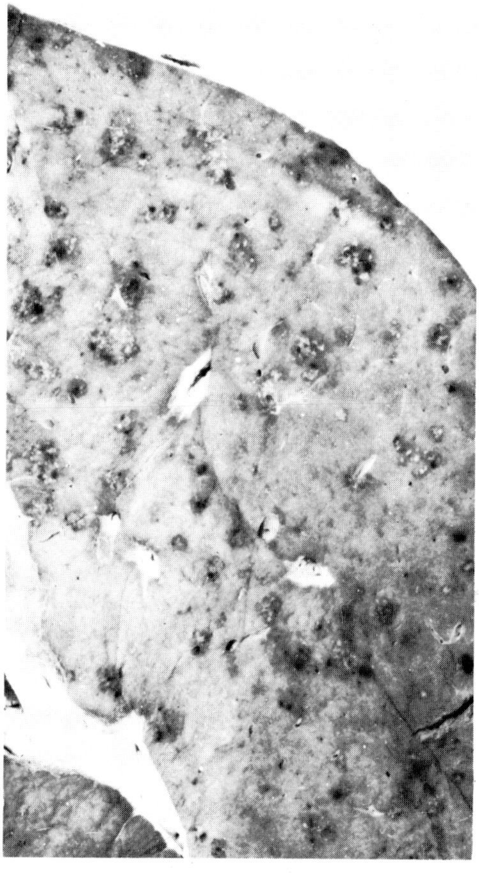

FIG. 8-23. *"Sawdust" on the cut surface of the liver of a fattened steer.* × 1.2.

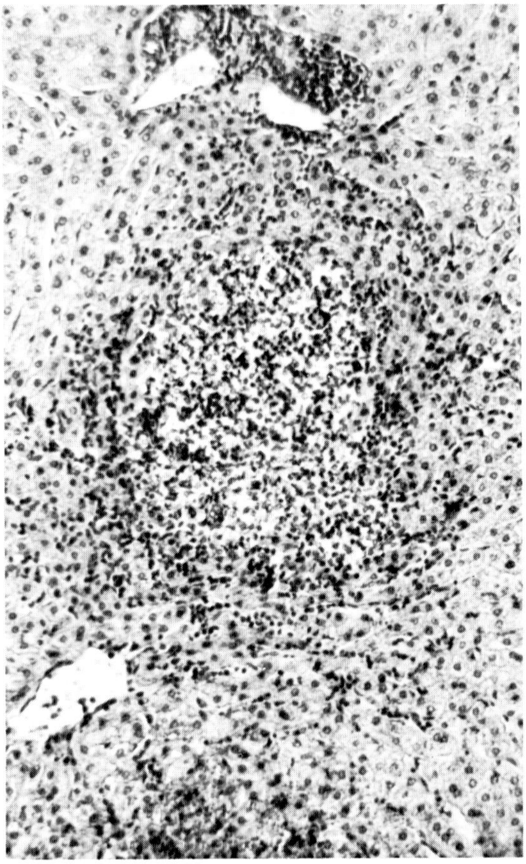

FIG. 8-24. *"Sawdust" in the liver of a fattened steer. H&E stain.* × 191.

angiectasis, sawdust can heal after an undetermined period of existence.

Both telangiectasis and sawdust probably predispose liver to abscesses by forming an anaerobic medium in which S. *necrophorus*, should it gain entrance, causes necrosis and eventually abscesses.

Clinical Signs and Postmortem Lesions. Telangiectasis and sawdust are both asymptomatic conditions. They are encountered at necropsy and at the time of postmortem examination at slaughter. Telangiectasis is observed as single or multiple reddish-black spherical foci, usually 1 to 5 mm in diameter. The foci may be distributed throughout the organ; superficial ones are visible through the capsule. Sawdust is similar to telangiectasis except the foci are gray. Telangiectasis and sawdust may coexist in the same liver and in juxtaposition within the same tissue lesion.

Telangiectasis and sawdust are not unwholesome as human food. Livers containing a large amount of either telangiectasis or sawdust are condemned for human food because of unesthetic appearance and because of suspicion of unwholesomeness and discrimination by consumers. Such condemned livers can be utilized for animal food.

Microscopically, telangiectasis contains dilated sinusoids filled with congested partially hemolyzed blood. Careful study of young lesions may reveal glycogen deposits, atrophy of some hepatic laminae and necrosis of some hepatic cells. In sawdust, congested blood is hemolyzed, and neutrophils, lymphocytes and mononuclear macrophages are present in the lesions.

Diagnosis. Neither telangiectasis nor sawdust is diagnosed clinically. The postmortem diagnosis is based on gross appearance. Confirmation can be obtained from histopathologic studies of affected liver tissue.

Prevention and Treatment. The only known means of reducing the incidence is by deceleration of the rate of fattening, a process not compatible with industrial and economic objectives of beef cattle fattening.

References

Anderson, A. C.: The Pathogenesis of Telangiectasis in the Bovine Liver. I. The Incidence of Telangiectasis. AJVR, *16* (1955a): 27–33.

——— II. Histopathological and Microbiological Studies. AJVR, *16* (1955b): 217–236.

——— III. Experimental Telangiectasis. AJVR, *16* (1955c): 237–239.

——— IV. Discussion and Summary. AJVR, *16* (1955d): 240–245.

Federal Meat Inspection. Statistical Summary. Consumer and Marketing Service. USDA. 1967–1969.

Getty, R.: Focal Hepatitis in Cattle. AJVR, *7* (1945): 437–449.

Jensen, Rue, Frey, P. R., Cross, F. and Connell, W. E.: Telangiectasis, "Sawdust" and Abscesses in the Livers of Beef Cattle. JAVMA, *110* (1947): 256–261.

Bovine Pancreolithiasis

(PANCREATIC CALCULOSIS)

Pancreolithiasis is the formation of single or multiple carbonaceous stones within the excretory ducts of the pancreas. While this condition is uncommon in animals in general, many sporadic cases reported have been in individual cattle. Twenty-eight case reports were assembled and compared from the German literature (Kast, 1962). In most cases clinical signs were vague and inconstant and none were diagnosed clinically (Fitch, Boyd and Billings, 1919). Three surveys of slaughtered cattle disclosed the following incidences of pancreolithiasis: 2 cases in 50,000 animals (Laxen, 1911), 4 in 5,000 (Solomon, 1933) and 4 in 50,000 (Wypychowski, 1937).

The cause of pancreolithiasis has not been studied. The stones have been analyzed chemically, however, and show the following approximate composition: calcium carbonate 90.5%; calcium phosphate 5.2%; magnesium carbonate trace amounts; fat and proteins 2%; and other 1.3%. Presumably each stone results from the precipitation of salts from the pancreatic juice around crystallization nuclei, some of which are desquamated cells. Growing by accretion, some stones remain small and unobstructive, while others occasionally obtain a diameter sufficient to occlude the pancreatic duct. In case of obstruction, secretion is retained within the pancreas and eventually the acinar tissue atrophies. If a duct ruptures, the secretion with its enzymes escape into surrounding tissue and the lipase causes necrosis of adipose tissue. As a result of obstruction of the main pancreatic duct, the pancreatic enzymes, including trypsinogen, lipase, lecithinase, amylase, sucrase, and maltase, do not enter the small intestine. While the intestinal juice also contains lipase, maltase, sucrase, lactase and amylase, the amount without the pancreatic juice is insufficient for complete digestion and a high fecal content of fat and carbohydrate is the result.

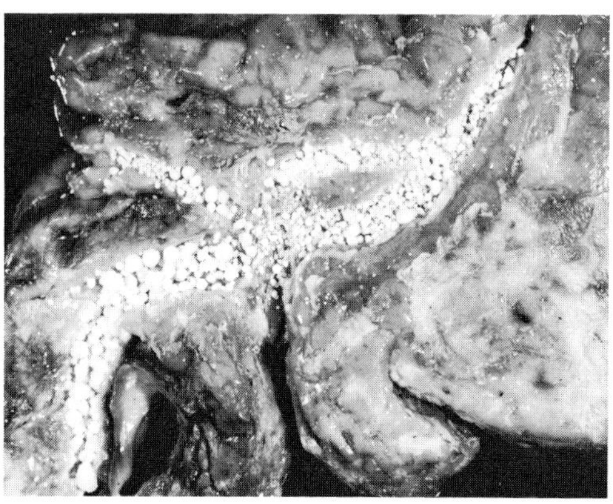

FIG. 8-25. *Pancreatic ducts filled with calculi.* × 0.5.

Since pancreolithiasis is seldom, if ever, diagnosed clinically, the stones are found unexpectedly at postmortem inspection following slaughter or at necropsy following death from an intercurrent disease. The pancreatic duct and its branches may be distended with as many as 1,500 firm, white, discrete and spherical or angular stones varying from 1 to 10 mm in diameter. Occasionally the wall of the duct is thickened and firm from chronic inflammation. In case of rupture of a duct, necrosis of adipose tissue is discernible.

References

Fitch, C. P., Boyd, W. L. and Billings, W. A.: Pancreatic Lithiasis of Cattle. Cornell Vet., *9* (1919): 68–73.

Kast, von A.: Pancreolithiasis Beim Rind. Berlin und Münchener., *75* (1962): 265–266.

Laxen, B.: On Pancreolithiasis. Dissertation. Hannover. 1911.

Salomon, S.: Primary Solitary Carcinoma of the Pancreas. Berl. Tierärzl. Wosch., *49* (1933): 230.

Wypychowski, E.: Pancreatic Stones of Cattle. Przeyl. Wet., *52* (1937): 19–20.

Polioencephalomalacia

(FORAGE POISONING; CEREBROCORTICAL NECROSIS)

Polioencephalomalacia, a non-infectious disease of feedlot and pasture cattle as well as sheep, is characterized by multiple foci of necrosis in the cerebral cortex. In Pennsylvania the disease has been described as focal necrosis in the cerebral cortex and in Britain, Germany and France, as cerebral corticonecrosis. These clinical and pathological terms, though originating from different geographic areas, apparently designate the same disease. Until the cause is determined, polioencephalomalacia, a descriptive term for necrosis of the gray matter of the brain, seems appropriate.

Polioencephalomalacia and infectious embolic meningoencephalitis, the two most prevalent neurologic diseases of feedlot cattle, result in severe economic damages to producers. These losses, although not measured, come from mortality, reduced feed-use efficiency, prolongation of fattening, and expensive treatments.

Review of Literature. The disease was first described in Colorado and neighboring western states in both cattle and sheep (Jensen, Griner and Adams, 1956). Since then it has been observed in eastern United States (Elliot, 1958), Britain (Howell, 1961; Spence *et al.*, 1961; Terlecki and Markson, 1960), New Zealand (Hartley and Kater, 1959) and Australia (Daly, 1968). While sheep only were included in the New Zealand study, it seems highly probable that the disease also exists in the cattle of that country. Descriptions of the disease in each of the geographic areas, in both cattle and sheep, revealed strong similarity in symptomatology and pathologic changes.

While many outbreaks have been studied carefully, the cause has not been determined. Bacterial cultures from affected brain yielded no consistent and significant organisms (Howell, 1961; Terlecki and Markson, 1960). Experiments to transmit the disease by parenteral inoculation of brain tissue from affected to normal animals were also unsuccessful. Chemical analyses of brain and other organs were negative for selenium, lead and arsenic. Force-feeding of contents of the alimentary tract from affected animals, as well as suspected water and plants from areas where the disease developed, to normal animals produced no change. Since neurons are highly susceptible to hypoxia and hypoglycemia, bloods from animals in early stages of the disease were tested for methemaglobin, sulfmethemoglobin and cyanmethemoglobin, which was not present in detectable amounts, and for blood sugar which was present in normal amounts (Jensen, Griner and Adams, 1956). *Clostridium perfringens* type D toxin was found in the small intestines in 3 of 21 sheep affected with the disease (Hartley and Kater, 1959). In one outbreak in Hereford bulls, 5 animals were affected; 1 died and 4 recovered; all showed typical symptoms, and the dead animal evinced typical neuropathologic changes. Several weeks following recovery of the 4 animals, the sera were tested quantitatively for the various types of antitoxin from *Cl. perfringens*. None of the antibody titers were above normal (Jensen, Griner and Adams, 1956).

Accidentally, feedlot cattle were fed pellets consisting of 44% linseed meal, 44% cottonseed meal and 12% sulfur. One hundred fifty-seven animals died. In the majority of fatal cases the course was short. Some animals, however, lived 7 to 10 days and exhibited symptoms and lesions similar to polioencephalomalcia (Tobiska and Jensen, 1946). This observation led to experimentation to determine if hydrogen sulfide causes polioencephalomalacia. Ruminal insufflation of sheep with sublethal doses of hydrogen sulfide did not produce characteristic signs or lesions (Griner, 1964).

In Britain, clinical observations lead to the theory that polioencephalomalacia is caused by an acute deficiency of thiamine. Eleven calves 4 to 8 months of age manifested signs of the disease; one animal, recumbent and comatose, was considered moribund. Following treatment with large doses of thiamine, given intramuscularly, all recovered (Davies, Collings, Venn and Bridges, 1965). This successful treatment was repeated by other clinicians with similar results (Daly, 1968; Little and Sorenson, 1969). In a supporting experiment, a calf was weaned to a thiamine-deficient semi-synthetic milk diet and administered thiamine antagonists, Pyrathiamine and Amprolium; subsequently, the animal developed polioencephalomalacia (Pill, Davies, Collings and Venn, 1966). A still more detailed investigation performed biochemical tests on 13 natural cases. An abnormally high and prolonged rise in blood pyruvate levels followed the intravenous administration of glucose, and these levels declined rapidly after injections of thiamine. At necropsy, thiamine levels in tissue of the cerebral cortex and liver were abnormally low (Pill, 1967). In seeking an explanation for the deficiency, thiaminase of ruminal fluids was measured in cases of polioencephalomalacia and in cases of other diseases. Thiaminase levels were higher in animals with polioencephalomalacia by a factor of 2 to 18 (Edwin and Allcroft, 1968).

Occurrence. Polioencephalomalacia occurs in both feedlot and pastured cattle of both sexes whose age varies commonly from 3 months to 4 years. In Colorado, the age of highest incidence is 12 to 18 months for feedlot animals. In geographic areas where cattle are entered in the feedlot at younger ages, the age for high incidence of disease may be among still younger animals. The disease also occurs in feedlot and pasture sheep. Seasonally, it is more common in feedlot cattle during winter months of January, February and March. This seasonal occurrence may be due to the presence of more cattle in fattening pens. The annual incidence for both feedlot and pasture cattle also varies. During the 1940's and 1950's the incidence was much higher than during the late 1960's. Geographically, the disease exists in the western and eastern regions of the United States, in Britain, New Zealand, Australia and Europe.

Etiology and Pathogenesis. The specific and certain cause of polioencephalomalcia is not known. According to one theory, however, an acute deficiency of thiamine is an important causative factor of cerebral corticonecrosis, as it is known in Britain. Although largely empirical and clinical, the supporting evidence for this theory is the successful treatment of affected cattle. Even some advanced moribund cases in coma have responded favorably to the treatment. The high and prolonged blood levels of pyruvate following intravenous administration of glucose and the rapid fall of pyruvate levels

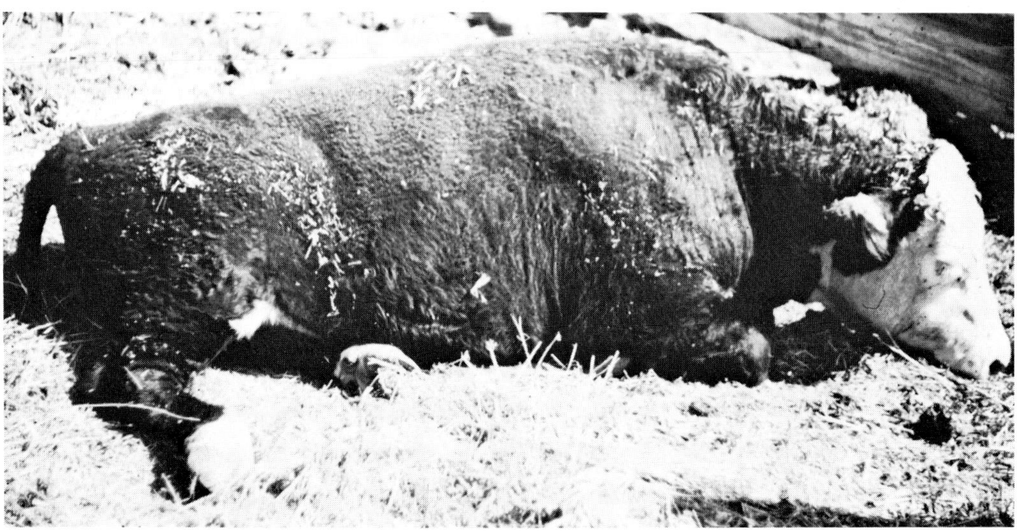

FIG. 8-26. *Feedlot steer comatose from polioencephalomalacia.*

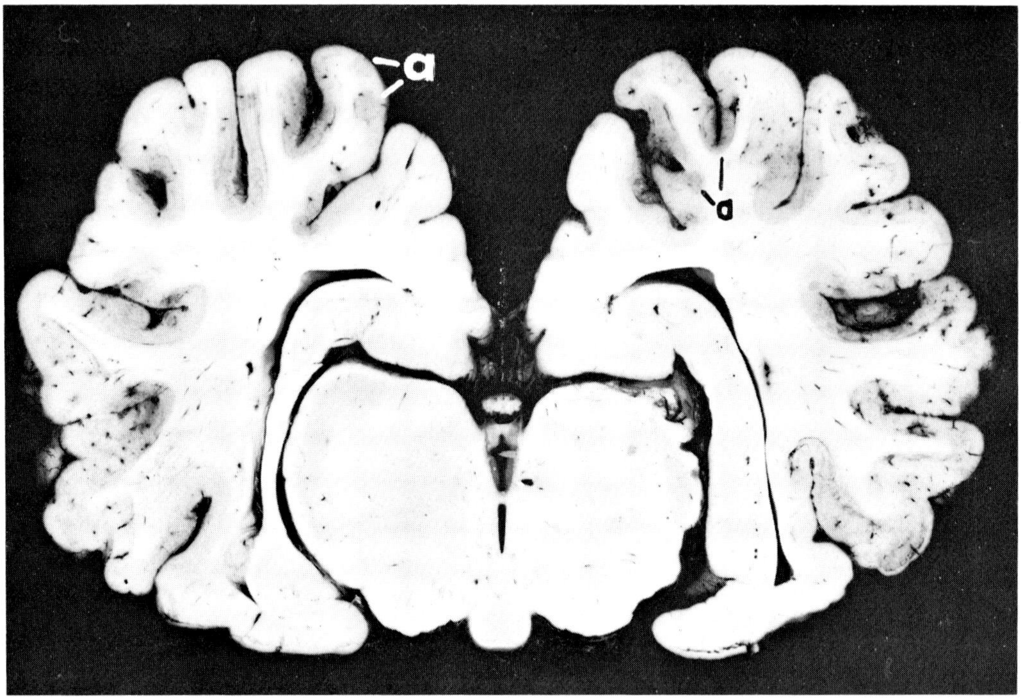

FIG. 8-27. *Cross section of brain from a steer which died from polioencephalomalacia. a. Foci of necrosis in cerebral cortex.* × 1.2.

after injection of thiamine strongly adds to the validity of the interpretation. The mechanism by which the thiamine deficiency develops is poorly understood because the dietary intake of thiamine appears to be more than adequate. Within the rumen, concentrations of thiaminase may destroy the vitamin before absorption can take place. Because thiamine has a central role in metabolizing carbohydrate, a deficiency of this vitamin results in blood accumulations of pyruvate and theoretically causes cerebral edema and neuronal necrosis. The metabolic disturbances damage and necrose neurons. These cellular changes in the region of the calcarine sulcus, an area of visual cortex, result in impaired vision. In recovered animals, the necrotic tissue has been removed by lysis and phagocytosis, leaving cysts in some areas, and meninges in direct contact with white matter in others. Presumably, recovered animals are susceptible to recurrence.

Because of the nature of the pathologic

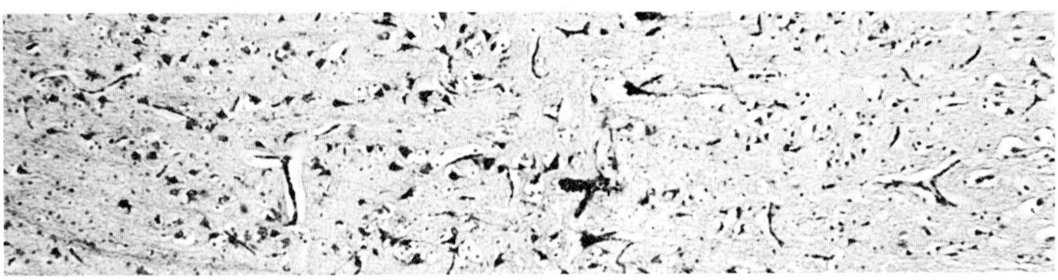

FIG. 8-28. *Section through cerebral cortex from an animal with polioencephalomalacia. Outer laminae are necrotic; inner laminae (left) are viable. Nocht's stain.* × 75.

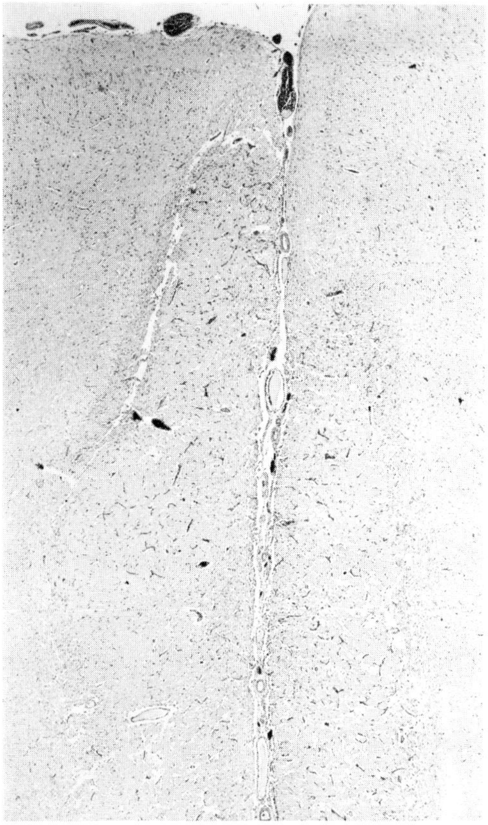

FIG. 8-29. *Necrosis in cerebral cortex from a fatal case of polioencephalomalacia. Nocht's stain.* × 13.

changes in the brain, many veterinarians have supported the hypothesis that the disease is caused by acute hypoxia or acute intoxications. Researchers, however, have not detected methemoglobin, sulfmethemoglobin or cyanmethemoglobin in animals in early stages of disease development. Pesticides recently used can, as specific causes, be eliminated because the disease was common during years before they were used. Since neuronal degeneration and necrosis are end results from cell injury, many adverse factors including unknown intoxications and hypoxies, may be contributing causative factors.

Since the cause is yet unknown, this important disease merits intensive research and until the cause is identified, prevention is impossible and treatment the only means of control.

Clinical Signs and Postmortem Lesions. The disease exists in two degrees: severe and mild. Feedlot cattle usually are affected with the severe degree. Often affected animals are found dead without clinical signs having been observed. In early stages of the disease, when discovery of sick individuals in a herd is difficult, affected animals can be identified by their excitability, their incoordination, their impaired vision and their propensity to remain towards the center of the herd. Continuous driving for 15 to 20 minutes often accentuates the signs and facilitates detection. In advanced stages affected animals separate from the herd. Some cattle are affected suddenly. They back away from feed bunks, display twitching of muscles of the ears and

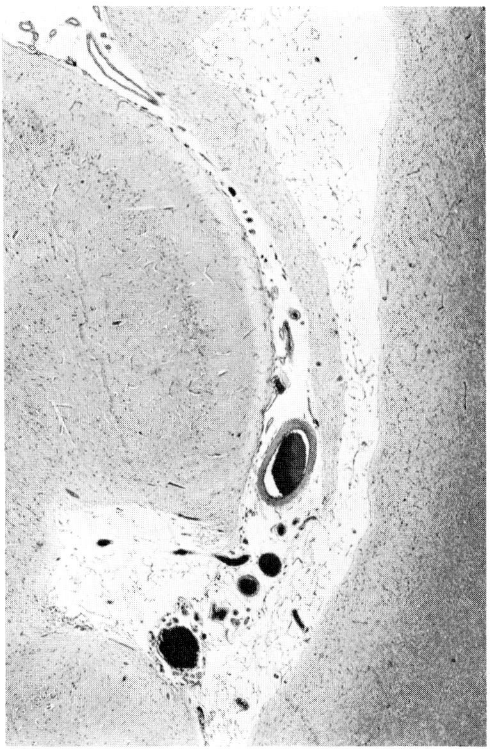

FIG. 8-30. *Cyst in cerebral cortex of an animal which recovered clinically from polioencephalomalacia 3 months earlier. Weil's stain.* × 18.

eyelids, and sometimes of the limbs. Convulsions may occur. During the short period of ambulation the animal is disoriented, blind and physically weak. Walking may be in circles. Temperature is normal except during and following convulsions when it may rise slightly. Pulse and respiratory rates are accelerated. After a few hours, prostration and coma supervene. During the time of coma, the limbs make thrashing movements and the head is in opisthotonis. Amaurosis, medial strabismus and nystagmus are common. After several days of illness the cerebrospinal fluid pressure exceeds 200 mm of water, the normal value, and the cell content, mostly lymphocytes, varies up to 100 per cmm. Death usually occurs within a few days. Morbidity usually is low, but may go as high as 50%. The mortality rate of affected animals is very high.

The mild form of the disease often occurs in pasture cattle and develops within 7 to 10 days following change from overgrazed to lush pasture. Affected animals are partially or totally blind, normal in temperature, physically weak and anorexic. Partial paralysis of throat muscles impairs deglutation and causes salivation. Diarrhea is intermittent. Affected animals often push with the head against solid objects and walk in circles. Prostration and coma may develop. Morbidity varies up to 50%; the mortality rate for affected animals is approximately 50%.

In non-fatal cases recovery is possible but slow. Although clinical improvement follows neuron recovery and organismal adaptation,

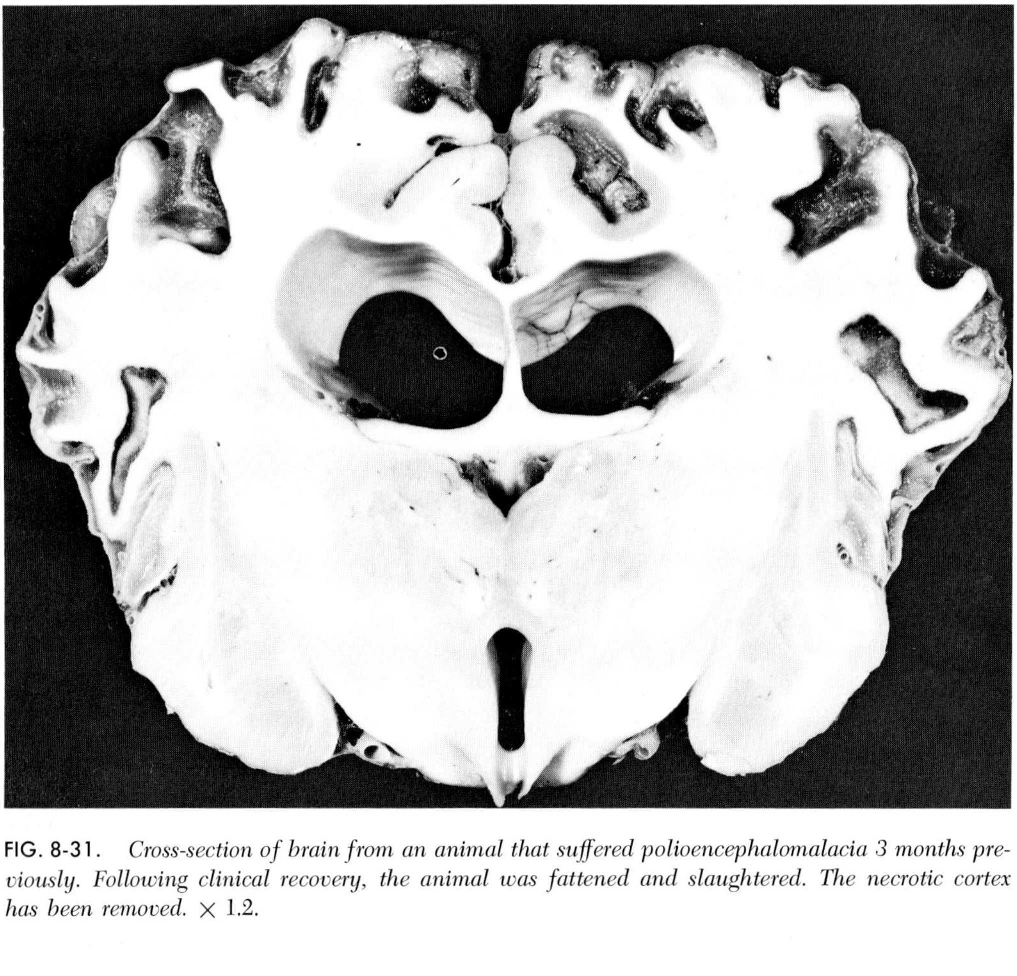

FIG. 8-31. *Cross-section of brain from an animal that suffered polioencephalomalacia 3 months previously. Following clinical recovery, the animal was fattened and slaughtered. The necrotic cortex has been removed.* × 1.2.

impaired vision persists. Fattening can be resumed and marketing finally effected.

At necropsy, lesions are limited to the brain. Swelling in this organ may push the cerebellum into the foramen magnum and cause meningeal hemorrhages. Fresh or unfixed brains are excessively soft in affected areas of the cerebral cortex. Gross sections reveal multiple foci of necrosis of gray matter, especially in the coronal, suprasylvian, lateral, calcarine, and ectosylvian sulci and adjacent gyri. In some animals focal necrosis is located also in the thalami. After 2 to 3 days of illness the cortical foci are yellowish, measure 1 to 10 x 1 to 8 mm, and a cleavage line separating the necrotic from viable tissue is evident. Hemorrhage may occur in necrotic areas of the thalami and the amount of cerebrospinal fluid is increased.

In clinically recovered cases the brain is reduced in size and lateral ventricles are dilated. The necrotic gray matter has been lysed or removed. This focal decortication often places meninges in direct contact with white matter of gyri and results in widened sulci. Cortical cysts, 1 to 2 mm in diameter, may be present. All gross changes are best delineated after fixation of the entire brain in 10% formalin.

Histopathologic changes vary with stages of development. In early stages the necrotic tissue is laminar in extent but intact. Perineuronal and perivascular edema are prominent. Necrotic neurons are shrunken and usually eosinophilic, although some neurons are basophilic. Nuclei are pyknotic, karyorrhexic or absent. At margins of the lesions, both necrotic and viable neurons are present. After 2 to 3 days of illness the discrete focal lesions are readily delimited. The necrotic tissues including neurons, are beginning to liquify and compound granular cells accumulate at the margins. Some endothelial cells of capillaries enlarge and give indication of multiplication.

In clinically recovered brains, all necrotic tissue has been removed and may be replaced by cortical cysts whose lumens contain a network of capillaries and whose walls consist of astrocytes and astrocytic fibrils. If necrosis extended through all cortical layers, the leptomeninges will be in direct contact with the proliferated fibrocytes and fibrils.

Diagnosis. Sudden onset, normal body temperature, cortical blindness, nystagmus, strabismus, disorientation, hyperesthesia, convulsions and coma clinically typify polioencephalomalacia. In addition, the cerebrospinal fluid has pressure above 200 mm of water and cell content, usually lymphocytes, from 5 to 40 cells per cmm. Confirmation can be obtained at necropsy by identifying typical lesions.

The differential diagnosis requires careful consideration of infectious embolic meningoencephalitis, listeriosis and acute lead poisoning. In infectious embolic meningoencephalitis, an acute febrile disease, cerebrospinal fluid contains more than 200 cells, mostly neutrophils, per cmm. Postmortem lesions include single or multiple infected infarcts up to 10 mm in diameter. Listeriosis, also a febrile disease, often results in unilateral facial paralysis and circling ambulation. Acute lead poisoning is nonfebrile and usually of short course. The cerebrospinal fluid contains no cells. Chemical analysis of blood and/or feces may reveal increased levels of lead.

Prevention and Treatment. Until the cause is discovered, little can be done to prevent the disease. In some outbreaks additional cases can be prevented by a complete change of diet and water. Treatment of affected animals consists of intramuscular or intravenous injections of 1 to 2 gm of thiamine hydrochloride. Methylene blue administered at the rate of 1 to 2 gm intravenously helps in detoxification. In addition, generous amounts of fluid and glucose should be administered intravenously. Because of reduced capacity of affected animals to swallow, fluid and nutriment should be pumped into the stomach.

References

Daly, F. J.: Polioencephalomalacia: Response to Thiamine Treatment in Sheep and a Cow. Aust. Vet. J., *44* (1968): 394.

Davies, E. T., Pill, A. H., Collings, D. F., Venn, J. A. J. and Bridges, G. D.: Cerebrocortical Necrosis in Calves. Vet. Rec., *77* (1965): 290.

Edwin, E. E., Lewis, G. and Allcroft, R.: Cerebrocortical Necrosis, A Hypothesis for the Possible Role of Thiaminases in its Pathogenesis. Vet. Rec., *83* (1968): 417.

Elliott, G. A.: Focal Necrosis in the Cerebral Cortex of the Bovine: A Histopathologic Study. Vet. Ext. Quart., Univ. Pa., *150* (1958): 75.

Griner, L. A.: Personal Communications. (1964).

Hartley, W. J. and Kater, Joan C.: Polioencephalomalacia of Sheep. New Zealand Vet., *7* (1959): 75–80.

Howell, J. McC.: Polioencephalomalacia in Calves. Vet. Record, *73* (1961): 1165–1168.

Jensen, Rue, Griner, L. A. and Adams, O. R.: Polioencephalomalacia of Cattle and Sheep. JAVMA, *129* (1956): 311–321.

Little, P. B. and Sorenson, D. K.: Bovine Polioencephalomalacia, Infectious Thrombolic Meningoencephalitis, and Acute Lead Poisoning in Feedlot Cattle. JAVMA, *155* (1969): 1892–1903.

Pill, A. H., Davies, E. T., Collings, D. F. and Venn, J. A. J.: Experimental Reproduction of Lesions of Cerebrocortical Necrosis in a Calf. Vet. Record, *78* (1966): 737–738.

Pill, A. H.: Evidence of Thiamine Deficiency in Calves Affected With Cerebrocortical Necrosis. Vet. Rec., *81* (1967): 178–180.

Spence, J. B., Stevens, A. J. and Saunders, C. N.: Cerebrocortical Necrosis in Sheep and Cattle. The Clinical Syndrome. Vet. Record, *73* (1961): 28–34.

Terlecki, S. and Markson, L. M.: Cerebrocortical Necrosis in Cattle and Sheep. Vet. Record, *73* (1960): 23–27.

Tobiska, J. W. and Jensen, Rue: Livestock Poisoning Caused by Sulfur in Combination With Protein Concentrates. Colorado A & M News, Sept. 1946.

Spondylitis

(SPINAL ABSCESSES; POSTERIOR PARALYSIS)

An acute infectious but non-contagious disease, spondylitis is characterized clinically by posterior paralysis and pathologically by infection of one or few vertebral bodies. Various species of bacteria contribute to the cause of the disease. Because its incidence is relatively low, the disease has little economic importance to the total cattle industry, but serious monetary losses from prolonged courses of expensive treatment and a high mortality rate may accrue to a single producer.

Review of Literature. Only a very few natural cases, but no formal investigations of bovine spondylitis, have been reported. One 7-year-old Guernsey cow and two other cattle, each with some posterior paralysis, were observed. In the Guernsey, an epidural abscess and spinal cord necrosis were located at the fifth and sixth thoracic vertebrae. *Corynebacterium pyogenes* was isolated from lesions of the three animals (Saunders and Roberts, 1950). Over a period of 10 years a series of bovine necropsies contained ten cases of spondylitis (Colorado State University, 1948–1964). Their statistics are presented in Table 29. The high incidence among Herefords reflects regional numerical superiority of the breed.

Occurrence. Although pertinent confirming statistics are not available, spondylitis occurs sporadically and probably equally among all breeds and sexes. While older animals may be affected, cattle under 3 years of age are more susceptible. Unaffected by neither stage of fattening nor of season, the disease has been reported in the western and eastern parts of the United States, but probably exists wherever a major cattle industry occurs.

Etiology and Pathogenesis. *Corynebacterium pyogenes* and *Spherophorus necrophorus* have been isolated from infected vertebral bodies and adjacent meninges, and other species of bacteria are, in some cases, also present. The possible hematogenous origin and exclusive localization of infection in the vertebral bodies motivated scientists to postulate mechanical bone injury as a predisposing factor.

While the pathogenesis has not been determined experimentally, a sequence of de-

TABLE 29 *Bovine spondylitis at Colorado State University*

Age		Sexes		Breeds		Location	
Years	Cases	Name	Cases	Name	Cases	Vertebrae	Cases
1	4	M	7	Hereford	7	C	1
1	3	F	3	Angus	1	T	6
2	3			Holstein	1	L	3
				Brown Swiss	1		

velopmental events can be conjectured. Causative bacteria, in small numbers, enter the systemic blood circulation from a peripheral lesion and are transported to all organs including the skeleton. In some cattle, the causative bacteria may theoretically be carried to the vertebrae by migrating larvae of *Hypoderma* spp. Possibly as a result of predisposing injury, the organisms localize in the osseous, periosteal, or cartilagenous discal tissue of the vertebral body. Metabolic products from the growing bacteria extend necrosis in the vertebral body. During early stages of lesion development, the infectious processes may also extend to adjacent vertebrae and to the dura mater of the spinal cord. In late stages, tissue defenses may arrest the spreading infection and form an abscess. Increased pressure around a segment of spinal cord and absorbed neurotoxic metabolites may interrupt impulse conductivity, cause necrosis and result in paralysis posterior to the infection. Continued use of the weakened vertebrae in attempting ambulation may cause spontaneous fracture. In most cases the bone and cord damage is irreversible, the paralysis progressive, and the termination fatal.

Clinical Signs and Postmortem Lesions. Following an indefinite but probably short incubation period, the body temperature rises and ranges between 103°to 105° F. Walking movements are incoordinated and decelerated. In early stages, clinical sign detection is facilitated by forcing animals to walk or run continuously for several minutes. After a short course, the disease progresses to paralysis posterior to the lesion and later, prostration. Unless the infection is located in the anterior cervical vertebrae, the animal remains mentally alert. With infection in the posterior thoracic, lumbar, or sacral vertebrae, forelimb movements are vigorous and the abscesses may be detected by rectal palpation. Hematological studies usually reveal a moderate leukocytosis. Frequently clinical abnormalities are not observed prior to prostration.

With a low sporadic incidence, the disease has a clinical course of 5 to 14 days and invariably terminates fatally. The unwillingness of owners to tolerate the prostration of the animal or the long course of the disease often results in euthanasia. When submitted for slaughter early in the course and when body temperature is normal, the infected part is condemned as food, while the balance of the carcass, if otherwise normal, is judged satisfactory. At necropsy, the lesions are limited to the vertebrae and included spinal cord. When located in the thoracic vertebrae, where it is most commonly, the lesion is single, but may involve the vertebrae anterior and/or posterior to the original infection. An abscess may have formed ventral to the infected vertebra. Sagittal sectioning of the vertebrae reveals the gray or yellow necrotic bone of the vertebral body and extension of the infection to the epidural tissue and dura mater. Hyperemia, hemorrhage and exudate may be apparent on the external surface of the dura mater. The spinal cord may also show hyperemia, necrosis and hemorrhage. Occasionally the infected vertebrae are fractured. Causative bacteria can be isolated usually from the infected tissue.

Histopathologically, the infected tissues

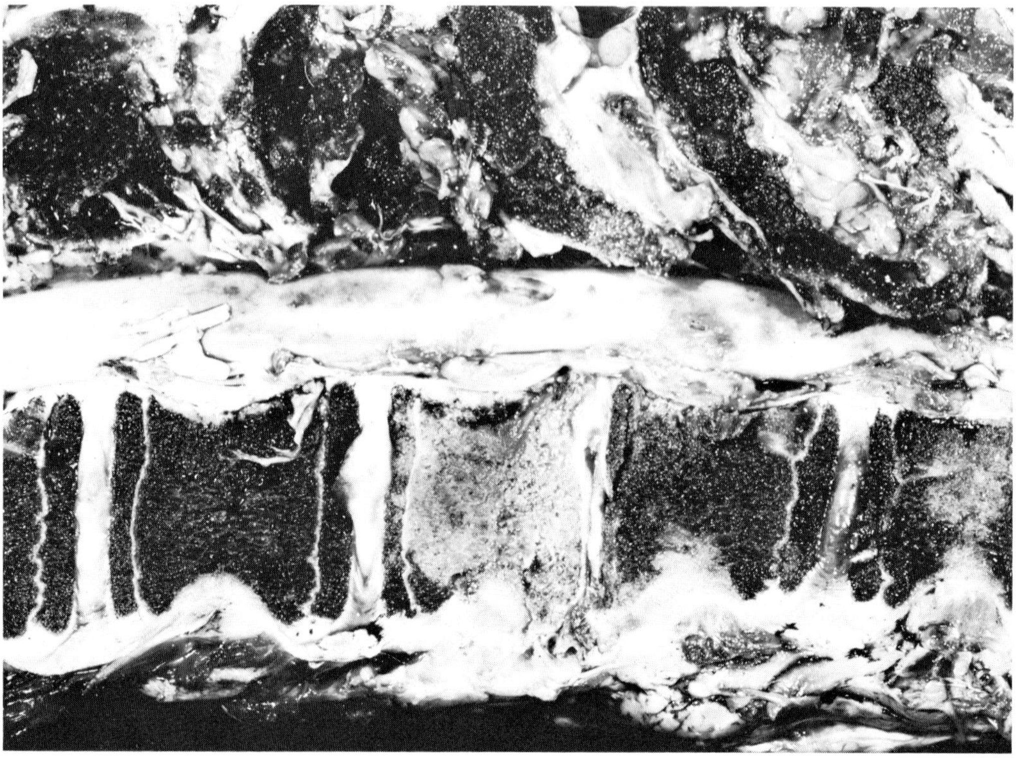

FIG. 8-32. *Sagittal section of thoracic vetebrae showing necrosis of vertebral bodies.* × 0.8.

show necrosis and inflammation. The bone contains colonies of bacteria and an abscess may be forming. In the dura mater the exudate is limited to the external surface. Neurons of the gray matter and/or myelinated tracts of the white matter may be degenerated or necrosed. Hemorrhage into the necrotic cord is common.

Diagnosis. The clinical identification of spondylitis is based on typical signs and postmortem lesions. Important signs include fever, rapidly developing posterior paralysis, and sporadic incidence. Occasionally, the abscesses can be palpated through the rectum. Confirmation of the original diagnosis is readily obtained at necropsy. Sagittal sectioning of all vertebrae with a saw or cleaver may be necessary to locate the site of the infection.

The differential diagnosis requires consideration of listeriosis, sporadic bovine encephalomyelitis, polioencephalomalacia and trauma. Listeriosis is characterized by circling ambulation, unilateral facial paralysis, coma and often a higher incidence than spondylitis. In sporadic bovine encephalomyelitis, the prostration and paralysis are accompanied by coma, peritonitis, pericarditis and pleuritis. Cattle with polioencephalomalacia are not febrile but are blind, and when prostrated, comatose. Animals paralyzed from spinal trauma often have a clinical history of exposure to possible injury through transportation or from sexual riding.

Prevention and Treatment. Because details of the cause and pathogenesis have not been determined through research, a method for preventing spondylitis is not known. The control of *Hypoderma* spp. may prevent some cases of spondylitis. Treatment is ineffective. Following an early diagnosis, the affected animal should be slaughtered for recovery of investment.

References

Colorado State University Necropsy Records. 1948–1964.
Griner, L. A.: Personal Communications. 1964.
Saunders, L. Z. and Roberts, S. J.: A Case of Posterior Paralysis in a Cow. Cornell Vet., *40* (1950): 283–286.

Calculosis

(URINARY CALCULI; WATERBELLY)

Calculosis, a non-infectious disease of cattle, is characterized by the formation within the urinary tract of concretions composed of matrix and salt crystals and by the occlusion of an excretory duct. Calculus is an aggregation of colloidal matrix with crystals of mineral salts deposited in and on the matrix. Normal urine contains matrix and ions of salts in solution. Economically, the disease causes an annual loss of approximately $4 million (Losses in Agriculture, 1965).

Review of Literature. Calculi consist of inorganic salts deposited in an organic matrix. The mechanism for the formation of calculi has been studied extensively in ruminants, as well as in other animals, and people. Both matrix and salts have been investigated carefully. Chemically, the matrix consisted of a mixture of preformed polyelectrolytes, including proteins, mucoproteins and peptides (Udall and Chow, 1969). One experiment compared the urinary polyelectrolytes from lambs being fattened on grain concentrate with lambs maintained on a diet of alfalfa. The urine from fattening lambs contained more peptides, and these compounds showed a higher capacity for binding inorganic cations, especially magnesium (Chow, Hamar and Udall, 1968). The quantity of urine protein and peptides and the number of calculi in feedlot lambs were increased by feeding high concentrate rations (Packett and Coburn, 1965) and by subcutaneously implanting diethylstilbesterol (Udall and Jensen, 1958; Udall and Chow, 1965). Another macromolecular substance, the urine peptides, showed a strong potential for binding calcium and magnesium ions (Chow, Hamar and Udall, 1968). While it has been suggested that the stress from exposure of animals to inclement weather also increases the urine content of mucoprotein (Udall, Seger and Chow, 1965), little supporting evidence has been obtained.

In ruminants normal urine has been analyzed for ions. Cations of magnesium, potassium and sodium were abundant, while those of calcium were scarce. The anions were chloride, sulfate, phosphate and silicate (Newson, Tobiska, and Osland, 1943). It has been postulated that chloride and sulfate ions normally are bound to the mucoprotein and that this blocks further ion binding and the formation of crystals (Udall, Deem and Maag, 1958).

Experimentally, calculosis has been prevented by force-feeding sodium chloride to the extent of 4 to 10% of the dry matter of the ration. This resulted in marked diuresis, and dilution of the urine was assumed to prevent the precipitation (Elam, Schneider and Ham, 1957; Udall, 1959; 1962). Careful investigations indicated that the high ash content of a ration caused increased consumption of water and diuresis (Udall, Seger and Chow, 1965). In one significant experiment, two lots of animals were each fed rations whose total ash content were equal. In the one ration, however, much of the ash consisted of sodium chloride. During the period of experimentation, both lots experienced diuresis to the same degree. The animals receiving the sodium chloride did not develop urinary calculi. This experiment suggested that the sodium chloride, and not diuresis, protected against the formation of calculi (Udall and Chow, 1965).

Occurrence. While calculi may form equally in the urinary tracts in males and females, they readily are excreted without obstruction in females. Occlusion of the urethra occurs commonly in castrated males from 6 to 24 months of age. The incidence is greater during fall and winter months, especially in periods following cold inclement weather. Geographically, the disease is more common in semi-arid regions, and consequently, incidence is high in the western and southwestern regions of the United States and in western Australia.

Etiology and Pathogenesis. Urinary calculi, complex in structure and development, are caused by the interaction of many factors: diet, hormones, and environment. The cause of excretory duct occlusion and the disease, calculosis, adds anatomical and pathological factors.

Because of the economic need to finish and market cattle in a minimum time, the fattening diet has a high ratio of concentrate to roughage. In some cases, the ratio is as high as 15 or 20 to 1. The grain concentrates, having high phosphorus content, provide that element in excess of animal needs and the diets in which phosphorus exceeds 0.6% of the ration contribute to a high incidence of calculi. High concentrate diets also result in a higher percent of low molecular weight urine peptides and these substances, because of strong ion binding potential, favor calculi development. Diets having a high proportion of grain concentrate, especially those including sorghum, are known to be calculus provoking, while diets of alfalfa are non-calculus provoking. Compressing the feed into pellets further enhances its capability for causing calculi.

The use of diethylstilbesterol as a feed additive or as a tissue implanted pellet markedly increases the urinary polyelectrolytes, including peptides, proteins and mucoproteins, and the number of calculi. In feedlot lambs an incidence of 20% calculosis has followed diethylstilbesterol implantation; whether or not this high disease potentiality exists for cattle is conjectural.

During late fall months, especially November and December, ambient temperature fluctuations may be sudden, wide and accompanied by rain or snow. The stresses from these environmental factors contribute to the cause of calculosis, and, a series of cases within a single feedlot may frequently follow these climatic events.

A predisposing factor is the abnormally small diameter of the urethra in steers. The castration of male calves at early age results in underdevelopment of the penis and urethra and, consequently, smaller calculi, as they move with urine from the bladder, occlude the urethra.

Bovine urine is a complex solution containing protein, mucoprotein, peptides and many ions including chloride, sulfate, phosphate, silicate and carbonate anions, and magnesium, sodium, potassium, ammonium and calcium cations. These are the substances from which calculi are formed. The proportions of components vary widely within the same animal at different times and among animals of the same feedlot. Each calculus formed consists of organic matrix containing salt crystals. Following careful demineralization, the delicate matrix has the same shape as the original calculus.

While extensive research has been performed on the subject, no consensus about the mechanism for calculus formation has been determined. During recent years, however, several hypotheses have been presented. According to one interpretation, calculus formation, a physical and chemical process, proceeds in two stages: First, peptides, proteins and mucoproteins aggregate to form an organic matrix. Containing both positive and negative charges, the matrix binds both anions and cations. In the urine of feedlot cattle magnesium cations bind to the matrix at points of negative charge and complex ammonium phosphate anions bind to points of positive charge. The spatial pattern of ion binding creates centers for

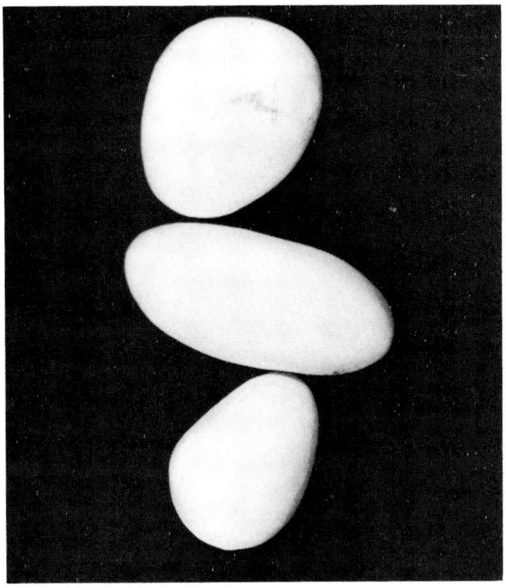

FIG. 8-33. *Smooth surfaced phosphatic calculi.* × 2.7.

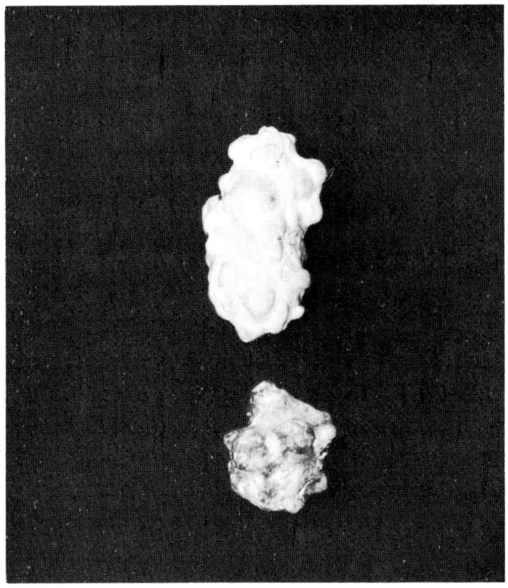

FIG. 8-34. *Spiny silicacious calculi.* × 2.7.

crystalization. Secondly, crystals of mineral deposit in the matrix, and by accretion the mass grows to form variable sized calculi of magnesium ammonium phosphate. The mass of mineral and matrix is highly insoluble.

The feeding of sodium chloride results in chloride anion execretion through the kidneys. In the urine where calculi are forming the chloride anions bind to the matrix at points of positive charge. The resulting mineral-matrix mass dissolves in urine and is excreted without calculus formation.

Calculi may form at any anatomical point along the urinary system from the renal calyces to the urinary bladder. From the point of formation, calculi tend to be transported along the system by flow of urine. Calculi of small diameter move freely through ducts, but the entrance of one stone into a duct of similar diameter frequently results in obstruction. Inflammation and swelling around a lodged stone causes tight closure of the ductal lumen. Proximal to the obstruction, urine accumulates, generates pressure, and may rupture the organ. Rupture of the urinary bladder discharges urine and possibly other calculi into the peritoneal cavity. From here urea and other constituents are reabsorbed into the blood and may accumulate to toxic and fatal levels. Rupture of the urethra proximal to the point of obstruction discharges urine into the subcutaneous tissue of the abdomen, and from here one or more sinuses may drain to the exterior.

Clinical Signs and Postmortem Lesions. Steers affected with calculosis exhibit anorexia, lateral ossilating movements of the tail and physical evidence of abdominal pain. Efforts are made repeatedly, but unsuccessfully, to urinate. The prepucial hair is dry and often filled with crystals. Over the ischial arch the urethra is dilated and pulsating. Rectal palpation discloses distention of the urinary bladder. Following rupture of the urinary bladder, the abdomen mainfests fullness and the animal becomes depressed and prostrated from uremia. Abdominal centesis reveals the urine in the body cavity. In case of rupture of the urethra, the subcutaneous tissues of the posterior abdomen are filled with urine which may discharge to the sur-

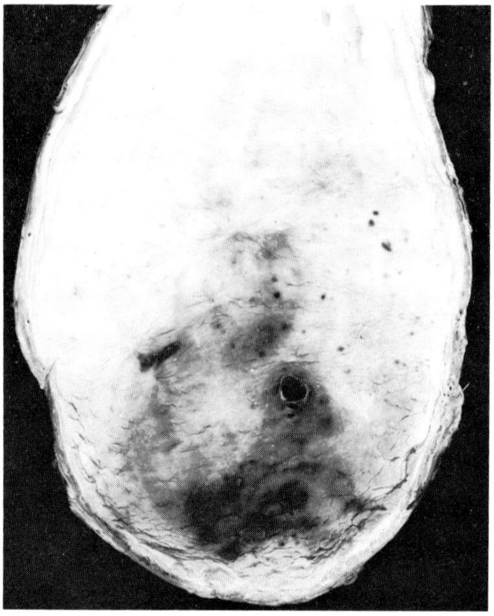

FIG. 8-35. *Urinary bladder ruptured at fundus from urethral occlusion by a calculus.* × 0.7.

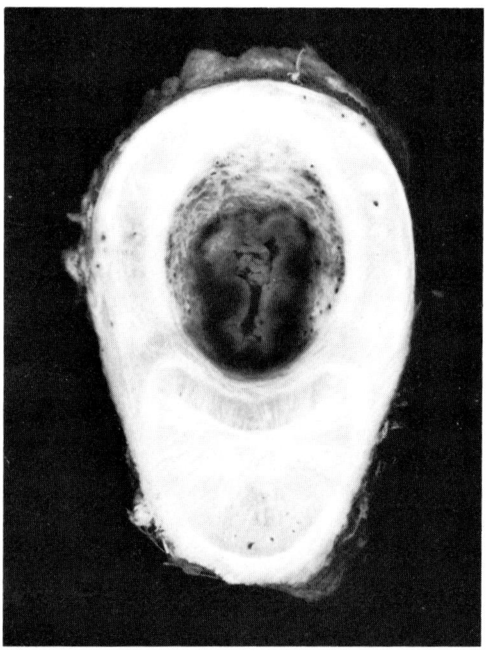

FIG. 8-36. *Cross section of penis proximal to occlusion of the urethra by a calculus. The mucosa of the urethra is necrotic and hemorrhagic.* × 2.7.

face through a fistula. Encrustation of the muzzle often results from severe uremia. Respiration is rapid and shallow.

At necropsy, an occluding calculus is found at the proximal curve of the sigmoid flexure. Around the calculus and proximally into the urinary bladder the urethra is inflamed, necrotic and hemorrhagic. In case of rupture, the inflamed bladder shows the rent which may be covered by a film of fibrin. The abdominal cavity contains large volumes of urine. Additional calculi may be found in the lumen of the bladder and in the abdominal cavity. Single or multiple calculi may also be found in calyces of the kidneys. In case of rupture of the urethra, urine fills the subcutaneous tissues of the abdomen and a fistula from the urethra to exterior may be present. Peritonitis from secondary infection with *Escherichia coli* is often present.

The calculi from urine of feedlot cattle are firm, smooth and spherical. Variable in number and size, they are white to gray in the bladder, and those occluding the urethra may be stained with blood. Chemical analysis shows that the mineral consists mostly of magnesium ammonium phosphates and constitutes 95% of the calculus weight. Calculi forming in cattle whose diet consists of grass are spiny and contain silicate minerals. Incompletely mineralized calculi are soft or elastic in consistency.

At emergency slaughter of animals with a ruptured bladder or urethra, the carcass emits an urinous odor and is unsuitable for human food.

Diagnosis. Clinical diagnosis is based on the characteristic signs. Pathognomonic are the distention and pulsation of the urethra over the ischial arch, distention of the urinary bladder, and unsuccessful attempts to urinate. Blood analysis indicates a level of blood urea nitrogen from normal to 175 mg%. After rupture of the bladder the abdomen fills and distends with urine which may be removed by needle centesis and identified. Following rupture of the urethra the subcutis of the posterior abdomen is infiltrated with urine.

The differential diagnosis requires consideration of ascites, bloat, acute indigestion and pneumonia. Ascites as a part of generalized edema often is caused by failure of the right side of the heart. The ascitic fluid does not possess the characteristics of urine. In bloat the rapidly developing abdominal distention is concentrated on the left side. Acute indigestion is associated with borborygmus which can be detected by auscultation. Pneumonia is usually a febrile disease with dyspnea and nasal discharge. Auscultation of the thorax discloses solidification of parts of the lungs. The above mentioned diseases, confusable with calculosis, do not interfere with normal urination.

Prevention and Treatment. Calculosis can be prevented by including sodium chloride in the ration to the extent of at least 4% of the total dry matter or by feeding ammonium chloride to the extent of 2% of the concentrate feed. Treatment may be applied either before or after rupture of the bladder. In partially fattened cattle the diagnosis is made occasionally before rupture of the bladder occurs. In this case, either urethrotomy or centesis of the bladder are beneficial. Urethrotomy is performed proximal to the point of occlusion and the urine is drained through the incision. Centesis of the bladder is achieved by passing a large needle and a firm non-collapsible tube through the rectum into the bladder. Drainage of the bladder provides temporary relief. Following either of the surgical operations, the animal should be slaughtered as soon as is feasible for salvage of the carcass value.

Most cases of urinary calculosis, unfortunately, are diagnosed after the bladder has ruptured. Treatment of such cases requires drainage of urine from the abdominal cavity by repeated centesis and urethrotomy. In approximately one-third of the ruptured bladders, the rent is small and healing is spontaneous. The bladder can be repaired by laparotomy and surgical closure of the rent. Antibiotics should be administered to control peritonitis. Following rupture of the urethra and infiltration of the subcutis with urine, treatment consists in urethrotomy for drainage of urine from the bladder and multiple skin incisions for drainage of urine from the tissues.

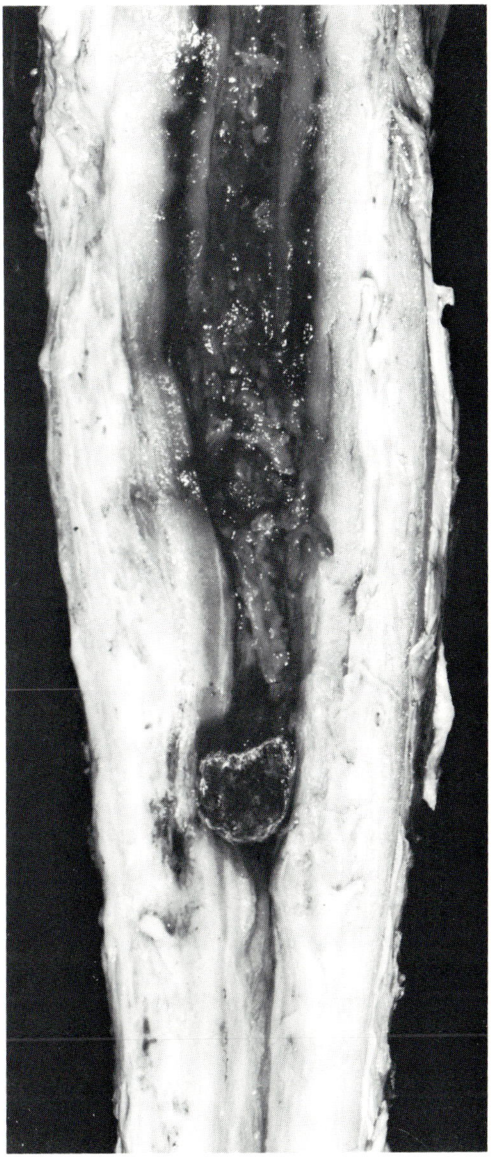

FIG. 8-37. *Opened urethra occluded by a calculus. Proximal to the calculus the urethra is necrotic and hemorrhagic; distal to the calculus the urethra is normal.* × 1.7.

In calculosis, multiple stones are usually formed and occlusion of the urethra tends to recur. Therefore, marketable animals should be slaughtered to obtain the carcass value as soon as recovery from the disease has occurred.

References

Boyce, W. H., Garvey, F. K. and Norfleet, C. M.: Ion Binding Properties of Electrophoretically Homogenous Mucoproteins of Urine in Normal Subjects and in Patients with Renal Calculus Disease. J. Urology, 72 (1954): 1019–1031.

Boyce, W. H., Pool, C. S., Meschan, I. and King, J. S.: Organic Matrix of Urinary Calculi. Acta Radiologica, *50* (1958): 543–560.

Boyce, W. H. and King, J. S.: Crystal-Matrix Interrelations in Calculi. J. Urology, *81* (1959): 351–365.

Chow, F. H., Hamar, D. W. and Udall, R. H.: Studies on Urolithiosis. XI. Interaction of Urine Polyelectrolytes and the Inorganic Ions. Investigative Urology, *5* (1968): 557–567.

Cornelius, C. E., Moulton, J. E. and McGowan, B.: Ruminant Urolithiasis: I. Preliminary Observations in Experimental Ovine Calculosis. AJVR, *20* (1959): 863–871.

Elam, C. J., Schneider, B. H. and Ham, W. E.: Incidence of Dietary Sodium Chloride on Incidence of Urinary Calculi in Sheep. Proc. Soc. Exp. Biol. & Med., *95* (1957): 769–772.

Losses in Agriculture, ARS, USDA. Aug. 1965. Agricultural Handbook No. 291.

Mia, A. S. and Cornelius, C. E.: Ruminal Urolithiasis. VI. Fractionation of Ovine Urinary Biocolloids by Gel Filtration. Investigative Urology, *1* (1964): 439–445.

Newsom, I. E., Tobiska, J. W. and Osland, H. B.: Effect of Rations on the Production of Urinary Calculi in Sheep. Tech. Bull. 31, 1943. Colo. Agri. Exp. Station.

Packett, L. V. and Coburn, S. P.: Urine Proteins in Nutritionally Induced Ovine Urolithiasis. AJVR, *26* (1965): 112–119.

Udall, R. H., Deem, A. W. and Maag, D. D.: Studies on Urolithiasis I. Experimental Production Associated with Feeding in Steers. AJVR, *19* (1958): 825–829.

Udall, R. H., and Jensen, Rue: Studies on Urolithiasis. II. Observation in Feedlot Lambs Following Implantations of Diethylstilbestrol. JAVMA, *133* (1958): 514–516.

Udall, R. H.: Studies on Urolithiasis. III. Control by Force Feeding of Sodium Chloride. AJVR, *20* (1959): 423–425.

———: Studies on Urolithiasis. IV. The Effects of the Ration on the Predisposition as Measured by Urinary Mucoproteins. AJVR, *20* (1959a): 426–429.

———: Studies on Urolithiasis. V. The Effects of Urinary pH and Dietary Sodium Chloride on Urinary Excretion of Proteins and the Incidence of Calculosis. AJVR, *23* (1962): 1241–1245.

Udall, R. H., Seger, C. L. and Chow, Fu-Ho Chen.: Studies on Urolithiasis. VI. The Mechanism of Action of Sodium Chloride in the Control of Urinary Calculi. Cornell, Vet., *60* (1965): 198–203.

Udall, R. H. and Chow, Fu-Ho Chen.: Studies on Urolithiasis. VII. The Effects of Sodium, Potassium, or Chloride Ions, in the Control of Urinary Calculi. Cornell Vet., *55* (1965a): 538–544.

———: *The Etiology and Control of Urolithiasis in Advances in Veterinary Science and Comparative Medicine.* Vol. 13. 1969. Academic Press, Inc., New York City, N. Y.: pp 29–57.

Eosinophilic Myositis

(SARCOSPORIDIOSIS; SARCO)

Eosinophilic myositis, a subacute or chronic asymptomatic disease, is characterized by inflammatory foci in the voluntary muscles and heart, and is of unknown cause. A disease of highly fattened beef cattle, it causes economic losses through condemnation at postmortem inspection of entire carcasses because of widely disseminated foci of inflammation or parts of carcasses from localized inflammation. Statistics on the incidence of eosinophilic myositis are available for slaughtered cattle. From 1967–69 an average of more than 28 million cattle were slaughtered in the United States annually. Of this number, 0.01% were affected to some degree with the disease. Economic losses result from condemnation of affected carcasses and parts of carcasses.

Previous investigations of disease of muscles have revealed two morphologic types: uncomplicated eosinophilic myositis and granulomatous eosinophilic myositis. Since evidence is lacking for the subdivisions, we are considering the two alleged types as one disease.

Review of Literature. Eosinophilic myositis has been recognized for many years. As is indicated in records of the Meat Inspection Division of the United States Department of

Agriculture, the incidence has gradually increased in recent decades. During 1967 through 1969 nearly 28 million cattle were slaughtered annually. Of these 1 animal per 10,000 was affected with eosinophilic myositis (Federal Meat Inspection Services, 1967–1969).

In California, however, the incidence was 1 case per 3,000 slaughtered cattle (Maddy, 1955). A study in Colorado extending over 3 years and involving 612,762 slaughtered cattle indicated the overall incidence was 1 case of eosinophilic myositis per 3,500 animals; in heifers, 1 case per 1,553 cattle; and in steers, 1 per 4,417. The difference between sexes was statistically significant. The steers and heifers affected with the disease came from 65 feedlot enterprises; of these, only 8 enterprises contained affected cattle on 2 or 3 consecutive years (Reiten, Jensen and Griner, 1966).

Based on the type of morphologic lesions, the disease has been classified into two forms: (1) eosinophilic myositis in which large numbers of eosinophils accumulate in tissue where muscle fibers are being destroyed, and (2) sarcosporidial myositis in which eosinophils and granulomas occur. An early investigator, (Beller, 1924) believed that eosinophilic myositis is caused by the protozoan *Sarcocystis fusiformis.* More recently, however, the importance of the role of *S. fusiformis* has been refuted and the possibility of allergy as a cause hypothesized (Cohrs, 1962). By some investigators the ganulomatous form of eosinophilic myositis is still assumed to be caused by *S. fusiformis.*

Until recently most scientists classified *S. fusiformis* as a protozoan which parasitizes voluntary and cardiac muscle (Levine, 1961). The life history was considered to be direct without the necessity of an intermediate host (Scott, 1943). Some investigators recently obtained evidence that *S. fusiformis* is an Asperigillus-like fungus. The organism from swine muscle was cultured in artificial media where it acquired the morphologic characteristics of a fungus; and when the cultures or infected tissues were fed to 50 healthy swine, 25 developed sarcosporidiosis. The control animals remained uninfected (Spindler and Zimmerman, 1945). Further investigations of the morphology of *Sarcocystis* in swine muscle suggested that the septa subdividing the cysts into compartments have the characteristics of hyphae of fungi (Spindler, 1947). Beginning 15 days after inoculation artificially infected swine excreted infective spores in feces and urine. When these excretions were fed to experimental animals, sarcosporidiosis developed (Spindler and Zimmerman, 1946). In general, however, protozoologists have not concurred in classifying *Sarcocystis* as a fungus.

Attempts to incriminate *Trichinella spiralis* as a cause were not conclusive (Kennedy, 1955).

In searching for a means to diagnose eosinophilic myositis in living cattle, researchers compared muscle aqueous extract, serum and urine from 50 diseased heifers with 50 normal heifers. Because of their high sensitivity, disc electrophoretic analyses for protein differences were made. While slight differences were observed in some diseased animals, they were not consistent and, consequently, not diagnostically useful (Tengerdy and Imes, 1967).

While eosinophilic myositis has been found primarily in fat beef cattle (Maddy, 1955; Reiten, Jensen and Griner, 1966), it was also encountered as a generalized infection in a heifer, resulting in muscular weakness and emaciation (Bowler, 1948).

Occurrence. Eosinophilic myositis occurs in highly fattened steers and heifers 1 to 2 years of age as well as western range cows but rarely in dairy cattle. In the United States the incidence has been determined with considerable accuracy for slaughtered cattle. Throughout the entire United States the annual incidence of eosinophilic myositis in slaughtered cattle is approximately 0.01%; but in the western region the incidence is three times the national figure. In California it is 0.03%. In Colorado a sample of 612,762 fat steers, heifers and cows was examined carefully at slaughter. Of these animals, 173 (0.03%) contained a sufficient amount of eosinophilic myositis for condemnation of carcasses, or parts of carcasses, and the incidence was significantly higher in heifers and cows slaughtered during summer months than in any other groups. The disease had no propensity to recur in cattle of feedlots where cases were previously maintained. In addition to the United States, the disease has been diagnosed in Europe. In both geographic areas, a disease with similar lesions has been observed in muscles of swine, sheep and dogs.

Etiology and Pathogenesis. The cause of eosinophilic myositis is unknown. Hypersensitivity has been postulated, but not confirmed, nor even seriously studied, as a possible cause.

Sarcocystis fusiformis, a protozoan parasite, has been suspected by some investigators as a cause. The active form of the organism, the trophozoite, is banana-shaped and measures 6 to 15 × 2 to 4 μ. Colonies of the trophozoites form cysts inside voluntary and cardiac muscle cells of most cattle. Each cyst is longitudinally fusiform and often measures several millimeters in length. Produced by parasite and/or host, the cyst wall has internally extending septa which compartmentalize the cavity. Nests of trophozoites occupy the compartments. Sarcocysts occur in normal cattle, as well as in animals with eosinophilic myositis. In animals affected with eosinophilic myositis, the cysts are randomly distributed in and away from lesions. Because of these observations the theory that sarcosporidia causes eosinophilic myositis has low credibility.

The life history is simple and direct. Mature cysts eventually release individual trophozoites into the blood which carries them to the wall of the alimentary tract, or to the urinary system. By unknown means the trophozoites enter the lumen of the alimentary tract and mix with feces, or they enter the lumen of the urinary system and mix with urine. In either alimentary or urinary system they are excreted as spores to the exterior where, presumably they become infective, through contamination of feed and water, to the same or different animals, especially of the same species. Following ingestion, the spores become trophozoites which penetrate the wall of the alimentary tract, enter blood vessels and are carried to the muscles. As an ameboid-shaped organism, the trophozoite penetrates the sarcoplasm of the muscle cell and multiplies by binary fission. A wall is formed by either parasites and/or host around the trophozoites.

Since the cause of eosinophilic myositis is undetermined, the pathogenesis is unknown. Presumably, however, an inflammatory reaction begins around degenerated or altered muscle cells. Early in the process the cellular infiltrate consists of eosinophils. Within the focus of reaction many muscle cells atrophy. Presumably, small foci of reaction eventually heal. Extensive and numerous lesions in the myocardium may lead to failure of affected chambers.

Clinical Signs and Postmortem Lesions. Except for unusual cases, eosinophilic myositis is asymptomatic. Rarely the myocardium is affected sufficiently to cause failure of a chamber, but occasionally generalized involvement of a skeletal muscle causes weakness and dysfunction. Hemograms prepared from heart blood from slaughter-diagnosed cases have not indicated consistent eosinophilia or other diagnostic change.

Usually the disease is observed at postmortem inspection of slaughtered cattle, or at necropsy of animals dead from intercurrent diseases. Lesions are located within the heart, tongue, crura of the diaphragm and masseter muscles. Less commonly, other voluntary muscles, such as the longissimus dorsi, psoas, thigh and shoulder muscles are affected. Individual lesions are round or elliptical and vary up to 1 mm in diameter. Occasionally the lesions are manifested as streaks between muscle fibers. In color they are yellow-green or grey and may be single or multiple and widely disseminated. Numerous confluent foci form a large lesion many inches in diameter. In old or healed cases, the lesions are gray in color and firm in consistency.

The histopathology varies with stages of development. Early, one or more striated muscle cells are hyalinized and fragmented. In early lesions large numbers of eosinophils, which cause the gross discoloration, surround

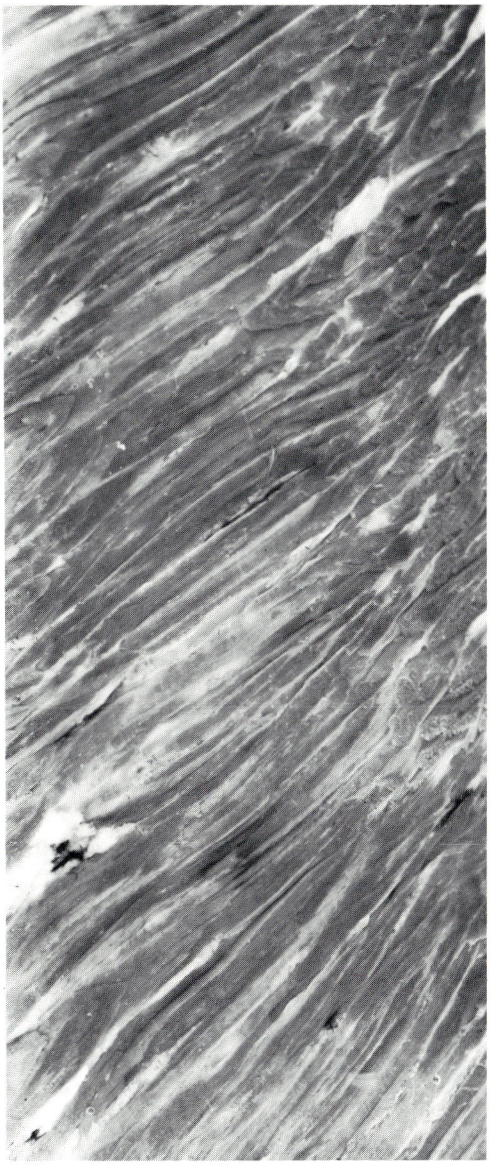

FIG. 8-38. *Eosinophilic myositis in muscle of a steer.* × 2.0.

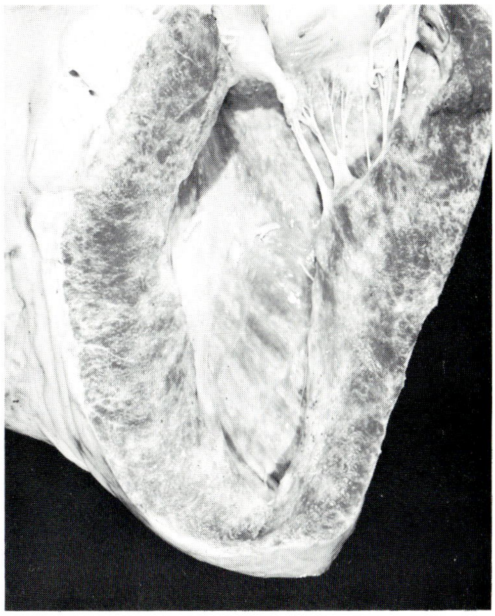

FIG. 8-39. *Eosinophilic myositis in heart of a steer.* × 0.3.

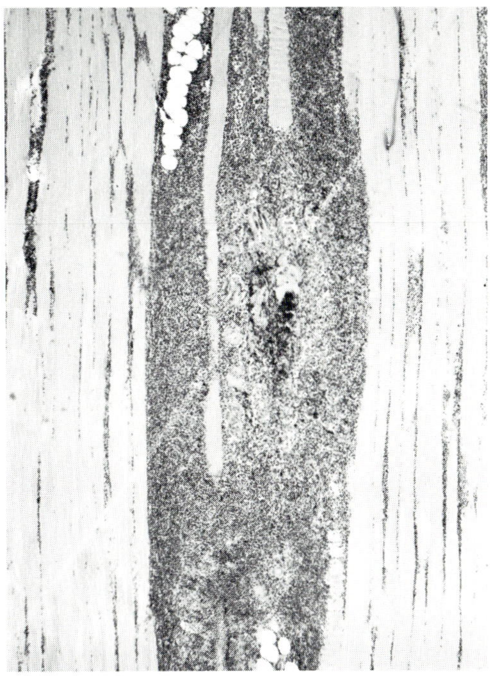

FIG. 8-40. *Eosinophilic myositis in muscle of steer. Nocht's stain.* × 36.

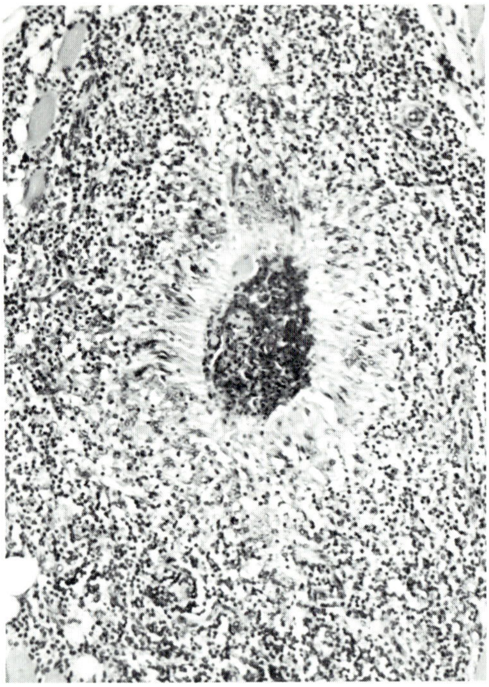

FIG. 8-41. *Granulomatous eosinophilic myositis. Nocht's stain.* × 104.

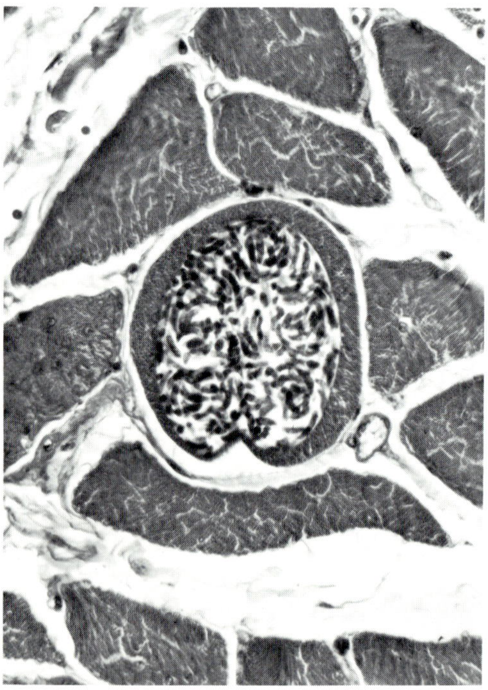

FIG. 8-42. *Sarcocystis fusiformis in a muscle cell. H&E stain.* × 317.

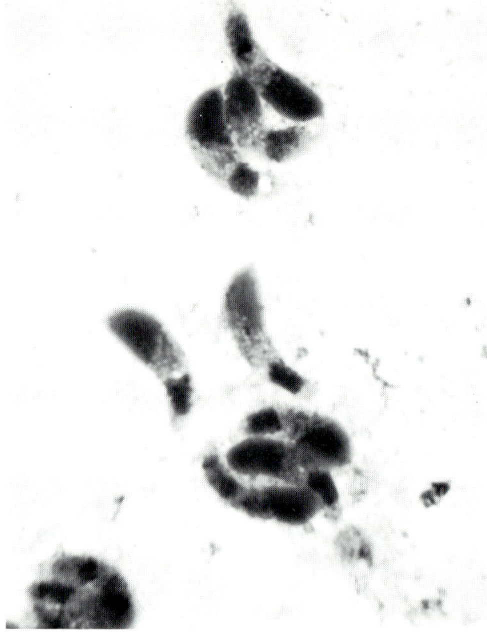

FIG. 8-43. *S. fusiformis. Giemsa stain.* × 1412.

the affected muscle fibers and invade the sarcoplasm. The endomycium is infiltrated, and some adjacent muscle cells surrounded by inflammatory cells may atrophy. Sarcolemmal nuclei from some injured muscle cells proliferate and form syncytia. In lesions of long standing, many lymphocytes, mononuclear macrophages, and some proliferated fibrocytes are combined with the eosinophils. The connective tissue and exudate eventually replace many muscle cells. Granulomas which are often present consist of a central mass of hyalinized necrotic muscle cell fragments and dead leukocytes surrounded by a zone of eiptheloid cells. Calcification may have occurred. More peripheral are fibrocytes, lymphocytes and the eosinophils. Cysts of S. *fusiformis* are distributed at random throughout normal and diseased muscles. In old or healed lesions the eosinophils are replaced by fibrocytes and a modest number of lymphocytes and mononuclear macrophages.

Although the affected muscle is innocuous as food, but is yellow-green in color, consumers suspect unwholesomeness and, therefore, discriminate against the product; consequently, limited lesions are excised and condemned while the remaining part of the carcass is satisfactory for human food. Carcasses in which the lesions are numerous and widely disseminated are condemned for human food.

Diagnosis. Because of the absence of clinical signs and the lack of biochemical or serologic tests, eosinophilitic myositis is never diagnosed clinically. Diagnosis is established on the basis of gross appearance at the time of postmortem examination of slaughtered animals and at necropsy. The detection of few and small lesions requires considerable experience and careful discernment. A diagnosis based on gross appearance can be confirmed histopathologically.

The differential diagnosis requires consideration of suppurative myositis, cysticercosis, trichinosis and metastatic lymphosarcoma. Suppurative myositis is the formation of single or multiple small abscesses. The exudate is semifluid, and pyogenic bacteria can usually be isolated in the laboratory. In cysticercosis, each cyst measuring up to 10 mm in diameter, contains a white opaque scolex of the larva of *Taenia saginata*. Trichinosis, rare in beef cattle, causes uneven muscular opacity, and larvae of *Trichinella spiralis* can be observed microscopically in muscle cells. Metastatic foci of lymphosarcoma in voluntary muscles are manifested as soft grey tissue within and between muscles. Elsewhere in the animal tissues the primary neoplasm, and possibly other metastatic foci, are discernible.

Prevention and Treatment. Since the cause and means of transmission are unknown and since the disease is asymptomatic, prevention and treatment are yet to be developed.

References

Beller, K. F.: Uber eine parasitare Musskelerkrankung unserer Haustiere. Ein Beitrag zur Biologie und Pathogenitat der Sarkosporidien, Ztschr. fur Infektionskrank., Parasitare Krank., und Hyg. der Haustiere. *26* (1924): 53.

Bowler, G. E.: Sarcosporidiosis in a Cow. JAVMA, *13* (1948): 266.

Cohrs, P.: Nierberle und Cohrs. *Lehrbuch der Speziellen Pathologischen Anatomie der Haustiere.* Vierte Auglage. Gustav Fischer Verlag. Stuttgart. (1962): 914–920.

Federal Meat Inspection. A Statistical Summary. Consumer and Marketing Service U.S.D.A., 1967, 1968, 1969.

Hadlow, W. J.: Disease of Skeletal Muscle. Chapter in: Innes, J. R. M. and Saunders. L. Z. *Comparative Neuropathology.* Academic Press. New York (1962): 147–243.

Kennedy, P. C.: Experimental Bovine Trichinosis: An Attempt to Produce Eosinophilic Myositis of Cattle. Cornell Vet., *45* (1955): 128–152.

Levine, N. D.: *Protozoan Parasites of Domestic Animals and of Man.* Burgess Publishing Co. Minneapolis. (1961): 318–325.

Maddy, K. T.: Sarcosporidiosis. North Am. Vet., *36* (1955): 455–457.

Reiten, A. C., Jensen, Rue and Griner, L. A.: Eosinophilic Myositis (Sarcosporidiosis; Sarco) in Beef Cattle. AJVR, *27* (1966): 903–906.

Scott, John W.: Life History of Sarcosporidia, With Particular Reference to *Sarcocystis tenella.* University of Wyoming Agric. Exper. Station Bull. 259, (February 1943): 1–64.

Spindler, L. A.: A Note on the Fungoid Nature of Certain Internal Structures of Meischner's sacs (Sarcocystis) from Naturally Infected Sheep and Duck. Proceed. Helminthological Soc. of Washington, *14* (1947): 29–30.

Spindler, L. A. and Zimmerman, H. E.: The Biological Status of *Sarcocystis.* J. Parasitology, *31* (1945): supplement 13.

Spindler, L. A., Zimmerman, H. E., Jr. and Jaquette, D. S.: Transmission of *Sarcocystis* to Swine. Proceedings Helminthological Soc. of Washington, *13* (1946): 1–11.

Tengerdy, R. P. and Imes, G. D.: Disc Electrophoresis of Body Fluids in Cattle With Eosinophilic Myositis. AJVR, *28* (1967): 875–878.

Bovine Lymphosarcoma

(LYMPHOCYTOMA; MALIGNANT LYMPHOMA; LYMPHOBLASTOMA; LEUKOSIS ENZOOTICA BOVIS; LEUKOSIS; LEUKEMIA; PSEUDOLEUKEMIA; LYMPHADENOSIS)

A chronic neoplastic disease, bovine lymphosarcoma is characterized by malignant proliferations of lymphoid cells, by progressive cachexia and by a high mortality rate. Diffuse or nodular, the neoplastic growths are gray, soft and often multicentric in origin. Since the disease is uncommon, sporadic and usually affects mature cattle, it has minor economic importance to the United States cattle industry, especially the cattle fattening enterprises. While the incidence in breeding herds may be significant, only few feedlot cattle are affected. Some losses, however, result from the emaciation and the eventual death of affected animals. In some respects the disease resembles leukemia of mice and leukosis of chickens.

Review of Literature. During the last two decades various aspects of bovine lymphosarcoma have been reported and studied, and records of the federal meat inspection services have indicated that within the United States lymphosarcoma is probably the second most common neoplasm of cattle. From 1967 through 1969, an average of 28.7 million adult cattle and 3.9 million calves were slaughtered annually; of these, lymphosarcoma occurred in 17 per 100,000 adults and in 2.7 per 100,000 calves (Federal Meat Inspection, 1967–1969). In Denmark, the disease was not uniformly distributed in the adult cattle from Zealand, Holland and Jutland. While the average national incidence was 4.1 cases per 100,000 cattle in some counties the incidence was less than 1 case per 100,000, and in other counties 40 cases per 100,000. In 25 observed herds, lymphosarcoma occurred only after introduction of new cattle, and the initial cases occurred as long as four years after the new addition (Bendixon, 1957).

Following their study of many affected individuals and herds, researchers made these categories of the disease: (1) The enzootic form with multiple-cases per herd and often with a history of animal introductions within 4 years, and (2) the sporadic form occurring in cattle under 18 to 20 months of age and showing skin lesions (Bendixon, 1960; 1960a). By use of a series of hemograms, peripheral blood lymphocytosis was observed in various stages of the disease (Bendixon, 1960; Marshak *et al.*, 1962; Theilen *et al.*, 1961). Using this hematological technique as an aid in diagnosis a "leukosis key" was developed. Hemograms were prepared and, for the disease, each animal was classified as normal, suspicious or positive (Gotze, 1954). Positive lymphocytosis in a clinically healthy animal was indicative of a pretumorous disease stage. In one investigation, application of the technique to 18 multiple-case herds indicated 6 herds with some generalized lymphocytosis, 3 with partial, and 9 with none; while in 9 lymphosarcoma-free herds, 2 indicated generalized lymphocytosis and 7 none. The investigators concluded that generalized lymphocytosis is not found exclusively in lymphosarcoma (Hare *et al.*, 1964).

From a study of its many causal aspects, veterinarians have reasoned that lymphosarcoma probably is an infectious disease. Evidence supporting this conclusion has come from epizootiological, serological and electron microscopic investigations. In a study to determine patterns of its transmission, 10 calves from cows hemotologically positive for lymphosarcoma were removed at birth from dams and raised on premises where no other cattle were maintained. The calves received neither colostrum nor milk from dams but were raised on artificial diets. Of these animals, one died from lymphosarcoma at age 479 days. Three others became hematologically positive to the disease at 194, 207, and 619 days of age (Bederke, Tolle and Schmidt, 1968). In another study, fetuses from lymphosarcomatous cows were delivered by cesarean section, denied dam colostrum and milk and raised in isolation. Two of these calves developed the disease (Straub, 1966).

Data from pedigree analysis of 6 multiple-case herds indicated an aggregation of cases within cow families and a high statistical significance for distribution of the disease. In one herd, Guernsey and Holstein cattle had been maintained together for 20 years but during a subsequent 3-year period, 5 Holstein and no Guernsey animals developed the disease. While some of the information from these studies suggested genetic susceptibility, much of the data admittedly fit a hypothesis of vertical transmission of an infectious agent (Marshak *et al.*, 1962). Detailed investigations in Germany supported several facts determined from previous experiments: Lymphosarcoma remained within affected herds for more than 20 years, even though new bulls were used for breeding; genetically unrelated animals introduced into affected herds developed the disease; and some herds remained disease-free while genetically related herds were affected (Bottger, 1956). In one study to determine the cause of the disease, investigators isolated a virus-like agent from cows having lymphosarcoma. When inoculated into bovine embryonic spleen cell cultures, the agent caused syncytial formation among the cells. An antigen prepared from the infected cell cultures produced immunodiffusion when tested against serum from both lymphosarcomatous cows and apparently normal cows. Fluorescent conjugates prepared with precipitating sera stained infected cells while nonprecipitating sera failed to do so (Malmquist and Van Der Maaten, 1969). However, other investigators using cell cultures have been unable to isolate virus-like agents from rapidly growing lymphosarcomatous tissue (Lieberman and Wittman, 1965).

Using electron microscopy, veterinarians have found additional evidence that virus-like agents may be one factor in the cause of bovine lymphosarcoma. For example, centrifuged milk samples from lymphosarcomatous cow herds and samples from a pool tank were examined ultrastructurally and were found to contain virus-like particles having diameters varying from 60 to 110 m μ; similar samples from 8 lymphosarcoma-free herds contained no identifiable particles (Dutcher, Larkin and Marshak, 1964). Tissue biopsies from lymphosarcomatous cows contained particles resembling virus (Dutcher *et al.*, 1967), and cultures of bovine embryonic spleen cells inoculated with lymphosarcomatous tissue revealed virus-like particles in the cell membrane (Malmquist and Van Der Maaten, 1969).

At necropsy, neoplasm was primary in the lymph nodes and metastatic in the heart, kidneys, abomasum, uterus and spinal cord (Marshak *et al.*, 1962). In 17 cases cytologic studies of lymph nodes and cell cultured leukocytes showed hypodiploid or hyperdiploid chromosomal changes (Hare *et al.*, 1964).

Occurrence. While all breeds, sexes and ages of cattle are susceptible to lymphosarcoma, the disease aggregates in come cow families and specific bull descendants, and occurs most commonly in ages 4 to 8 years. Sporadic cases may occur at all ages and are found in many herds. Except in fattening retired cows and bulls, the disease is uncommon in feedlot cattle of the usual ages, 6 months to 2 years. Unaffected by season, the disease occurs in all regions of the United States and in other cattle-raising countries. In Denmark and Germany, it commonly occurs, but cases are unevenly distributed, and by herd testing and slaughter of affected individuals the disease has been eliminated from some herds.

Etiology. The full cause of bovine lymphosarcoma is unknown. Many facts, however, suggest that a virus-like agent is at least one factor in the cause. Both clinical and laboratory evidence support the viral hypothesis. Vertical transmission maintains the causative agent and the disease within lines or families of cattle for long periods. Infected herds develop cases of lymphosarcoma while genetically related lines may remain clean. The disease may enter a herd by introducing new, presumably carrier, animals. In the laboratory, virus-like agents have been isolated from lymphosarcomatous tissue and grown in cultures of bovine embryonic spleen cells. Virus-like particles have also been found in centrifuged milk samples. Using electron microscopy as a research tool, virus-like particles have been found in tissue biopsies, infected cell cultures and in centrifuged milk. Virus-like particles from milk vary in diameter from 60 to 110 m μ. Since the virus has been found in both lymphosarcomatous cows and apparently healthy cows, its role as a causative agent is disputable.

While lymphatic leukemia in mice and

leukosis in poultry, both viral diseases, are characterized by neoplastic proliferation of lymphocytes, no data have been advanced suggesting that these and bovine lymphosarcoma are etiologically related.

Pathogenesis. Since the cause of bovine lymphosarcoma is unknown, the pathogenesis is incompletely understood. Presumedly, the causative agent, possibly complex but including a virus, transmits from infected dam to susceptible fetus within the uterus or to the calf through infected colostrum and milk. During a prolonged pretumorous period, the causative agent acts directly on lymphoid tissue and stimulates neoplasia at one or more points. With primary proliferation in the lymphoid tissue, the sinusoids become occluded; the germinal centers are destroyed and replaced with neoplastic lymphocytes and lymphoblasts. Affected lymph nodes enlarge. During early disease stages the neoplastic cells are restricted to the nodal parenchyma, but eventually the nodal capsule is invaded and surrounding tissue infiltrated. Commonly neoplastic cells metastasize to other organs. Myocardium, bone marrow, abomasal wall, kidneys, postorbital fat, pelvis and spinal epidural tissues are often affected. Muscle, skin, liver, nerves and other organs are susceptible, but less commonly invaded. The metastatic growths pressurize and destroy cells, and the invaded organs lose some or all functions. Growths may be nodular or diffuse. In the blood, lymphocytosis may be transitory or permanent, mild or severe. In advanced stages, some peripheral lymph nodes may be conspicuously enlarged.

The virus-like agent apparently is transmitted from infected cows to fetuses. Transmission may occur within the uterus at the time of birth or through the milk subsequent to birth. By this means families of cows remain infected, and the commercial trade of individual animals carrying the virus spreads the disease to other herds.

Clinical signs vary according to the extent of injury to the secondarily invaded organs. Degrees of failure of bone marrow, heart and spinal cord are manifested. When emaciation develops, death is invariable.

Whatever its nature, viral or unknown factors, the causative agent persists for decades within an affected herd and susceptible cattle introduced into the herd may develop the disease. The transfer of individual cattle from affected to clean herds may spread the disease, and 4 years may lapse from the time of introducing new animals until cases of lymphosarcoma in the previously clean herd appear.

Clinical Signs and Postmortem Lesions. After a period of slow and insidious development, bovine lymphosarcoma presents variable signs. Despite ready availability of ample feed and water, the rate of gain in body weight is slow and eventually becomes a loss. Body temperature, while usually normal, may slightly elevate temporarily and repeatedly. Some of the lymph nodes, pal-

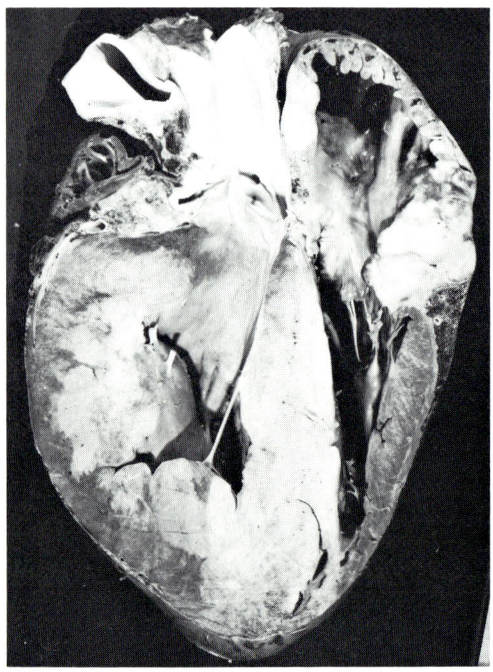

FIG. 8-44. *Bovine heart affected with lymphosarcoma. The right atrium, septum and left ventricle are infiltrated.* × 0.4.

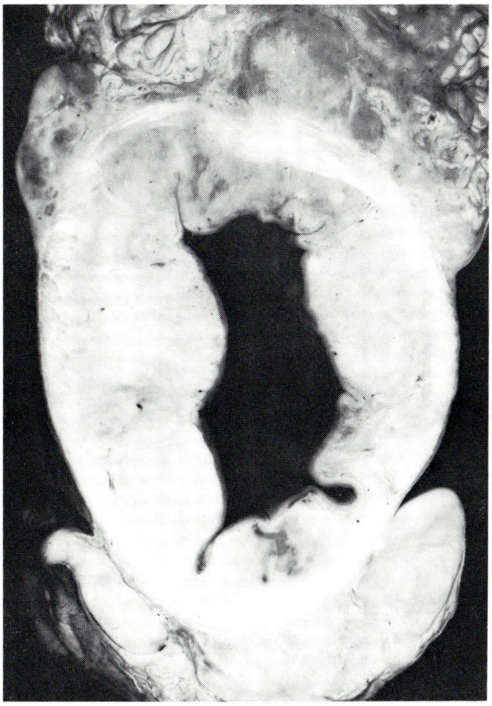

FIG. 8-45. *Gross cross section of bovine abomasum thickened by infiltration of malignant lymphocytes.* × 0.6.

pable from the exterior and per rectum, are enlarged either unilaterally or bilaterally. Enlarged parotid, prescapular or prefemoral nodes are often conspicuous, but readily movable by palpation. Unilateral enlargement of a prescapular node may cause deflection of the head and neck to the opposite side, and enlargement of the postorbital nodes causes exophthalmia. In some cases posterior paralysis, from spinal involvement, is an early sign.

Additional signs depend on the metastatic involvement of other organs. Invasion and destruction of the bone marrow results in normocytic anemia with subnormal hemoglobin levels and paleness of visible mucous membranes. The preparation of a series of hemograms usually reveals at least temporary and frequently terminal lymphocytosis. Leukocyte counts vary from normal numbers to 300,000 per cu mm with an abnormally high percentage of lymphocytes. Invasion of the myocardium results in tachycardia, indistinct heart sounds, and physical weakness. Compression of specific heart segments, or of the venae cavae, may cause generalized passive congestion and extensive edema. Infiltration of the abomasal wall seldom causes luminal obstruction, but may result in ulcers and luminal hemorrhage. Invasion of the spinal epidural space with compression of the cord or infiltration of spinal ganglia and spinal nerves is a common cause of incoordinated movements and partial or complete paralysis, especially of the posterior limbs.

Chemical examination of the blood may show elevation of the serum glutamic-oxaloacetic transaminase and serum lactic dehydrogenase levels (Marshak *et al.*, 1962).

While sporadic cases may occur in any herd, the case incidence within a herd is low and usually zero. In the United States, the average annual incidence in slaughtered adult cattle is 18 cases per 100,000 animals and in calves 2 cases per 100,000. Reports from Denmark indicate an average incidence of 4.1 cases per 100,000 cattle. The course is usually prolonged and may extend over several months. All cases die.

At necropsy, the carcass is usually emaciated and anemic. Groups of lymph nodes are often enlarged by a factor of five or more, and the descending order of frequency is mandibular, prescapular, prefemoral, supramammary and sublumbar nodes. Capsules are tight, and uniformly gray, soft, tissue bulges from the cut surfaces. If the capsule has been invaded, surrounding tissues may be affected and adhesed to the nodes. Heart, abomasum and spinal cord are the three common organs of infiltration. The myocardium, often infiltrated in the right atrium, right ventricle and septum, is thickened and pale. Circulatory interference may have caused generalized passive congestion and edema. Nodules of neoplastic tissue in the spinal epidural space may cause local compression, disfigurement and atrophy of the cord. The abomasal wall may be thickened and firm from neoplastic infiltration. Kidneys, liver, muscle, nerve trunks and other organs may

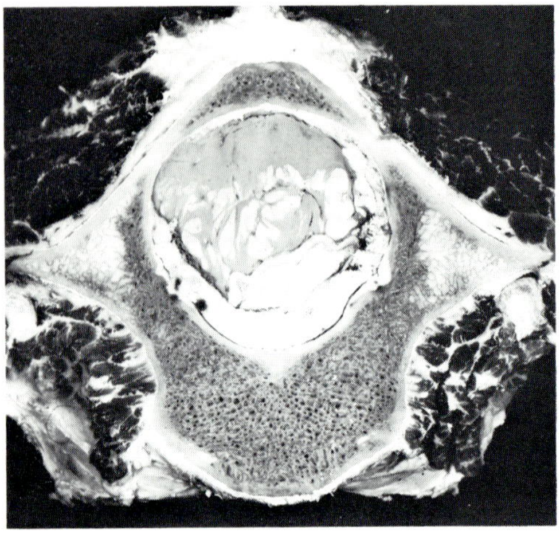

FIG. 8-46. *Gross cross section of bovine cervical vertebra showing compression of the spinal cord from metastatic lymphosarcoma in epidural space.* × 0.7.

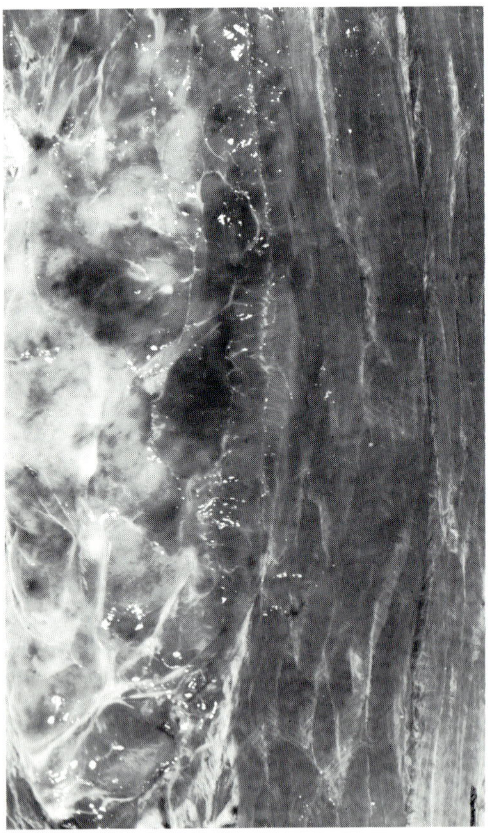

FIG. 8-47. *Voluntary muscle infiltrated with metastatic lymphosarcoma.* × 1.0.

be affected, but the brain rarely is damaged.

Histopathologically, the neoplasm consists of a delicate stroma and two cell types: (1) lymphocyte 8 to 10 μ in diameter with a central nucleus and clumps of chromatin, and (2) lymphoblast 12 to 15 μ in diameter with at least one prominent nucleolus in the nucleus. Mitoses are common, and in any organ the neoplastic cells infiltrate, destroy and replace many normal cells.

Diagnosis. The clinical identification of bovine lymphosarcoma is based on enlargements of groups of lymph nodes. Rectal palpation may reveal internal enlargements. In some stages of the disease, hemograms indicate marked leukocytosis with more than 77% lymphocytes. Confirmation can be obtained by biopsy of affected nodes and the location of the characteristic neoplastic lymphocytes and/or lymphoblasts. At necropsy both primary and metastatic neoplasms can be located.

The differential diagnosis requires consideration of chronic purulent infections, such as metritis and arthritis, metastatic neoplasms and various causes of paralysis such as spondylitis. The chronic infection in afferent tissue or organs of an enlarged group of lymph nodes usually can be detected by careful examination. A primary malignancy with metastatic foci in a lymph node is also frequently detectible, especially if the primary growth is afferent to a peripheral lymph node. Spondylitis, mechanical injuries to the spinal cord and peripheral nerve damages are not associated with marked enlargements of groups of lymph nodes. Enlarged nodes can be biopsied for histopathologic examination.

Prevention and Treatment. In Denmark, enzootic lymphosarcoma is considered an infectious, reportable disease and multiple-case herds are quarantined against sale of cattle except for slaughter. By this procedure, the rate of disease spread is reduced and clean herds are protected against exposure to possible carrier animals. No other means of prevention and no effective treatment have been developed. Cases diagnosed in early stages of the disease should be submitted to slaughter for recovery of investment. At slaughter visibly affected organs are condemned. If the neoplasm is localized, the healthy part of the carcass, if otherwise normal, is satisfactory for food. If metastases are systemic and widespread, the entire carcass is condemned.

References

Bederke, G., Tolle, A. and Schmidt, F. W.: Placental Transmission of Bovine Leukosis. Zentralb. Vet. Med. Reihe, *15* (1968): 782–793.

Bendixen, H. J.: Studies on Leukosis in Cattle. I. Occurrence and Distribution of Cattle Leukosis in Denmark. Nord. Vet-Med., *9* (1957): 1–33.

———: Studies on Leukosis in Cattle. II. The Clinical Diagnosis of Leukosis in Cattle. Nord. Vet-Med., *10* (1958): 273–301.

———: Investigations Concerning Bovine Leukosis in Denmark. III. Clinical Symptoms of the Transmissible Enzootic form and the Sporadic Form. Dtsch. Tierarztl. Wschr., *67* (1960): 169–173.

———: Untersuchungen uber die Rinderleukose in Denmark. Dtsch. Tierarztl. Wschr., *67* (1960a): 55–63.

Bottger, T.: Causes of Neoplastic Forms of Bovine Leukosis. Dtsch. Tierarztl. Wschr., *63* (1956): 332–336.

Dutcher, R. M., Larkin, E. P. and Marshak, R. R.: Virus-like Particles in Cow's Milk From a Herd With a High Incidence of Lymphosarcoma. U. S. National Cancer Institute, *33* (1964): 1055–1059.

Dutcher, R. M. *et al.*: Evidence in Support of a Virus Etiology for Bovine Leukemia. Cancer, *20*(1967): 851–856.

Federal Meat Inspection.: Statistical Summary. C&MS-54 (1967, 1968, 1969).

Gotze, R., Rosenberger, G. and Ziegenhagen, G.: Leukosis in Cattle. Hematological and Clinical Diagnosis. Mh. Vet. Med., *9* (1954): 517–526.

Hare, W. C. D., Marshak, R. R., Abt, D. A., Dutcher, R. M. and Croshaw, J. E.: Bovine Lymphosarcoma. A Review of Studies on Cattle in Eastern United States. Canad. Vet. J., *5* (1964): 180–198.

Jarplid, B.: Studies on the Site of Leukotic and Preleukotic Changes in the Bovine Heart. Path. Vet., *1* (1964): 366–408.

Lieberman, H. D. U. and Wittman, W.: Etiologic Studies of Bovine Leukemia. 2. Tissue Culture. Arch. Exp. Veterinarmed., *19* (1965): 1383–1404.

Malmquist, W. A., Van der Maaten, M. J. and Boothe, A. D.: Isolation, Immunodiffusion, Immunofluorescence, and Electron Microscopy of a Syncytial Virus of Lymphosarcoma and Apparently Healthy Cattle. Cancer Research, *29* (1969): 188–200.

Marshak, R. R., Coriell, L. L., Lawrence, W. C., Croshaw, J. E., Schryver, H. F., Altera, K. P. and Nichols, W. W.: Studies on Bovine Lymphosarcoma. I. Clinical Aspects, Pathological Alterations, and Herd Studies. Cancer Research, *22* (1962): 202–217.

Papparella, V.: Electron Microscopy of the Virus of Lymphatic Leucosis of Cattle. Zooprofilassi, *14* (1959): 254–256.

———: Sensitivity of Guinea Pigs to the Causal Agent of Bovine Leucosis. Acta Med. Vet., Napoli, *5* (1959a): 157–176.

Straub, O. C.: Preliminary Results in Study of Vertical Transmission of Bovine Leukemia. Wermer-Gren Center Int. Symposium Series., *6* (1966): 239–243.

Theilen, G. H., Schalm, O. W. and Gilmore, V.: Clinical and Hematological Studies of Lymphosarcoma in a Herd of Cattle. AJVR, *22* (1961): 23–31.

Foot Rot

(**INFECTIOUS PODODERMATITIS; FOUL CLAW; FOUL-IN-THE FOOT**)

Foot rot, an acute or chronic infectious disease of cattle, is characterized by lameness from swelling and necrosis of the interdigital and coronary skin, and is caused, in part, by *Spherophorus necrophorus*. This disease, seldom fatal, causes economic loss by reducing body weight of fattened cattle, by requiring treatment, labor and drugs, and by delaying marketability.

Review of Literature. While foot rot has been recognized as a disease of cattle since the beginning of the twentieth century, it has recently, because of high incidence, assumed greater importance and in some regions has been rated as a disease of primary importance (Griner, 1964). Clinically, it has been studied extensively and a satisfactory means of treatment has been developed (Adams, 1960; Kingman and Stansbury, 1944). In addition, the pathologic changes for both the acute and chronic stages have been determined. The etiology, although studied intensively, has not been determined adequately. Many investigators have concurred in the opinion that S. *necrophorus* is present in the lesions and is responsible for most clinical signs and pathologic changes (Flint and Jensen, 1951; Kingman and Stansbury, 1951). Most investigators, however, share the view that probably S. *necrophorus* is a secondary invader and enters the tissue following some primary injury (Flint and Jensen, 1951; Roberts, 1946). Some observers have postulated that traumatic injury from impact with stones, frozen mud and penetrating foreign bodies constitute the primary lesion (Frank, 1959). Others, however, have noted that the disease may spread rapidly to as much as 90% of a pen of cattle under conditions which provide no opportunity for traumatism and, therefore, have postulated that the primary cause is a contagious agent, such as a virus, which has eluded identification (Griner, 1964). Most scientists have agreed that the bacteria invade the interdigital skin from the surface (Flint and Jensen, 1951; Greenough, 1962). Furthermore, the inoculation of viable S. *necrophorus* into the medial volar digital artery produced lesions unlike foot rot. The application of tissue from infected feet to scarified skin of normal feet, however, failed to produce the disease (Flint and Jensen, 1951; Gupta, Fincher and Bruner, 1964). The assumption that the lesions are points of entry for S. *necrophorus* to cause liver abscesses is erroneous. Also the similarity of foot rot to lesions caused by *Chorioptes bovis* has been pointed out (Monlux *et al.*, 1961).

Occurrence. Foot rot is responsible for 40 to 60% of all diseases of bovine feet. While the disease occurs in all types of adult cattle, both on the range and pasture and in confinement, epizootics occur in feedlot cattle, 1 to 2 years of age, with an incidence up to 90%. Sixty percent of the lesions are in hind feet. Both sexes and all breeds are susceptible. The disease, however, has not been transferred to other species of animals. While the disease may occur during all months, its incidence is higher from December through March. It exists geographically in all major cattle producing countries.

Foot rot of sheep is entirely distinct and unrelated to foot rot of cattle.

Etiology and Pathogenesis. The primary cause of epizootic foot rot is unknown. In the occasional or sporadic case, the primary cause may be a traumatic injury to the interdigital skin by impact with stones, frozen manure, metallic bodies or lacerating plant fibers, such as serrated grass leaves and awns. Regardless of their nature, the primary causes mechanically injure or devitalize the interdigital skin. In epizootic foot rot they appear to spread rapidly throughout cattle of a pen and to retain viability in the environment.

The secondary cause, S. *necrophorus*, is widely distributed in feedlot manure and soil, and consequently inhabits the skin surface of all bovine feet of both healthy and diseased cattle. In addition to foot rot, the organism is the secondary cause of calf diphtheria and liver abscesses. The organism has no ability to attack or penetrate healthy and intact skin or mucous membrane. However, it readily grows through injured skin and penetrates the derma and other non-covering tissues where it becomes pathogenic and causes extensive necrosis, a characteristic from which it acquired its specific name. Highly pleomorphic, S. *necrophous* in young active lesions and in new growing cultures is filamentous, non-branching, non-sporforming, granular, variable in width and gram-negative in staining, while in old lesions and in old cultures it becomes coccoid and rod-shaped. Although not easily cultured on artificial media, the organism grows under strictly anaerobic conditions on solid media, such as blood agar, and in liquid media, such as Roseneau's brain broth with a pH between 7.0 and 8.4. It produces acid and gas by fermenting glucose, maltose and glycerol, but does not ferment xylose, rhamnose, mannose, raffinose, inulin, dulcitol, dextrin, erythritol, sorbitol or inositol. The endotoxins probably contribute to the cause of tissue necrosis. Being highly susceptible to many adverse factors, the organism is killed in 15 minutes by temperature of 55° C, and it is easily killed by most standard disinfectants.

Whatever the primary causative agent of epizootic foot rot, it spreads rapidly among a susceptible pen of cattle. It causes injury, even though slight, to the interdigital skin and the skin adjacent to the coronary band. Omnipresent in manure, S. *necrophorus* penetrates the skin at points of injury. In the derma this bacterium is highly pathogenic. Multiplying rapidly, it causes necrosis and acute inflammation. In most cases the infection is limited to the soft tissues and after a course of 7 to 10 days, complete healing occurs. In a small number of animals, however, the infection spreads dorsally and laterally into one or both adjacent coffin joints. In this event the arthritis becomes chronic and endures for long periods. Exudate discharges through a sinus to the exterior and

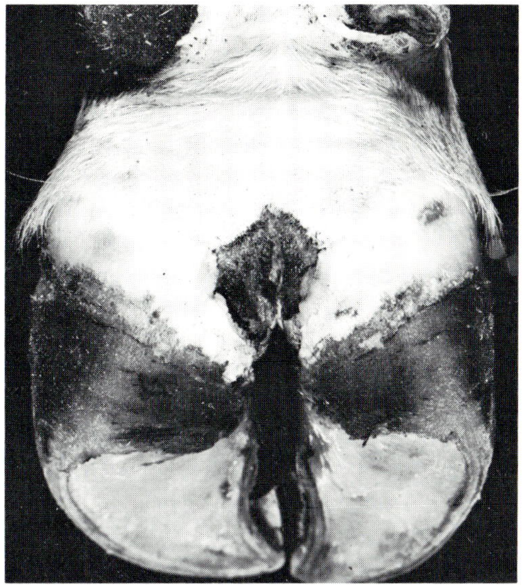

FIG. 8-48. *Posterior surface of a foot with acute foot rot. Necrosis extends from the interdigital skin onto the posterior surface.* × 0.7.

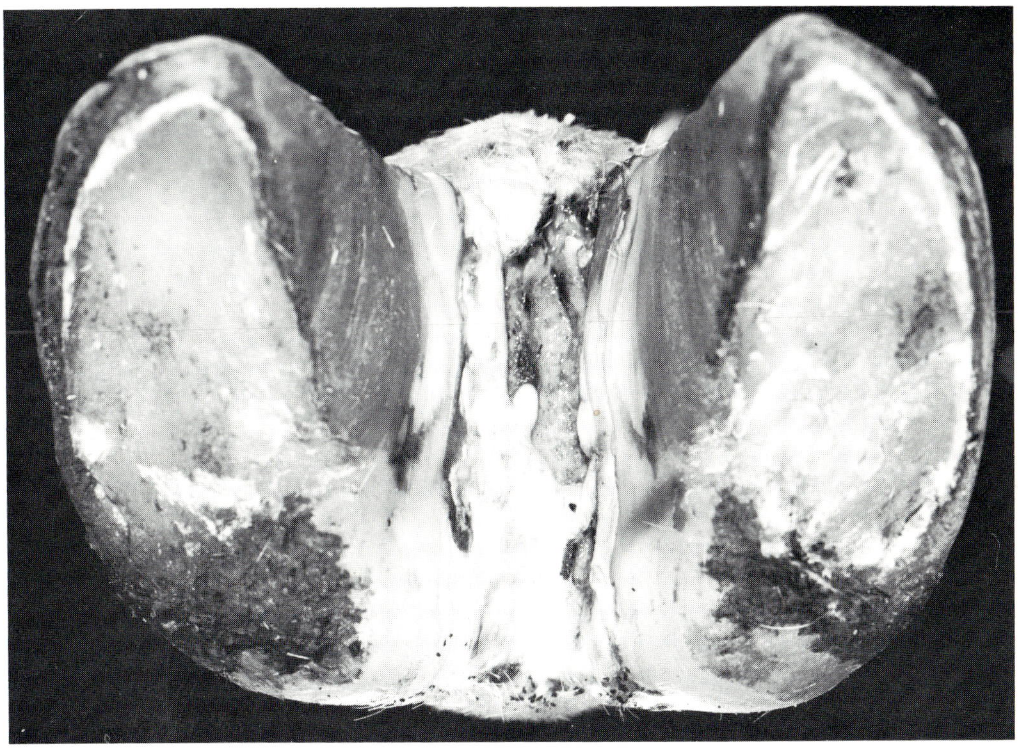

FIG. 8-49. *Interdigital tissue of a foot with acute foot rot. The skin is necrotic and ulcerated.* × 1.1.

granulation tissue may proliferate around the sinus. Healing eventually occurs by ankylosis of the infected joint. Much of the lameness results from increased pressure from swelling inside the hoof.

The acute infection rarely penetrates proximally, but when this happens a phlegmonous infection of the entire limb may occur. This complication, unless treated, may be fatal.

Postulations that liver abscesses are caused by S. *necrophorus* which enters the blood vascular system through such peripheral lesions as foot rot and calf diphtheria are not tenable. Organisms which enter the veins in lesions of foot rot are carried directly to the lungs where they may cause lung abscesses. Any organisms which filter through the lungs are carried over the systemic arterial system to all organs where abscesses may form. In general, cattle with abscessed liver do not concurrently contain abscesses of the lungs or other organs. Consequently, the bacteria causing liver abscesses must enter the liver through the portal blood after penetrating the wall of the alimentary tract.

Additional critical research to determine the primary cause of foot rot is needed. Until such information is available an effective means for prevention cannot be instituted.

Clinical Signs and Postmortem Lesions. Body temperature varies from normal to 105° F. Lameness develops suddenly and may affect multiple feet of one animal. Although most diseased feet are lame, some feet with little or no swelling may escape lameness. Non-pigmented skin of the interdigital space and coronary band is reddened. Swelling may extend dorsally as far as the fetlock joint. Close examination of the feet reveals moist necrosis of the involved skin and this lesion is often visible between the claws and at the posterior and anterior surfaces. In early stages the necrosis is superficial. In more advanced stages necrosis extends into the derma between the digits and often onto the digits around the coronary band on the anterior and posterior surfaces. Detachment of necrotic tissue may leave an ulcer. In chronic cases one digit may be enlarged and firm and contain a fistula which discharges exudate from the coffin joint to the surface of the interdigital space or near the coronary band. Palpation may reveal thickening of the second phalanx. Morbidity varies up to 90%; mortality of affected animals is low.

At necropsy or slaughter, feet in acute stages of foot rot exhibit necrosis, varying from superficial to deep, of the interdigital tissue. The necrotic tissue, firm and brown, is surrounded by acute inflammation and edema. In chronic stages, infected tissue extends into the coffin joint which contains exudate and often a fistulous tract. Exostosis may have developed around the infected joint. In animals recovered from chronic foot rot, the involved coffin joint cavity is occluded by cartilage. The transverse diameter of the second and third phalanges may be increased from exostosis.

When observed histopathologically, early acute stages manifest coagulative necrosis, extending for variable distances into the derma of the interdigital tissue, and also acute inflammation surrounding the necrosis. The dead tissue contains an abundance of filaments of S. *necrophorus* and often other species of bacteria.

Diagnosis. Foot rot is diagnosed clinically on the basis of typical signs and lesions. In epizootic foot rot, many animals become lame within a short period. Acute lameness with swelling involves single or multiple feet of a single animal. Interdigital skin is necrotic and swollen. Individual feet should be cleaned and examined carefully for lesions. Radiography is useful in diagnosing arthritis and exostosis of chronic foot rot.

Differential diagnosis requires consideration of traumatic injury, laminitis, interdigital papilloma and mycosis of the coronary skin. Trauma is common; the hoof is often lacerated or penetrated by foreign bodies, such as nails and wire. A careful examination of the lame foot should reveal the injury and often the cause. In case of laminitis the foot,

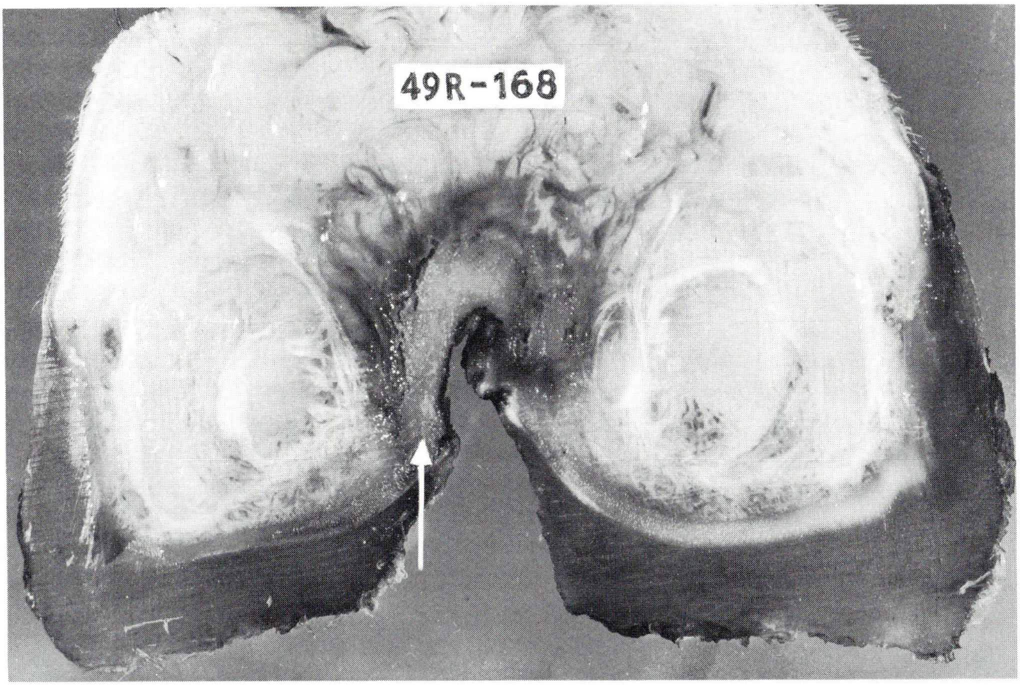

FIG. 8-50. *Frontal section of a foot with acute foot rot. The interdigital necrotic tissue is surrounded by inflammation and edema.* × 1.3.

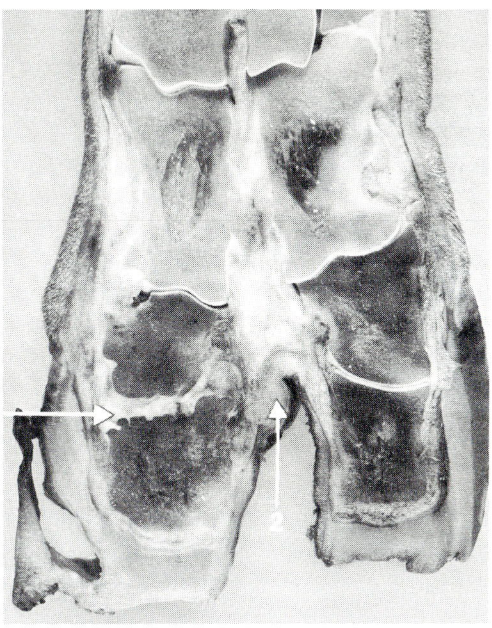

FIG. 8-51. *Frontal section of a foot following healing of chronic foot rot. The left coffin joint cavity is occluded. Exostosis has formed around the second and third phalanges.* × 0.8.

tender to pressure over the hoof walls and soles, does not contain the lesions of foot rot. Interdigital papilloma is a proliferative mass located between the digits. In mycotic dermatosis the skin at the coronary band becomes scaly, thickened and dry. These first three entities usually involve a single foot of a single animal and are distinguished from foot rot by the absence of necrosis of the interdigital skin.

Prevention and Treatment. The incidence of foot rot can be reduced in many cases by avoiding excessive moisture within the standing areas of the pens. Concrete standing pads at the feeders and around watering troughs provide drainage. Powdered lime placed along standing areas has been used to reduce infection. Objects capable of traumatizing the feet should be removed from the pens. Despite planned sanitation and careful management, a high rate of morbidity often occurs in outbreaks of the disease. While unproven in efficacy, organic iodide compounds have been used widely as prophylactic agents. They are mixed with salt in the proportion 1 part of iodide compound to 9 parts of salt and are offered continuously to the animals throughout the fattening period. Or, prevention has been achieved by continuously feeding the drug at a daily rate of 60 mg per animal for cattle weighing under 600 pounds and 120 mg per animal for cattle weighing over 600 pounds.

Treatment may be for individual animals or for entire lots. If the number of cattle affected is small, individuals are treated intravenously with (1) sulfamethazine or sulfathiazole at the rate of 1 grain per pound of body weight per day, or (2) oxytetracycline or chlortetracycline intravenously at the rate of 5 mg per pound of body weight per day. A combination of antibiotic and sulfonamide may be used. Frequently a single treatment is adequate. If the incidence of foot rot within a lot is high the entire group is treated by (1) medicating the feed with oxytetracycline or chlortetracycline at the daily rate of 1 mg per pound of body weight for 7 days, followed by one-half the dose for 7 days more, or (2) medicating the drinking water with sulfathiazole or sulfamethazine at the rate of 1 pound per 100 gallons of water for 2 to 3 days, followed by one-half the dose for an additional 2 to 3 days. Chronic lesions can be treated by curetting the infected tissue and applying tincture of iodine or medicated ointment.

References

Adams, O. R.: Foot Rot in Cattle. JAVMA, *136* (1960): 589–599.

Flint, J. C. and Jensen, Rue: Pathology of Necrobacillosis of the Bovine Foot. AJVR, *12* (1951): 5–13.

Frank, E. R.: *Veterinary Surgery*, 6th ed., Burgess Publishing Co., Minneapolis, (1959): 212–213.

Greenough, P. R.: Observations on Some of the Diseases of the Bovine Foot. Vet Record, *74* (1962): 1–9.

Griner, L. A.: Personal Communications. (1964).

Gupta, R. B., Fincher, M. G. and Bruner, D. W.: A Study of the Etiology of Foot Rot in Cattle. Cornell Vet., *54* (1964): 66–77.

Kingman, H. E. and Stansbury, W. M.: Treatment of Necrophorus Infections of Cattle with Sulfapyridine. North Am. Vet., *25* (1944): 671–674.

Kuznetsov, G. S.: *Hoof Diseases of Domestic Animals*. Governmental Publishing House for Agricultural Literature, Leningrad. (1957).

Monlux, W. S., Roun, E. S., Diesch, S. J. and Hunt, J. A.: Foot Rot and a Mucosaltype Disease. JAVMA, *138* (1961): 379–381.

Roberts, S. J.: Observations on Various Phases of Dairy Cattle Practice. North Am. Vet., *27* (1946): 284–287.

Smith, H. A. and Jones, T. C.: *Veterinary Pathology*, 3rd ed., Lea & Febiger, Philadelphia (1966).

High Mountain Disease

(BRISKET DISEASE; ALTITUDE DISEASE)

An insidious circulatory malady, high mountain disease is characterized by pulmonary arterial hypertension; by hypertrophy, dilitation and failure of the heart; and by generalized edema. It occurs in cattle residing at altitudes 5,000 feet or higher and is caused by prolonged breathing of hypoxic air. Although not a major bovine disease, the condition affects small numbers of cattle grazing mountain pastures and ranges but even fewer animals in feedlots of the high plains. Economic losses result from unthriftiness of clinical and subclinical cases, inefficient use of forage and concentrate feeds and deaths of severely affected cattle. The wide geographic distribution of the disease in mountainous regions where cattle production is a major industry results in considerable total loss to the industry.

Because people respond to residence at high altitude in a manner similar to the way cattle respond and because they are affected with a similar malady, referred to as Monge's disease, bovine high mountain disease has high scientific interest and has been investigated intensively during the second half of the twentieth century.

Review of Literature. According to the memories of ranchers, high mountain disease may have occurred in Colorado cattle as early as 1889. The first formal description, however, was in 1915 when researchers studying the disease concluded that affected animals suffer from cardiac hypertrophy, dilitation and failure; that the disease is caused by inadequate oxygen in high altitude air; and that the condition may be heritable (Glover and Newsom, 1915). Later the same disease was recognized and studied in cattle living in the high Andes Mountains of South America. Clinical signs and cardiac changes were similar to the disease in North America (Caparó, Capeira and de la Vega, 1955). Recognizing that heart changes were localized in the right ventricle, researchers postulated that atmospheric hypoxia causes pulmonary changes which increase resistance to circulation through the lungs and that the increased work leads to hypertrophy, dilitation and failure of the right ventricle (Pierson and Jensen, 1956).

With some recognition of cardiac involvement, researchers concentrated their studies on the heart. In one experiment 119 bovine hearts—41 from clinical cases of high mountain disease, 39 from normal cattle residing at high altitude and 39 from cattle residing at low altitude—were investigated. Each ventricle was dissected from the septum, and component parts were weighed separately. Weight ratios of right ventricle (RV)/total ventricular mass (T), left ventricle (LV)/total ventricular mass and septum/total ventricular mass were analyzed. The mean weight ratio of 0.435 for RV/T in diseased hearts significantly differed from the mean weight ratio of 0.251 for RV/T in normal hearts. The difference in measurements confirmed suspected hypertrophy of the right ventricle (Alexander and Jensen, 1959). In a more formally designed experiment, 20 Hereford cattle from a single source were randomly distributed in two lots. Animals of lot 1 were maintained at 5,000 feet altitude, and animals of lot 2 at 10,000 feet altitude, but both lots were fed the same diet. At four intervals during the 7-month experiment, pulmonary arterial pressures were measured on each animal, and at termination of the experiment all cattle were slaughtered. Mean weight ratio of 0.324 for RV/T in high altitude hearts was significantly higher than mean weight ratio of 0.243 for RV/T in low altitude hearts. Hypertrophy of the right ventricle was evident in all cases (Alexander, Will,

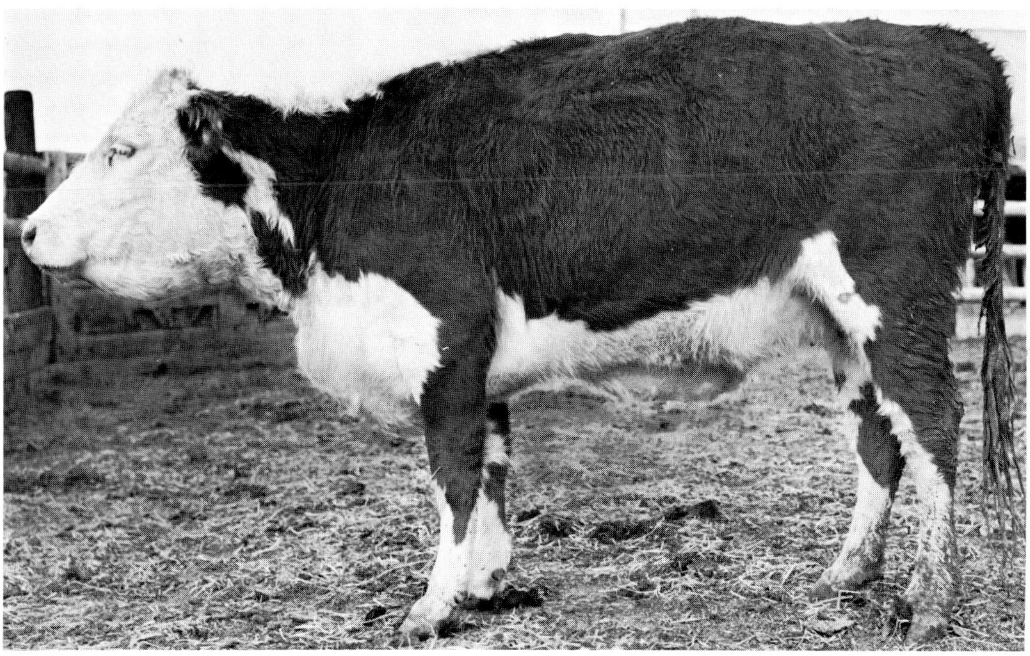

FIG. 8-52. *Animal with high mountain disease, showing diarrhea, and edema of intermandibular space, brisket and abdomen.*

Grover and Reeves, 1960). In order to determine histopathologic changes, the researchers measured the transverse diameters of 1,000 randomly selected cardiac cells from the ventricles of both diseased and normal hearts. Statistical analyses indicated that cells of the right ventricle of diseased hearts are significantly larger than cells of the right ventricle of normal hearts (Sera and Jensen, 1950). The effects of altitude on hearts of other species were also determined. When hearts of 59 guinea pigs raised at an altitude of 14,900 feet were weighed and compared with hearts of 83 guinea pigs raised at sea level, the high altitude hearts were significantly heavier (Tappan and Reynafarje, 1956). Among people acclimatized to altitude of 13,000 feet, 8 of 30 autopsies contained hearts having hypertrophy of the right ventricle (Castrode and Iglesias, 1956). Radio-

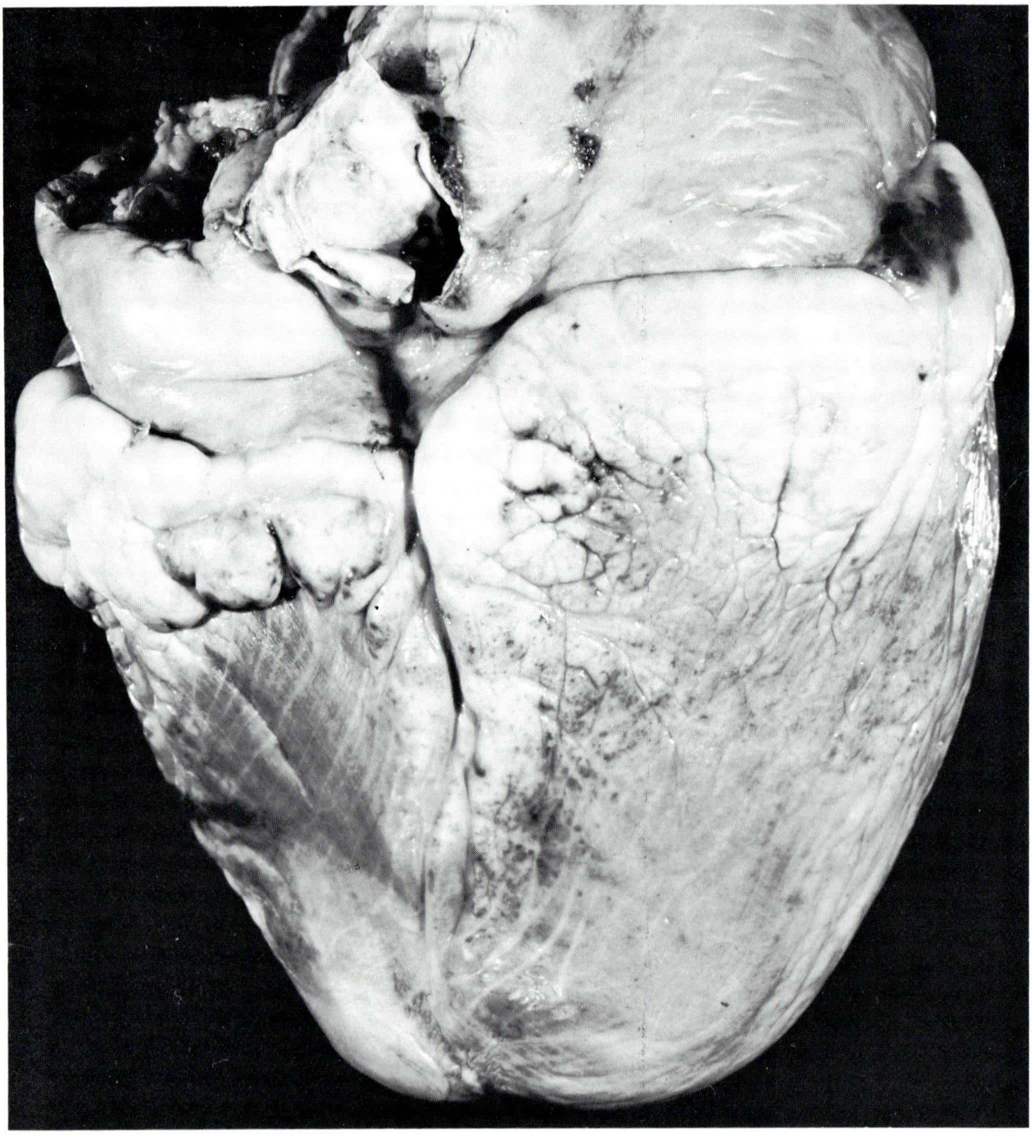

FIG. 8-53. *Dilated and hypertrophied right ventricle of heart from an heifer affected with high mountain disease.* × 1.0.

graphs on 400 people living at altitude of 14,700 feet evinced 69% with enlarged hearts, and of these 67% had prominence of the right ventricle (Rotta, 1947).

Physiologic studies have been highly productive in understanding high mountain disease. When cats were used experimentally, the anaethetized animals breathed 10 to 11% oxygen in nitrogen, and this hypoxic mixture of gases invariably caused immediate increase in the mean pulmonary arterial pressure of the experimental animals (Euler and Liljestrand, 1946). In one study, actual clinical cases of bovine high mountain disease were moved from the range to the laboratory. In the experimental animals, the mean pulmonary arterial pressures were higher than those in normal cattle (Hecht *et al.*, 1959). In an experiment referred to above, 10 Hereford cattle were maintained at altitude of 5,000 feet and 10 at 10,000 feet. Both groups received the same diet throughout the 7 months of experimentation. The mean pulmonary arterial pressure was measured on each animal at beginning and termination, and at two intermediate intervals. The beginning pressures were similar in both lots and averaged 27 mm Hg. At termination of the experiment, the low altitude cattle had average pressure values of 27 ± 4.4 mm Hg, while the cattle at high altitude had average pressure values of 63 ± 29 mm Hg. Animals having the 3 high pressures developed clinical signs of the disease. Weight ratios of right ventricle/total had a positive correlation to mean pulmonary arterial pressure (Alexander, Will, Grover and Reeves, 1960). In general, researchers have agreed that humans and all other species of mammals develop pulmonary arterial hypertension from breathing hypoxic air (Aviado, 1960).

To seek reasons for pulmonary arterial hypertension, the pulmonary vessels of both normal and diseased cattle were studied. Among 24 cattle with clinical high mountain disease, hypertrophy of the medial muscle of muscular arteries and arterioles was a common change. Other lesions included proliferation of the tunica adventitia, intimal

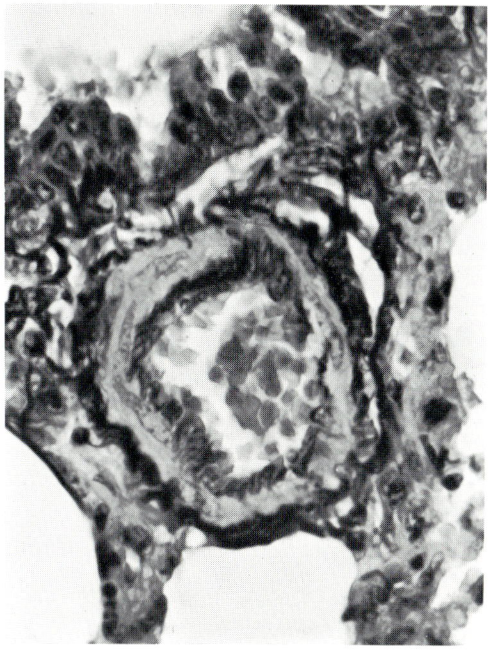

FIG. 8-54. *Arteriole in terminal bronchiole of normal steer. Verhoff Van Giesson stain.* × 620.

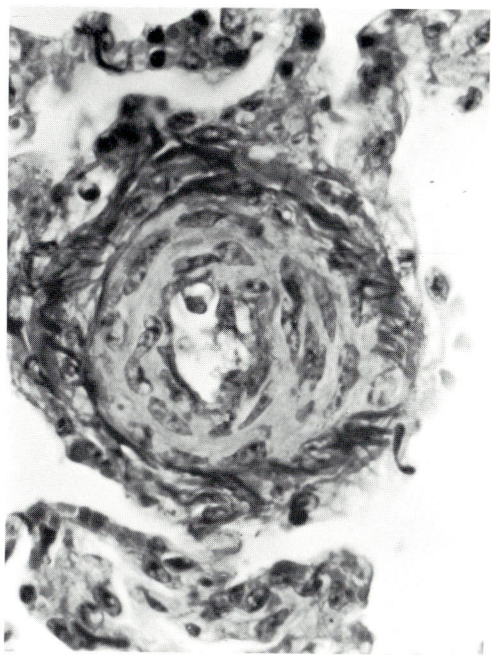

FIG. 8-55. *Arteriole in terminal bronchiole of steer with high mountain disease, showing medial muscular hypertrophy. Verhoff Van Giesson stain.* × 620.

elastosis and fibrosis, and thrombosis (Alexander and Jensen, 1963; 1963a).

In a study to determine the possible inheritance of susceptibility to high mountain disease, two groups of cattle, one susceptible and the other resistant, were assembled. All animals, both male and female, in the susceptible group had resided at high altitude, had developed the disease and recovered when they were relocated at low altitude. Members of the resistant group, both male and female, were healthy animals selected from a herd residing at 9,000 feet altitude. The pulmonary arterial pressure was measured for a large number of cattle, and those individuals having average pressures of 27 mm Hg were selected for the group. The two groups were bred separately, and the resulting calves were used experimentally. Eleven resistant calves and 9 susceptible calves were relocated to altitude 10,000 feet. After 30 days the mean pulmonary arterial pressure for the resistant calves was 29 ± 2 mm Hg and the susceptible group 54 ± 4. These data suggested strong possibilities for some heritability (Alexander and Will, 1969).

Occurrence. High mountain disease occurs in all sexes and breeds, but not uniformly. Beef breeds, especially Herefords and Angus, are the common types used to graze high altitude ranges and pastures. According to producer records some families among the Hereford and Angus breeds have a higher than normal incidence, and some producers have shown genetic relationship between many animals developing the disease. Among animals transported from low altitude to high altitude for grazing, or fattening, the incidence is higher than among those indigenous to high altitude. The overall incidence among all cattle residing at altitudes of 5,000 feet or higher varies from 0.5 to 2%.

Cattle 6 months to 2 years of age suffer the highest incidence. During these ages the most susceptible animals develop the disease and are removed from herds. The natural selection leaves older groups with higher mean resistance.

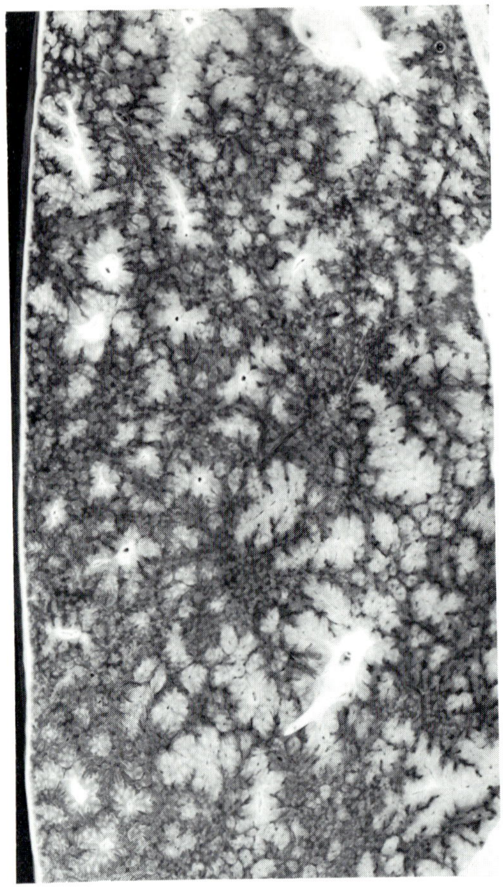

FIG. 8-56. *Cut surface of liver from a steer affected with high mountain disease. The dark network is reticulofibrous tissue filled with blood.* × 0.7.

Most cases of clinical high mountain disease are encountered during late summer and autumn months. New cases are often observed following a storm in which ambient temperatures reach below average seasonal levels.

Geographically, high mountain disease develops wherever cattle are maintained for any purpose at altitudes of 5,000 feet or higher. The Rocky Mountains of Colorado, New Mexico, Montana, Utah and Wyoming and the mountainous parts of western Canada of North America and western countries of South America are common locations of the disease. Cases have also been found on cattle ranges of Mount Kenya.

Many species of domestic animals appear to be resistant to high mountain disease but people show susceptibility to a similar condition.

Etiology and Pathogenesis. The fundamental cause of high mountain disease is prolonged breathing of hypoxic air by genetically susceptible cattle. The potency of hypoxia, as a disease producing situation, varies directly with altitude from 5,000 to 10,000 feet and higher. After 4 to 6 weeks residence at altitude of 10,000 feet Hereford cattle develop a statistically significant increase in mean pulmonary arterial pressure. After a few months cases of clinical disease may form. Under experimental conditions, the hypoxia produced in an hypobaric chamber and produced by dilution of air with nitrogen results in the same physiopathologic effects.

Secondary causes enhancing the effects of hypoxia are numerous. Lung conditions, such as bacterial pneumonia, verminous pneumonia from *Dictyocaulus viviparus* and alveolar emphysema, increase resistance to circulation. Sudden climatic storms with meteorologic reduction of atmospheric pressure and the lowering of ambient air temperature seems to constrict pulmonary vessels and produce new cases of disease. Factors requiring greater cardiac output, such as the performance of physical work from walking, running and struggling, may also contribute to the total cause.

Although some important aspects in the pathogenesis are not understood, many factors are known. Prolonged breathing of hypoxic air by genetically susceptible cattle stimulates continuous, or possibly repeated episodes of, contraction of the media of muscular arteries and arterioles in the pulmonary lobules. The exact mechanism of this action is not known, but it may be through chemical receptors. Contractions of the medial muscle appears to eventually result in hypertrophy. Subsequently, the intima of some vessels thickens, mineralizes, and in some cases, thromboses. These vascular changes, separately and in combinations, reduce the diameters of vessel lumens and markedly increase the resistance to circulation through the lungs.

Responding reflexly, the right ventricle, attempting to maintain adequate circulation through the lungs, performs more work. Myocardial cells hypertrophy, the ventricular mass enlarges and the ventricular cavity expands. As a result of hypertrophy the heart may be fully able to perform the new work load; if so, the ventricle has compensated for the resistance to pulmonary circulation and no clinical signs of disease form. If, however, resistance to pulmonary flow is excessive, the right ventricle, even after hypertrophy, may not be able to sustain the amount of work required for circulation; in this event, cardiac decompensation or failure gradually develops. Passive congestion becomes generalized. Tissue hypoxia develops. Increased permeability to plasma proteins in the capillary walls and enhanced venous capillary pressure cause fluids to pass as edema from plasma into body cavities and tissues. In the liver, congestion and hypoxia around central veins of lobules cause central zonal necrosis and replacement of hepatic cells with reticular and collagenous fibers. In fatal cases death results from circulatory failure.

During early stages of the disease, quiet relocation of affected animals to low altitude frequently results in recovery. The greater partial pressure of oxygen relaxes pulmonary vessels which reduces work required of the right ventricle, and recovery occurs. Return to the higher altitude, however, usually causes recurrence of the disease.

Clinical Signs and Postmortem Lesions. Developing insidiously among affected animals, cases of high mountain disease present clinical signs of congestive heart failure. Unthriftiness and depression develop early. Gains in body weight are slow and may be replaced by losses. As the disease progresses, the pectoral region enlarges from subcutaneous edema which rapidly advances anteriorly along the ventral part of the neck into the intermandibular space and posteriorly along the ventral abdominal wall. Jugular veins distend and may present distinct cardiac pulsations. The abdomen enlarges because of the accumulation of ascitic fluid. Hydrothorax diminishes lung sounds and, along with hydropericardium, obscures heart sounds. Although usually normal, body temperatures may fluctuate upward from infectious complications, such as pneumonia and enteritis. As edema extends into the alimentary tract profuse diarrhea with dark-colored feces develops. Affected cattle fatigue easily from forced exertion and have difficult and oral breathing. Elbows may be abducted to facilitate breathing. Visible mucous membranes may be cyanotic. Hemograms may indicate from 10 to 15% increase in number of erythrocytes. Catheterization of the heart reveals an increase in mean pulmonary arterial pressure from normal values of 25 to 30 mm Hg to 80 to 100 or more mm Hg. Relocation of cases to significantly lower altitudes often results in clinical improvement or recovery. The clinical course varies from 1 to 12 weeks.

Although the primary pathologic changes are in the lungs, these organs often contain no gross lesions. Occasionally, however, cases of high mountain disease contain factors which contribute causally to the disease; these include chronic alveolar emphysema, broncopneumonia, and verminous pneumonia in adult cattle, and thrombosis of branches of the pulmonary artery and bronchopneumonia in cattle up to 6 months of age. With cardiac enlargement of the right ventricle, the apex may be dextrotranslocated, and the entire organ may be rounded. Dissection indicates dilitation and hypertrophy of the right ventricular wall, moderator bands and chordae tendinae. As a result the right AV valves may be insufficient. The weight ratio of right ventricle/total ventricular mass may be changed from normal value of 0.251 ± 0.01 and a range of 0.214 to 0.284 to 0.435 ± 0.087 and a range of 0.308 to 0.554. The pulmonary artery and venae cavae are distended. With generalized edema, subcutaneous tissues along the ventral part of the neck and abdomen, intermuscular connective tissue and the mesentary are heavily edematous. Hydrothorax, ascites and hydropericardium are prominent. Along the alimentary tract, edema is severe. Abomasal plicae, the submucosa of the abomasum and intestines, and the mestenteric attachments are thickened from edematous fluid. Hemorrhaging ulcers may be present, especially in the abomasum. Enlarged, firm and cyanotic, the conspicuous liver changes often attract unwarranted attention.

Histopathologic changes are both primary to the disease cause and secondary to passive congestion. In the lungs primary changes are in the muscular arteries and arterioles. In these vessels obvious thickening of the medial muscle appears to be hypertrophy, but the thickening may result in part from fixation in a state of contraction. In addition some vessels contain elastosis, fibroelastosis, mineralization and thrombosis of the intima. Thickening of the adventitia occurs around many arteries. Changes secondary to pulmonary lesions are generalized. Myocardium of the right ventricle, and to some extent the septum, is hypertrophied. Cells and fibers of connective tissue, especially of the subcutis and submucosae, are spatially separated by fluid. Veins are congested throughout dependent tissues. In the liver lobules hepatic veins and sinusoids of the central zone of lobules are distended with blood. In advanced cases of the disease, hepatic cells of the central zone have been replaced with collapsed normal reticular fibers and proliferated collagenous fibers. Circulating blood filters through the connective tissue mesh.

Diagnosis. High mountain disease can be diagnosed on clinical evidence of congestive failure of the right ventricle in cattle residing at altitude of 5,000 feet and higher. Subcutaneous edema along the ventral part of the neck, thorax and abdomen, distension and pulsation of the jugular veins and eventual diarrhea are indicative signs. Mean pulmonary arterial pressure of 80 mm Hg, or higher, as determined by catheterization, is especially important. At necropsy, a weight ratio of right ventricle/total ventricular mass of 0.308 to 0.554, in the absence of other causes, and medial muscular hypertrophy, intimal sclerosis, and adventiatial proliferation of pulmonary muscular arteries and arterioles provide diagnostic confirmation.

Pulmonary factors adding to the primary cause may be present. These conditions include verminous pneumonia, bacterial bronchopneumonia and pericardial adhesions. The parasitism can be determined by finding characteristic embryonated eggs of *Dictyocaulus vivipara* in feces. Bronchopneumonia and pericardial adhesions and chronic alveolar emphysema can be detected through skillful auscultation of the thorax.

The differential diagnosis requires consideration of compressive neoplasms in, or near, the heart, cardiac developmental anomalies and myocardial infections. Metastatic neoplasms, such as lymphosarcoma, may compress the pulmonary artery or the right ventricle and produce signs of right ventricular failure. The primary neoplasm may be detected and identified in more accessible locations such as peripheral lymph nodes. Developmental anomalies may produce characteristic bruits. Abscesses in the septum or right ventricular wall and traumatic pericarditis may evoke fever and leukocytosis. Traumatic pericarditis results from penetration by nails or pieces of wire from the lumen of the reticulum through the wall of the reticulum and the diaphragm into the pericardial sac. Species of bacteria, mechanically carried by the metallic body, cause infection throughout the sac. Fibrinous exudate accumulates on the serous surfaces and fluid exudate and gas form in the sac. In prolonged cases, adhesions between pericardium and epicardium may form and impose extra work on the heart. Affected cattle are anorexic and constipated.

Prevention and Treatment. Whenever possible, the pedigrees of cases of high mountain disease should be determined. Within some herds one or few bulls may sire most cases of the disease; if so, elimination of the sire may reduce the number of disease cases. Although the possibility of breeding disease resistant cattle appears possible, more research is required before this practice can be recommended.

Treatment of high mountain disease should be directed towards three fundamental considerations: (1) decreasing the load on the heart, (2) increasing cardiac efficiency, and (3) eliminating fluids. An effective and economic procedure is to transport, with minimal animal exertion, affected animals to significantly lower altitude. Approximately 50% of cases respond to this practice. Exertive restraint should be avoided. As soon as restraint can be tolerated, treatment with parenteral digitalis and supportive oxygen is beneficial. Recovered animals should be fattened and marketed without return to higher altitude.

References

Alexander, A. F. and Jensen, Rue: Gross Cardiac Changes in Cattle with High Mountain (Brisket) Disease and in Experimental Cattle Maintained at High Altitudes. AJVR, *20* (1959): 680–689.

———: Pulmonary Vascular Pathology of Bovine High Mountain Disease: AJVR, *24* (1963): 1098–1111.

———: Pulmonary Vascular Pathology of High Altitude-Induced Pulmonary Hypertension in Cattle. AJVR, *24* (1963a): 1112–1122.

Alexander, A. F., Will, D. H., Grover, R. F. and Reeves, J. T.: Pulmonary Hypertension and Right Ventricular Hypertrophy in Cattle at High Altitude. AJVR, *21* (1960): 199–204.

Alexander, A. F. and Will, D. H.: Progress Report, Genetic Aspects of High Altitude Adaptation in Cattle. U. S. Public Health Service. Nat. Inst. of Health (1969).

Aviado, D. M.: The Pharmacology of the Pulmonary Circulation. Pharm. Rev., *12* (1960): 159–239.

Caparó, A. C., Capeira, M. and de la Vega, E.: Mal de Montana Cronico en Vacunos. Anales de la Facultad de Medicina, 38: No. 2, Second Trimester, 1–10, 1955.

Castro, J. C. de and Iglesias, B.: Preliminary Report on Anatomic Studies at High Altitudes, U. S. Dept. of the Air Force, School of Aviation Medicine, Report No. 55-97, 1956, p 6.

Euler, U. S. von and Liljestrand, G.: Observations on the Pulmonary Arterial Blood Pressure in the Cat. Acta Physiologica Scandinavica, *12* (1946): 301–320.

Glover, G. H. and Newson, I. E.: Brisket Disease. Colo. Ag. Exp. Station Bulletin 204, January 1915.

Hecht, H. H., Lange, R. L., Carnes, W. H., Kuida, H. and Blake, J. T.: Brisket Disease. I. General Aspects of Pulmonary Hypertensive Heart Disease in Cattle. Trans. Assoc. Am. Physicians, 72 (1959): 157–172.

Pierson, R. E. and Jensen, Rue: Brisket Disease in: *Diseases of Cattle. A Textbook and Reference Work.* Evanston, Ill. Am. Vet. Publications, 1956, p. 717–723.

Rotta, A.: Physiologic Condition of the Heart in Natives of High Altitudes. Am. Heart J., 33 (1947): 669–676.

Sera, R. and Jensen, Rue: Unpublished Data, Colorado State University, 1950.

Tappon, D. V. and Reynafarje, B.: Tissue Pigment Studies in Altitude Adaptation. U. S. Dept. of the Air Force, School of Aviation Medicine, Report No. 56-97, 1956.

Vitamin A Deficiency

(AVITAMINOSIS-A; NIGHT BLINDNESS)

A chronic and insidious disease, vitamin A deficiency is characterized by unthriftiness, night blindness, diarrhea, edema and convulsions, and its nutritional cause is an inadequate supply of metabolizable vitamin A. Occurring at both subclinical and clinical stages, vitamin A deficiency is most often found in cattle raised in the arid western states where low rainfall limits the availability of green carotene-rich forage and where cattle are maintained in feedlots for 6 or more months. In feedlot cattle subclinical vitamin A deficiency, although unmeasured, probably is common and results in significant monetary losses to the feedlot industry. Economic losses rise from decreased feed consumption, low rates of live weight gain, low efficiency in feed utilization, prolonged feeding periods, increased susceptibility to infectious disease and condemnation of carcasses at slaughter.

Review of Literature. The occurrence of vitamin A deficiency has been observed and studied in the United States (Huber and Smith, 1963) and in England (Abrams *et al.*, 1961) where the signs and lesions of the disease were similar for both dairy and beef types of cattle. Broad sequential studies, from the research conducted in the United States, on requirements of feedlot cattle for vitamin A, have resulted in recommendations for increasing amounts (Committee on Animal Nutrition. National Research Council, 1958; Ibid., 1963).

The levels of vitamin A and carotene in plasma and liver vary with the rate of intake. On average Montana pasture, the plasma of normal 1- and 2-year-old beef cattle contained an average of 93 to 100 IU of vitamin A per 100 ml and only slight monthly variations were noted. The mean carotene levels ranged, however, from 223 to 252 micrograms per 100 ml of plasma and the monthly variance was high; March contained the lowest and May and June, the highest levels. As determined by tissue biopsies, the livers of normal cattle contained 83 to 168 IU of vitamin A per gram of fresh tissue. For calves, heifers and steers, plasma levels of vitamin A below 33 IU per 100 ml and liver content less than 33 IU per gram of fresh tissue were considered dangerously low (Huber and Smith, 1963; Jungherr, Helmboldt and Eaton, 1949; Pope, Baker and Macvicar, 1961).

In feedlot cattle the dynamics of liver-stored vitamin A and ingested carotene have also been studied. In research conducted at Colorado State University, 120 Hereford steers, transferred from pasture to the feedlot, were assigned to 5 equal lots. The animals of lot 1 were slaughtered at 0 days on feed and the other lots at 40-day intervals. All lots were fed the same ration consisting of alfalfa, corn silage, corn, bran and cotton seed meal. The diet provided for each animal an average daily consumption of carotene as follows: First 40-day period 469,000 mcg; second 40-day period 317,000 mcg; third 40-day period 237,000 mcg; and the fourth 40-day period 205,000 mcg. At the time of slaughter, the average content of vitamin A per gm of liver was as follows: At 0 days on feed 171 IU; at end of first 40 days 79 IU; at end of 80 days 40 IU; at end of 120 days 18 IU; and at the end of 160 days 6 IU. At the end of each 40-day period the average hepatic store per animal had been reduced by approximately 45% from the end of the previous 40-day period (Frey and Jensen, 1946; 1947).

For some conditions, the instability of vitamin A and carotene has been determined, and researchers know that the movement of these substances through the fore stomachs of cattle has caused the destruction of considerable amounts. Incubation for 9 hours of vitamin A and carotene in ruminal fluids caused a reduction of 35% of the carotene and 40% of vitamin (King, Lohman and Smith, 1962). Dietary nitrates consumed with vitamin A and carotene also resulted in destruction. In experimental rats, the inclusion of nitrite in their diet caused rapid depletion of both vitamin A and vitamin E (O'Dell, Erek, Flynn, Garner and Munrer, 1960). Abnormally high concentration of both nitrites and nitrates in forage from heavy soil fertilization and drought has been suspected as a contributor to vitamin A deficiency. The manner by which animals develop the deficiency is unknown, but the nitrates may have caused less active isomers in the plant, in the alimentary tracts (Huber and Smith, 1963) or in the wall of the small intestine (Thompson, Ganguly and Kon, 1949).

In cattle clinical signs and pathologic changes from vitamin A deficiency have been described for both naturally occurring and experimentally induced disease. In an early report (1935) night blindness in calves was ascribed to atrophy of the optic nerves at the points where they traversed the foramina. In 24 natural cases, the atrophy was assumed to be caused by compression from constriction of deformed bone (Moore, Huffman and Duncan, 1935). A similar interpretation of the cause of optic nerve atrophy resulted from studying the natural disease on three English farms (Abrams, Bridge, Palmer and Spratling, 1961). In a controlled experiment, however, dimensions of the optic foramina of affected cattle were not significantly different from those in normal control cattle. In this experiment, the optic nerve atrophy appeared to result from twisting of the nerve near the foramina, from an increase in cerebrospinal fluid pressure, and from some malformation of the foramina (Blackmore, Ottany, Sellers, Eden and Moore, 1957). Edema of the optic disc and bleaching of the tapetum lucidum, as observed with the ophthalmoscope, were early signs of impaired vision (Huber and Smith, 1963).

In studies using rats as experimental animals rather than cattle, hepatic vitamin A depletion resulted in a series of retinal changes. First, the blood level diminished to near zero. Then rhodopsin, a compound in the pigmented epithelium, declined; this alteration initiated night blindness. Finally, both opsin and rhodopsin were lost and the rods deteriorated. The administration of vitamin A during the depleting process reversed the changes (Dowling and Wald, 1958). In young experimental rats, vitamin A deficiency interfered with endochondral growth of bones and resulted in long bones becoming short and thick and in vertebral and cephalic bones becoming disproportionately heavy (Wolbach, 1947). Whether or not these findings about the relationship of rats to vitamin A deficiency can be assumed for beef cattle is conjectural, but the probability of similarity is high.

Occurrence. In feedlot animals subclinical or clinical vitamin A deficiency is found in: (1) cattle entering fattening pens soon after weaning and fed for 6 to 12 months or longer for show exhibition or market on a diet low in carotene; (2) cattle 1 to 2 years of age entering the feedlot after a summer of drought, having low stores of vitamin A in the liver, and being fattened on a diet low in carotene; and (3) cattle raised and fattened on feed with a high content of nitrate from heavy soil fertilization or from drought stunting. Usually the deficiency develops during winter and early spring months when access to fresh carotene containing feed is most remote. All ages, breeds, and sexes are susceptible. In the United States cattle raised in the arid western and southwestern states are most commonly affected. Animals of other arid countries also develop the disease. Cattle fattening on a high concentrate diet appear to require a greater than normal intake of vitamin A and with a daily supply of 20,000 to 40,000 IU per animal may show deficiency when feeding continues beyond 120 days.

Etiology. Vitamin A deficiency is caused by inadequate intake of vitamin A from the alimentary system prior to and during fattening. Deficiency results from low hepatic stores in animals entering the feedlot, from consumption of diets low in carotene and/or from destruction or interference to absorption by nitrites and other possible anitmetabolites. The requirements of feedlot cattle of various ages and sizes for vitamin A are presented in Table 30. In determining the needed vitamin A intake in the diet, consideration should be given to the probable hepatic stores acquired from pre-feedlot grazing. The requirements can be supplied from carotene, vitamin A, or a combination of both. The requirements for vitamin A vary somewhat among individual animals. In general, however, needs are enhanced by nitrates in feed and water, inadequate dietary protein and phosphorus, thyroid hyperfunction, diethylstilbestrol administration, high concentrate ration and high ambient temperature.

Pathogenesis. Components of the bovine diets contain variable amounts of carotene, and animals inefficiently convert the ingested carotene to usable vitamin A. While moving through the fore stomachs 40 to 80% of orally administered vitamin A is destroyed; this loss may result from microbial and nitrate action on the unstable vitamin A. In the wall of the small intestine carotene is converted to vitamin A alcohol, absorbed, changed to ester form as a protein complex and transported through the lymph and blood. Surpluses beyond immediate metabolic needs are stored in the liver, and depending on the amount of absorbed vitamin A, the hepatic store is constant, elevated or diminished. A constant and critical blood level is maintained by varying the hepatic store.

Prolonged inadequate absorption of vitamin A results in a sequence of predictable changes in cattle. At first the hepatic vitamin A is withdrawn to maintain normal blood level of 100 to 150 IU per 100 ml of plasma.

TABLE 30 ***Recommended amounts of vitamin A for feedlot cattle***

Type of Animal	Animal Weight lb	daily intake/animal* Carotene mg	or	Vitamin A IU
Calves	400	75		30,000
finishing	600	78		35,000
as short	800	100		40,000
yearlings	1,000	125		50,000
Finishing yearlings	600 to 1,100	125		50,000
Finishing 2-yr. olds	800 to 1,200	125		50,000

* In addition each animal may be given 0.5 to 1 million IU of injectable vitamin A.

When the liver becomes depleted the blood level also diminishes, and tissue demands for vitamin A are not satisfied. As plasma vitamin A lowers to 40 to 50 IU per 100 ml, clinical signs of deficiency begin to develop. In the retina, rhodopsin, a red pigment containing vitamin A aldehyde, diminishes and night blindness begins. Further loss of rhodopsin causes deterioration of the outer segments of the rods of the outer nuclear layer. Early correction of the deficiency reverses the ocular changes.

From vitamin A deficiency, other changes also occur. Because of the accelerated rate of secretion or from a decelerated rate of absorption, the pressure of the cerebrospinal fluid augments. Higher pressure on the central nervous tissue results in nervousness, incoordinated movements and convulsions of increasing frequency. In addition, edema of the limbs, brisket and abdomen forms. Advanced and extreme cases develop generalized edema, a condition referred to as anasarca, but the mechanism for the fluid accumulation has not been elucidated.

Besides the symptoms and lesions of vitamin A deficiency in adult animals, additional adversities affect growing cattle. In calves interference to endochondral bone growth at epiphyses results in heavy shortened bones with skeletal crowding of parts of the central nervous system. In calves and young adults epithelial cells of the conjunctivae excessively keratinize, and epithelial cells of the parotid salivary duct and of the uterine glands undergo metaplasia to stratified squamous cell types. These combined changes increase susceptibility of affected animals to infectious diseases such as pneumonia, metritis, cystitis and conjunctivitis.

Clinical Signs and Postmortem Lesions. Evidences of deficiency vary with disease development and with individual cattle. During early stages animal appetites wane, food intake diminishes, hair coats roughen and rates of gain in body weight reduce. Night blindness develops and is evident during dusk and dawn, when the animals collide with objects in unfamiliar locations. Ophthalmoscopic examination reveals papilledema and bleaching of the tapetum lucidum. In more advanced stages, exophthalmia, excessive lacrymation, mild corneal opacities and permanent blindness are apparent. Subcutaneous edema of the limbs and profuse diarrhea are intermittent but with progressively longer periods in evidence. Prostrative convulsions, each of several minutes duration and often provoked by excitement and forced movements, become progressively frequent and are accompanied by weak, incoordinated and staggering movements. Pressure of the cerebrospinal fluid is usually above 100 mm of aqueous saline solution. Cattle suspected of vitamin A deficiency usually present herd histories of origin from areas of summer drought and of fattening on a diet obviously low in carotene, or one of components stored for more than 1 year. Chemical analysis reveals a low level of carotene in the diet and less than 50 IU of vitamin A per 100 ml of plasma. While the number of herds with subclinical or borderline deficiency may be high, the incidence of advanced deficiency is low. Within an affected herd different

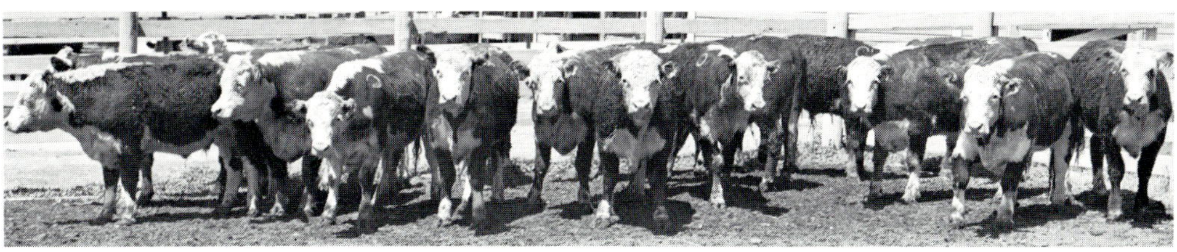

FIG. 8-57. *Vitamin A deficient steers showing roughened coats, diarrhea, exophthalmia, and limb edema. Convulsions were repetitive in some animals.*

animals may show different signs and only uncommonly does any one animal present all disease signs. The mortality rate resulting directly from the deficiency is low but may be elevated from predisposition to intercurrent infections.

At necropsy, few additional lesions are discernible, excepting those from possible intercurrent infections as pneumonia. The orbital portion of the optic nerves are tortuous and, near the optic foramina, atrophic. While some investigations indicated an association of urolithiasis with vitamin A deficiency, the causal relationship is in doubt.

Histopathologic studies disclose changes in some epithelial structures. The conjuntival epithelium is excessively cornified and epithelium of the uterine glands and excretory ducts of the parotid salivary gland may show degrees of metaplasia from cuboidal and columnar cells to stratified squamous types.

Diagnosis. The clinical identification of borderline vitamin A deficiency is difficult and seldom achieved. Overt clinical deficiency, however, is based on the presence of typical signs in cattle with plausible herd histories. Signs of crucial importance are: ocular papilledema and conjunctival epithelial cell cornification, both discernible in early stages; for the herd, unthriftiness and low rates of gain in body weight; for individual cattle, night blindness, diarrhea, convulsions and limb edema. Confirmation of the diagnosis can be obtained by finding less than 50 IU of vitamin A per 100 ml of plasma and less than 30 IU per gram of fresh liver by biopsy or at necropsy. Often the plasma level remains normal until the hepatic supply is depleted.

The differential diagnosis requires consideration of infectious keratoconjunctivitis and cardiac circulatory disturbances. While pinkeye may have a high case incidence within a herd, as does vitamin A deficiency, keratojunctivitis causes deep corneal ulceration and is not accompanied by the nervous signs of vitamin A deficiency. Cardiac infections of the right side and some congential anomalies result in generalized passive congestion and edema of the neck and brisket. These single cases in a herd are not accompanied by other signs of vitamin A deficiency. Plasma and hepatic levels of vitamin A can be measured and used for establishing a definitive diagnosis.

TABLE 31 *Vitamin A equivalent in feedstuffs*

Feedstuff	*Vitamin A Equivalent 1000's IU/lb.*
Alfalfa hay, pre-bloom	337
Alfalfa hay, early bloom	86
Alfalfa hay, mid bloom	22
Alfalfa hay, late bloom	25
Alfalfa hay, past bloom	19
Alfalfa leaves meal, dehyd.	112
Alfalfa silage	20
Alfalfa meal, dehyd.	56
Barley grain	trace
Beet pulp with molasses, dried	trace
Beet sugar top, silage	7
Clover, alsike, hay	124
Clover, ladino, hay	111
Corn cannery waste, silage	3
Corn dent silage, dough stage	7
Corn yellow dent, gr 2	1
Fescue, meadow hay	47
Grass-legume unsp. silage	50
Grass-legume, silage with molasses pres.	52
Lespedeza hay, pre-bloom	111
Oat hay	67
Oat silage	29
Pea vine silage	24
Prairie hay, mid-bloom	22
Prairie hay, late bloom	17
Prairie hay, past bloom	6
Sorghum fodder	14
Sorghum silage	7
Soybean hay	24
Soybean, silage	17
Timothy hay, mid bloom	35
Timothy silage	23
Vetch hay	305
Wheat hay	72
Wheat straw	2

Prevention and Treatment. Bovine vitamin A deficiency can be prevented by supplying an adequate amount of vitamin A and/or carotene. When admitted to the feedlot, cattle should be evaluated for probable hepatic stores of vitamin A. On the basis of hepatic stores and of carotene content of feed, the vitamin A requirements of the animals, as presented in Table 30, should be supplied. The sources of dietary carotene in vitamin A equivalents are shown in Table 31. If necessary, vitamin A concentrate supplement, in the form of gelatinized vitamin A palmatate, can be added to the diet. A part or all of the requirement can also be supplied as injectable vitamin A given intramuscularly.

Except for animals in early stages of the disease, treatment for vitamin A deficiency is unsatisfactory. Cattle in early stages should be given a diet with high carotene and/or vitamin A content. Heavy doses of injectable vitamin A can also be administered parenterally. Animals in advanced stages of deficiency should be marketed early for recovery of investment. At slaughter, edematous parts and entire carcasses are unsatisfactory for food and are condemned. Non-edematous parts, if otherwise normal, are suitable for food.

References

Abrams, J. T., Bridge, P. S., Palmer, A. C. and Spratling, F. R.: Apparent Hypovitaminosis A in Young Cattle in East Anglia. Vet. Rec., *73* (1961): 683–690.

Blackmore, F., Ottany, C. W., Sellers, K. C., Eden, E. and Moore, T.: The Effects of a Diet Deficient in Vitamin A on the Development of the Skull, Optic Nerves, and Brain of Cattle. J. Comp. Path. & Therap., *67* (1957): 277–288.

Chung, A. C. and Houck, J. C.: Connective Tissue. IX. Effects of Hypervitaminosis A Upon Connective Tissue Chemistry. Proc. Soc. Exp. Boil. & Med., *115* (1964): 631–633.

Committee on Animal Nutrition. Nutrient Requirements of Beef Cattle. National Academy of Sciences. National Research Council. Publication 579. (1958).

———. Nutrient Requirements of Beef Cattle. Revised Edition. National Academy of Sciences. National Research Council. Publication 1137. (1963).

Davis, C. L., Elliot, R. F. and Lassiter, C. A.: The Effect of Lecithin, Choline, and Methionine on the Vitamin A and Carotene Plasma Levels and Liver Stores of Young Calves. J. Dairy Sc., *39* (1956): 440–447.

Frey, P. R. and Jensen, Rue.: Depletion of Hepatic Reserves of Vitamin A and Carotene in Cattle. J. Nutrition, *32* (1946): 133–141.

———: Depletion of Vitamin A Reserves in the Livers of Cattle. Science, *105* (1947): 313.

Huber, W. G. and Smith, G. S.: Field Aids in the Diagnosis of Bovine Vitamin A Deficiency. Vet. Med., *58* (1963): 875.

Jungherr, E. L., Helmboldt, C. F. and Eaton, H. D.: Experimental Vitamin A Deficiency in Young Dairy Cattle. J. An. Sc., *8* (1949): 641.

Marsh, H. and Swingle, K. F.: The Calcium, Phosphorus, Magnesium, Carotene, and Vitamin A Content of the Blood of Range Cattle in Eastern Montana. AJVR, *21* (1960): 212–221.

Moore, L. A., Huffman, C. F., and Duncan, C. W.: Blindness in Cattle Associated With Constriction of the Optic Nerve and Probably of Nutritional Origin. J. Nut., *9* (1935): 533–551.

O'Dell, B. L., Erek, Z., Flynn, L., Garner, G. B. and Munrer, M. E.: Effects of Nitrite Containing Rations in Producing Vitamin A and Vitamin E Deficiency in Rats. J. An. Sc., *19* (1960): 1280.

Pope, L. S., Baker, F. H. and Macvicar, R. W.: Vitamin A Studies With Beef Cattle. Okla. Ag. Exp. Station Bulletin B-578 (1961).

Thompson, S. Y., Ganguly, J. and Kon, S. K.: The Conversion of *B*-Carotene to Vitamin A in the Intestine. Brit. J. Nutrition, *3* (1949): 50–78.

Wolbach, S. B. J.: Bone & Internal Surg. *29* (1947): 171.

Riding

(BULLING STEERS; BULLER STEERS)

"Riding," a term describing abnormal sexual activity among steers, is characterized by their repeated and persistent mounting of one or more other steers. The activity may be simulated feminization or simulated masculinization and is either temporary or permanent. In feminization, the more common form of riding, the affected steer sexually attracts other steers and tolerates being ridden; while in masculinization the affected steer aggressively and repeatedly mounts other steers, or heifers and cows if available, and unsuccessfully attempts copulation. The cause is unknown. Because the incidence within herds is high, but unmeasured, the condition has significant monetary importance. Economic losses result from herd unrest, physical injury, condemnation of parts of carcasses at slaughter, occasional deaths, reduction of liveweight gains, expenditure of vigilant labor time and the need for special management practices, such as isolating and restraining pens.

Occurrence. Among steers sexual riding is common wherever aggregrates of cattle are assembled. In feedlots, however, the condition occurs more often and intensely, and all steer fattening enterprises are affected at all seasons. While the disease may occur in steers of all ages, animals weighing approximately 700 pounds or more show a high incidence and the behavior may be manifest at any stage of fattening. Geographically, the condition occurs throughout the United States and in other countries where large numbers of steers are assembled in a common fattening pen.

Etiology and Pathogenesis. The causes of riding have not been experimentally investigated, are inadequately understood and many factors may be involved in the complex behavior. The consumption of large amounts of feed concentrates, crowding within pens, idleness and the lack of exercise may be predisposing and contributing factors. The emission of estral odors by a few individual steers may be the exciting cause of simulated feminization, and these odors may result from recent subcutaneous implantation of estrogen pellets and/or the development of diseases. Animals affected with acute indigestion, urinary calculosis, coccidiosis, liver abscesses and those recently subjected to surgery, may emit odors or evince behavior which attracts and invites mounting by other steers.

In simulated masculinization one or few steers are persistently preoccupied with riding other steers. In some animals incomplete castration may result in the retention in the animal of some functional Leydig cells which synthesize and secrete androgenic hormone. The testosterone formed in this manner stimulates libido. An occasional steer may be masculinized by secretion of excessive amounts of adrenal androgen. But in most affected steers the physiological or pathological sources of stimulation and the direct causes of the mounting activity are unknown.

A knowledge of the hormone chemistry and physiology in steers, although desperately needed, has not been investigated. Accurate information on the subject would help explain the cause of riding and other abnormal behaviors, and it might also elucidate the action mechanism for some feed additives and growth stimulators and provide a sound scientific base for their use. Basic physiological information may suggest a rational preventive and therapeutic treatment for riding.

In dry pens herd agitation from excessive riding causes air contamination with dust from soil and manure. Inhalation of these contaminants may contribute to the cause and exacerbation of respiratory diseases, such as rhinitis, sinusitis, calf diphtheria and pneumonia.

Clinical Signs. In the simulated feminization form an individual steer becomes sexually attractive to other steers. The affected animal is mounted on the buttocks repeatedly by other steers of the pen. The riding results in variable amounts of abrading and denuding of the skin over the posterior part of the animal, especially the tail head and tuber coxas but may include the costal and gluteal regions. The abraded and sometimes necrosed skin and contused subcutis, muscles, and tubercoxal bursas become hyperemic, swollen and painful. The affected animal rapidly weakens, fatigues and prostrates. In the victimized animals, possibly affected with other diseases, the primary disease becomes aggravated and more complicated. Unless severely affected steers are removed from the pen, provided protection against other steers, and given adequate veterinary attention and nursing care, the injury is aggravated and may result in death. The course of the disorder is variable. Mild cases may endure a few minutes, and severe ones for many days or for the entire time of association with the original pen of cattle.

In the simulated masculinization form the

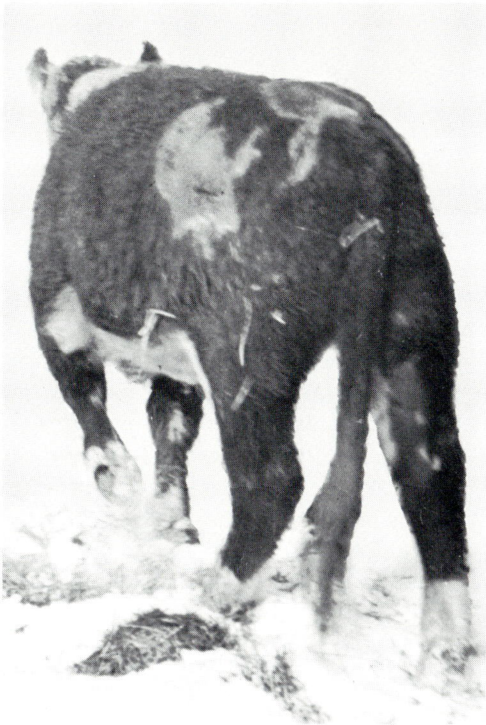

FIG. 8-58. *Denuded and lacerated skin from riding.*

affected animal persistently and indiscriminately mounts other steers. This highly erratic behavior may endure for a few hours or several days and in some cases for the duration of time the animal is associated with the cattle pen where the condition was initiated. In animals affected for prolonged periods, the rate of gain in body weight is diminished, not only for the masculinized steer, but for the entire pen.

Diagnosis. Riding in either the simulated feminization or masculinization forms is diagnosed on the basis of animal behavior and the development of abraded skin lesions. The act of repeated riding is usually observed by the animal caretaker. The skin abrasions and denudation may be observed simultaneously with the behavior or subsequent to the riding. The lesions must be distinguished from such skin diseases as mange and ringworm. The acute dermatitis from riding is characterized by surface abrasions and hemorrhages and by subcutaneous swelling and contusions. The microscopic study of skin scraping will help confirm an uncertain diagnosis.

Prevention and Treatment. Following analysis of its causes, the simulated feminization form is treated for correction. If the riding is secondary to some other disease, the animal should be isolated from the herd and the primary disease rationally treated. Following recovery from the primary disease, the animal can be returned to the original feedlot. If the riding is caused by hormone pellet implantation in the subcutaneous tissues, the affected animal should be isolated from the pen and given either of two courses of treatment. In the first type of treatment, 500 mg of repositol progesterone is injected subcutaneously and the animal is returned to the original pen of cattle, 48 or more hours after the progesterone administration. In the second type of treatment the implanted hormone pellet is surgically excised and 500 mg of repositol progesterone are administered intramuscularly. The treated animal should be kept in isolation for at least 48 hours before being returned to the original pen of cattle. Cases of simulated feminization for which no apparent cause is discernible are treated by isolation and alteration of body odors. Many of the sprays or dips used as acaricides and insecticides are satisfactory for this purpose. If a pen of cattle contains four or more animals affected with simulated feminization, the entire lot should be sprayed or dipped. Another recommended dip or wash for affected animals consists of the following mixture (Dewar, 1951): equal parts of phenol, glycerin, oil of eucalyptis and oil of asafetida. During isolation, contusions, hematomas, cellulitis, fractures and tubercoxal bursitis should be properly treated. After isolation and treatment affected animals should be returned to the original feedlot during times of feeding when animal attention is not directed to the returning steer. Some severely affected steers, instead of returning to the original pen, may be placed with pens of heifers, or in separate pens for bullers, for completion of fattening. Isolation alone corrects approximately 50% of cases.

Cases of simulated masculinization are also treated by isolation. If castration appears to be incomplete, the remaining testicular tissue and the distal portions of the spermatic cords can be excised.

Reference

Dewar, J. K.: *Questions and Answers.* American Veterinary Publications, Inc., Wheaton, Illinois. 1951. pp. 33–34.

Estrus Control and Therapeutic Abortion

Feedlot heifers and to a lesser extent cows, have a high capacity for converting feed at a rapid rate into good quality beef and for this reason are preferred by some producers. However, both pregnancy and estrus decrease the beef-making capacity and tend to negate the advantage. With the exception of spayed heifers, both conditions occur commonly among pens of female cattle because pregnancies may exist either with or without knowledge of the seller or buyer at the time heifers and cows are purchased for fattening. Even in heifers guaranteed to be open, existing pregnancies may be discovered during the course of fattening. Because advanced pregnancies in marketed beef cattle decrease the percentage of carcass yield at slaughter and increase the volume of live weight discarded at the time of slaughter, meat packing enterprises, in order to compensate for the losses, are forced to purchase fattened heifers and cows at discount prices. Parturition during the fattening period interrupts the fattening process, causes loss of some body weight and disqualifies the affected animal for slaughter for days. Often cattle in advanced stages of pregnancy and cattle evincing recent parturition are removed from the fattening pens for other types of management and use. While in many respects, pregnancies in feedlot cattle are undesirable, they have the advantage of preventing animal agitation and unrest.

Because estrus may occur at approximately 21-day intervals in nonpregnant heifers and cows, a large pen of open heifers has some individuals in heat almost constantly. During the 8- to 30-hour estral period, the affected animals are preoccupied with sexual activity, and the process reduces feed consumption and live-weight gains. In addition, many cohabitating animals participate in sexual riding, and the result is general disturbance among many of the animals in the whole pen. By recognizing the disadvantages of pregnancy and estrus in feedlot cattle, veterinarians and other scientists have developed methods and practices whereby estrus can be prevented or pregnancies interrupted.

Review of Literature. Estrus is that part of the female sexual cycle when copulation is acceptable and when ovulation occurs. The possibility of controlling estrus by determining and applying principles of hormone physiology and chemistry has been recognized and attempted. Progestogens, a group of sterol compounds, exert an inhibitory effect on ovulation and estrus. One of these, melengestrol acetate (MGA), is especially efficacious. When administered orally to heifers MGA has been 900 times more potent and when given intravenously 10 to 15 times more potent than medroxyprogesterone, a related compound (Zimbleman and Smith, 1966). MGA has also been used to stimulate growth. In one experiment, two lots of heifers were fed for 161 days on a standard fattening ration. Control cattle of lot 1 received no feed additive, while lot 2 received in the ration an oral dose of 0.4 mg of MGA/animal/day. Heifers of the control pen averaged gain in body weight of 2.66 pounds/animal/day, while the heifers treated with MGA averaged 2.79 pounds/animal/day, an increase of 5% over the control pen. In addition, the heifers receiving the MGA manifested no estrus and its associated unrest (Matsushima, McCann and McLaren, 1969). In four earlier experiments conducted at commercial feedlots and using 2,106 heifers, the growth stimulating effects of melengestrol and diethylstilbestrol were compared. In each trial, heifers receiving MGA averaged higher daily gains in body weight and were more settled in behavior than were heifers receiving diethylstilbestrol (Matsushina, Weichenthal and Heeney, 1967).

During the late 1940's when calving in feedlot heifers became a financial and biological problem, several methods for inducing abortion were tried. Diethylstilbestrol in vegetable oil was given intramuscularly in various doses to pregnant heifers, but results were unsatisfactory. In 1950 when administered to ewes to induce early estrus, the relationship of estradiol to abortion was accidentally discovered. During the process of treatment, estradiol was given inadvertently to some pregnant ewes and within 1 week following the drug administration they aborted their fetuses (Mackey, 1950). Knowing that estradiol not only induced early estrus but caused abortion was insight to method for inducing bovine abortions, and in an initial test each of two pregnant heifers given an injection of 100 mg of diethylstilbestrol in propylene glycol also aborted (Burch, 1952).

To obtain more precise information on efficacy of diethylstilbestrol as an abortifacient, two formal experiments were conducted. In the first (Mackey, 1955), five lots of feedlot heifers containing 435 animals, some of which were pregnant, were studied. Animal weights ranged from 500 to 800 pounds and pregnancy stages varied from 2 to 8 months. All animals, both pregnant and non-pregnant, were each injected with 100 mg of diethylstilbestrol in propylene glycol. Of these, 87 (20%) aborted within 30 days after treatment. In the second experiment (Hill and Pierson, 1958) 2,760 feedlot heifers in 26 pens were examined and of these 761 were pregnant. Each of the pregnant heifers was given diethylstilbestrol, the dose ranging from 100 to 175 mg and varying directly with the stage of pregnancy. Eighty % of all treated heifers aborted, but 89% with gestation varying from 120 to 210 days aborted. Abortions occurred from 3 to 25 days after injection with a peak arriving between the tenth and twelfth day; the larger dosage did not increase the abortion rate. Twenty-one days after the first injection each unaborted heifer was given a second dosage; the amount was 25 mg greater than the first injection. After 3 additional weeks 50% of the heifers receiving the second dose had aborted.

Application of Estrus Inhibitor. Following receipt of heifers or cows at the feedlot, each animal should be examined for pregnancy. In order to obtain good management, open heifers and pregnant heifers should be placed in separate pens. The diet of the non-pregnant heifers should include a protein supplement made into a pellet. A formula for the pellet may include the following ingredients: 60% cottonseed meal, 3.5% wheat shorts, 5% iodized salt, 4% dicalcium phosphate, 11% urea (45% N), 2.5% dried molasses, 14% calcium carbonate and sufficient MGA to provide a daily dose of 0.4 mg per animal. The pellets should be fed throughout the entire fattening period, but as long as MGA is included it provides growth stimulation and estrus inhibition. Before using MGA, clearance for the intended route of application should be ascertained from the Food and Drug Administration, and the required drug withdrawal period prior to slaughter should be complied with. In the event that market demands for breeding heifers, rather than feeding cattle, change, the altered disposition of heifers being fattened may be reversed by adjustment of the ration and discontinuance of the use of MGA. Following withdrawal of the drug, estrus should occur within 48 to 120 hours, and at least 50% conception rate can be expected from artificial insemination at the first estrus.

Application of the Abortifacient. Upon entrance into the feedlot pens, heifers and cows with some pregnant, should be permitted to rest and adjust to the feedlot environment. Cases of shipping fever and other diseases or injuries from transportation should be appropriately treated and the cattle slowly introduced to the diet of high concentrate feed.

At the end of the first 3 weeks when most adjustments have been made, the use of abortifacients can be initiated, and either of two courses of treatment can be followed: (1) the injection of all heifers and/or cows with the abortifacient or (2) the injection of pregnant heifers only. The procedure of injecting all heifers has many undesirable aspects and is usually not recommended. The injected estrogen in non-pregnant heifers causes near simultaneous estrus in most of the animals, and this in turn, results in unrest, agitation, sweating, riding, lowered feed consumption, diminished gains in body weight, agitated pen dust and respiratory distresses. If this procedure is utilized, feedlot owners should be advised of its disadvantages and informed that cattle in the third trimester of pregnancy are not susceptible to diethylstilbestrol as an abortifacient.

The second method, injection of pregnant animals only, is practical and scientifically sound but requires restraining equipment such as the squeeze chute. Each animal is identified and by rectal palpation the stage of gestation for each pregnancy is determined. Animals in the third trimester of pregnancy should be separated from the other animals and maintained on non-fatening diet until after calving or marketed as replacement cows in breeding herds. The pregnant animals with gestations not exceeding 6 months are susceptible to abortifacients and should be injected with diethylstilbestrol according to the dosage given in Table 32.

TABLE 32 ***Dosage of diethylstilbestrol in propylene glycol***

Gestation Days	*Diethylstilbestrol mg*
up to 150	100
151 to 210	125 to 150

After the administration of the abortifacient, the feedlot animals should be observed carefully, cases of abortion recorded, and all aborted fetuses removed from the pens and buried or burned. If at the end of 30 days the abortion rate is low, the remaining cases of pregnancy, as determined by rectal palpation, should be reinjected. Abortion is caused by strong uterine contractions stimulated by the diethylstilbestrol.

Results from the Abortifacient. Following the administration of diethylstilbestrol, abortions occur from 3 to 30 days, and the peak of abortion rate is reached 10 to 15 days after injection. Pregnancies in 80 to 90% of heifers whose gestation does not exceed the second trimester are expected to abort.

Cattle in the more advanced stages of pregnancy show a propensity for complications following abortion. The udder develops to noticeable dimensions but recedes after 60 days. Placentas may be retained and require manual removal. Prolapse of the vagina and/or rectum may occur. Retained dead fetuses may become emphysematous and require manual removal, and treatment of metritis may be needed. Following abortion the treated animals may show a superior rate of gain in body weight over untreated cattle (Hill and Pierson, 1958).

During the process of inducing abortions, precautions should be exercised: swine should be removed from the feedlot to avoid the development of traumatic anovulvitis; cattle injected with diethylstilbestrol should not be slaughtered for food within 30 days of the time of drug administration; and the drug should not be administered to lactating cattle whose milk is used for human consumption.

References

Burch, G.: Pitman-Moore Co., Indianapolis. Personal communications. 1952.

Mackey, D. R.: Greeley, Colorado. Personal communication. 1950.

———: Therapeutic Abortion in Feedlot Cattle. California Veterinarian, *8* (1955): 33–34.

Matsushima, J. K., Weichenthal, B. A. and Heeney,

M. W.: Melengestrol Acetate. Colorado Farm and Home Research, *17* (1967 No. 2): 10–11.
Matsushima, J. K., McCann, C. P. and McLaren, R. J.: MGA and Stilbesterol for Feedlot Heifers. Beef Nutrition Research, Colorado State University Report. Feb. 28, 1969, pp. 15–16.
Hill, H. J. and Pierson, R. E.: Repositol Diethylstilbestrol as an Abortifacient in Feedlot Heifers. JAVMA, *132* (1958): 507–512.
Zimbleman, R. G. and Smith, L. W.: Control of Ovulation in Cattle with Melengestrol Acetate. I. Effect of Dosage and Route of Administration, II. Effects on Follicular size and Activity. J. Reprod. And Fertility, *11* (1966): 185–201.

Traumatic Anovulvitis

An acute non-contagious disease, traumatic anovulvitis is characterized by lacerations of the vulva, anus and perineum and by secondary infection of these areas. In these organs the primary injuries are usually superficial and inconsequential, but secondary invasions of them by numerous contaminating bacteria from manure and soil may cause severe wound infections which often spread to surrounding tissues and organs. Since the disease occurs uncommonly, it has minor economic importance to the cattle industry, but occasionally high incidence within an affected herd causes losses to an individual producer. Economic losses come from reduced rates of gain in live weight, occasional death, expensive treatments and possibly delayed marketing of fat animals.

Review of Literature. The literature on traumatic anovulvitis is limited to case reports within the United States. The disease has been described in feedlot cattle in western (Pierson and Hill, 1956) and mid-western (Aitken, 1956; Kinsley, 1929) states and in dairy cattle (Little, 1932) of the eastern states. The incidence varied from 40 to 98% of the animals within a herd. While the disease usually occurs in females, the anus of male animals has been affected (Little, 1932).

The specific cause of the disease has been suggested but not proved. The nature of the lesions led some investigators to suspect malicious injury (Little, 1936). The frequent association of affected cattle with swine and the improvement following separation of cattle from swine led others to infer swine perpetration by biting (Aitken, 1956; Pierson and Hill, 1956). Numerous species of bacteria isolated from the infected wounds have been independently incapable of producing the lesions.

Occurrence. A disease of cattle only, traumatic anovulvitis is encountered mostly in feedlot heifers. Cows may also be affected but steers rarely develop anal lesions. Geographically, they often occur where cattle and swine cohabitate. Since the cattle fattening and swine producing industries are fully developed, and often are simultaneously pursued on the same farms in the mid-western states, the disease is found more often in that area. Season and stage of cattle fattening appear to have little influence on the incidence.

Etiology and Pathogenesis. Lacerations of the vulva, anus and perineum are self-inflicted and swine-inflicted. Intensive itching of the anatomical area may come from allergic reactions and possibly from dermatitis, and affected cattle find sharp projections, such as nails, wire and bolts, on fences and watering and feeding equipment and vigorously rub against these objects to relieve the itching. In doing so, the tissues abrade and lacerate. Repetition of the process may result in considerable damage and inoculation of contaminating bacteria into the wounds.

Swine, cohabitating with feedlot cattle and dependent on cattle manure for part or all of their food, occasionally bite perineal organs of the cattle, and the bites inflict either superficial or deep lacerations. The hogs seek grain in the newly deposited feces of reclining cattle. To stimulate defecation the hog roots the bovine perineal region, and a few animals bite the vulva and surrounding skin. Protruding placental membranes from recent bovine abortions and uterine discharges strongly motivate the biting pigs. A few swine gradually acquire a biting vice and at each opportunity attack reclining cattle. The lacerations may be single or multiple and superficial or deep.

The deep incisions commonly become contaminated with bacteria from the soil, the mouths of swine and the skin and feces of the cattle. Bacterial species of the genera *Corynebacterium, Spherophorus, Staphylococcus, Streptococcus, Escherichia* and *Clostridium* are commonly involved. Ischemia from the irregular lacerations and growth of contaminating bacteria cause necrosis and inflammation. The infection may spread to include both lacerated and healthy tissues, but in most cattle, however, the spreading is arrested early and healing occurs. The animals may succumb from spread of the infection into the pelvic organs, including the urethra and urinary bladder, and from systemic intoxication. Most animals, however, recover completely without complications.

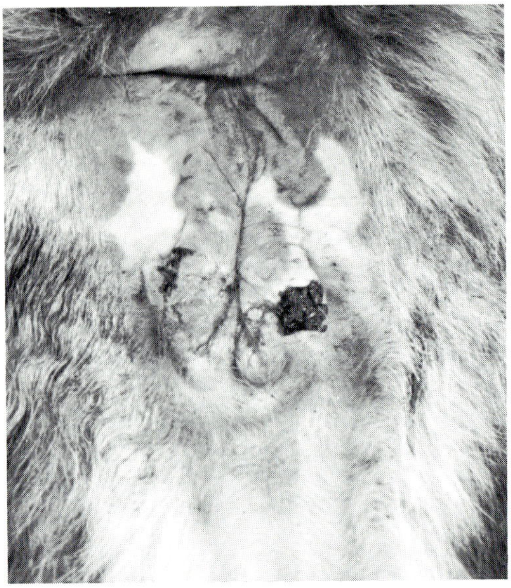

FIG. 8-59. *Traumatic vulvitis in a feedlot heifer.* × 0.4.

Clinical Signs and Lesions. Soon after laceration, hemorrhage as well as the wounds may be evident and noted by the herdsman. Following the secondary infection the body temperature may range from 103° to 105° F, and severely affected animals may show anorexia, gauntness and depression. The tail is extended and urination painful. Straining may be prominent.

The lesions show variable amounts of necrosis, exudate and swelling. In mild cases, the superficial lacerations are covered with a dried crust. In severe cases, the deep and infected lacerations contain large amounts of necrotic tissue and inflammatory exudate which often obscures the original trauma involving the vulvar labia, commissures, clitoris and external urethral oriface, as well as the perineum and anus. Rarely does the infectious process cause severe swelling or extend deeply into the extragenital pelvic tissues. In healing stages the swelling subsides and the exudate forms a dried crust.

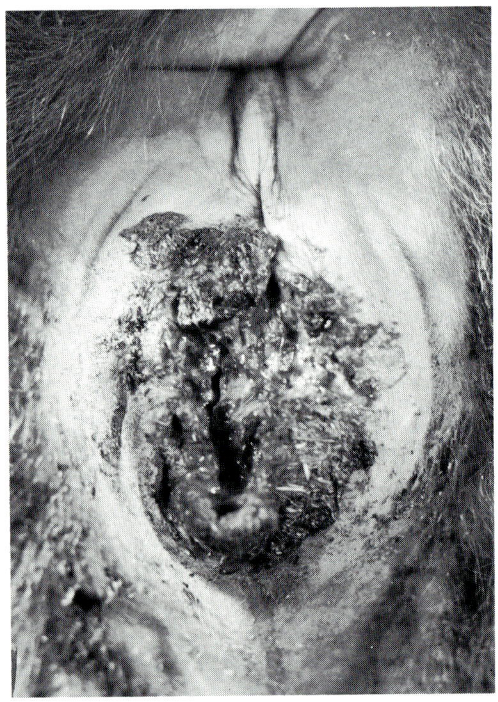

FIG. 8-60. *Traumatic vulvitis with severe secondary infection.* × 0.5. (*Courtesy of Dr. R. E. Pierson.*)

While the incidence within a herd may be

sequential and distributed over many weeks, most outbreaks develop a near simultaneous incidence as high as 98% of a herd. The course may extend over 7 to 14 days, but the mortality is negligible.

Diagnosis. Traumatic anovulvitis is diagnosed from gross lesions within a herd having a history of severe itching and rubbing or of close cohabitation with swine. In case of self-inflicted trauma, the affected animals seem preoccupied with scratching, and they devote considerable time to the process. In cattle containing swine-inflicted lesions, the actual biting is insidious and difficult to detect. Considerable time and attention may be required to identify culpable individuals. The differential diagnosis requires consideration of accidental injury, complications following parturition or late induced abortion, contagious pustular vulvoaginitis and allergic reactions. Accidental trauma, usually involving only a single animal, may result from rubbing against fences and feedlot equipment. In fat cows and heifers, parturition or late abortion often cause severe genital lacerations which may become secondarily infected and necrotic. The clinical history and evidence of recent birth enable differentiation of the malady from traumatic anovulvitis. Contagious pustular vulvovaginitis, a manifestation of viral bovine rhinotracheitis, is characterized by pustules and acute swelling of the vulvar mucosa, but the disease does not affect the skin of the perineum, and it does not occur in cattle immunized against viral bovine rhinotracheitis. Histopathologic sections may reveal the presence of characteristic inclusion bodies. In the laboratory the virus may be isolated and identified. In allergic vulvitis the itching perineal tissues are acutely swollen and edematous. Relief from signs comes within 12 to 24 hours from the administration of antihistamines or cortical steroids.

Prevention and Treatment. The self-inflicted lacerations can be prevented by removing all traumatizing objects from access to the cattle. Fences should be inspected at frequent intervals for projecting nails, barbed wire, bolts and sharp wooden splinters. Water fountains and other equipment should be kept harmless by removing all cutting edges and puncturing projections.

The primary lacerations from swine bites can be avoided by excluding swine from cattle feedlots. Presumedly, most lacerations are inflicted by one or few pigs, and only the identification and elimination of the biting animals prevent the development of additional cases. Identification of the guilty pigs, however, requires constant and prolonged vigilance which often is expensive in time and may be unsuccessful.

After separating swine from the cattle, severely affected heifers may require treatment for control of the secondary infection. The wounds should be cleaned and treated topically with disinfectants. Sulfathiazol, sulfapyridine or antibiotics are effective for parenteral application.

References

Aitken, W. A.: Anovulvitis in Heifers. JAVMA, *129* (1956): 73.

Kinsley, A. T.: Anovulvitis and Posthitis in Cattle. Vet. Med., *24* (1929): 493.

Little, R. B.: Anovulvitis in Cattle. Vet. Med., *27* (1932): 432–434.

Pierson, R. E. and Hill, H. J.: Necrotic Vulvitis in Feedlot Heifers. JAVMA, *129* (1956): 71–73.

Traumatic Bursitis

An acute but non-infectious disease, traumatic bursitis is characterized by enlargement and distension of the sternal, supraspinous and tuber coxal bursas. Bursas are closed collapsed cavities containing a small amount of viscid fluid. Inconstant in existence and location, they are more commonly present in adult cattle than in young animals. The bursal wall consists of outer connective tissue and an inner membrane. The membrane contains many fibrocytes and capillaries. The bursas are located at points of friction and are interposed between opposing surfaces. Usually they are between a bony prominence and an over-riding tendon, muscle or skin. The bursa with lubricating fluid enables free movement of the two opposing surfaces. Since the disease is not only uncommon but seldom incapacitating, it has little economic importance to the cattle-fattening industry. A high incidence, however, within a single herd may adversely affect an individual producer. The prolongation of treatments, depressed market prices of visibly affected animals and trimming of carcasses at slaughter result in minor economic losses.

Occurrence. While all sexes and breeds appear equally susceptible to bursitis, the different bursas are predisposed to injuries at specific ages. Animals approximately 6 months of age show a high incidence of sternal bursitis because of discongruity between the small animal body-size and the feeding and watering equipment found in average feedlots. Because of sexual riding propensities of the age group, many cases of tuber coxal bursitis develop among 2-year-old steers and heifers. Even though the condition may occur anytime during fattening, most cases develop within 3 to 4 weeks after admission to feedlots.

Etiology and Pathogenesis. Traumatic bursitis is caused by repeated injuries, usually mechanical, to the bursa. Tuber coxal bursitis results from sexual riding. Some steers are repeatedly mounted by other steers; and estral heifers, by other heifers. In the process of mounting, the feet of the aggressive animal may strike and injure one or both tuber coxae. The bursas and adjacent soft tissues become contused, and the skin abraded and lacerated.

Sternal and supraspinous bursitis are caused by repeated mild injuries. The use of feeding and watering equipment not suitable to the bovine vertical dimensions may require small cattle to reach too high for either feed or water; and in their attempts, they inflict mild injury to the bursa located over the anterior part of the sternum. The top rail of feed bunks may be placed too low for large cattle, or they may be placed on the cattle side of the posts. While feeding, cattle may push against the rail and contuse the supraspinous bursa. Hemorrhage and necrosis may occur in the bursal cavity and soft tissues.

Regardless of anatomical location, the injured bursa secretes excessive amounts of synovium, which enlarge and distend the sac. Hemorrhage into the fluid and necrosis of tissue aggravate the lesion. Early discontinuance of the injuries may result in reabsorption of the synovium and in healing. Continuation of the trauma, however, may result in chronic bursitis with thickening and mineralizing of the bursal wall; in this case, healing may require surgical opening and excision of the bursa. In some cases, the affected tissues become secondarily infected with pyogenic bacteria which convert the bursitis into an abscess.

Additional basic studies on the anatomy of bursas are acutely needed. At the present time, the development, location, constancy, size and morphology of bursas are inadequately known. Most anatomists agree that tubercoxal and supraspinous bursas occur in specific locations, but the size, shape and constancy of the structures are in dispute. Because of its inconspicuousness and possible inconstancy the sternal bursa is not generally recognized, and some anatomy books do not mention its existence. New information would increase the understanding of bursitis.

Clinical Signs and Lesions. After a variable period and a differing number of injuries, enlarged bursas become spherical, circumscribed and soft, and they measure 2 to 10 inches in diameter. Body temperature, appetite and behavior of the animal remain normal. In early stages of development, the enlarged bursas are inconspicuous and their detection may require palpation; in advanced stages, they are visually noticeable. In old and advanced lesions, the bursa may be firm or may have ruptured and discharged synovium onto the skin surface.

Dissection at surgery, or necropsy, reveals

the sharply delimited sac and surgical opening discloses the cavity containing 100 to 1,000 ml of pale yellow synovium. Some bursas contain fragments of necrotic tissue and masses of fibrin within the synovium. The inner surface of the bursal sac wall is smooth excepting at points of severe injury and necrosis. Histopathologically, the wall contains lymphocytes and mononuclear macrophages. Phagocytized pigment from hemoglobin may be present, and blood capillaries numerically increased.

Within a geographic region, the herd incidence approximates 1 to 2%, and the individual morbidity rate within affected herds varies from one or two animals to 50% of the herd. The mortality rate is negligible, and unless the cause is removed before the lesions become large, the disease course extends over many weeks or months. When affected animals are submitted for slaughter, the diseased bursas are excised and condemned, but the remaining carcass, if otherwise healthy, is satisfactory for food.

Diagnosis. Traumatic bursitis is diagnosed from the observation of enlarged and softly distended sternal, supraspinous or tuber coxal bursas, occurring in cattle with normal appetites and body temperatures. The diagnosis can be confirmed by passing a needle into the lesion and by finding synovium in the cavity.

The differential diagnosis requires consideration of large abscesses, massive hematomas and, in the case of sternal bursitis, brisket edema from cardiac defects. Abscesses from foreign bodies and hematomas from injuries will, by needle centesis, show the presence of pus or blood respectively. In brisket edema from cardiac disease, the affected animal is physically weak, and thoracic auscultation may reveal abnormal heart sounds.

Prevention and Treatment. Feedlot cattle should be carefully observed for developing abnormalities. To avoid tuber coxal bursitis, feminized steers and estral heifers, often victims of sexual riding, should be isolated until the riding propensity has been corrected. When cattle enter feedlots, they should be segregated into lots of similar-sized animals, and for easy and efficient animal use, feeding and watering equipment should be adjusted to the height of the animals. The top neck rail of the feeding equipment should be placed, with reference to the cattle, on the opposite side of the posts and at the proper height. This placement avoids injury to the supraspinous bursa. In order to avoid injury to the sternal bursa, the lower neck rails should also be adjusted to the height of the animals. As animals grow in height, adjustment of equipment may be necessary.

Treatment varies according to the stage of bursitis development. In early stages affected cattle should be protected against additional injuries by adjusting feeding and watering equipment. Without repeated injury, the extra synovium frequently reabsorbs, and individual treatment may not be necessary. In early stages, when the bursa is small, discontinuing the causative injuries and ad-

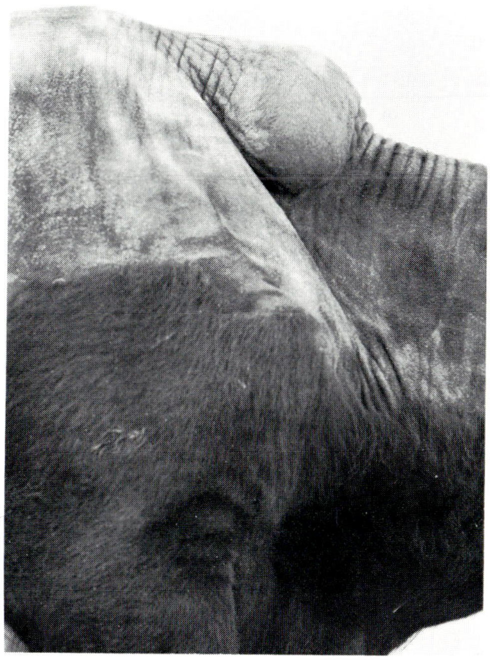

FIG. 8-61. *Supraspinous bursitis from repeated injuries on feeding equipment.*

ministering reposatory cortical steroids may result in cure.

Animals in advanced stages of bursitis require individual surgical treatment. The enlarged bursa is liberally incised, the synovium completely drained, and fibrin and necrotic tissue removed. To prevent recurrence, the lining membrane of the cavity is excised or destroyed by cauterizing with 20% tincture of iodine. Repeated cautery may be necessary. The wound is treated daily with topical applications of Scarletol, solutions of urea in propylene glycol or solutions of sulfonamides. Healing of the open wound is gradual and may extend over 1 month.

9

The problem of pollution from cattle feedlots

Since 1950 the United States generally and some individual states specifically have experienced a new cycle of concern over the increasing pollution of water and air. The decline in quality of these resources has reached the point of endangering the health and welfare of people, fauna and flora, and of jeopardizing continuing development of natural resources and industrial enterprises. The major sources of water pollutants have been municipal sewages and industrial wastes; the major sources of air pollutants have been the gaseous emissions from combusting fossil fuels in engines of automobiles and in engines for generating power and heat for public use. To these sources a third major contributor to both air and water contamination has been added—the pollutants from agricultural activities. Livestock enterprises have annually generated two billion tons of wastes, and to those wastes, cattle feedlot operations have contributed major quantities of solids, liquids and gases. Public concern over the problem has resulted in the enactment of state and national laws for effecting abatement and control of all pollutants of water and air. The legislation gives financial assistance to researchers to help discover scientific principles and develop practical methods for degrading and disposing of feedlot wastes. Following development of a satisfactory disposal technology, feedlot operators will be expected to adopt and use the new systems. The high costs of the research and development will be shared by the beneficiaries, both public and private.

Review of Literature. Historically, the cattle fattening industry evolved as a seasonal farm operation in which field crops and residues were used to feed and fatten small numbers of cattle during winter months. Gradually, however, small seasonal feedlots have been replaced by large and continuously operating enterprises. The high plains region of the United States experienced such a change. From 1962 through 1968 the number of cattle fattened in feedlots having a capacity of less than 1,000 animals increased by 22%, while during the same period the number of cattle fattened in feedlots having a capacity of more than 1,000 animals increased by 211% (Statistical Reporting Service, 1968). Commonly, the large capacity feedlots located and developed near municipalities. Furthermore, the increasing demand for beef meat has enhanced the problem. The amount of beef consumed per capita increased from

63.4 pounds in 1950 to about 114 pounds in 1970, and the demand is estimated to reach 125 pounds by 1980 (Seaborg, 1970).

Any form of nitrogen entering water or air by surface runoff, by percolation through soil, and by volatilization from a surface was regarded as possible pollution (Stewart, 1969). Quality standards for human drinking water limited the nitrate-nitrogen content to 10 ppm (= 45 ppm nitrate) (American Public Health Assn., 1965). Feedlot runoff was investigated for pen surfaces and for animal unit concentrations (Gilbertson *et al.*, 1969; McCalla *et al.*, 1969). Runoff contained concentrations of ammonia nitrogen ranging from 16 to 140 mg/l and of suspended solids from 1,500 to 12,000 mg/l. The chemical oxygen demand was from 3,000 to 11,000 mg/l. Concentrations of contaminants were greater during summer months from animal pens having paved surfaces and high cattle densities (Lipper, 1969).

By percolation into earth beneath feedlots, forms of nitrogen were found to enter the soil profile and ground water. In Missouri, studies of ground water samples indicated great variance in content of nitrate-nitrogen. Water samples from beneath livestock feeding operations were significantly higher than were samples from beneath field crops (Smith, 1965). An extensive study of the problem was conducted in the South Platte River Valley of Colorado where intensive farming is practiced and where most of Colorado's feedlot industry is located. The semi-arid valley is underlain with ground water table that varies from 10 to 65 feet beneath the surface. Soil cores from the surface to water table or bedrock were obtained from 47 feedlots, 28 irrigated fields and 21 dryland-cropped fields. The average total amount of nitrate-nitrogen in the soil profile to a depth of 20 feet was for different land uses as follows: alfalfa, 79; native grassland, 90; cultivated dryland, 261; irrigated fields excluding alfalfa, 506; and feedlots, 1,436 pounds per acre. Beneath feedlots the 20-foot profile content of nitrate-nitrogen varied from near zero to over 5,000 pounds per acre. In general, profiles low in nitrate were too low in oxygen for nitrate to accumulate. Low oxygen levels may have resulted from concomitantly high levels of organic carbon which created a high biological oxygen demand. In most cores the concentration of nitrate-nitrogen decreased with depth from the surface. Core hole water samples also varied in solute content. Water from beneath feedlots contained larger amounts of nitrogen and organic carbon than other water samples. Water from beneath 28 irrigated fields contained an average of 0.2 ppm nitrogen, while 29 samples from beneath feedlots contained an average of 4.5 ppm or 22 times greater concentration (Stewart, Viets and Hutchinson, 1968; Stewart, Viets, Hutchinson and Kemper, 1967).

In addition to nitrate contamination of water from percolation through soil and surface runoff, feedlots as a source of air pollution, have also been investigated. Using laboratory models, the effect of soil moisture on volatilization of ammonia was studied. In one experimental model the soil was initially moist, but in the other model it was initially dry. The addition of bovine urine at the rate of 5 ml per 21 CM^2 at 2-day intervals to moist soil resulted in less than 25% of the added nitrogen being volatilized as ammonia and 65% converted to nitrate. The addition of the same amount of urine at 4-day intervals to initially dry soil resulted in evaporization of essentially all water between urine applications and in 90% of added nitrogen being converted to ammonia and volatilized into the atmosphere (Stewart, 1970). With evidence that urinary nitrogen is volatilized as ammonia, the scientists further investigated both the movement of the compound in air and its deposition in the environment. Ammonia traps were set up at variable distances around feedlots and, for comparison, in areas containing no feedlots. The amount of ammonia absorbed in the traps varied directly with size of feedlot and inversely with distance from feedlot. Wind direction, of course, influenced distribution of the ammonia. A lake located a considerable distance from a feedlot annually absorbed from the air approximately 0.9 kg of ammonia nitrogen per acre, while a lake located 0.4 km from a large feedlot absorbed 16.6 kg per acre, an increase by a factor of 18. The investigators concluded that ammonia volatilized from feedlots contributed to significant nitrogen enrichment to nearby surface water (Hutchinson and Viets, 1969). In addition to ammonia, many other volatile odorous compounds from manure have been identified: hydrogen sulfide, sulfur dioxide, skatole, fatty acids, alcohols, aldehydes, ketones, esters, amines, mercaptans, nitriles, aromatics and alkyl halides (Loehr, 1968; Moorman, 1965).

Throughout the nation public sentiments in municipalities and states have urged private citizens, as well as officials of industry and government, to protect water and air, two vital public resources, against unnecessary pollution. In response to these public demands the Congress, as well as some state legislatures, enacted protective legislation for conserving resources. Beginning with the basic Act in 1956 and continuing with subsequent Amendments in 1961, 1965 and 1966, the Congress approved legislation for protecting and conserving the nation's present and future water supply. The legislative purpose was to abate pollution and improve the quality of water. The law made federal grants available to public and private agencies for obtaining new information on the subject and for developing scientifically sound and feasible municipal, state and interstate programs. Recognizing the primary rights and responsibilities of states for protecting the water, the Act required states to classify waters according to uses and to establish, within a specified time, quality standards for each category. In the event of state failure to enact standards acceptable to other affected states and to the Secretary of the Interior, the federal government was authorized to intervene and by itself establish acceptable standards for enforcing program compliance for maintaining standards (Federal Water Pollution Control Act, 1956–1966). Based on the finding that urbanization, industrial development and increasing use of motor vehicles was enhancing air pollution and endangering the public health and welfare, the Congress, as well as some individual states, has enacted a series of corrective measures. In 1955 the Department of Health, Education and Welfare was authorized to assist states and municipalities, which had primary rights and responsibilities for protecting air and water against pollution, in developing appropriate correctional programs. Despite conscientious efforts by city and state officials, air pollution worsened and resulted in additional legislation that reaffirmed state and local responsibilities and provided federal grants for air pollution control programs (Clean Air Act, 1963). By 1967 further and significant deterioration in air quality was obvious and, alarmed at this change, the Congress enacted more restrictive measures. The new law directed the Department of Health, Education and Welfare, in cooperation with states and other agencies, to designate geographic regions for developing air quality standards and to collect supportive technological data for air quality standards. The law further directed that, when technologically feasible, the states adopt acceptable air quality standards and implement programs for abating and preventing air pollution. In case state programs failed, the Department of Health, Education anf Welfare was authorized to invoke court action to enforce compliance (Air Quality Act, 1967). Feedlot location and management related to both water and air pollution.

Feedlot Manure. Consisting of a mixture of feces, urine, hair and added bedding, feedlot manure varies in composition with the diet. The starting ration commonly contains a high percentage of roughage, but the percentage of concentrate is increased gradually and rapidly to a ration containing a high percentage of concentrate. In general, wet manure contains approximately 85% moisture and 15% solids; from the solids approximately 10% volatile solids, 4% ash and 0.05% ammonium nitrogen can be obtained. In addition to moisture and solids, manure contains vast numbers of microorganisms, some pathogenic, and often some viable weed seeds. In decomposing manure the pH ranges from 8 to 9 and the ammonia content and COD value are high, but the salt concentration is increased.

Although feedlot cattle are fattened on a diet containing a high percentage of concentrate, the volume of manure, varying with size and health of animal, is great. One steer weighing 900 pounds daily produces approximately 43 pounds of feces and 17 pounds of urine of 60 pounds of manure. Thus each animal-year of feeding produces approximately 11 tons of manure. At the present time most cattle are fattened in feedlot enterprises each having a capacity of 1,000 or more animals and three sets, comprising 3,000 cattle, are fattened annually; these animals produce approximately 11,000 tons of wet manure.

The logistics of managing this volume of manure requires careful planning. Several alternative methods have been developed. One practice is to mound the manure towards the center of the pen. Fermentation within the mound generates heat and, during times of low ambient temperatures, produces a warm dry surface where cattle can rest in comfort. Enlarged by continuous additions, the mound may persist for indefinite time. The disadvantage to this method is that the mound reduces available pen space and consequently lowers the animal capacity of the pen, and thus increases the capital investment in the enterprise. Another practice is to remove manure from pens 1 to 3 times annually and stockpile the material at some convenient location. In semi-arid regions the surface dries rapidly and forms a seal that reduces volatilization of malodorous compounds. A disadvantage to this procedure is the cost of extra handling of the manure. Whenever feasible and convenient, the stored and decomposed manure from either pen mound or stockpile can be returned as fertilizer to the soil of crop fields. Each ton contains approximately 5.8 pounds N, 3.6 pounds P_2O_5 and 6.2 pounds K_2O.

Water Pollution. Fresh feces contain protein, and urine contains urea, creatinine, creatine, hippruic acid and allantoin. The amino groups of these nitrogenous compounds in manure are converted by bacteria to ammo-

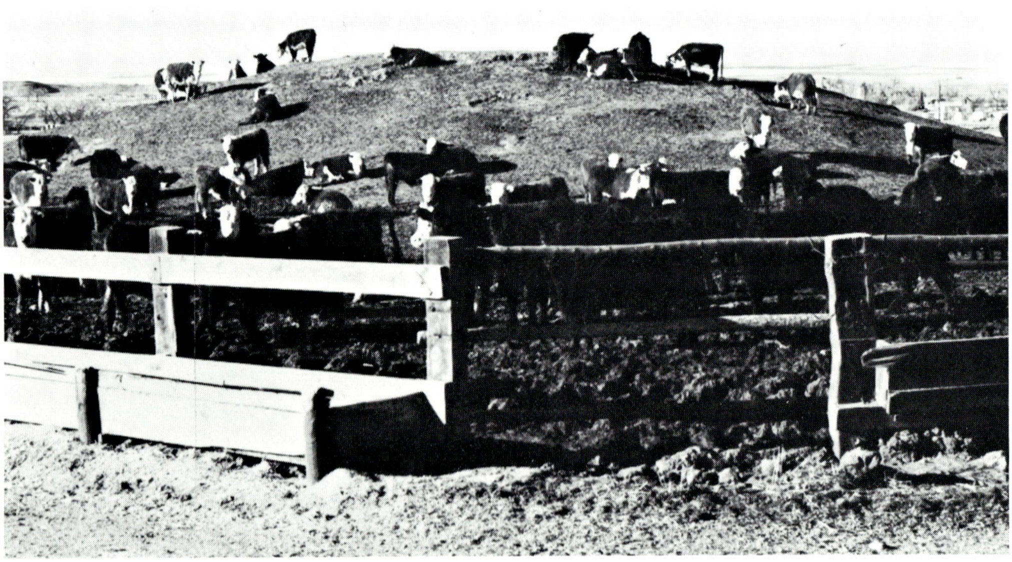

FIG. 9-1. *Manure mound in a feedlot.*

nia, then to nitrite, and finally to nitrate. The nitrates may move either as runoff into surface water of streams, rivers and lakes, or they may percolate through pervious earth materials into the soil profile and ground water. Nitrite, derived from oxidation of ammonia or reduction of nitrate, is toxic to people, especially infants, and animals. Ingested nitrite may convert hemoglobin to methemoglobin, a stable compound, that has little capacity for transporting oxygen.

Feedlot runoff water commonly accumulates below sloping surfaced cattle pens. Derived from clean surface water flowing into pens and from natural precipitation, the runoff contains a load of ammonium nitrogen, sediment and pathogenic bacteria, including *Salmonella dublin, S. typhimurium* and possibly *Leptospira pomona.* The content of ammonia nitrogen varies up to 140 mg/1 and of suspended solids up to 12,000 mg/1; these substances have a chemical oxygen demand of 3,000 to 11,000 mg/1.

Federal and state statutes prohibit the discharge of contaminated runoff water into clean public waters. In order to protect waters against pollution and to comply with regulations, specific rules and precautions should be exercised by feedlot owners. Cattle enclosures, alleyways and manure stockpile areas should be graded to provide drainage and thus avoid collection of fluids and sludges in pens. Flowing clean water should be diverted from entering contaminated areas. Appropriate conveyance channels should be constructed to carry all runoff fluids from animal pens, alleyways and manure storage areas into evaporation and retention basins.

A satisfactory feedlot disposal system consists of evaporation basins and/or retention basins. An evaporation basin is a sealed pond for holding contaminated runoff for evaporation of the water. As a means of runoff disposal, evaporation is feasible only in areas where the annual average rate of evaporation exceeds the annual average rate of precipitation. The evaporative capacity of a basin equals the annual average evaporation minus the annual precipitation. The surface area of an evaporation basin must have sufficient drying capacity to evaporate all precipitation likely to fall on the entire cattle pens, alleyways and manure storage areas during one average year. Basin depth must be sufficient to retain the precipitation plus 2 feet for storage of solids and 1 foot for freeboard. Residues must be removed and transferred to crop soil land or to land fill as often as is necessary to maintain basin capacity.

Retention basin, a sealed pond for holding contaminated runoff, must provide a means for transferring the contents to a disposal area. The volume of the basin must be sufficient to retain all runoff and sediment from the precipitation anticipated to fall on animal pens, alleyways and manure storage areas during the largest 24-hour storm of a 10-year period. Depth must provide the necessary volume plus 2 feet for solids and 1 foot freeboard. The basin contents must be removed by irrigation channels, tank trucks or sprinkler systems to crop soil or other approved disposal areas at approximately 15-day intervals.

The sloping sides and flat bottom of both evaporation and retention basins must be sealed and so constructed as to prevent leakage, spillage and uncontrolled discharge in any way; the entire structure must be fenced against animal intrusion and gated for cleaning and maintenance.

Data on annual precipitation and evaporation can be obtained from the State Water Pollution Control Commission.

Nitrates of manure may percolate into the soil and ground water beneath feedlots. The soil profile to a depth of 20 feet beneath feedlots varies in nitrate nitrogen from none to as much as 5,000 pounds per acre. Paved pen surfaces and dry impervious soil pen surfaces reduce percolation of dissolved nitrates, but pervious moist soil at pen surfaces allows percolation to occur. The nitrate-nitrogen within the soil may enter the ground water aquifer and raise the nitrogen content to an average of 4.5 ppm which amount is 22 times greater than the nitrogen in average ground water beneath crop fields. The water from ground water wells near feedlots may contain excessive amounts of nitrogen. Ground water in general, however, is little affected because of the small percentage of surface area used as feedlot.

Air Pollution. Feedlots also are of concern as a source of air pollution. Ammonia and other odorous compounds emanate from the manure and animals. The added nitrogen can be volatilized as ammonia; from moist soil surfaces the amount of volatilization can be 25%; from dry soil surfaces the amount of volatilization may be as much as 90%. By air movements, the ammonia is dispursed to the surrounding environment and is absorbed into water surfaces of lakes and ponds and may contribute to a significant nitrogen enrichment of water and possibly of soil. Ammonia and other malodorous compounds, including hydrogen sulfide, sulfur dioxide, skatole, amines, mercaptans and aromatics, volatilize into the air and create objectionable circumstances for nearby communities. The effect of prolonged breathing of these air contaminants on people and animals has not been determined. Cattle themselves are exposed to the highest concentrations, but in them adverse effects have not yet been identified. Cattle, however, remain in the feedlot and inhale the gases for usually around 120 days. Individuals of neighboring communities breath lower concentrations for much longer periods. Although odors may be reduced by stockpiling manure and by practicing good principles of sanitation, adequate control cannot be achieved until extensive research and development, some now in progress, have been completed. As soon as technological research provides the necessary information and methodology for control, local, state and federal statutes certainly will be enacted and enforced.

References

Air Quality Act of 1967. Public Law 90–148. 90th Congress, S. 780.

American Public Health Association, Inc., New York. *Standard Methods for the Examination of Water and Waste Water.* 12th Edition (1965).

Federal Water Pollution Control Act. Public Law 84-660 as amended in 1961 (PL 87-88), by the Water Quality Act of 1965 (PL 89-234) and by Clean Water Restoration Act of 1966 (PL 89-753).

Gilbertson, C. B., McCalla, T. M., Ellis, J. R., Cross, O. E. and Woods, W. R.: Beef Feedlot Wastes: Characteristics of Runoff, Solid Wastes and Nitrate Movement on Dirt Feedlots as Affected by Animal Density and Feedlot Slope. J. Water Pollution Control Federation, (1969).

Hutchinson, G. L. and Viets, F. G.: Nitrogen Enrichment of Surface Water by Absorption of Ammonia Volatilized From Cattle Feedlots. Science, *166* (1969): 514–515.

Lipper, R. I.: Design for Feedlot Waste Management—History and Characteristics. Presented at Seminar, "Design for Feedlot Waste Management" Topeka, Kan. (1969).

Loehr, R. C.: Effluent Quality from Anaerobic Lagoons Treating Feedlot Wastes. J. Water Pollution Control. Fed., *39* (1967): 384–391.

———: Anaerobic Lagoons: Considerations in Design and Application. Trans. Am. Soc. Ag. Eng., *11* (1968): 320–322.

McCalla, T. M., Ellis, J. R., Gilbertson, C. B. and Woods, W. R.: Chemical Studies of Runoff Following Rainfall and Snowmelt from Cattle Feedlots. Agronomy Abstr., (1969): 84–85.

Minor, J. R., Baumann, E. R. Willrich, T. L. and Hazen, T. E.: Pollution Control—Feedlot Operations. J. Water Pollution Control Fed., *42* (1970): 391–398.

Moorman, R.: Controlling Odors from Cattle Feedlots and Manure Dehydrating Operations. J. Air Pollution Control Assoc., *15* (1965): 34–35.

Seaborg, D.: Beef Cattle: The Next Ten Years. Livestock and Meat Situation. ARS, USDA (May, 1970): 32–35.

Smith, G. E.: Nitrate Problems in Water as Related to Soils, Plants and Water. Univ. of Missouri Special Report #55 (1965): 42–52.

Statistical Reporting Service. Number of Cattle Feedlots by Size Groups and Number of Fed Cattle Marketed 1962–1967. SRS-14. July 1968.

Stewart, B. A.: Volatilization and Nitrification of Nitrogen from Urine Under Simulated Cattle Feedlot Conditions. Environmental Science and Technology, *4* (1970): 579–582.

Stewart, B. A., Viets, F. G. and Hutchings, G. L.: Agriculture's Effect on Nitrate Pollution of Ground Water. J. Soil and Water Conservation, *23* (1968): 13–15.

Stewart, B. A., Viets, F. G., Hutchings, G. L. and Kemper, W. D.: Nitrate and Other Water Pollutants Under Fields and Feedlots. Environmental Science and Technology, *1* (1967): 736–739.

Wadleigh, C. H.: Wastes in Relation to Agriculture and Forestry. U.S.D.A. Misc. Publ. 1065. March 1968.

Index

Page numbers in *italics* refer to illustrations; page numbers followed by t refer to tables.